LOW BACK PAIN

Mechanism, Diagnosis, and Treatment

FIFTH EDITION

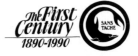

LOW BACK PAIN

Mechanism, Diagnosis, and Treatment

FIFTH EDITION

JAMES M. COX, D.C., D.A.C.B.R.

Director, Cox Low Back Pain Clinic
Fort Wayne, Indiana
Postgraduate Faculty Member
National College of Chiropractic
Lombard, Illinois
President Emeritus and Director
International Chiropractic Academy on the
  Study of Back Pain, Inc.
Diplomate
American Chiropractic Board of Radiology

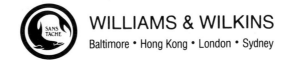

WILLIAMS & WILKINS
Baltimore • Hong Kong • London • Sydney

Editor: Jonathan W. Pine, Jr.
Associate Editor: Linda Napora
Designer: Dan Pfisterer
Illustration Planner: Ray Lowman
Production Coordinator: Raymond E. Reter

Copyright © 1990
Williams & Wilkins
428 East Preston Street
Baltimore, Maryland 21202, USA

Accurate indications, adverse reactions, and dosage schedules for drugs are provided in this book, but it is possible that they may change. The reader is urged to review the package information data of the manufacturers of the medications mentioned.

Printed in the United States of America

First Edition 1975
Second Edition 1978
Third Edition 1980
Fourth Edition 1985

Library of Congress Cataloging in Publication Data

Cox, James M.
　　Low back pain: mechanism, diagnosis, and treatment / James M. Cox.—5th ed.
　　　p.　cm.
　　Includes bibliographies and index.
　　ISBN 0-683-02152-4
　　1. Backache.　2. Chiropractic.　I. Title.
　　[DNLM: 1. Backache.　2. Chiropractic.　WE 755 C877L]
RZ265.S64C69　1990
617.5′64—dc20
DNLM/DLC
for Library of Congress
　　　　　　　　　　　　　　　　　　　　　　　　　　89-9022
　　　　　　　　　　　　　　　　　　　　　　　　　　CIP

89 90 91 92 93
1　2　3　4　5　6　7　8　9　10

Foreword

Browsers leafing through the pages of this book might think to themselves: Why should I spend my time or money on it? What can I learn from it? How will it help me? Perhaps the single most outstanding reason for believing that the time and money would be well spent is the fact that the book's author has been a full-time private practitioner all his professional life. He writes from the perspective of one whose livelihood for a quarter century has depended on his ability to help thousands of his patients get better. He shares with his readers the clinical experience that comes only from seeing large numbers of patients, year after year, for many years. He writes as one who knows full well that patients care only about what works, what gets results—about what you, the practitioner, can do for them. They don't want to hear about your handicaps, difficulties, or problems, your scope of practice or interprofessional rivalries. They aren't impressed by glibness, unctuousness, pomposity, or cant. They're deaf to excuses. If you can help them, they'll recommend you to others; if you can't, they won't recommend you to anyone. And they'll look for someone else who can help them.

Just a few years ago, anyone resorting to manipulation for a "bad back" would, most of the time, have ended up in a chiropractor's office. And if the first chiropractor didn't help, more often than not the patient would seek out another. Medical manipulators were few and far between. Each generation of osteopaths was manipulating less than the one preceding it. As manipulators, chiropractors didn't have much competition then. Even the marginal practitioner might eke out a living. In recent years, all that has changed. Nowadays there are all sorts of professionals and paraprofessionals claiming to perform what they call "spinal manipulative therapy"—or "SMT" for short. Individuals, institutions, and professions that a decade or so ago scorned manipulation and those who practiced it are today holding themselves forth as authorities on the subject. The newcomers claim that they can do everything chiropractors can, that they can do all these things better, and that they can do more besides—things that chiropractors are prohibited from doing.

At the same time that chiropractors find themselves confronted with the competition of all these latecomers to spinal manipulation, they also find themselves having to contend with the demands of third-party payers that their services be "cost effective"—just being efficacious is no longer enough. Since in the modern world the preponderance of payments to all practitioners are made by private and public insurers who insist on cutting costs, any practitioners who do not attempt to upgrade their standard of care while holding costs down may lose their patients to those who do.

I began by setting forth Dr. Cox's eminent qualifications for writing a book that would be useful to practitioners desirous of providing optimal care for their patients with low back pain. I will conclude by noting that (a) Dr. Cox has called upon experts to write chapters dealing with leg length inequality, the sacroiliac joint, scoliosis, laboratory evaluation, and neurosurgery; (b) he has continued his practice of bringing to his readers' attention those recent journal articles from the clinical and basic sciences that are significant for understanding the mechanism of low back pain and for undertaking the diagnosis and treatment thereof; and (c) as in the four previous editions, Dr. Cox writes in a style readers can easily follow and thereby turns what could have been a chore into a pleasure.

William Bachop, Ph.D.
Professor of Anatomy
National College of Chiropractic
Lombard, Illinois

The fifth edition of *Low Back Pain: Mechanism, Diagnosis, and Treatment* has been expanded to include five guest authors. The author, James M. Cox, D.C., D.A.C.B.R., has rewritten the entire text to reflect the chiropractic, biomechanical, diagnostic, and therapeutic adjustive procedures that have evolved since the fourth edition was published. The textbook is now a multidisciplinary treatise on the care of the low back pain patient, from history to rehabilitation. Emphasis is placed on the conservative manipulative adjustive chiropractic approach to the subject of low back pain.

Dr. Cox has utilized a data base that has been developed from literature searches into all aspects of biomechanics, diagnosis, and treatment of low back pain. He has correlated these data with his clinical research and the treatment of patients suffering from low back pain. This approach, research findings coupled with patient management, provides the practitioner with a treatment plan that is based on patients' needs. The rationale for treatment selection is based on research findings from all disciplines.

The textbook has been written for the practitioner, irrespective of discipline, who struggles daily with the dilemma of low back pain patients; this work has been written to assist in the decision-making process. As the incidence of low back pain reaches epidemic proportions, it becomes imperative that all clinicians become aware of the various available treatment approaches.

The first chapter details the growth and acceptance of chiropractic, from its early leaders and educators to the present awareness of and interest in the benefits of chiropractic adjustive procedures. The philosophy of chiropractic is also discussed, as well as the role of chiropractors in today's health care delivery system.

Chapter 2, "Biomechanics of the Lumbar Spine," formulates the foundation for the entire text by describing current concepts relative to pain production and therapeutic relief.

Chapter 3, "Neurophysiology of Nerve Root Compression," discusses the effects on the nerve involved, as well as the changes in the innervated part. The long-held tenet in chiropractic science concerning disease states due to neurological insults is supported.

In Chapter 4, Dana Lawrence, D.C., succinctly shares his knowledge of the biomechanics, diagnosis, clinical effects, and treatment principles of the short leg syndrome.

Chapter 5, "Sacroiliac Joint," was written by Drs. Dana Lawrence and Chae-Song Ro. The challenges of understanding the biomechanics, neurology, changes with aging, diagnosis of abnormal motion, and subsequent treatment of aberrant states of the sacroiliac joint are discussed.

Transitional segments, described in Chapter 6, are considered by many authorities to be the most difficult low back problems to stabilize. In addition, they have the highest recurrence rate. The literature is reviewed and treatment parameters are presented for this condition, which affects 6% of the population.

The basic cause of low back or sciatic conditions is narrowing (stenosis) of the course of the nerve root from the cauda equina through the intervertebral canal. Chapter 7 defines and describes the areas and types of stenosis. In addition, the clinical presentation is discussed. Systems of marking plain films are presented, along with imaging modalities used for the diagnosis.

Donald D. Aspegren, D.C., has written the chapter on scoliosis, covering the use of electrical stimulation for conservative care and the effectiveness of various approaches, with special emphasis on the benefits of chiropractic flexion distraction manipulation coupled with electrical stimulation.

Chapter 9, "Diagnosis," includes a fixed-choice examination form. The form starts with the history and follows through to the treatment selection and plan. The latest diagnostic procedures, including magnetic resonance imaging (MRI), computerized tomography (CT), contrast-enhanced MRI and CT, myelography, and discography, are presented. This chapter takes all of the diagnostics and places them into a clinical decision-making algorithm that leads to a correlative diagnosis. Fifteen categories of low back pain are presented, along with the diagnostic criteria. The diagnosis is correlated from the fixed-choice examination form.

In Chapter 10, David J. Wickes, D.C., presents a systematic approach to ordering laboratory tests for patients with low back pain and sciatic conditions.

Chapter 11 provides an update on facet syndrome.

Chapter 12, "Care of the Intervertebral Disc," provides an explanation of the pain sensitivity of the disc and progresses through the research into the regenerative properties that are being studied concerning the intervertebral disc.

Spondylolisthesis and the identification of the degree of instability are presented in Chapter 13.

Rudy Kachmann, M.D., provides a neurosurgeon's perspective in Chapter 14.

The last chapter, "Care of Other Specific Low Back Conditions," presents problems encountered in daily practice—i.e., degenerative scoliosis, degenerative disc disease, compression fracture, failed back surgery syndrome, muscle weakness of the pelvic area, postural complexes due to foot mechanical defects—and their effect on the lumbar spine.

Upon completion of the 15 chapters, the practitioner and/or student will have a comprehensive understanding of the lumbar spine. This text fills a major void in the healing arts. It will benefit all who read it and the increasing numbers of patients who seek their help for relief of low back pain.

Allen Parry, D.C., Director
Postdoctoral and Related
*   Professional Education*
Logan College of Chiropractic
Chesterfield, Missouri

Preface

The fourth edition of this book was published in 1985, and its preface said that conservative care of the patient with low back pain was growing in importance, since surgical care had a very limited part in the total scenario of lumbar spine treatment. The last 5 years of research for this fifth edition have only served to bear out this observation.

This volume broadens the scope of diagnosis and conservative care of the lumbar spine by providing an update on research from the past 5 years in this subject. Five guest authors are included to cover specific areas of interest in their respective specialties: laboratory evaluation, sacroiliac joint mechanics and treatment, scoliosis, leg length inequality, and neurosurgical opinion of the low back pain patient. My role was to rewrite and expand the other 10 chapters to outline the role of chiropractic in today's health care delivery scheme, especially as it has evolved to encompass the responsibility for seeing one-third of patients suffering from low back pain. This is an awesome responsibility for such a young discipline.

The chapter on laboratory evaluation, for the first time in chiropractic, allows the reader-physician to follow a decision-making algorithm in interpreting symptoms and correlating them with the proper laboratory procedures and their interpretation to arrive at the diagnosis. This succinct outline for laboratory diagnosis has been too long in evolving in chiropractic. Every physician in practice will want this knowledge.

The sacroiliac joint has long been a topic of debate as to its mobility and pain-producing capabilities. Drs. Ro and Lawrence have intertwined the anatomy, mechanics, and treatment of sacroiliac joint problems into a never-before-written treatise on this important element in low back pain.

Scoliosis is handled by conservative procedures until surgical indications are manifested. Dr. Aspegren outlines the clinical parameters for utilizing electrical stimulation, bracing, manipulation, and finally surgery in this youth-afflicting disease. This chapter is indicative of the maturation of the chiropractic profession into mainstream healing.

The short leg syndrome is a long-debated subject. Dr. Lawrence furnishes the data from his extensive library on the subject so that you can make logical decisions on when and how to treat this malady.

Dr. Kachmann shares the neurosurgeon's view of the low back pain and sciatica patient, from the examination and diagnostic testing stages to the ultimate surgical stage. He shares his views on conservative care by chiropractors and explains how he sees the integration of the two disciplines in caring for the patient with low back pain.

Finally, this author (J.M.C.) has the responsibility of covering the current biomechanical knowledge of the low back and correlating it with the chiropractic care of the intervertebral and posterior element aspects of pain.

This text is meant to be a strong decision-making aid to the practitioner who treats low back pain patients. It is my intent that it help the physician to better care for the patient.

James M. Cox, D.C., D.A.C.B.R.

Acknowledgments

Writing a textbook requires the mental and physical strengths of many people. Starting with the principal author, there must be the desire to advance science and the relief of mankind's ailments. Behind the author must be an understanding family, beginning with a wife like mine. Judi is one person who lives the principle that everyone should be encouraged to attain his or her potential. She has tolerated the lack of family support by me that this book has required, realizing its importance. The book is as much her achievement as mine, for without her, none of this would be possible. To my children, Julie, Jill, Jim, and Jason, goes my love and promise to always support them as they have supported this venture.

Chiropractic has been rewarding for me, and this book allows me to give back something. Foremost for recognition is my stepfather, John Rodman, D.C., who first interested and encouraged me to seek chiropractic as a life's work. What wonderful guidance he afforded. The greatest chiropractic leader of all time was Joseph Janse, D.C., President of the National College of Chiropractic for most of his life. This man instilled the awareness that honesty and knowledge could groom a profession. He encouraged our profession when it needed it most. To him I owe the fact that this book exists.

To all my colleagues and friends who encouraged this effort, I will always feel gratitude. In particular, Theresa Roussel is to be singled out for her days of work in collating, correcting, and typing this manuscript.

Finally, I thank God for the inspiration and strength to conceive and produce this work.

James M. Cox, D.C.

Contributors

Donald D. Aspegren, D.C.
Director
Kipling Chiropractic Center
Lakewood, Colorado

Postgraduate Faculty
New York College of Chiropractic
Glenhead, New York

James M. Cox, D.C., D.A.C.B.R.
Director, Cox Low Back Pain Clinic
Fort Wayne, Indiana

Postgraduate Faculty Member
National College of Chiropractic
Lombard, Illinois

President Emeritus and Director
International Chiropractic Academy on the
    Study of Back Pain, Inc.

Diplomate
American Chiropractic Board of Radiology

Rudy Kachmann, M.D.
Private practice—Neurosurgery
Fort Wayne, Indiana

Dana J. Lawrence, D.C.
Editor, Journal of Manipulative and Physiological
    Therapeutics
Director, Department of Editorial Review and
    Publication

Professor
Department of Biomechanics and Chiropractic
    Technique
National College of Chiropractic
Lombard, Illinois

Chae-Song Ro, M.D., Ph.D.
Professor
Department of Anatomy
National College of Chiropractic
Lombard, Illinois

David Wickes, D.C.
Professor and Chairman
Department of Diagnosis
National College of Chiropractic
Lombard, Illinois

Contents

Chiropractic Today

James M. Cox, D.C., D.A.C.B.R.

Chiropractic practice is an expression of life itself—a fulfillment and commitment to society. No greater treatise could be written than to be remembered, in some small way, as an architect of chiropractic in your time.

        —James M. Cox, D.C.

CHIROPRACTIC'S LONG-AWAITED ACCEPTANCE

We are approaching the 100th anniversary of chiropractic.

Since publication of the last edition of this book, more excitement, growth, and clinical acceptance of chiropractic principles have occurred than in the past 95 years of the profession's existence. Let's explore proof of this statement.

Wiltse (1) may have put it best in the North American Spine Society's 1985 presidential address when he said that we must remember that many of the great healing advances have been made by people outside of medicine. History is replete with instances of this. For instance, midwives were scorching the cloth they laid over the umbilicus of newborns centuries before Lister or Semmelweis were heard of.

Wiltse further commented that perhaps medical doctors can take a lesson from history in dealing with spinal manipulation. The explanation given as to how manipulation works may be quite wrong by medical doctors' ideas, but its practitioners must be doing something right, or ten million people a year would not be filling their offices. The medical profession needs to at least learn about manipulation.

Medicine is very eager to learn what chiropractic has to offer human suffering, so it is para-

mount that chiropractors continue to study to be in the mainstream of manipulation. Wiltse (1) went on to say, on another topic, that he believes that every spine surgeon's office can be a research center. We live in a moment in history when many of the offices are made up of several, often five or six, surgeons. These large groups offer wonderful opportunities for clinical research, sometimes even better than a university setting.

Again, we in chiropractic have utilized the individual chiropractic office as the foundation of research. Most past research and technical advances in chiropractic have emanated from the private offices of chiropractors. To prove this, visualize such names as Gonstead, Illi, Nimmo, DeJarnette, Janse, Rich, Goodheart, Harper, Logan, Lee, Wunsch, and hundreds of others. Chiropractic has shown that it had the foresight and the premise to move forward. Such success in any profession, against such strong opposition, is rare.

Chiropractic—Number One Medical Alternative

White (2) reports in *Medical Economics* that one-third of the patients who answered a survey had consulted a nonphysician. More than one in three respondents had sought treatment from a nonphysician. A few had actually defected from conventional medical care altogether, like the Missouri woman who wrote: "My chiropractor *is* my regular doctor. He refers if I need something he can't provide." Or the young Oregon woman who said that she went to both a chiropractor and a naturopath because "I want natural healing whenever possible. I don't have a regular doctor."

Most patients went to a nonphysician in rebellion against their doctor, in anger or in frustration. A disturbing 36% said they tried a nonphysician or a nonosteopath because their regular physician couldn't help them. To their minds, the medical doctor either wouldn't help or wasn't qualified to treat their problems.

No question about it, the nonphysicians are making sure that patients know about their "special expertise," and many physicians apparently are not. A young Florida woman explained her decision to go to a nonphysician this way: "I saw a chiropractor because my doctor doesn't handle nutrition" (2). A Pennsylvania jogger didn't even consult her doctor about an injury, she said, because "an area chiropractor has specific athletic-injury training. He was more qualified than my physician to treat me" (2).

Of the 36% of the patients who sought treatment from a nonphysician, 68% saw a chiropractor.

An Idaho mother of two asserted that physicians "prescribe pills that mask symptoms but don't cure the problem. I get healthier, less expensive care from a chiropractor." (2).

Struggle between Traditional Medicine and Chiropractic

Coburn (3) describes and analyzes the social history of chiropractic in Canada to partially test a thesis regarding changes in the dominance of the medical profession. He earlier sketched its achievement of dominance, which occurred by World War I; its consolidation of power, which lasted until after World War II; and the early signs of a decline in its dominance, signalled by the 1962 doctors' strike in Saskatchewan.

One test of the historical sequence described, and particularly the recent signs of decline in medical power, is to examine one of orthodox medicine's major competitors, chiropractic. To what degree has medicine been successful in its opposition to chiropractic?

The development of chiropractic in Canada shows its early survival and recently, in the 1960s and 1970s, its increasingly popular use and official recognition. Particularly important in its recent success was the establishment of a college in

Canada in 1945 and the partial inclusion of chiropractic under government health insurance in the 1970s.

While chiropractic has gained acceptance and recognition, it has sacrificed many of its earlier claims to be an alternative healing art, and to some degree chiropractic has become "medicalized." Medicine, however, has also been forced to make concessions. Despite total medical opposition, chiropractic survives. The recent successes of chiropractic tend to confirm an earlier thesis of the beginnings of the decline of medical dominance and to show that medicine, while dominant, was never hegemonic.

However, chiropractic did not produce medicine's current difficulties. Rather, medicine is being challenged directly by state power and pressures to rationalize health care and is being affected indirectly by the class struggle. Chiropractic itself owes much of its own early success to support by the working class and working class organizations such as unions (3).

As a test case, chiropractic is important in a number of respects. First, it is the occupation that has most directly challenged and competed with medicine as an alternative healing system. Second, it is an occupation that has survived the most strenuous efforts of the medical profession to destroy it. Third, the struggle between chiropractic and medicine is an ongoing one, which covers the crucial period of the past 20 to 25 years, the time in which, we argue, medicine has experienced a relative decline in power (3).

In the writings on professionalization, there is almost universal agreement that chiropractic was previously "marginal," "deviant," or "nonprofessional" but that it has gained in professional attributes and in legitimacy and is now more like a profession or actually is a profession. For example, Walter Wardwell (4), one of the first sociologists to study chiropractic, at first viewed it as a marginal profession because of its lack of legal standing, low status, and so forth. However, his later writings imply that chiropractic has been increasing its legitimacy and decreasing its marginal role. A number of writers have followed Wardwell's lead. For example, Cobb (5) states that chiropractic has shifted from a position of deviance to one of popular demand for services and for public pressure on legislators. Several doctoral dissertations in the United States also support the contention that chiropractic is developing from a healing sect to a healing art, or from an occupation to a profession. One contradictory conclusion is given by Sternberg (6), on the basis of a study of chiropractic students at a New York State chiropractic college. Sternberg (6) claims that chiropractic is destined to disappear because of the incompatibility of the predominant chiropractic solo mode of practice with the increasingly bureaucratic and group-organized American health care system (3).

Growth of Manipulative Physicians' Numbers

In the last 90 years, manual medicine has gained popularity in the United States. There are approximately 19,000 osteopathic physicians and 23,000 chiropractors currently practicing this type of therapy. Revenues in excess of $1.3 billion are collected yearly in fees from 130 million patients seen by chiropractors alone. Approximately 3,000 students graduate from 15 osteopathic and 16 chiropractic schools each year. The 15 osteopathic colleges are educationally equal to medical schools. Five of these are state funded and interrelated with state universities. Out of a required curriculum of in excess of 5,200 hours, osteopathic graduates must complete 200 credit hours in the specific field of manipulative medicine and an additional 400 to 700 elective hours. Within the first 3 years, a chiropractic graduate must complete 780 credit hours in chiropractic diagnosis and therapy. The 4th year is devoted to internship in a clinic under the direction of a licensed chiropractor (7).

Why Patients Seek Chiropractic Care

Silver (8) states that it has been known for some time that chiropractic has a constituency of its own and that clients of chiropractors are not using this therapeutic modality solely because orthodox medical practitioners are absent or unavailable. He cites the danger to the medical profession of losing out in this public policy struggle. There are testimonies to the potential benefits of chiropractic. Word-of-mouth dissemination of miraculous cures appears in the press, attributed to athletes who have found chiropractic manipulation helpful; thereby, chiropractors get to be athletic team doctors. Orthopedists, in private conversations, confess to referring patients to chiropractors. This author saw a patient only yesterday who was referred by her neurologist. Being shocked at this referral by a medical

doctor, the patient told me that the neurologist said that, even though it would not be popular with his colleagues, he had gone to a chiropractor and had been greatly helped. In the area of muscle and joint disorders, not so well explored by the medical profession as some other disease and discomfort areas, a natural arena for chiropractic activity exists.

Silver (8) points out that, in the 1980s, the issues have not been so clear, the facts not so obvious against chiropractic. First, many other healing practices similar to chiropractic are today more or less accepted into the orthodox medical practice system. He imagines that if chiropractic, rather than acupuncture, had been brought out of China to a palpitating American public less than 10 years ago, it might have fascinated and conquered the lay and professional community with its miraculous effects as did acupuncture. Orthodox medicine is bitterly attacked for its often heedless, even mindless, use of dangerous and useless drugs, technology, and surgical procedures. The World Health Organization promotes traditional healing and derogates orthodox medicine for the developing world as too much, too soon, and too expensive.

Silver (8) states that he thinks chiropractic will continue to be funded by governmental agencies. Chiropractic is undergoing significant change and adaptation. At present, there are 13 schools accredited by an accrediting body recently approved by the United States Office of Education, with three more schools about to open. Students are required to have at least 2 years of prechiropractic college followed by 4 years in a chiropractic college. A recent study of one school showed the average student, for whom chiropractic represented a second career, to be somewhat older than the corresponding medical student. The students, like the practitioners, tend to be white, male, and of lower middle and working class origins. Approximately 25% of the classes in school today are female.

Silver analyzes the chiropractor's approach to treating the patient and finds that the chiropractic doctor assumes that the burden of health resides with the patient and that it is within the patient that the motivation and potential for health exist. The chiropractic philosophy is that, since the power of maintaining health is located within each person, a person's own attitudes and life-style are important factors that contribute to health status. Therefore, cooperation on the part of an active patient is part and parcel of chiropractic treatment.

This is not only a totally different view of the sick role; it is also one that is more in line with current social views of what the doctor-patient relationship should be. It sets its face against the active doctor-passive patient concept.

Wardwell, cited by Silver (8), is convinced, from his most thorough study of chiropractic, that chiropractic will be accepted as a reimbursable healing activity and that this will be good for patients and practitioners alike. Health professionals have an obligation to review the situation of chiropractic in the light of current practices, patient responses, and developing policies. What is in the best interest of the patient?

Demand For Chiropractic Care Is Strong

According to the United States Department of Health and Human Services, in the nation's most comprehensive compilation of health care statistics, entitled *Health—U.S.* (9), consumer demand for chiropractic services is strong. Data indicate that patient demand over the past 5 years has kept pace with the growth of the number of chiropractors in the United States. The publication's (9) 1983 figures showed an estimated 28,500 doctors of chiropractic practicing in the United States, compared with 23,000 in 1979. During this same period, chiropractic income grew from $1.4 billion to $2.0 billion. Although the number of chiropractors has increased dramatically since 1979, patient demand and spending by the patients themselves as well as by public and private insurance sources have kept pace.

This growth is particularly impressive in light of the fact that chiropractic has traditionally been sustained economically by the marketplace, rather than by government subsidy. Unlike hospitals and medical doctors, who receive on the average more than 60% of their income from federal, state, and local government programs funded by taxpayers, chiropractic care has, for the most part, been paid for from the patients' own pocketbooks—even when alternative sources of care were available at subsidized rates, or even free (9).

Profile of a Chiropractic Patient

Deyo (10) states that over $8 billion is spent annually for medical care of back pain (excluding disability and indirect costs). Little is known about how the various types of practitioners are used by the public in the care of back pain, or how frequently each is sought. To answer these questions, data from the second National Health and Nutrition Examination Survey was analyzed from 1976 to 1980. This included a sample representing the civilian, noninstitutionalized population of the United States, including 27,801 subjects. Of these people, 13.8% reported having had at least one episode of low back pain lasting more than 2 weeks. Seventy-five percent of these patients reported pain within the last year, with 33% having pain of less than 1 month's duration, 33% having pain lasting 1 to 5 months, and 33% having pain lasting 6 months or longer, with the remainder unable to remember.

Of patients having back pain for at least 2 weeks, 84.6% of them sought professional care. There were important racial, regional, and educational differences in the use of various types of practitioners. The most common source of care was the general practitioner, followed by the orthopedic surgeon; the next most common source of care was the chiropractor, with nearly one-third of low back pain sufferers having sought care from the chiropractor.

The use of chiropractors and osteopaths was much higher among whites than among other racial groups. Chiropractors are used much more often in the West than in other regions of the country. Subjects with back pain living in the Northeast were much less likely to obtain care from either a general practitioner or a chiropractor than subjects in other regions of the country. Poorly educated subjects were more likely to obtain care from a general practitioner than were well-educated subjects, and they were also less likely to obtain care from an orthopedist and internist. Deyo (10) stated that, perhaps counterintuitively, there was no substantial difference among educational groups in the use of chiropractic care. Deyo found the racial difference in the use of chiropractors an unexpected finding. He explained the interest in chiropractic by white, well-educated patients as being due to possible marketing practices, geographic distribution, reimbursement strictures, or cultural differences in the perception of chiropractors. Regardless of the reason, the fact remains, in this author's mind, that one-third of well-educated persons seek chiropractic care for their low back pain problems.

Does Chiropractic Substitute for Less Available Medical Services?

To answer this question, a study was done in a medically underserved rural area to study health care utilization before and after a significant increase in medical manpower. There was a slight increase, rather than a decrease, in the use of chiropractic services associated with the growth in the physician manpower pool. The level of access to physicians was not a significant predictor of chiropractic utilization (11). This is substantiated by the proportion of chiropractic users who also had visited a physician that same year: 76.3% in 1972 and 81.3% in 1977, suggesting that members of this study were actually triaging themselves to different kinds of health practitioners for different complaints or problems. Further support comes from the discovery that perceived access to physicians' services did not correlate with chiropractic utilization.

A New Zealand Study

In New Zealand, public hospitals have long surgical waiting lists, and therefore it is almost impossible to get nonurgent surgery done in hospitals without a long wait. This is emphasized by the fact that health insurance is one of the fastest growing industries in New Zealand (12). With continuing cutbacks in government expenditure in implementation of the "user pays" principle, it seems that there will be increasing reliance on health insurance. Those planning private health facilities know full well that as long as the public system continues to deteriorate, a significant proportion of the population will pay insurance premiums for the best care, no matter what the premium. This author notes how well this recent 1986 study in New Zealand correlates with the above-cited study finding that patients go to chiropractors even though the majority pay their own bills. It is an indication that people seek chiropractic care with the secondary thought of having the fee paid for by a third party payer (12).

A Commission of Enquiry into Chiropractic in New Zealand (13) made the following summary: "Chiropractors are the only health practitioners who are necessarily equipped by their education and training to carry out spinal manual therapy.

"Chiropractors should, in the public interest, be accepted as partners in the general health care system. No other health professional is as well qualified by his general training to carry out a di-agnosis for spinal mechanical dysfunction or to perform spinal manual therapy: and the responsibility for spinal manual therapy training, because of its specialized nature, should lie with the chiropractic profession. Part time or vacation courses in spinal manual therapy for other health professionals should not be encouraged."[a]

Not All Medical Doctors Are Adequately Trained to Treat Low Back Pain

An example of the interest in chiropractic and the use of manipulative technique appeared in 1983 in the *Medical Journal of Australia* in answer to a medical doctor's request for enlightenment on why medical practitioners refer patients to chiropractors (14). The secretary of the Australian Association of Musculoskeletal Medicine answered the question by stating that there are several reasons why some doctors refer patients with back pain to nonmedical osteopaths or chiropractors. He stated that undergraduate training often does not adequately prepare medical graduates for examining and treating patients who have the common mechanical causes of back pain, and that physiotherapists and increasing numbers of doctors realize from listening to their patients that manual therapy can provide relief from back pain. He further stated that 11 controlled clinical trials indicate that manipulation is of benefit in managing acute low back pain. Feeling that chiropractors have not published such work, he wrote that such research validates the quality of manual therapy available within the medical profession. He then ended by stating that doctors need to realize that chiropractic therapy is available within the medical profession from those who have completed courses in spinal manipulation. Further, these patients will receive not only the same skilled manipulation, but, in addition, will be treated by practitioners with hospital and clinical experience with a broad armamentarium of treatment modalities in addition to manual therapy.

Who Should Practice Spinal Adjusting?

In the debate going on over who should control and practice spinal manipulation, the question of

---

[a] From Report of the Commission of Enquiry: Chiropractic in New Zealand. Presented to the House of Representatives by His Excellency the Governor-General. New Zealand, Hasselberg, Government Printer, 1979.

referral by medical doctors to chiropractors has been addressed from other viewpoints (14). Included in the debate were the thoughts of a hospital representative who felt that there was overwhelming evidence, provided by inquiries from around the world, supporting the concept of cooperation between medicine and chiropractic. He suggested that all general practitioners form a professional relationship with a registered chiropractor in their area. Not only would they be surprised by the results in neuromusculoskeletal problems, but they would also be surprised by the willingness of the patient to attend. A recommendation was made that both professions begin preliminary talks to form a better working relationship throughout Australia. The patient would benefit most from such cooperation.

Another reply to the question dealt with the tales of chiropractors making erroneous diagnoses with disastrous therapeutic results. However, the reverse situation also happens. Several cases were cited, including an elderly man with a crushed fracture of the thoracic vertebra, a nurse with pulmonary tuberculosis, and a middle-aged woman with a palpable abdominal neoplasm, whose diagnoses had all been missed by medical practitioners prior to their seeing chiropractors. Chiropractors, in each case, through suitable examination, made the correct diagnosis and the appropriate referral before treatment was instituted (14).

This author would state that certainly chiropractors are well-trained physicians in the diagnosis and treatment of spinal problems. Not to understand that is to fail to read the catalogs of the colleges of chiropractic, to see the licensing examinations required for practitioners in the United States, and to see the postgraduate education attended by chiropractors today.

COMPARATIVE COST OF CHIROPRACTIC CARE

Chiropractic as Nonhospital Care

Chrysler Corporation did a study to determine the cost and average length of stay for admissions to hospitals for nonsurgical back pain from 1980 to 1983 (15). The decision was made by Chrysler to focus on the top eight hospitals that constituted almost 40% of the cost problem. A detailed audit by Blue Cross-Blue Shield Michigan auditors, using the HDI (Health Data Institute) appropriateness criteria, determined that fully 70% of the cases in those hospitals, constituting 85% of the hospital days, failed to meet any criteria justifying the admission.

Audit findings at all eight hospitals were unacceptable, but admissions for nonsurgical back pain to three hospitals were almost completely inappropriate. Chrysler presented evidence to the hospitals that 95% of the patients whose cases were studied were admitted with a diagnosis of back spasm, backache, or sciatica. There was a markedly low incidence of severe illness. On the other hand, 73% had no neurological abnormalities at any time during their hospitalization. Only 4% of patients were nonambulatory. Moreover, very few of these patients previously had tried home bed rest. Based on these data, Chrysler's goal was to effect a change in evidently wasteful physician and hospital patterns.

One practice that particularly had to be challenged involved the use of traction as a treatment regimen. Traction serves as an excuse for hospitalization and is a contributing factor to the excessive lengths of stay associated with these unnecessary hospitalizations for back pain. It commonly has been used for treatment of both lumbosacral sprain syndrome and disc herniation. However, HDI research disclosed that traction has never been shown to be efficacious for either condition (15). Despite these facts, traction was used in 70% of the Chrysler cases studied.

Another overused practice with both cost and quality of care implications that had to be addressed was the administering of electromyograms. The medically unjustifiable use of this test was a significant problem at all hospitals studied. The HDI research showed that electromyography's legitimate role in the management of back patients is limited. For example, in the patient who is a candidate for surgery, the test occasionally may be helpful in localizing the nerve root involved with disc herniation. In the vast majority of cases, however, the electromyogram adds nothing to the clinical assessment.

Chiropractic is nonhospital-based care and meets the criteria desired by corporations and insurance companies.

Cost of Low Back Care

Brown (16) reported the average length of hospital stay and average cost for herniated disc treatment methods (Table 1.1). We can see that the

Table 1.1.
Average Costs for Herniated Disc Treatment[a]

Procedure	Average Length of Hospital Stay (days)	Average Total Cost
Chemonucleolysis	2.3	$1,549.02
Disc excision	6.6	$4,203.21
Myelography and Chemonucleolysis	4.3	$1,905.48
Myelography and disc excision	9.6	$5,427.67

[a]Data taken from Brown M: *Intradiscal Therapy, Chymopapain or Collagenase.* Chicago, Year Book, 1983, p126.

cost of medical procedures is an area where chiropractic can be effective.

Sweezy (17) reported that the cost of outpatient care for low back pain patients amounts to 1.5 days of hospital cost when low back pain and arthritis are being treated.

Camp (18) reported that in Oregon the costs per patient for treating intervertebral disc protrusions by surgery were as follows:

• Fifty-four chemonucleolysis patients, $16,228;
• Forty-four laminectomy patients, $13,486;
• Thirty-seven microsurgical patients, $10,465.

The disability costs for these patients amounted to the following:

• Chemonucleolysis patients, $36,000;
• Laminectomy patients, $29,000;
• Microsurgery patients, $18,000.

This certainly is a good example of the cost of back surgery and the costs to insurance and industry for the disability.

These health care statistics are rather surprisingly elevated to enormous costs when one considers that it is estimated that the health costs could triple by the year 2000 (19). The report states that spending on health care in America will reach 15% of the gross national product by the end of the century, up from 10.9% now.

Health care costs are expected to more than triple by the year 2000, from the current $458 billion to $1.5 trillion (19). The changes are due to the way health care services are used, rather than the aging of the population. The report also attributed the expected increase to the nation's reliance on expensive new medical technologies. The marked increase in health care costs after age

65 is also a factor. Considering the present costs cited by Camp for the care of low back pain in Oregon, that would escalate such charges to well over $100,000 per patient for surgical care in lumbar disc herniations. Certainly a frightening thought!

Snook (20) stated in 1980 that 25% of back cases accounted for 90% of the total cost of treatment. One-third of the cost of treatment is for medical cost, and disabilities are the remaining two-thirds (Fig. 1.1). Interestingly, hospital costs comprise one-third of the medical dollar, in spite of the fact that only 30% of the injured are hospitalized. Physicians' fees comprise one-third of the medical expense. Workmen's Compensation reports state that back injuries average 21% of all compensable work injuries. It is estimated that $2.7 billion per year is paid for care of back pain in the United States. Liberty Mutual Insurance Company, in 1980, paid $217 million for compensable back pain, almost $1 million for each working day (20). Total workmen's compensation costs for back pain in the United States each year can be estimated at $4.6 billion.

To evaluate the impact of back injury on industry, Spengler (21) conducted a retrospective analysis of injuries among hourly employees of a large industrial manufacturer in western Washington. The Boeing Company provided injury information on 31,200 employees for a 15-month period from July 1, 1979, to September 30, 1980. Of the 4645 injuries reported, 900 were back injuries. Claims related to back injuries constituted 19% of all workers' compensation claims but were responsible for 41% of the total injury costs, or approximately $1 million.

Back Pain Absorbs a Disproportionate Amount of Expense

Burton (22) states that low back disorders typically represent no more than 30% of insurance

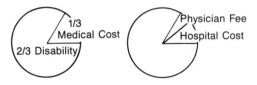

Figure 1.1. *Left,* Breakdown of treatment costs for back pain. *Right,* Breakdown of medical costs for back pain.

claims, but they account for more than 60% of health claim payments, particularly to industrial workers. This disproportionate relationship identifies the management of low back disease as the most inefficient application of health care funds and strongly suggests the need for much closer scrutiny and consideration in the future. He states that the health care profession is still seeking a cost-effective, conservative method for management of disc herniations. He states that his gravity lumbar reduction therapy is probably the most cost effective. He cites statistics from the Minnesota Department of Labor and Industry indicating that the average direct medical cost of treating a patient with disc herniation is $23,000. Actual costs are far higher, since they also reflect lost wages, lost productivity, insurance payments, and job retraining. He states, as opposed to the $23,000 typical case management of disc herniation, that the total cost for his inpatient program of traction reduction averages $3,400. This also saves the cost of postsurgical failure because of its efficiency and low risk potential.

Chiropractic Is Not Always the Least Expensive Care

This author does not think it is prudent to lead the reader to think that chiropractic is necessarily the cheapest form of low back care. Depending upon the problem, the extent of treatment must be determined. A study in West Virginia by the Workman's Compensation Fund examined 200 cases of back and neck injuries treated by chiropractors and 200 by physicians and osteopaths in 1980 and 1981 (23). The study was initiated at the request of chiropractors. It was pointed out that treatment and compensation for back injuries drained between $20 billion and $30 billion from the American economy every year. Workman's Compensation in West Virginia makes no recommendation to injured workers about choice of health care providers and does not deny payment to any providers licensed by the state.

Sixty licensed chiropractors were included in the study sample, and 10 of these had individual payments nearly $1000 greater than the average payment, which meant an average payment of more than $2000 per case. Chiropractors treated compensation patients for an average of 58 days, whereas medical doctors treated theirs an average of 38 days. Chiropractors kept their 200 patients off the job for a total of 11,556 days, and

medical doctors kept their 200 away from work for only 7746 days. Patients treated by chiropractors received an average of $1887 in disability benefits from Workman's Compensation, and those treated by physicians got only $1100 (23).

The average payment to a chiropractor was $1276; to a medical doctor, only $545. Total fees paid to chiropractors for their 200 cases totaled $255,139—234% of the $108,918 paid to medical doctors.

CHIROPRACTIC EFFECTIVENESS SEEING BROAD APPLICATION

Laying on of Hands

The laying on of hands as a method of healing has had its enthusiasts and skeptics through the ages, but recent studies appear to support the theory that electromagnetic fields may emanate from living tissue in one person and may produce demonstrable clinical improvement in another (24).

In fact, the studies have prompted the National Institutes of Health to award a 3-year grant to investigate the technique's effect on anxiety in patients scheduled for heart surgery. Dr. Janet Quinn, director of medical-surgical nursing at the University of South Carolina, has already begun gathering data on the ability of "therapeutic touch"—the contemporary name for the laying on of hands—to lower anxiety levels in cardiac patients. The research is based on a transfer of energy, biomagnetism, from the therapist to the patient.

In the trial, trained therapists used mental focusing techniques and a circling of their hands in outward movements about 6 inches from the patient's solar plexus. Untrained controls mimicked the therapists without being aware of the experiment's objective. Dr. Quinn noted a 17% reduction in anxiety in patients undergoing noncontact therapeutic therapy (NCTT), measured by testing participants with the standard self-evaluation questionnaire before and after exposure (24).

I do not attempt to seem esoteric, but to show one direction in healing that may involve chiropractic concepts. Some researchers have found that stress and anxiety can compromise the body's natural immunity from disease by suppressing natural killer cell activity. Medical sociologist Inger Corless (24) is currently conducting studies of AIDS and leukemia patients at the University of California, San Francisco, before and after NCTT. Dr. Corless says the patient group was selected for the study of the effect of NCTT on lymphocyte activity because of the large number of blood tests they undergo.

Dr. Bernard Grad (24), a biologist and associate professor at the Allan Memorial Institute of Psychiatry of McGill University in Montreal, has shown that mice genetically predisposed to leukemia respond favorably to such changes in magnetic fields. "The results [of such exposure] showed, without doubt, that the magnetic fields reduced the incidence of lymphatic leukemia in these animals," he says (24).

Endorphin Increase Following Manipulation

The role of spinal manipulation in the relief of pain is becoming clearer and more demonstrable as time passes. One approach to this study is through the effect of manipulation on the neurochemical mechanisms of antinoception. Chief among these is β-endorphin, which has been found to produce a wide range of beneficial effects, especially analgesia.

The results of the study demonstrated a small, but statistically significant, increase in serum β-endorphin levels in the experimental group at 5 minutes postintervention. The levels in the placebo and control groups demonstrated a steady decrease that was distinct from the response in the experimental group. With reservations regarding the sample size, the findings appear to demonstrate a small but unexpected increase of serum β-endorphin in response to a single cervical manipulation. This finding allows us to hypothesize that the pain-relieving effect of manipulation is, in part, due to a short-term increase in β-endorphin levels (25).

The findings from clinical trials and clinical experience agree that manipulation works best on pain of short duration. Its effectiveness tends to be all or nothing. Most published trials have shown that patients treated by manipulation improved more quickly (26) than untreated controls.

Manual Palpation for Spinal-Visceral Involvement

An interesting article concerning upper cervical subluxation as an occurrence with Crohns's disease was reported by Duke University Medical Center (27). They report a previously healthy 21-year-old black woman in whom erosive cervical spine disease with C1-C2 subluxation spontaneously developed. Various investigations led to the discovery of Crohn's disease, a heretofore unreported association. Thus, clinically silent or undiagnosed inflammatory bowel disease should be considered in the cause of atlantoaxial subluxation. This author feels this to be a most interesting association between spinal subluxation and organic disease. Furthermore, this is an association chiropractors have claimed and treated in the past 95 years of their existence.

Manual palpation of the spine for diagnosing possible viscerosomatic or somatovisceral disease was discussed in a study of 108 patients in the cardiac service of a hospital (28). A palpatory examination was conducted of segmental vertebral motion and muscle tension over the transverse processes at the T1-T5 area of the left side. The results for 108 patients in the cardiac service that were examined were compared with those of a group of patients with gastrointestinal disease who were observed to have similar evidence of somatic dysfunction but at vertebral levels associated with the autonomic nerve supply of the particular viscera involved. The palpatory findings were found to have a predictive value of 75% for indicating the presence of cardiac disease (28).

In another study, it was found that 43% of 72 patients with significant coronary stenosis had thoracic osteophytes, compared with the same finding in only 15% of patients with normal coronary arteries. It was concluded in this study (29) that the presence of thoracic osteophytosis is a specific indicator of coronary atherosclerosis 85% of the time and that further investigation was necessary to confirm the association.

EXTENT OF THE PROBLEM OF LOW BACK PAIN

Kelsey et al. (30, 31) state that there are 2.5 million low back injured and 1.2 million low back disabled adults in the United States. Furthermore, low back pain is the diagnosis in 10% of all chronic health problems. Impairments of the back are the most frequent cause of activity limitation in persons under 64 years of age. In subjects aged 25 to 44 years, a decrease in work capacity was caused by low back pain. An average of 28.6 days per 100 workers was lost each year, and there was an average of 9 days of confinement to bed. Each year, 113,000 laminectomies and disc excisions, as well as 34,000 other lumbar spine operations, are performed.

Frymoyer et al. (32, 33) report a retrospective and cross-sectional analysis in the United States of 1,221 males, 18 to 55 years of age, who had enrolled in a family practice facility from 1975 to 1978. Almost 70% had had low back pain. Extrapolating to the 50 million working American males in the age group 18 to 55, it was calculated that 17 million work days are lost annually. These patients had significantly more leg complaints, sought more medical care and treatment, and had more lost time from work when compared to people without low back pain. Patients with severe low back pain require care from health care practitioners, and a variety of medical treatments are required. Table 1.2 presents Frymoyer's listing of the type of health care services and treatment utilized by men with low back pain.

Rowe (34–36) reports that low back pain was the second most common excuse for sickness absence, second only to upper respiratory illness, among employees at a plant in New York City over a 10-year period. Thirty-five percent of sitting workers and 47% of workers with physically heavy jobs had made visits to the medical department because of low back pain during the 10-year period. Recurrences were frequent, occurring in about 85% of the people.

Low Back Pain Is Second Most Feared Disease

This author remembers hearing John Frymoyer state at the Challenge of the Lumbar Spine, 1986, that low back pain was the second most feared disease among men, second only to cancer. He further estimated that low back pain costs from $16 billion to $60 billion each year and that, in 1984, there were over 250,000 lumbar surgeries performed with a 15% failure rate. He stated that there are 40,000 reoperations per year.

Various occupations have been studied to predict the incidence of herniated lumbar intervertebral discs or sciatica. A study (37) was done of 592 men and women who had been discharged from a hospital with this diagnosis and were followed for 11 years. These cases were compared with 2140 controlled studies matched individually for sex, age, and place of residence. Subjects who, at the initial examination before the follow-up, had reported a history of back pain or sciatica were excluded. In men, the risk of being hospitalized due

Table 1.2.
Health Care Services and Treatment Utilized by Men with Low Back Pain[a]

Health Care Practitioner	Percentage Moderate ($n=565$)	Percentage Severe ($n=288$)
Family physician	30.5	66.7
Orthopedic surgeon	8.8	32.3
Neurosurgeon	2.7	9.5
Osteopath	7.0	23.8
Chiropractor	12.7	27.5
Physiotherapist	3.8	16.1
Other	5.0	12.1

[a]Data taken from Frymoyer JW, Pope MH, Constanza MC, Rosen JC, Goggin JE, Wilder DG: Epidemiologic studies of low-back pain. *Spine* 5(5):419–423, 1980.

to herniated lumbar disc or sciatica was lowest in professional and related occupations, significantly higher in all other groups, and highest among blue-collar workers in industry and among motor vehicle drivers. The variation in the risk between occupational groups of women proved less but was nevertheless still apparent. However, in women, but not in men, the risk was significantly associated with self-assessed strenuousness of work (37).

Tall men are found to account for a disproportionately large proportion of sickness caused by low back pain. This has been true in the mining industry, the steel industry, and the military (38).

Back pain, particularly the low back, has plagued humanity for thousands of years. Descriptions of lumbago and sciatica are found in the Bible and in the writings of Hippocrates (39). It is estimated that today, in the United States, 75 million people suffer from back pain, and there are 7 million new victims each year. Of these, 5 million are partly disabled and 2 million are unable to work at all. Eighty percent of people in the United States will suffer from this affliction some time in their lives (40).

The financial cost of low back pain is enormous. Five billion dollars will be spent in the United States this year on the diagnosis and treatment of low back pain, and another $10 billion will be spent on disability compensation, lawsuits, and worker's compensation. The cost for treatment of low back pain is higher than the cost for treatment of heart disease or the cost from traffic accidents. Ninety-three million work days will be lost annually in the United States due to low back pain. The incidence of low back pain increases faster than that of any other ailment of the human race (41).

Second Leading Group of Patients Seeking Care

It has been estimated that patients with low back complaints comprise the second largest diagnostic group seeking care from family physicians and make one-third of all orthopedic outpatient visits (42). Breen (43) points out that, of patients seeking chiropractic care for the first time, 53% complained of low back pain; 20% of lower leg pain; and 18%, of thigh and knee pain. Yet no universally recognized treatment exists for this common problem. Consequently, patients with low back pain not only frequently seek assistance from more than one specialist but also often receive conflicting advice as to the appropriate management of their condition (44).

RISK INDICATORS FOR LOW BACK TROUBLE

Four hundred forty-two men and 478 women, aged 30, 40, 50, and 60 years, were studied to identify possible indicators for first-time low back pain experience, recurrence, or persistence during a 1-year follow-up period. For men, the most important indicators for recurrence or persistence for low back trouble were intermittent claudication, restlessness, or other discomfort in the lower limbs; frequent headaches; and living alone. For women, the corresponding indicators were rumbling of the stomach and feeling of fatigue. For first-time experience of low back trouble, the indicators identified a frequent pain in the top of the stomach, previous hospitalizations and operations, daily smoking, and a long distance from home to work. It was stated that the results suggest that the population likely to experience future low back trouble does not enjoy good general health even prior to the first low back pain episode. In turn, this may lead to a greater psychosocial pressure on these patients (45).

Eighty-six percent of women who had been pregnant were found to have suffered from low back pain during pregnancy, and 51% experience aggravation of their low back pain during menstruation (46).

Epidemiology of work factors of low back pain was measured in men and women. In males, five variables had a direct relationship to low back pain: less overtime, more monotony, frequent lifting, heavy physical activity, and a high level of tension or worry at the end of the day. In females, three variables were directly correlated to the occurrence of low back pain: less responsibility, a high level of worry or tension at the end of the day, and extreme fatigue at the end of the day (47). A statistically significant increased risk of back injury is found in employees younger than 25 years of age, although their claims tend to be low in cost. Older employees have a lower injury rate, although there is a significantly increased risk of incurring high-cost back injury in older employees. The 31- to 40-year-old age group was most susceptible to high-cost back injury, and new employees tended to have a significantly increased risk of back injury. Women had fewer injuries than men but a statistically significant increased risk of becoming a high-cost injury claim. There was also a correlation between the incidence of back injuries and poor employee appraisal rating performed by the employee's supervisor within months before the injury (48).

The prevalence of alcohol problems with chronic low back pain finds alcohol abuse significantly more frequent among male low back patients (49). The use of analgesics and sedatives was not related to the degree of alcohol consumption. Alcohol problems were not found to influence the rehabilitation process negatively, probably because the rehabilitation program was not directed to the back only. The current study found that alcohol abuse and low back pain commonly occur together. It could not be decided, however, whether (a) alcohol abusers have more physical low back pain disorders; (b) alcohol abusers use the complaint of low back pain more commonly as a more socially accepted reason for missing work; or (c) chronic low back pain sufferers are driven to greater levels of alcohol consumption. In any case, accompanying alcohol abuse does not lessen the response to treatment of low back pain.

Seventy-six patients with chronic low back pain were asked to complete a pain disability index and a family history pain checklist. A significant positive relationship was found between the severity of chronic pain disability and the number of chronic pain conditions in the patient's families of origin and genesis. These findings support the position that pain disability is learned from family members, but controlled research is needed before dismissing genetic and other factors (50).

FACTORS ASSOCIATED WITH THE DIAGNOSIS AND TREATMENT OF LOW BACK PAIN

Congenital Anomalies

Many authors discuss the incidence of congenital anomalies in association with low back pain. Montgomery (51), who performed a thorough search of the literature, states that the use of pre-employment x-rays has been based upon the hypothesis that developmental abnormalities predispose to an increased incidence of low back injuries. The preponderance of evidence, however, indicates that this hypothesis is not substantiated. Snook et al. (52) point out that the common selection techniques such as medical histories, examinations, and x-rays are not an effective control for low back injuries. Employers who use these selection techniques have just as high an incidence of injuries as have employers who use no selection techniques.

X-ray Examinations Questioned

Reuler (53) states that the majority of adults will have at least one episode of acute low back pain, which will likely resolve regardless of treatment. Lumbar spine radiographs are overused, and there is little scientific support for many of the therapeutic interventions advocated. Even for those patients with symptomatic herniated discs, only a small fraction will ultimately require surgical intervention (53).

Low back pain is the most expensive ailment in the 30- to 60-year age group, and the most common reason for workman's compensation payments. It is second only to upper respiratory infection as the most common cause of absenteeism in industry. It is estimated that 7 million lumbosacral spine x-rays are performed annually, at an estimated cost of $825 million. Studies have shown that few lumbosacral examinations reveal important findings (54).

X-RAYS OF NO VALUE IN DETERMINING LOW BACK PAIN PRESENCE

When chiropractors and medical doctors interpreted lumbar spine radiographs in patients who had never had low back pain and patients who were having mild to severe low back pain, conclusions were reached that spinal radiographs were of no value in determining the presence or absence of low back complaints and had no value in epidemiological studies (55).

Troup (56) states that there are few epidemiologically established methods for identifying people who are susceptible to a first attack of back pain, though once back pain has been reported, recurrence may be predicted. Not too much is absolute in the cause and prevention of work-related back injuries. It is stressed that x-ray examination has very little value as a predictor of who will be at risk for back injury. Functional physical tests that do have some value in identifying who will be at risk of low back injury include lumbar flexibility, back extensor muscle endurance, general physical fitness, and osteopathic palpatory techniques. Once back pain has occurred, the following clinical signs correlate with the risk of reinjury to the back: restriction of pain-free straight leg raising, positive testing for nerve root tension, inability to sit up, pain or weakness on resisted hip flexion, and back pain on passive lumbar flexion.

Postural Faults Not Found to Lead to Spinal Pain

An epidemiological study examined the relationship between postural discrepancies and the subsequent development of back and neck pain in females who were members of the graduating classes of 1957, 1958, and 1959 of an eastern United States women's college. Posturally, symmetry was gathered from two sources: (a) measurements made from posture pictures taken early in the freshman year of college and obtained from each woman in the study; and (b) subjective evaluations made by the physical education department faculty at the time of examination. Information on the development of back and neck disorders during the subsequent 25 years was obtained by a questionnaire. Three parameters of postural asymmetry were examined from the posture picture measurements: elevation of one shoulder, elevation of one hip, and deviation of the spine from the midline of the body. Neither these parameters nor the physical education department evaluation was associated with a subsequent report of low back pain, mid back pain, or neck pain (57).

X-rays Not Recommended to Diagnose Spinal Pain

Deyo (58) states that for patients with low risk of systemic illness, lumbosacral films can be omitted or delayed without causing patient anxiety, dissatisfaction, or dysfunction. Furthermore, this strategy may reduce future expectations of x-ray use and costs of care.

X-rays are not now recommended for three major reasons:

1. The x-rays do not predict who will have low back problems.
2. Individuals receive radiation to reproductive organs, which is not beneficial to their health.
3. An asymptomatic and only radiologically evident finding that would not affect work can nevertheless prevent an applicant from getting a particular job. This may infringe on his/her civil right of equal opportunity for employment and may even affect future insurability.

Finneson (59) states that there is no higher incidence of transitional vertebrae in the backs of those seeking care for low back pain than there is in the normal population. Wigh and Anthony (60) point out that of 200 patients operated on for lumbar disc herniations, 42 had a lumbosacral transitional vertebra. In none of the 42 patients was there myelographic evidence of herniation of such a disc. This certainly raises the question, addressed in the chapter on transitional segments, of how best to treat Bertolotti's syndrome (61). Semon and Spengler (62) point out that there is no significant difference in time loss between athletes with spondylolysis and those without it. Lenz (63) found that 86.6% of patients with spondylolisthesis showed favorable results under chiropractic manipulation of a flexion-distraction type.

Stenosis, it is believed, enhances the symptoms of disc protrusion and necessitates surgery in patients with a prolapsed disc (64). Martin (65) found, however, that back pain preceded leg pain in only three of 16 patients with a prolapsed disc. Furthermore, in patients with a recurring prolapsed disc necessitating repeat surgery, stenosis was found at the level of surgery. This raises two questions: Does back pain preceding leg pain indicate protrusion, and does leg pain without back pain indicate prolapse? Rothman and Simeone (66) state that in patients with a prolapsed disc

there may be a sudden onset of sciatica and a sudden abatement of back pain. It is not clear what role stenosis, lateral recess, and central stenosis play in the etiology of neurogenic intermittent claudication. Eisenstein (67) points out that the lower limit of normal in the sagittal diameter of the vertebral canal is 15 mm. Ullrich et al. (68) point out that the smallest normal sagittal canal diameter is 11.5 mm with stenosis. Therefore, some differing opinions exist as to the lowest normal sagittal diameter of the vertebral canal.

FACET INVOLVEMENT

A description of severe disabling low back pain is given in a patient whose radiographs show near-normal facet structures. Spinal fusion of patients with low back pain showed the excised facet joint surfaces to have some of the histological changes seen in chondromalacia patellae and in osteoarthritis of other larger joints. The most frequent change was focal full-thickness cartilage necrosis or loss of cartilage with exposure of subchondral bone, but osteophyte formation was remarkably absent in all specimens. It was suggested that there are both clinical and histological similarities between the facet arthrosis syndrome and chondromalacia patellae. Facet arthrosis may be a relatively important cause of intractable back pain in young and middle-aged adults (69).

Among the theories regarding the possible mechanisms involved in osteoarthrosis of the articular facet joints is a theory based on preliminary histological evidence of an extensive vascular supply to the osteoarthritic cartilage at the lumbosacral zygapophyseal joints (70).

Disc space narrowing causes a marked increase in peak pressure between opposed facets in the zygapophyseal joints, and it is known that there is an association between osteoarthrosis of these joints and osteophytic lipping of vertebral bodies. However, osteoarthrosis of these zygapophyseal joints need not always occur at the same level as intervertebral disc degeneration. Vascularization of the articular cartilage of the facet joint in minor osteoarthrosis may be a source of pain, since the blood vessels in the hypervascular area are innervated by vasomotor nerves.

This increased vascular supply may indicate an attempt at cartilage repair and may indicate further that low back pain of a vascular origin could be experienced by patients with minor osteoarthrosis.

Salicylate and Nonsteroidal Antiinflammatory Drug Effects

Discussing the vascularization of joints in degenerative osteoarthrosis, the effects of salicylate and nonsteroidal antiinflammatory drug effects on cartilage must be reviewed. Both of these drugs decrease the synthesis of glycosaminoglycan, causing the lowered proteoglycan content found in osteoarthritic cartilage (71).

Newman (72), in a retrospective investigation of the relation between the use of nonsteroidal antiinflammatory drugs and acetabular destruction in primary osteoarthritis of the hip, found that regular intake of these drugs was noted in 31 of 37 patients with acetabular destruction. This was further disturbing because of the difficulty in achieving satisfactory hip replacements in patients with severely damaged acetabula.

HYDROCORTISONE EFFECTS ON CARTILAGE

Similarly, the intramuscular injection of hydrocortisone has been found to accelerate the aging process of the nucleus pulposus of the intervertebral disc. Degenerative changes occur earlier in the periphery of the nucleus pulposus than in the central region and develop earlier in mice treated with higher doses of hydrocortisone than in mice treated with lower doses. This could be of significance in the treatment of humans with hydrocortisone (73).

Hydrocortisone treatment results in a decrease in cartilage plate thickness, leading to degenerative changes. Such suppression of the growth of the spinal column, often seen in children, may be the result of long-term steroid treatment (74).

FACET WEIGHT BEARING

Normal facet articulations carry from 3 to 25% of the superimposed body weight. If the facet joints become arthritic, the load can become as high as 47% (75). Further, the transmission of compressive facet load occurs through contact of the tip of the inferior facet with the pars of the vertebra below. The overloaded facet joint will cause rearward rotation of the inferior facet, resulting in stretching of the joint capsule. This increased facet load is due to a decreased disc height. The final hypothesis is that excessive facet loads stretch the joint capsule and can be a cause for low back pain (75).

The question as to what causes the onset of pain and instability, the facet or the disc, remains unanswered. Mooney and Robertson (76) performed lumbar facet injection on 100 consecutive patients with lumbago and sciatica and found that one-fifth of these patients received long-term relief and one-third received partial relief. Carrera et al. (77) point out that the distance between adjacent points on articular facets of 40 apparently normal joints was 2 to 4 mm. They therefore considered a joint space of less than 2 mm diagnostic of articular cartilage thinning. Carrera (78) injected anesthetic and steroid into the facet joints of 20 patients and found that six patients reported continued relief of pain after 6 to 12 months, seven experienced complete return of pain several days to 6 months later, and seven derived no benefit from the block. Dory (79) found that when anesthetic or steroid was injected into 70 lumbar joints in 27 patients, the articular capsule nearly always burst, and the leaking medium provided an explanation of how the injected anesthetics worked in the relief of low back pain. The leakage occurred in the lateral aspect of the joints where branches of the posterior ramus of the spinal nerve pass, and medially where it enters the epidural space and, sometimes, the intervertebral foramen.

Chynn et al. (80) reported that in spinal stenosis, the superior articular process is more sagittally oriented. Furthermore, their study indicates that plain films are of great usefulness in the diagnosis of lumbar spinal stenosis, contrary to the opinion of some authorities who believe that such plain films are of little value. In many cases, clinical presentation and the careful analysis of plain films are sufficient to reach an almost certain diagnosis.

Lora and Long (81) found that radicular radiation of pain is not generated by stimulation of the nerves in and around the facets, but widespread referral of sensation even into the leg is possible. This referral of sensation, however, characteristically had a diffuse nonradicular character, was difficult for the patient to localize, and did not go below the knee in any patient.

Hypermobility

Van Akkerveeken et al. (82) found that when the annulus fibrosus and posterior longitudinal ligament were unstable due to tearing or stretching, there was a posterior and rotatory displacement of the vertebral bodies upon one another on extension. We utilize this technique in diagnosis to determine the stability of facet syndrome, and we correlate it with recurrent and totally relievable low back pain. Patients having 3 mm or less movement of the posterior body plate margins in relation to their adjacent vertebrae are considered to have stable functional spinal units; however, those showing over 3 mm of movement, one upon the other, are said to have unstable facet syndromes. The superior segment of an unstable facet segment may move either anteriorly, as a degenerative spondylolisthesis, or posteriorly, as a retrolisthesis subluxation, depending upon the plane of articulation of the zygapophyseal joints. Retrolisthesis is more common at the L5 level and degenerative spondylolisthesis at the L4 segment. Further details on these entities will be covered in Chapter 11, "Facet Syndrome," and Chapter 13, "Spondylolisthesis."

Tropism

In a study of 82 patients with low back and sciatic pain, this author (83) found that 23% revealed tropism at the level of the disc lesion. Ehni and Weinstein (84) state that 20% of the normal population have stenosis. Cyron and Hutton (85) state that articular tropism results in the manifestation of lumbar instability as joint rotation, with this rotation occurring toward the side of the more oblique facet, where it will create additional stress on the posterolateral annulus fibrosus; this will be the side of the nuclear protrusion. Determination of tropism on plain radiographic study versus computed tomography study will be discussed in Chapter 2 from the results of a research study performed in this author's low back pain clinic.

Straight Leg and Well Leg Raising Signs

Breig and Troup (86) state that medial hip rotation is associated with increased tension and neurological dysfunction of the lumbosacral roots. We apply medial hip rotation with the straight leg raising sign to make this evaluation. Furthermore, Hudgins (87) states that the crossed straight leg raising (well leg raising) sign is indicative of a herniated lumbar disc in 97% of patients, even with a negative myelogram. We also apply this sign for clarification. In Chapter 9, "Diagnosis," the significance of pain location on straight leg raising, that is, whether it is located in the low

back, leg, or both, will be covered based on two research studies.

Rotational Motion of the Lumbar Spine

Farfan (88) points out that, in the laboratory, as little as 3° of forced rotation of the intervertebral joint produces damage to the disc and facets. The outer fibers of the annulus are stretched and may be torn off the end plate. The inner annulus becomes separated and loose if forced rotation is continued. Virgin (89) observed that compression was not a factor in causing nuclear protrusion. He found that, when a longitudinal incision was made in the posterolateral part of the annulus all the way to the nucleus, under compression the nucleus did not change its shape or escape. It was only under rotation that the loud snapping sounds were heard as the annular fibers tore. These sounds were similar to the loud snapping sounds known to occur with the sudden onset of backache. Lumsden and Morris (90) found that approximately 6° of rotation occurred at the lumbosacral joint during maximal rotation and that rotation at the lumbosacral joint was not measurably affected by tropism. Maigne (91) states that no rotation is possible in the lumbar spine because of facet orientation and form, and that flexion and extension are essentially all that are permitted in the lumbar spine.

The ultimate role of rotation in chiropractic practice must, therefore, be fully evaluated. Certainly it is a problem, as most disc injuries coming to malpractice are the result of various lumbopelvic moves made in the side posture position (92).

Validity of Lateral Bending Studies in Diagnosing Disc Lesion

Controversy exists on this subject and will be addressed fully in Chapter 2, "Biomechanics," and Chapter 9, "Diagnosis." Gainer and Nugent (93) state that lumbar disc herniation is one of the most common causes of back pain and is usually easily diagnosed by a history and physical examination. The use of lateral bending studies of the lumbar spine is extremely important to the chiropractic physician in the differentiation between medial, lateral, and subrhizal disc herniations, contained or noncontained, as well as in the establishment of postreduction findings of improvement. Weitz (94) states that the lateral bending sign studies have diagnostic reliability

1. Twenty of 39 patients (51%) with an unequivocal clinical picture of a ruptured intervertebral disc unrelieved by conservative care had good or excellent results after rotatory manipulation of the spine under anesthesia.
2. The appearance of these patients' myelograms before and after manipulation, whether positive or negative, was unchanged.
3. Ten of the 27 patients with positive myelograms had good to excellent results 3 years or more after manipulation.
4. Patients without a demonstrable myelographic defect consistently did better after manipulation than those with a defect.

Comparison of Allopathic and Chiropractic Treatment

Woolley (109) interviewed workmen's compensation-covered patients in Utah to compare the outcome when treated by allopaths versus chiropractic medicine practitioners. One hundred and ten patients treated by medical doctors and 122 patients treated by chiropractors were interviewed.

Major areas of difference found in the study related to the number of treatment visits and duration of treatment. The patients were seen, on the average, about 13 times by chiropractors as opposed to approximately seven times by medical doctors. However, the treatments by the medical doctor took over 9 weeks, as opposed to 6.5 weeks for chiropractors. This averages out at 1.2 visits per week for medical doctor-attended patients versus 2.5 visits per week for the chiropractor-attended patients.

Deyo (110) states that traction stretches the back so that the vertebrae are pulled away from each other, and roentgenographic studies have suggested that spinal traction is capable of distracting vertebrae and diminishing disc protrusion in patients with herniated discs. The best study he cited was that of Larsson et al. (111), which suggested an advantage for the particular technique of autotraction over the use of a corset at 1 week, but not at 3 months of follow-up.

A number and variety of contraindications to joint manipulation are directly related to the skill of the manipulator, the techniques used, and the philosophy of practice. For instance, the traditional manipulator using a forceful lumbar torque or a high-velocity thrust might consider an acute injury or prolapse of the disc a contraindication, whereas a practitioner of oscillation would be more likely to proceed as long as the techniques for reducing the patient's pain were not aggravating any of the objective signs, such as loss of skin sensation and reflex change (112).

Traction Principles in Manipulation

The following points are essential to the administration of therapeutically effective lumbar traction (113):

1. The traction force must be great enough to effect a structural change (movement) at the spinal segment. Cyriax (114) reported a visible separation with sustained traction of 55 kg for 15 minutes. Other studies have reported measurable separation in the lumbar spine at weights ranging from 37 to 91 kg. Judovich (113) advocated a friction-free force equal to one-half of the patient's body weight as a minimum to cause therapeutic effects in the lumbar spine. It is not necessary that the first treatment be administered at that weight, and it must be remembered that the minimum weight necessary to cause measurable separation will not always be enough to produce satisfactory results. It is important in every case that the patient's reaction and the results of the treatment be assessed; adjustments can then be made until satisfactory results are achieved. The weights required to effect damage to the vertebral structures have also been studied. Most often cited is the study by Ranier, in which fresh cadavers were used. According to DeSeze and Levernieux (115), Ranier found that a force of 182 kg was necessary to produce a rupture of the dorsolumbar spine (T11, T12). Harris (113) indicated that enormous traction forces were necessary to cause damage to the lumbar spine, with the breaking load possibly as high as 364 kg.

2. A split table is necessary to eliminate friction. As mentioned previously, it is the effective traction force on the spine that is important, and any friction involved must be considered. A split table essentially eliminates friction.

3. The patients must be able to relax.

The traction mode (sustained or intermittent) selected will depend on the condition and comfort of the patients. Disc protrusions are usually treated more effectively by sustained traction or longer hold-rest periods (60-second hold, 20-second rest) of intermittent traction, whereas joint dysfunction and degenerative disc disease usually respond to shorter hold-rest periods of intermittent traction.

When disc protrusion is treated by spinal traction, the treatment time should be short. As the disc space is widened, the intradiscal pressure is decreased. This is a beneficial effect and, according to Saunders, explains the demonstration by Matthews of movement of contrast medium into the disc space. It seems that this decrease in pressure will only equalize pressure with that of the surrounding tissue. When the pressure is equalized, the "suction" effect on the protrusion is lost. If this has occurred and the patient is released from traction, the intradiscal pressure could, at least theoretically, increase in relation to that of the surrounding tissue. If this is the case, increased pain may appear after treatment. Saunders has not observed this adverse reaction in intermittent treatments of less than 8 minutes. Often, the first treatment is only 3 to 5 minutes long.

Unilateral Lumbar Distraction Principles

Unilateral lumbar traction can be administered effectively by hooking only one side of the pelvic harness to the traction source. It can be especially effective when traction is indicated and a stronger force is desired on one side of the spine, for example, in unilateral joint dysfunction. Unilateral lumbar traction may also be effective in the treatment of patients with disc protrusion who have "protective scoliosis." Patients who have protrusion lateral to the nerve root may lean away from the side of symptoms for relief. When patients with protective scoliosis are placed in conventional bilateral traction, the scoliosis straightens, which may cause increased pain. The traction does not appear to be beneficial. Conversely, if the scoliosis can be maintained while the traction is applied, the treatment may be administered without increasing patient discomfort, thus enhancing the chances of achieving the desired results of the treatment (113).

A single, blind, randomized, controlled, clinical trial of rotational manipulation for low back pain of recent onset in 81 adults was carried out against a control treatment of minimal massage and low-level electrostimulation. The initial

status and outcome were measured on scales quantifying symptoms, activities of daily life, mobility, tenderness to palpation, aggravation of pain by coughing or sneezing, limitation of motion on testing, and forward flexion. On retest, there was no statistically significant difference between the improvement scores of the treated or control groups on any of the scales (116).

Chemonucleolysis Results

Fager has similar negative findings on a prominent surgical procedure called chemonucleolysis (117). He states that papaya in his life will be limited to the breakfast table. He goes on to state that he has seen marked disc narrowing following this procedure and he has nightmarish visions of the 6000 medical doctors, who were trained to inject the patients, performing this on 50 to 100 patients a year and producing an entirely new generation of iatrogenic back problems in the future, just as our generation has produced many of the present postsurgical failures by injudicious surgery.

Epidural Steroid Injection

Seventy-three patients with lumbar radicular pain syndromes were treated in perspective, randomized, double-blind fashion with epidural steroids. Patients had radiographic confirmation of lumbar nerve root compression, consistent with the clinical diagnosis of either an acute herniated nucleus pulposus or spinal stenosis. No statistically significant difference was observed between the control and experimental patients with either acute disc herniation or spinal stenosis. Use of epidural steroids, therefore, must be made with the realization that no clinical efficacy for this treatment has been found (118).

The Reduction of Disc Protrusion

Burton (119) has developed a system of gravity lumbar reduction of herniated nucleus pulposus which he feels addresses the following disc problems:

1. Disc "bulging," producing distention of the annulus and posterior longitudinal ligament. This entity produces pain by stimulating branches of the sinuvertebral nerve. A dorsal ramus pain syndrome typically referred to the low back, hips,

and knees is produced. Pain is rarely referred as far as the ankles.

2. A herniated disc, in which nuclear material extends beyond the annulus but is contained by the posterior longitudinal ligament (sometimes called a "roof disc"). Compression of a spinal nerve either exiting or traversing the interspace produces sciatic pain that radiates to the toes and feet and neurological findings that are associated with this compression.

3. A herniated disc in which nuclear material extends beyond the annulus and is beginning to erode through the posterior longitudinal ligament but has not yet become a free protrusion.

Experience has shown that when herniated disc material extrudes past the posterior longitudinal ligament (free protrusion) or migrates in the spinal canal (sequestered fragment), the application of gravity traction accentuates pain and neurological deficit rather than alleviating it. This is most important to document, because it signals the need to discontinue the gravity reduction program and consider more aggressive treatment modalities such as chemonucleolysis or surgery.

Cheap Care Is Not Always the Best Care

Snook (20) discusses treatment of patients from the standpoint of the insurance industry. He states that everyone knows that low back pain is a costly problem, but that cheap care is generally short-sighted and looks for a quick and simple medical solution to the low back problem. The goal is to get the patient back to the same job as quickly as possible, without regard to the type of job being performed. Cheap care often emphasizes the detection of malingerers and fails to recognize that physicians, lawyers, management, and unions can also interfere with return to work. Cost-effective care is synonymous with early intervention, conservative treatment (unless otherwise indicated), patient follow-up, education (for both the patient and the employer), and timely decisions regarding care management. Cost-effective care recognizes the value of early return to work as part of the therapy and utilizes such techniques as modified work and modified hours. Cost-effective care also recognizes the high rate of recurrence and tries to reduce it with job redesign or job replacement. The goal of cost-effective care is not only to return the individual to work, but to keep him or her there.

Low Back Wellness School

Moffet et al. (120) report that 92 chronic low back pain patients were randomly allocated to two groups to evaluate the effectiveness of a back school compared with an exercise-only regimen according to specified outcome variables. Data from 78 patients with 7 years mean duration of symptoms was analyzed. At 16 weeks, functional disability and pain level showed a significant difference, with back school patients continuing to make an improvement. Back school methods of managing low back pain make maximal use of limited resources and appear to be effective, especially in the longer term.

Another study (121) states that rehabilitation training in the treatment of low back pain gives the following benefits:

1. Pain elimination;
2. Stretching of the lumbar part of the spine and relieving of compressed nerve roots;
3. Strengthening of trunk muscles by forming a strong "muscle corset;"
4. Restoring good body posture, consequently restoring the stability of the spine.

This author utilizes low back wellness school in a 2-hour class held every 3 weeks in our clinic. Low back wellness school, therefore, is available to every new patient within, at the most, 3 weeks after starting treatment in our clinic. It consists of three portions: the first being teaching the patient the causes of low back pain; the second being instruction in ergonomic principles on how to bend, lift, and twist the back in daily living so as to cause minimal irritation; and the third consisting of showing the patient how to do the 12 Cox low back wellness exercises.

Each patient who goes through low back wellness school has a complete understanding of his or her low back problem, how to cope with it, how to do his or her part at home to limit aggravation of a weakened spine, and how to do the home exercises. The patient is able to assume the responsibility for his or her own care and soon comes to realize that recurrence is usually due to some foolish movement performed outside of the office. Back school allows us to shift the basic responsibility of a patient's back problem to the patient, rather than having the patient make the doctor assume the greatest, if not total, burden of the low back problem. Until the patient attends low back wellness school, he or she is not as involved in his or her back care as we would like.

Clinical Considerations

In a 2-year statistical study of 194 patients with acute disc syndrome, Valentini (122) found that 171 were successfully treated by chiropractic manipulation and 23 failed to respond to treatment. He believed that in patients with acute disc syndrome the aim of treatment should be the earliest possible reduction of the disc protrusion or adaptation of the protrusion and nerve root to a more specific coexistence. The treatment used was a side posture rotary adjustment performed in the free and painless direction toward the opposite side of the antalgic posture. In 71% of these patients, he also utilized a distraction technique.

Tindall (123) states that 200,000 lumbar disc operations are performed by neurosurgeons each year and that this represents the most common operation performed by the majority of neurosurgeons. Concerning the use of the electromyogram (EMG), he believes that it virtually never influences the decision involving the management of the patient and does not establish the diagnosis of a herniated lumbar disc. He also believes that protrusion or rupture of the nucleus pulposus is usually preceded by degenerative changes characterized structurally by radiating cracks in the annulus that weaken its resistance to nuclear herniation. The characteristic clinical features of back and leg pain are related to irritation and stretching of the sinuvertebral nerve by the bulging annulus and by direct pressure on the nerve root, respectively.

Eagle (124) states that among the world's 2 million doctors, there are only 20 who have devoted their careers exclusively to researching back pain. With a permanent pool of 2 billion patients who might benefit from advice or ministrations, the scope for further research is almost unlimited.

Cookson (125), writes rather pointedly that when the patient with low back pain is examined, three questions must be kept in mind. For us, the most important of these is: "Is this a disc lesion or one of the uncommon causes of backache?" (125). The list of authors who state that 90% of low back pain is caused by the intervertebral disc is quite lengthy.

At the 1975 Symposium on the Research Status of Spinal Manipulative Therapy, Nachemson (126) stated that new types of treatment for low back pain are introduced with some frequency in the medical field, tried for some time, and then proven or disproven by clinical trials in various places around the world. No such attempts have been made by chiropractors or osteopaths for nearly 100 years.

Goldstein (127) states that studies on the scientific basis of manipulative therapy should not be misread to mean only basic science studies. Studies on the scientific basis of manipulative therapy clearly include both basic studies in areas such as biomechanics, and clinical studies in areas such as the efficacy of therapy; "clinical studies are considered as much a part of research on the scientific basis of any therapy as is the understanding of the fundamental mechanisms underlying therapy" (127).

Disc Lesions in Children and Adolescents

The incidence of lumbar disc protrusion in children varies from 0.8% (128) to 3.2% (129) for surgically proven disc protrusions. Fifty-eight patients, ranging in age from 8 to 19 years, were followed for an average of 6.8 years after the onset of their lumbar disc protrusion. Trauma was not a significant etiological factor, but there was a high incidence of low back pain in relatives of affected patients. The clinical picture was similar to that seen in adults except for a relative paucity of neurological signs. Approximately 40% of the patients responded well to conservative treatment. Of the patients treated surgically, 50% had good results; these patients had short histories of low back and leg pain. The other half of the surgically treated patients with fair or poor results did have slightly longer histories, but there was no factor obviously affecting the outcome. It was felt that early admission to a hospital for a trial of conservative treatment should be offered for adolescents with a clinical picture of a prolapsed disc. Failure of the symptoms to resolve even in the absence of neurological signs should prompt radiculography with a view to surgical exploration (130).

Response of Patients to Chiropractic Care

Bronfort (131) reported the clinical course of low back pain during chiropractic treatment given to 298 patients in 10 different chiropractic clinics.

At the first contact with the chiropractor, the patient had a current episode of low back pain that had lasted less than 1 week in 30% of cases and more than 4 weeks in 51%. Sixty-five percent had radiating pain into the lower extremities; 38% were unable to work. Fifty-three percent of the patients had consulted a medical doctor or had received other types of treatment due to the current episode. Nineteen percent were referred to the chiropractor by the medical doctor.

After each period of registration, approximately 75% of the patients reported being free of symptoms or feeling much better.

Another study of 465 patients undergoing chiropractic care produced the following statistics (132).

1. In general, chiropractic measures are more effective in nonaccident (NA) cases than in accident (AC) cases in both male and female patients.
2. No single adjustment level (cervical, thoracic, lumbar, or sacral) shows any advantage over the others in low back pain case management.
3. In patient management, manipulative therapy in addition to nonmanipulative methods did not appear superior to only nonmanipulative approaches (nutrition, physical therapy, and counseling); this may be due to a physician's selection of therapeutic measures as opposed to random selection.
4. Female patients with NA-caused disorder responded better to chiropractic treatments when compared to those with AC-caused back pain problems.
5. Male AC patients responded better to chiropractic treatment than did female patients with AC-caused problems.
6. Among various age groups, no particular group is more associated with low back pain problems.
7. In general, there are proportionally more NA-caused cases than AC cases in both males and females.

The study suggests that the chiropractic conservative health care is effective in most cases of nonaccident-caused low back pain disorders (132).

Acceptance of Chiropractic by the Public

Patient acceptance of chiropractic care is demonstrated in a report by Parker and Tupling (133). Of 84 patients visiting a chiropractor for the first time, 82% had received previous treatment and failed to respond, nearly 60% gave a desire for

pain relief as the sole reason for their visit, and two-thirds affirmed that they visited the chiropractor as a last resort. At 10-week follow-up, however, all but 11% reported some improvement, and 74% were sufficiently satisfied with their treatment to affirm that they would return to a chiropractor if their condition recurred.

Parker and Tupling (133) also found that, at the initial consultation, patients who were asked to compare medical doctors and chiropractors with regard to interpersonal attitudes, technical skills, and social characteristics stated that they considered the chiropractor to be more expensive, less available, and less regarded by society than are general practitioners. At follow-up, however, patients judged chiropractors to be equal to general practitioners in technical competence but somewhat superior with regard to interpersonal characteristics. Parker and Tupling conclude that the chiropractor fulfills an emerging cultural need for a less technocratic medical system with an emphasis on holistic natural therapies and consideration of interpersonal needs. They suggest that "the chiropractor may be more attuned to the total needs of the patient than his medical counterpart" (133).

BACK SURGERY: AN EVALUATION

Chronology of the Study of Back Pain

Modern studies of the lumbar spine date back to the 1820s. In 1858, von Luschka described the anatomy of the disc (134). Dandy (135), in 1929, performed surgery on a lumbar spine from which he removed free fragments of herniated disc that had compressed the cauda equina; he noted that the lesion afforded an explanation of low back and leg pain. Mixter and Barr (136), in 1934, reported on the role of herniation of a lumbar disc in the etiology of sciatica. Their classic paper marked the beginning of the trend toward use of surgery in the relief of low back and leg pain. This trend has continued to the present, and as late as 1976, 450,000 back operations were performed in the United States during the course of one year (137).

Effects on and Cost to Patients

Dommisse and Grahe (138) state that 48% of 7391 patients operated on by 17 surgeons and reported in 23 publications had recurrence of symptoms (backache, sciatica, or both) within a year after back surgery. Burton (139) states that the long-term failure rate of back surgery has been variously reported as being between 10% and 40%. The number of persons with the failed back surgery syndrome (FBSS), characterized by intractable pain and functional incapacitation, must be significant. He concludes by stating that lumbar arachnoiditis, a definable pathological entity, appears to be present in failed back surgery syndrome patients to a much higher degree than was previously thought: "If for no other reason that the mere existence of lumbar arachnoiditis, it is clear that a major reappraisal of the present medical and surgical approach to lumbar disc disease is called for. The introduction of foreign bodies into the subarachnoid space for diagnostic determinations invariably involves some patient risk. Emphasis must be placed on the most innocuous myelographic agents. Emphasis must also be placed on the development of noninvasive means of diagnosing disease of the lumbar spine."[b]

CHIROPRACTIC: AN ANSWER TO THE PROBLEM

Biomechanical Causes of Disc Disease

Intervertebral disc disease represents one of the most complex of medical disorders. It has been hypothesized that when humanity's ancestors traded their arboreal existence for that of an erect biped, the stage may have been set for the later development of intervertebral disc disease. Apparently, the human is not designed to withstand the stresses and strains created by the erect posture and centered on the lumbosacral spine. Repeated small traumatic insults add to the increased susceptibility of the spine and discs to degeneration. Yamada (140, 141) studied intervertebral disc herniation in biped rats and mice. He noted that when there was a change in the mode of locomotion from the quadrupedal stance to the bipedal stance, that is, walking on the hind legs, the animals developed degenerated lumbar discs within 12 to 24 months. No degeneration occurred in the control group, however. Yamada also showed that there were great mechanical stresses on the sacroiliac portion of the

spinal column in bipedal animals, which, he believed, resulted in intervertebral disc herniation.

Turek (142) describes well the pathophysiology of the continuous and progressive degenerative changes of the intervertebral disc. The process may begin in a young person of 15 years of age with the onset of concentric cracking and cavitation of the annular fibers, proceed in the mature adult in the 3rd decade of life to swollen granular changes in the nucleus pulposus, and culminate in the middle and later years of life with the disc becoming a sudden mass. Turek further describes the thinning of the annular fibers to a thin fibrous ring, which is torn by the slightest force (142).

In addition to the stresses caused by erect posture during locomotion and by degeneration of the disc, there is the stress produced by lifting weight. Strait et al. (143) demonstrated that tremendous low back strain may be involved in forward trunk flexion. An 180-lb man flexed 60° at the trunk from vertical and holding a 50-lb weight in his hands exerts an 850-lb compression force on the fifth lumbar vertebra.

The Role of Chiropractic

Over half the patients seen by the chiropractic physician complain of low back pain. When this low back pain is associated with sciatic neuralgia, the chiropractic physician must determine whether there is a disc protrusion, the level of its involvement, and the therapeutic approach to be instituted. It behooves our profession, therefore, to develop an approach to the problem of disc protrusion that encompasses diagnosis without the use of contrast medium and therapy without the use of surgical repair, tempered by the possibility that ultimately a surgical approach may be necessary in a few cases.

We in chiropractic have an opportunity to demonstrate that we have "an idea whose time has arrived," namely, that the best treatment for the patient with low back pain caused by disc protrusion is the conservative approach of chiropractic manipulation as described in this textbook. For many years, we have heard much about the diagnosis of disc protrusion from routine x-ray study of the low back. As is true in most other diseases of humans, diagnosis cannot and does not depend on x-ray study alone—it requires the use of clinical, laboratory, x-ray, and other procedures to achieve the highest degree of accuracy, and yet this use so often is found want-

[b] From Burton CV, Wiltse LL: Guest editors' comments. *Spine* 3(1):1–23, 1978.

ing. The diagnosis of disc protrusion is no different. It requires careful clinical, orthopedic, neurological, and roentgenographic findings to determine the site, type, and severity of the lesion.

CLINICAL RESULTS UTILIZING COX FLEXION DISTRACTION IN LOW BACK PAIN PATIENTS[c]

A chiropractic multicenter observational pilot study to compile statistics on the examination procedures, diagnosis, types of treatment rendered, results of treatment, number of days of care, and number of treatments required to arrive at a 50% improvement and a maximum clinical improvement was collected on 576 patients with low back and/or leg pain. The purpose was to determine the congenital and developmental changes in patients with low back and/or leg pain, the combinations of such anomalies, the accuracy of orthodox diagnostic tests in assessing low back pain, ergonomic factors affecting onset, and, ultimately, the specific difficulty factors encountered in treating the various conditions seen in the average chiropractor's office. For all conditions treated, the average number of days required to attain maximum improvement was 43 and the number of visits 19. It was concluded that this study provided useful data for assessment of routine chiropractic office-based diagnosis and treatment of related conditions; however, further controlled studies are necessary for validation of specific parameters.

Chiropractic manipulation is primarily carried out in a clinical or private office setting devoid of institutionalization, a situation with both positive and negative results. It has positive results in that it minimizes cost factors to patients, since hospital care is not utilized. Furthermore, it demands that chiropractic physicians develop their diagnostic skills to as high a degree as possible. It has negative results in that the patient must be sufficiently ambulatory to go to a private office for care. This removes some from chiropractic care because of their need to be institutionalized.

Interest in the nonsurgical care of low back pain and leg pain is prominent in the world today, primarily because learned surgeons, realizing that the success of surgery is directly related to the selection of the patient, feel that the best of conservative means should be attempted before resorting to surgery. Some even go as far as to state that 2 to 3 months of conservative care should be given before surgery is utilized. The insurance agency, along with the chiropractic profession, has

long questioned the length of time and number of visits required to produce satisfactory clinical results in patients suffering from low back pain and sciatica. To get answers, further questions must be asked: What are the specific diagnosis in parients seeking chiropractic care? What is the average visitation frequency and number days of care required to arrive at 50% versus maximum chiropractic relief?

Accurate assessment of the types of low back pain conditions the chiropractor is treating are best collected in private chiropractic practices, inasmuch as this is the setting under which the vast majority of cases are handled. With this fact in mind, the International Academy on Chiropractic Low Back Pain Study, a nonprofit research institution, selected 23 doctors of chiropractic throughout the United States who agreed to follow a prescribed examination procedure on 20 consecutive low back pain and/or sciatica patients who were seen in their respective offices. The findingd from these examinations were compiled on standardized forms for computer analysis.

Materials and Methods

A standardized 293-variable questionnaire form (available from the author, J.M.C., by request) was used by each participating doctor in the examination and treatment of 20 or more consecutive cases of low back pain that came to his private office for care. This fixed-choice form provided for easy coding of data. This data was later analyzed by the Statistical Package for the Social Sciences (SPSS).

Ultimately, from the examination and questions, a diagnosis is made. The diagnosis identifies forms of disc lesion such as an annular tear, nuclear bulge, nuclear protrusion, or nuclear prolapse; or a condition of discogenic spondyloarthrosis, facet syndrome, spondylolisthesis, lumbar spine stenosis, iatrogenic surgical- or chiropractic-induced back pain, functional low back pain, sprain and strain, subluxation, tropism, transitional segment, and so forth. It may well be that the final diagnosis could be a combination of two or more of these diagnoses.

General Data

The mean age was 43.4 years, with the minimum 13 and the maximum 86 years of age; 331 patients were male and 231 were female, with 14 not reported on; 109 were single, 386 were married; 37 were divorced, and 23 were widowed. Average height was 67 inches, with a minimum of 33 inches and maximum of 83 inches. Average weight was 165.8 lbs with a minimum of 94 lb and a maximum of 295 lb. Ninety patients were ectomorphs, 320 mesomorphs, 108 endomorphs, and 58 not specified.

The most common chief complaint was low back pain (464 patients), with the second chief complaint be-

[c] This section, comprising the remainder of Chapter 1, was previously published as: Cox JM, Shreiner, S: Chiropractic manipulation in low back pain and sciatica: statistical data on the diagnosis, treatment, and response of 576 consecutive cases; *Journal of Manipulative and Physiological Therapeutics*, vol 7, issue 1, pp 1–11, © by the National College of Chiropractic, 1984.

ing leg pain (78 patients). The most common secondary complaint was low back pain in 65 and leg pain in 258.

Of those reporting, 302 stated that the pain was constant and 216 that it was intermittent. On a scale of 1 to 10, with 1 being the least intense and 9 being the most intense pain, the average pain intensity was recorded at 6; 246 recorded the pain as being insidious, and 283 stated that it was acute and traumatic. Forty-seven patients could not describe the pain in these terms.

Activity Causing Injury

Etiologically, 210 cases did not know of any specific activity causing their injury, while 45 reported injury when bending without lifting, 58 bending while lifting, 47 rotating and bending while not lifting. Forty-six stated that the pain started after a fall, and in 41 it was due to an accident. Sports were involved in the onset of pain in 63 cases, with running and jogging being the most common activity. Each low back diagnosis was further divided according to the activity that caused the injury, and it is interesting to note that people with discogenic spondyloarthrosis, in the majority of cases, did not know what activity caused their injury, while in the diagnosis of disc prolapse, the majority of patients could distinctly link it to a bending, lifting, and/or rotation injury.

Injury Factors

Of those patients reporting prior back pain, 244 cited years of previous incidence prior to their present complaint; 147 stated that they had no previous back pain, while 52 reported weeks or months of prior pain. The most common site of injury was the home, followed by the workplace. Two hundred sixty-nine patients stated that lifting was not involved in their injury, while in those who stated that lifting was involved, it was found that 83 were lifting less than 10 lb, 82 were lifting 11 to 30 lb, 28 were lifting 31 to 50 lb, 15 were lifting 51 to 80 lb, 15 were lifting 81 to 101 lb, and 16 patients were lifting 101 to 200 lb, with seven lifting over 200 lb at the onset of injury. Two hundred fifty-five stated that they had no night pain with the back problem, but 250 stated that they did. Eighteen of the patients had considered suicide due to the low back problem.

Pain Description

Of the 571 patients describing dermatome location, 112 stated that it was the S1 dermatome, 65 at L5, 23 at L4, 15 at L3, 73 at L5 and S1, 12 at L4 and L5. Fifty-two stated that the pain was in the right leg, 40 the left leg, 25 both legs, and one reported alternating leg pain; 211 patients reported only low back pain, 80 low back and right leg, 114 low back and left leg, and 48 had both low back and bilateral leg pain. The onset of back and leg pain was described as leg pain occurring before the back pain in 20 cases, and as the back and leg pain coming on simultaneously in 94 cases, while 222 patients stated that the leg pain followed the low back pain. The leg pain was described as sharp by 224, dull by 167, throbbing by 32, and as a traction or burning by 12. The leg pain was described as extending to the buttock in 276 patients, to the thigh in 208, to the knee in 185, to the calf in 134, to the ankle in 90, to the foot in 62, and into the toes in 35. Among those describing the skin sensation, the feeling most commonly described was numbness, followed by tingling, burning, and a feeling of "being asleep."

Walking aggravated the low back pain in 138 patients, the left leg in 66, the right leg in 53, and both legs in 24, while 233 patients had no aggravation of the low back or leg pain by walking. Déjérine's triad aggravated the back and leg pain in 51% of the patients and was negative in 49%. The posture that made the symptoms worse was sitting in 347 cases, flexion at the waist in 163, standing in 149, hyperextension at the waist in 84, and recumbency in 22. The posture that caused a remission of the symptoms was recumbency in 390 cases, standing in 58, and sitting in 51.

Previous Diagnostic and Treatment Results

Fifty-six patients had myelography performed previously, with 32 being positive, 21 negative, and three inconclusive. Eleven patients had computed tomography (Cat) scans, 13 had electromyography, three had discography, and one had an epidural venogram.

Prior Doctors Seen

Prior treatment before coming to the doctor involved in this project was by a medical doctor in 168 patients, a doctor of chiropractic in 90 patients, and a doctor of osteopathy in 13 patients; 69 patients, had been to both a medical doctor and a doctor of chiropractic, and eight had been to a medical doctor, a doctor of osteopathy, and a doctor of chiropractic, with 205 reporting having gone to no previous doctor.

Of those patients taking medication, 121 had no change, 33 were 25% improved, 31 were 50% improved, seven were 75% improved, and 13 were 100% improved, while eight stated that they were worse.

Twenty-seven patients had undergone low back surgery, 21 of them being laminectomy, four fusions, one microsurgery, and one an undefined procedure. The subjective relief of these patients at 1 year indicated that six of them felt worse, four felt no change, three felt 25% improvement, three felt 50% improvement, three felt 75% improvement, three felt 100% improvement; and five gave no report.

Of those patients receiving prior nonsurgical treatment, 153 cases had had manipulation; 10, epidural injections; two, chemonucleolysis; five, closed reduction; 87, physical therapy; and eight, acupuncture. Previous therapy had consisted of hot and cold in 83 cases, high-voltage galvanic in 17, low-voltage galvanic in 13, ultrasound in 60, traction in 32, massage in 21, trigger point in 10, and bracing in 31. Five patients had been to a low back pain school, eight had worn transcutaneous neuromuscular stimulation (TNS) units, four had psychological counseling, five had biofeedback, and two had a combination of these treatments. Of those reporting results from these therapies, 21 stated they were worse, 125 reported no change, 25 reported 25% improvement, 20 reported 50% improvement, and 25 reported 75 to 100% improvement.

Of patients having taken medication for their low back pain, 44 had taken anti-inflammatory drugs; 99, pain relievers; 55, muscle relaxants; four, tranquilizers; two, vitamin B_{12}; and 16, some other type of medication. The result obtained from this medication was stated to be worse in eight patients, no change in 121, 25% improvement in 33, 50% improvement in 31, 75% improvement in seven, and 100% improvement in 13; 29 patients did not report. Of 194 patients who reported a specific chiropractic technique as having been applied prior to having seen the doctors involved in this project, 38 of them stated that they had been in some way harmed through chiropractic manipulation.

Correlative Diagnosis of Low Back Pain Patients

Tables 1.3 and 1.4 reveal the diagnosis at the L4 and L5 levels as determined in these 576 cases. The total diagnoses may exceed 576 because one patient may have had more than one diagnosis. Of 126 L5 nuclear protrusions or prolapses, 61 occurred on the right side and 65 on the left. At the L4 level, where a nuclear protrusion or prolapse was found, 75 of the reported locations revealed 37 to occur on the right and 38 to occur on the left side.

Conditions Accompanying Disc Lesions

Correlation of L5 disc syndromes with presence of a second condition showed that 26% had accompanying facet syndrome, 17% accompanying stenosis, and 13% had tropism and discogenic spondyloarthrosis. Forty-six percent of those people suffering from an L4 disc syndrome also suffered from discogenic spondyloarthrosis at the L5 vertebra. Bertolotti's syndrome (L4 disc syndrome with L5 transitional vertebra) was seen in four patients.

Incidence of Stenosis

Slightly more than half the patients suffering from spinal stenosis exhibited signs of intermittent claudication. Fourteen percent of the patients with stenosis revealed retrolisthesis subluxation of L5 when the stenosis occurred at that level. Another 12% of the stenotic patients had retrolisthesis at two or more levels.

Patient Response to Chiropractic Manipulation

Table 1.5 shows overall patient response to chiropractic manipulation regardless of diagnosis. It should be noted that L5 disc conditions responded somewhat more favorably than did those at L4. *The mean number of days to 50% improvement, as measured both objectively and subjectively, was 14.4 (with a mean of 9.5 treatments), while the mean number of days to maximum improvement was 42.8 days (18.6 treatments).* Most patients required less than 10 treatments to achieve both 50% and maximum improvement (79% and 51% respectively). Maximum improvement is defined as the return of the patient to the pre-pain state, or the point at which treatment no longer renders relief. Three months is the usual maximum that any of these patients are treated, as it is felt that the maximum relief of pain is usually attained by then.

Discussion

The incidence of congenital anomalies does not appear to be any higher in those patients complaining of low back discomfort than in the normal population. The presence of such anomalies did not seem to produce less favorable treatment results. Treatment of anomalies of the low back required smaller numbers of treatments over longer periods of time, whereas treatment of acute disc protrusions required larger numbers of treatments for relatively shorter periods of time. This is due to the more acute and severe pain that accompanies the disc problems as compared to the anomalies. Stenosis is an example of an anomaly requiring a greater number of days for healing. Discogenic spondyloarthrosis without sciatica appears to respond most quickly to therapy.

Transitional segments at L5 had the slowest response to manipulative therapy, with only 21% of the cases showing maximum improvement within 10 days; however, transitional segments showed excellent response to manipulation. Transitional segments are the slowest to respond to manipulative care, yet have an excellent clinical result.

Note that L4 nuclear protrusion and spondylolisthesis responded more slowly than those conditions at L5 (Figs. 1.2 and 1.3). L5 disc protrusion and spondylolisthesis shows a sharper improvement rate within 10 to 20 treatments, and L5 spondylolisthesis shows a sharper incidence of improvement within 30 days as compared to L4 spondylolisthesis. L4 spondylolisthesis shows a much slower response than L5 spondylolisthesis in terms of days treated, as well as requiring a greater number of treatments to attain relief.

Days to Maximum Response

Linear response patterns were seen in facet syndrome (L4 and L5), nuclear protrusion (L4 and L5), and transitional segments (L5 only). Sprain, strain, spondyloarthrosis, and, most clearly, tropism response curves illustrate decaying exponential curves, indicating a more rapid rate to maximum improvement. Tropism, sprain, strain, and spondyloarthrosis show rapid improvement among this group of patients, with a majority achieving maximum improvement by 20 to 30 days (60% or greater of patients).

Comparisons between L4 and L5 levels for sprain,

Table 1.3.
L4 Diagnosis[a, b]

Dichotomy Label	Name	Count	Percentage of Responses	Percentage of Cases
Annular tear	x1	11	2.8	4.1
Nuclear bulge	x2	31	7.9	11.5
Nuclear protrusion	x3	79	20.3	29.3
Nuclear prolapse	x4	9	2.3	3.3
DSA	x5	72	18.5	26.7
Facet syndrome	x6	59	15.1	21.9
Spondylolisthesis	x7	15	3.8	5.6
Stenosis	x8	22	5.6	8.1
Iatrogenic	x9	2	0.5	0.7
Sprain, strain	x11	32	8.2	11.9
Tropism	x13	33	8.5	12.2
Transitional segment	x14	25	6.4	9.3
	Total responses	390	100.0	144.4

[a]From Cox JM, Shreiner S: Chiropractic manipulation in low back pain and sciatica: statistical data on the diagnosis, treatment, and response of 576 consecutive cases, *Journal of Manipulative and Physiological Therapeutics*, vol 7, issue 1, pp 1–11, © by the National College of Chiropractic, 1984.
[b]Value tabulated = 1.

Table 1.4.
L5 Diagnosis [a, b]

Dichotomy Label	Name	Count	Percentage of Responses	Percentage of Cases
Annular tear	y1	50	6.3	10.9
Nuclear bulge	y2	61	7.6	13.3
Nuclear protrusion	y3	107	13.4	23.4
Nuclear prolapse	y4	19	2.4	4.1
DSA	y5	122	15.3	26.6
Facet syndrome	y6	204	25.5	44.5
Spondylolisthesis	y7	20	2.5	4.4
Stenosis	y8	73	9.1	15.9
Iatrogenic	y9	3	0.4	0.7
Sprain, strain	y11	79	9.9	17.2
Tropism	y13	42	5.3	9.2
Transitional segment	y14	19	2.4	4.1
	Total responses	799	100.0	174.5

[a]From Cox JM, Shreiner S: Chiropractic manipulation in low back pain and sciatica: statistical data on the diagnosis, treatment, and response of 576 consecutive cases, *Journal of Manipulative and Physiological Therapeutics*, vol 7, issue 1, pp 1–11, © by the National College of Chiropractic, 1984.
[b]Value tabulated = 1.

strain, spondyloarthrosis, nuclear protrusion, and facet syndrome show little difference in these cumulative patient responses. Tropism response rate is greater for L5 than for L4, while stenosis response patterns are closely parallel up to 30 to 45 days. L5 stenosis shows more rapid improvements across the sample of patients.

Number of Treatments to Maximum Improvement

Due to incompatible summary categories of number of treatments, the response to treatment was plotted only for spondyloarthrosis, facet syndrome, nuclear protrusion, and spondylolisthesis. In all cases, these curves clearly show the decaying exponential pattern, with maximum improvement clearly being achieved in 30 treatments or less.

L4 and L5 spondyloarthrosis curves show little difference, with about 90% of the sample showing maximum improvement after 20 to 30 treatments (Fig 1.4). L4 and L5 facet syndrome again show little difference, with 80% improvement at 20 to 30 treatments and about 50% of the sample showing maximum improvement with 10 or less treatments. L4 and L5 nuclear protrusion response curves closely parallel each other after 20 to 30 treatments, but L5 nuclear protrusion response shows a more rapid improvement (over 70%) at

Table 1.5.
576 Patient Responses to Chiropractic Manipulation[a]

Excellent—275 (50%)
Very Good—74 (14%)
Good—60 (11%)
Fair—36 (6%)
Poor—22 (4%)
Surgery—17 (3%)
Stopped or did not start treatment—57(10%)
Exam, Not Treat—7 (1%)

[a]From Cox JM, Shreiner S: Chiropractic manipulation in low back pain and sciatica: statistical data on the diagnosis, treatment, and response of 576 consecutive cases, *Journal of Manipulative and Physiological Therapeutics*, vol 7, issue 1, pp 1–11, © by the National College of Chiropractic, 1984.

10 to 20 treatments compared with the L4 nuclear protrusion sample (Fig. 1.2).

Spondylolisthesis curves also are similar for both the L4 and L5 levels, but it appears that maximum improvement is achieved for the vast majority of the sample by 30 to 40 treatments (Table 1.5). Again, L5 spondylolisthesis patients showed a faster rate of improvement than did L4 patients.

Comparing these four diagnoses (spondyloarthrosis, facet syndrome, nuclear protrusion, and spon-

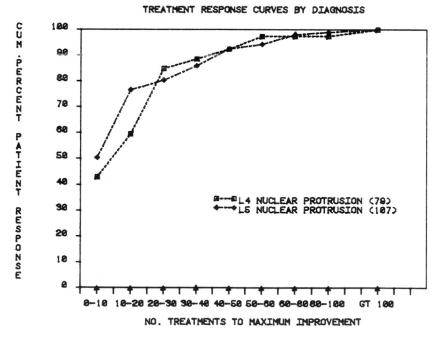

Figure 1.2. Treatment response curves for L4 and L5 nuclear protrusion. (Numbers in parentheses are numbers of patients.) From Cox JM, Shreiner S: Chiropractic manipulation in low back pain and sciatica: statistical data on the diagnosis, treatment, and response of 576 consecutive cases, *Journal of Manipulative and Physiological Therapeutics*, vol 7, issue 1, pp 1–11, © by the National College of Chiropractic, 1984.

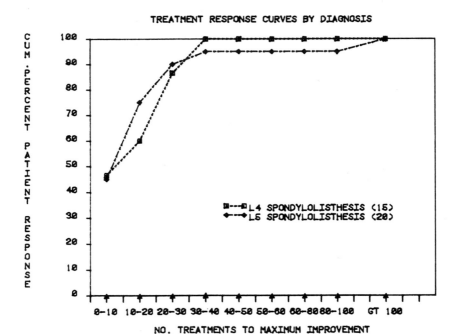

Figure 1.3. Treatment response curves for L4 and L5 spondylolisthesis. (Numbers in parentheses are numbers of patients.) From Cox JM, Shreiner S: Chiropractic manipulation in low back pain and sciatica: statistical data on the diagnosis, treatment, and response of 576 consecutive cases, *Journal of Manipulative and Physiological Therapeutics,* vol 7, issue 1, pp 1–11, © by the National College of Chiropractic, 1984.

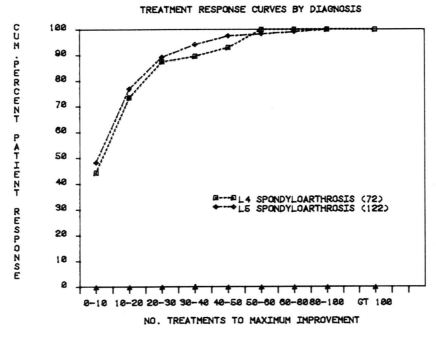

Figure 1.4. Treatment response curves for L4 and L5 spondyloarthrosis. (Numbers in parentheses are numbers of patients.) From Cox JM, Shreiner S: Chiropractic manipulation in low back pain and sciatica: statistical data on the diagnosis, treatment, and response of 576 consecutive cases, *Journal of Manipulative and Physiological Therapeutics,* vol 7, issue 1, pp 1–11, © by the National College of Chiropractic, 1984.

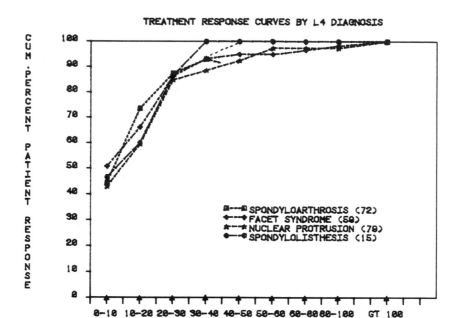

Figure 1.5. Treatment response curves for spondyloarthrosis, facet syndrome, nuclear protrusion, and spondylolisthesis at the L4 region. (Numbers in parentheses are numbers of patients.) From Cox JM, Shreiner S: Chiropractic manipulation in low back pain and sciatica: statistical data on the diagnosis, treatment, and response of 576 consecutive cases, *Journal of Manipulative and Physiological Therapeutics*, vol 7, issue 1, pp 1–11, © by the National College of Chiropractic, 1984.

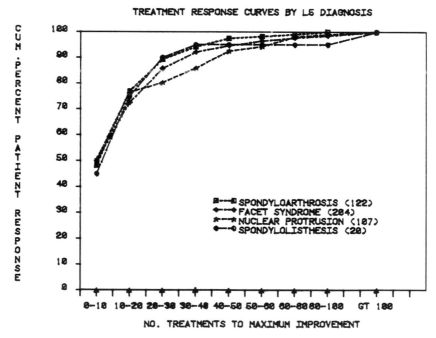

Figure 1.6. Treatment response curves for spondyloarthrosis, facet syndrome, nuclear protrusion, and spondylolisthesis at the L5 region. (Numbers in parentheses are number of patients.) From Cox JM, Shreiner S: Chiropractic manipulation in low back pain and sciatica: statistical data on the diagnosis, treatment, and response of 576 consecutive cases, *Journal of Manipulative and Physiological Therapeutics*, vol 7, issue 1, pp 1–11, © by the National College of Chiropractic, 1984.

dylolisthesis) at the L4 and L5 region reveals remarkably similar response curves for the number of treatments; overall, over 80% of these samples showed maximum improvement in 20 to 30 treatments. Nuclear protrusion in both L4 and L5 levels shows the slowest response curves after this treatment point (Figs. 1.5 and 1.6).

Conclusions

This descriptive investigation into treatment response by diagnosis and region, while illustrating clearly what can be expected using specific treatments, just begins to investigate some of the important questions. Future directions for this research include exploring additional correlates of response to treatment. Such relevant factors as previous medical history, and demographic characteristics such as age and sex, all may show a relationship to treatment and improvement, but statistical investigation must wait on some diagnoses until larger samples are gathered for each level and diagnosis. At this time, correlation and regression analysis into these related factors is necessary. Also at this time, the search for statistically significant differences of improvement rates can be explored.

It is realized that there are flaws in the research design that will be addressed in future larger collection efforts, and these collections are continuing. Furthermore, it is realized that the diagnosis of low back pain is still largely nonspecific in many cases. This study correlates the findings on x-ray, physical examination, and history in order to document trends or cogent factors in patients with low back or leg pain, while fully realizing that there are many nonspecific diagnoses of back pain.

References

1. Wiltse L: The presidential address: North American Spine Society, an amalgamation for progress. *Spine* 11(6):654, 1986.
2. White JS: The surprising swing to non-physicians. *Medical Economics* (May 30):55, 56, 63, 1983.
3. Coburn D, Biggs L: Limits to medical dominance: the case of chiropractic. *Sci Med* 22(10): 1035–1046, 1986.
4. Wardell W: Limited, marginal, and quasipractitioners. In Freeman H, Levine S, Reader LG: *Handbook of Medical Sociology*. Englewood Cliffs, NJ, Prentice-Hall, 1963.
5. Cobb A: Pluralistic legitimation of an alternative therapy system. *Med Anthrop* 1(4):1, 1977.
6. Sternberg D: Boys in plight: a case study of chiropractic students confronting a medically oriented society. Unpublished doctoral dissertation, New York University, Department of Sociology, 1969.
7. Dvorak J: Manual medicine in the United States and Europe in the year 1982. *Manual Medicine* 2: 3–9, 1983.
8. Silver GA: Chiropractic: professional controversy and public policy. *Am J Public Health* 70(4): 348–350, 1980.
9. Vital signs. *ACA J Chiropractic* (October):11, 1984.
10. Deyo RA, Tsui-Wu YJ: Descriptive epidemiology of low back pain and its related medical care in the United States. *Spine* 12(3):264–268, 1987.
11. Yesalis CE, Wallace RB, Fisher WP, Tulcheim R: Does chiropractic utilization substitute for less available medical services? *Am J Public Health* 70: 415–417, 1980.
12. Gray B: Two tier health system. *New Zealand Med J* (August 13):599, 1986.
13. Report of the Commission of Enquiry: Chiropractic in New Zealand. Presented to the House of Representatives by His Excellency the Governor-General. New Zealand, Hasselberg, Government Printer, 1979.
14. Chiropractic referral by medical practitioners (Editorial). *Med J Aust* (April 16):353–356, 1983.
15. Maher WB: Controlling low back pain costs at Chrysler. *Business and Health* (May):12–21, 1985.
16. Brown M: *Intradiscal Therapy, Chymopapain or Collagenase*. Chicago, Year Book, 1983, p 126.
17. Sweezy RL, Crittenden JO, Sweezy A: Outpatient treatment of lumbar disc sciatica. *West J Med* 145(1):43–46, 1986.
18. Camp P: Low back pain cost. *JAMA* 256(3), 1986.
19. Report from Department of Health and Human Services. *Fort Wayne News-Sentinel* (June 9):2A, 1987.
20. Snook S: In Pope MH, Frymoyer JW, Andersson G: *Occupational Low Back Pain*, New York, Praeger, 1984, pp 115, 117.
21. Spengler DM, Bigos SJ, Martin NA, Zeh J, Fisher L, Nachemson A: Back injuries in industry: a retrospective study. 1. Overview and cost analysis. *Spine* 11(3):241–245, 1986.
22. Burton CV: The gravity lumbar reduction therapy program. *J Musculoskeletal Medicine* 3(4):12–21, 1986.
23. Greenwood JG: Report on work-related back and neck injury cases in West Virginia: issues related to chiropractic and medical costs. *Florida Chiropractic Association Journal* (July-August):32, 1984.
24. Medical world news, July 22, 1985: The laying on of hands—energy from electromagnetic fields. *J Manipulative Physiol Ther* 9:76–77, 1986.
25. Vernon HT, Dhami MSI, Howley TP, Annett R: Spinal manipulation and beta-endorphin: a con-

trolled study of the effect of a spinal manipulation on plasma beta-endorphin levels in normal males. *J Manipulative Physiol Ther* 9:115–123, 1986.

26. Grayson MF: Manipulation in back disorders. *Br Med J* (December):293, 1986.

27. Jordan JM, Abeid LM, Allen NB: Isolated atlanto-axial subluxation as the presenting manifestation of inflammatory bowel disease. *Am J Med* 8:517, 1986.

28. Beal MC: A study of viscerosomatic reflexes. *Manuelle Medicin* 21(4), 1984.

29. Cox J, Gideon D, Rogers F: Incidence of osteophytic lipping of the thoracic spine in coronary heart disease: results of a pilot study. *J Am Osteopath Assoc* 82:837–838, 1983.

30. Kelsey JL, Pastides H, Bigbee GE: Musculo-skeletal disorders: their frequency of occurrence and their impact on the population of the United States. New York, Prodist, 1978.

31. Kelsey JL, White AA: Epidemiology and impact on low back pain. *Spine* 5(2):133–142, 1980.

32. Frymoyer JW, Pope MH, Costanza MC, Rosen JC, Goggin JE, Wilder DG: Epidemiologic studies of low-back pain. *Spine* 5(5):419–423, 1980.

33. Frymoyer JW, Pope MH, Clements JH, Wilder DG, McPherson B, Ashikaga T: Risk factors in low back pain. *J Bone Joint Surg* 65A:213–218, 1983.

34. Rowe ML: Preliminary statistical study of low back pain. *J Occup Med* 5(7):336–341, 1963.

35. Rowe ML: Disc surgery and chronic low back pain. *J Occup Med* 7(5):196–202, 1965.

36. Rowe ML: Low back pain in industry: a position paper. *J Occup Med* 11(4):161–169, 1969.

37. Heliovarra M: Occupation and risk of herniated lumbar disk or sciatica leading to hospitalization. *J Chronic Dis* 40(3):219, 1987.

38. Dales JL, MacDonald EB, Porter RW: Back pain: the risk factors and its prediction in work people. *Clin Biomechanics* 1:216–218, 1986.

39. Hippocrates, trans. by Withington ET: *Hippocrates.* London, vol 3, 1944. Cited in Lind G: Autotraction, treatment of low back pain and sciatica. Thesis, University of Linkoping, Linkoping, 1974, p 19. (Private publication available from library of author, J. M. Cox.)

40. Toufexis A: That aching back. *Time* 116(2):30–38, 1980.

41. *Medical Bulletin* (April 21), 1981.

42. Hall H: Logical approach to diagnosis of back pain. *Can Fam Physician* 21:79–83, 1975.

43. Breen AC: Chiropractors and the treatment of back pain. *Rheumatol Rehabil* 16(1):48, 1977.

44. Zylbergold RS, Piper MC: Lumbar disc disease: comparative analysis of physical therapy treatments. *Arch Phys Med Rehabil* 62:176, 1981.

45. Biering-Sorsenson F, Thomas C: Medical, social and occupational history as risk indicators for low back trouble in a general population. *Spine* 11(7):720, 1986.

46. Svensson HO, Anderson G, Hagstad A, Jansson PO: The relationship of low back pain, pregnancy and gynecologic disease. *Acta Orthop Scand* 56:334–359, 1985.

47. Svensson HO, Anderson G: The epidemiology of work factors related to low back pain in men and women. *Acta Orthop Scand* 56:344–359, 1985.

48. Bigos SJ, Spengler PM, Martin NA, Zeh J, Fisher L, Nachemson A: Back injuries in industry: a retrospective study. *Spine* 11(3):252–256, 1986.

49. Sandstrom J, Anderson GBJ, Wallerstedt S: The role of alcohol abuse in working: disability in patients with low back pain. *Scand J Rehabil Med* 16:147–149, 1984.

50. Pollard CA: Family history and severity of disability associated with chronic low back pain. *Psychol Rep* 57(3):813–814, 1985.

51. Montgomery CH: Preemployment back x-rays. *J Occup Med* 18:495–498, 1976.

52. Snook SH, Campanelli RA, Hart JW: A study of three preventive approaches to low back injury. *J Occup Med* 20(7):480, 1978.

53. Reuler JB: Low back pain. *West J Med* 143(2):259–265, 1985.

54. Kelen GD, Noji EK, Doris PR: Guidelines for use of lumbar spine radiography. *Ann Emerg Med* 15(3):245–251, 1986.

55. Frymoyer JW, Phillips RB, Newberg AH, MacPherson BV: A comparative analysis of the interpretation of lumbar spinal radiography by chiropractors and medical doctors. *Spine* 11(10):1020, 1986.

56. Troup JDG: Causes, prediction and prevention of back pain at work. *Scand J Work Environ Health* 10:419–428, 1984.

57. Dierk GS, Kelsey JL, Goel V, Panjabi MM, Walter SD, Laprade MH: An epidemiologic study of the relationship between postural asymmetry in the teen years and subsequent back and neck pain. *Spine* 10(10):872–877.

58. Deyo RA: Predicting disability in patients with low back pain. San Antonio, TX, University of Texas Health Service Center, *Clinical Research* 34(1):269A, 1986.

59. Finneson B: *Low Back Pain,* ed 2. Philadelphia, JB Lippincott, 1980.

60. Wigh RE, Anthony HF: Transitional lumbosacral discs: probability of herniation. *Spine* 6(2):168, 1981.

61. Keim HA, Kirkaldy-Willis WH: Clinical symposia. *Ciba Found Symp* 32(6):89, 1980.

62. Semon RL, Spengler D: Significance of lumbar spondylosis in college football players. *Spine* 6(2):172, 1981.

63. Lenz WF: Spondylolisthesis and spondyloptosis of

the lower lumbar spine: a macrostudy. *ACA J Chiropractic* 15:S107, 1981.

64. Ramani PS: Variations in the size of the bony lumbar canal in patients with prolapse of the lumbar intervertebral discs. *Clin Radiol* 27:302–307, 1976.

65. Martin G: Recurrent disc prolapse as a cause for lumbar disc lesion. *New Zealand Med J* 91:206, 1980.

66. Rothman RH, Simeone FA: *The Spine.* Philadelphia, WB Saunders, 1975, vol 1, p 452.

67. Eisenstein S: Measurement of the lumbar spinal canal in two racial groups. *Clin Orthop* 115:43–46, 1976.

68. Ullrich CG, Binet EF, Sanecki MG, Keiffer SA: Quantitative assessment of the lumbar spinal canal by computed tomography. *Radiology* 134:137–143, 1980.

69. Eisenstein SM, Parry CR: The lumbar facet arthrosis syndrome: clinical presentation and articular surface changes. *J Bone Joint Surg* 69B:3–7, 1987.

70. Giles LGF, Taylor JR: Osteoarthrosis in human cadaveric lumbo-sacral zygapophyseal joints. *J Manipulative Physiol Ther* 8:239–243, 1985.

71. Palmoski MJ, Brandt KD: Proteoglycan depletion, rather than fibrilation, determines the effects of salicylate and indomethacin on osteoarthritic cartilage. *Arthritis Rheum* 28:548–553, 1985.

72. Newman NM, Ling RSM: Acetabular bone destruction related to non-steroidal anti-inflammatory drugs. *Lancet* (July 6):11-14, 1985.

73. Higuchi M, Abe K: Ultrastructure of the nucleus pulposus in the intervertebral disc after systemic administration of hydrocortisone in mice. *Spine* 10(7):638–643, 1985.

74. Higuchi M, Kazuhiro A: Effects of hydrocortisone in the vertebral cartilage plate in mice: light and electron microscope study. *Spine* 10(4):297–302, 1985.

75. Yang KH, King AI: Mechanism of facet load: transmission as a hypothesis for low back pain. *Spine* 9(6):557–565, 1984.

76. Mooney V, Robertson J: The facet syndrome. *Clin Orthop* 115:149–156, 1976.

77. Carrera GF, Haughton VM, Syvertsen A, Williams AL: Computed tomography of the lumbar facets. *Radiology* 134:145–148, 1980.

78. Carrera CG: Lumbar facet joint injection in low back pain and sciatica. *Radiology* 737:665–667, 1980.

79. Dory MA: Arthrography of the lumbar facet joints. *Radiology* 140:23–27, 1981.

80. Chynn KY, Altman I, Shaw WI, Finley N: The roentgenographic manifestations and clinical features of lumbar spinal stenosis with special emphasis on the superior articular process. *Neuroradiology* 16:378–380, 1978.

81. Lora J, Long D: So-called facet denervation in the management of intractable back pain. *Spine* 1(2):121–126, 1976.

82. Van Akkerveeken PF, O'Brien JP, Park W: Experimentally induced hypermobility of the lumbar spine. *Spine* 4(3):236–241, 1978.

83. Cox JM: Low back pain: recent statistics and data in its mechanism, diagnosis and treatment from chiropractic manipulation. *ACA J Chiropractic* 13:S125–S138, 1979.

84. Ehni G, Weinstein P: *Lumbar Spondylosis.* Chicago, Year Book, 1977, p 19.

85. Cyron BM, Hutton WC: Articular tropism and stability of the lumbar spine. *Spine* 5(2):168–172, 1980.

86. Breig A, Troup JDG: Biomechanical considerations in the straight leg raising sign. *Spine* 4(3):242–250, 1979.

87. Hudgins WR: The crossed straight leg raising test: a diagnostic sign of herniated disc. *J Occup Med* 21(6):407–408, 1979.

88. Farfan H: A reorientation in the surgical approach to degenerative lumbar intervertebral joint disease. *Orthop Clin North Am* 8(1):9–21, 1977.

89. Virgin WJ: Experimental investigation into the physical properties of the intervertebral disc. *J Bone Joint Surg* 33B:607, 1951.

90. Lumsden RM, Morris JM: An in vivo study of axial rotation immobilization at the lumbosacral origin. *J Bone Joint Surg* 50A:1591, 1968.

91. Maigne R: Low back pain of thoracolumbar origin. *Arch Phys Med Rehabil* 61:389–394, 1980.

92. Harrison J: *Malpractice Alert.* International Chiropractor's Association 2(2), December 1981.

93. Gainer JV, Nugent GR: The herniated lumbar disk. *Am Fam Pract* 10(3):127–131, 1964.

94. Weitz EM: The lateral bending sign. *Spine* 6(4):388–397, 1981.

95. Porter RW, Miller CG: Back pain and trunk list. *Spine* 11(6):596, 1986.

96. Pilling JR: Water soluble radiculography in the erect posture: a clinico-radiological study. *Clin Radiol* 30:665–670, 1979.

97. Bachop WE: Controlled clinical trails, third party payers, and the fate of the chiropractor. *J Manipulative Physiol Ther* 3:95, 1980.

98. Aitken AP: Rupture of the intervertebral disc in industry: further observations and end results. *Am J Surg* 84:261–267, 1982.

99. Wood K: New approaches to treatment of back pain. *West J Med* 130(4):394–398, 1979.

100. Kessler RM: Acute symptomatic disc prolapse. *Phys Ther* 59(8):978–987, 1979.

101. Fahrni WH: Conservative treatment of lumbar disc degeneration: our primary responsibility. *Orthop Clin North Am* 6(1):93–103, 1975.

102. Nachemson A: The lumbar spine, an orthopaedic challenge. *Spine* 1(1):59–69, 1976.

103. Johnson EW, Fletcher FR: Lumbosacral radiculopathy: review of 100 consecutive cases. *Arch Phys Med Rehabil* 62:321–323, 1981.

104. Anonymous: Treatment of lumbar disc protrusion by automatic chiropractic traction instrument. Translated at the National College, Chicago, IL, 1982. (Available from library of author, J. M. Cox.)

105. Szepesi Z: Prevent sacroiliac degeneration. *Aches Pains* 2(9):15, 1981.

106. Hirschberg GG: Treating lumbar disc lesion by prolonged continuous reduction of intradiscal pressure. *Texas Med* 70, 1970.

107. Trief PM: Chronic back pain: a tripartite model of outcome. *Arch Phys Med Rehabil* 64(1):53–56, 1983.

108. Chrisman OD, Mittnach T, Snook GA: A study of the results following rotatory manipulation of the lumbar intevertebral disc syndrome. *J Bone Joint Surg* 46A:517–524, 1964.

109. Woolley FR, Kane RL: A comparison of allopathic and chiropractic care. In Buerger AA, Tobis JS (eds): *Approaches to the Validation of Manipulation Therapy.* Springfield, IL, Charles C Thomas, 1977, pp 217–223.

110. Deyo RA: Conservative therapy for low back pain—distinguishing useful from useless therapy. *JAMA* 250(8):1058–1059, 1983.

111. Larsson U, Choler U, Lidstrom A, Lind G, Nachemson A, Nilsson B, Roslund J: Auto-traction for treatment of lumbago-sciatica: a multicenter controlled investigation. *Acta Orthop Scand* 51:791–798, 1980.

112. Paris SV: Spinal manipulative therapy. (Available from library of author, J. M. Cox.)

113. Saunders HD: Use of spinal traction in the treatment of neck and back conditions. Chattanooga Publications (private publication), pp 3–24.

114. Cyriax J: *Textbook of Orthopaedic Medicine,* ed 7. East Sussex, England, Ballière-Tindall, pp 315–316.

115. DeSeze S, Levernieux J: Les tractions vertébrales: premiers éxtudes experimentales et résultats thérapeutiques dáprès un expérience de quatre années. *Semaine des hôpitales de Paris* 27:2085, 1951.

116. Godfrey CM, Morgan P, Schatzker J: A randomized trial of manipulation from low back pain in a medical setting. *Spine* 9(3):301, 1984.

117. Fager CA: The age-old back problem, new fad, some fallacies, from the Department of Neurosurgery, Tahey Clinic Medical Center. *Spine* 9(3):326, 1984.

118. Cuckler J, Bernini PA, Wiesel SW, Booth RE, Rothman RH, Pickens GT: The use of epidural steroids in the treatment of lumbar radicular pain. *J Bone Joint Surg* 67A:63–66, 1985.

119. Burton C: In Kirkaldy-Willis WH: *Managing Low Back Pain.* New York, Churchill Livingstone, 1983, p 193.

120. Moffett JA, Chase SM, Portek I, Ennis JJ: A controlled, prospective study to evaluate the effectiveness of a back school in the relief of chronic low back pain. *Spine* 11(2):120–122, 1986.

121. Milanowska K: Value of complex rehabilatory training in treatment of low back pain. Rehabilitation Department, Academy of Medicine, Poznan, Poland.

122. Valentini E: Acute lumbar disc syndromes under chiropractic care: a two year statistical study. Monteux, Switzerland, Swiss Chiropractic Association, 1979.

123. Tindall GT: Clinical aspects of lumbar intervertebral disc disease. *J Med Assoc Ga* 70:247–253, 1981.

124. Eagle R: A pain in the back. *New Scientist* (October 18):170–173, 1979.

125. Cookson JC: Orthopedic manual therapy: an overview. Part II. The spine. *Phys Ther* 59(3): 259–267, 1979.

126. Nachemson A: A critical look at the treatment of low back pain. In: *The Research Status of Spinal Manipulative Therapy.* NINCDS Monograph No 15, DHEW No 76–998. Bethesda, MD, National Institute of Neurological and Communicative Disorders and Stroke, 1975, pp 287–292.

127. Goldstein M: Research in spinal manipulation— reflections on processes, priorities and responsibilities. *J Manipulative Physiol Ther* 3:41, 1980.

128. Webb JH, Svien HJ, Kennedy RLJ: Protruded lumbar intervertebral discs in children. *JAMA* 154:1153–1154, 1954.

129. O'Connell JEA: Intervertebral disc lesions in childhood and adolescence. *Br J Surg* 47: 611–616, 1960.

130. Clarke NMP, Cleak DK: Intervertebral lumbar disc prolapse in children and adolescents. *J Pediatr Orthop* 3:202–206, 1983.

131. Bronfort G: Chiropractic treatment of low back pain: a prospective study. *J Manipulative Physiol Ther* 9:99–113, 1986.

132. Sheladia VL, Johnston DA: Efficacy of various chiropractic treatments; age distribution, and incidence of accident and non-accident-caused low back pain in male and female patients. *J Manipulative Physiol Ther* 9:263, 1986.

133. Parker G, Tupling H: The chiropractic patient: psychosocial aspects. *Med J Aust* 2:373–376, 1976.

134. Von Luschka H: *Die Holgelenke des Neuschlichen Korpes.* Berlin, George Reimer, 1858.

135. Dandy WE: Loose cartilage from intervertebral disc simulating tumor of the spinal cord. *Arch Surg* 19:660, 1929.

136. Mixter WJ, Barr JS: Rupture of the intervertebral

disc with involvement of the spinal canal. *N Engl J Med* 211:210–215, 1934.

137. Nordby E: *Am Med News* October 3), 1977.
138. Dommisse GF, Grahe RP: The failures of surgery for lumbar disc disorders. In Helfet AJ, Gruebel-Lee DM (eds): *Disorders of the Lumbar Spine*. Philadelphia. JB Lippincott, 1978, p 202.
139. Burton CV: Lumbar arachnoiditis. *Spine* 3(1): 24–29, 1978.
140. Yamada K: The dynamics of experimental posture: experimental study of intervertebral disc herniation in bipedal animals. *Tokushima J Exp Med* 8:350–361, 1962.
141. Yamada K: The dynamics of experimental posture: experimental study of intervertebral disc herniation in bipedal animals. *Clin Orthop* 25: 20–31, 1962.
142. Turek S. *Orthopaedics—Principles and Their Applications*. Philadelphia, JB Lippincott, 1956, chap 27, p 748.
143. Strait LA, Inman VT, Ralston HJ: Sample illustrations of physical principles selected from physiology and medicine. *Am J Physics* 15:375–382, 1947.

2

Biomechanics of the Lumbar Spine

James M. Cox, D.C., D.A.C.B.R.

The Individual Has Always Had To Struggle To Keep From Being Overwhelmed By The Tribe. To Be Your Own Man Is A Hard Business. If You Try It, You'll Be Lonely Often, And Sometimes Frightened. But No Price Is Too High To Pay For The Privilege Of Owning Yourself.

—Rudyard Kipling

Clinicians of all disciplines who treat low back problems meet a plethora of frustrations, challenges and disappointments, as well as both expected and unanticipated successful therapeutic outcomes. The reason must be the multifactorial etiology of pain in the low back. I chose to start this chapter with a smorgasbord of patient presentations to set the tempo for discussing the biomechanics of the low back.

Figure 2.1 illustrates the great challenge in low back complaints—a patient with low back pain with radiating sciatic radiculopathy; inability to bear weight; pain on coughing, sneezing or bowel movement; reflex change; and great fear and anxiety. The patient's x-ray (Fig. 2.2), except for an obvious sciatic list to the right side, is devoid of degenerative changes, which may be a certain part of her future, while the computed tomography (CT) scan seen in Figure 2.3 reveals good reason for her discomfort. This is an obvious diagnosis; unfortunately, most low back diagnoses are not so easily made.

Perhaps Figures 2.4 and 2.5 represent the above patient in 30 or 40 years. Certainly they represent a most challenging spine to a practitioner, whether his or her mode of treatment be drugs, surgery, manipulation, acupuncture, physiological therapeutics, or esoteric methods. This probably is the result of developmental and degenerative changes in response to life's abuse of the spinal system.

Figures 2.6 through 2.9 show end products of degenerative disc disease commonly encountered in clinical practice. Some degenerative spondylolisthesis cases are well controlled by conservative means, including manipulation (as shown in this text in chapter 14, "Spondylolisthesis"), while some require surgical stabilization, as shown in Figures 2.8 and 2.9.

Figure 2.10 shows an example of the congenital and developmental aspects of low back pain. The transitional segment, with its pseudoarthrotic changes, is followed by degenerative changes of the disc levels above. Figure 2.11 shows asymmetry of facet development, as illustrated by the overdeveloped right fifth lumbar superior facet with a facet-lamina contact resulting in bone-reactive hyperostosis.

Figure 2.12 shows a not uncommon patient. Scoliosis, with or without degenerative disc disease, is sometimes an easy case but sometimes requires surgical stabilization for relief.

Figures 2.13 and 2.14 show perplexing findings. Figure 2.13 is a CT scan showing the disc protrusion to occupy 38% of the sagittal diameter of the vertebral canal; it was performed while the patient was in severe low back and lower extremity pain. Figure 2.14 is a repeat CT scan per-

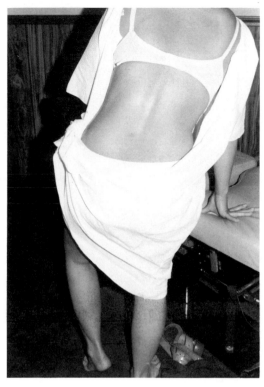

Figure 2.1. The great challenge in low back pain patients—this figure shows a patient with low back pain and radiating sciatic radiculopathy, leaning in a flexed position and unable to straighten the leg. This is a typical herniated nucleus pulposus case.

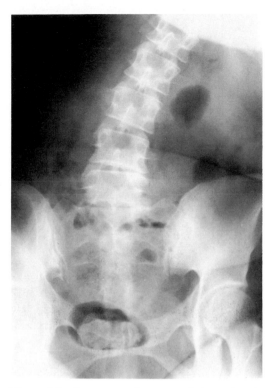

Figure 2.2. Posteroanterior x-ray of the patient in Figure 2.1. This is a Lovett reverse sciatic scoliosis in that the spinous processes rotate to the left convexity instead of to the right concave side. This is a typical rotation scoliosis seen in serious disc lesions.

formed when manipulative care had relieved the patient's symptoms; it shows no difference in the size of the disc protrusion. What is the explanation for this? We attempt to answer this question in chapter 3, which deals with neurophysiology of nerve root compression.

Figure 2.15 shows a condition seen with greater frequency by manipulating physicians—the aftermath of surgical facetectomy for relief of extreme lateral disc prolapse. The resultant unilateral collapse of the triple joint complex certainly creates new problems for the spine, as evidenced by the reactive bone changes on the left side with the left lateral flexion subluxation of L4 and L5.

Figure 2.16 shows a positive myelogram for an L5-S1 disc protrusion and certainly indicates upset kinematics in this patient's future.

Finally, the pathological causes of spine instability are seen in clinical practice. Figure 2.17 shows the flexion deformity of compression frac-

ture, and Figure 2.18 the unfortunate pathological fracture.

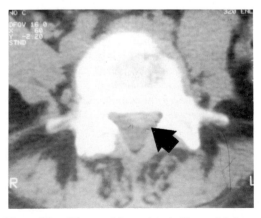

Figure 2.3. CT scan of the patient in Figure 2.1 shows a large left disc herniation at the L4-L5 disc level. All cases should be so easily Diagnosed!

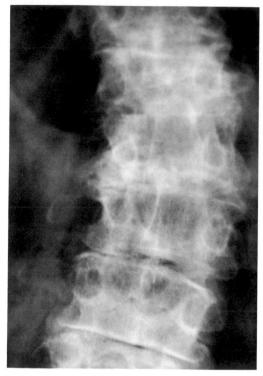

Figure 2.4. Degenerative spondyloarthrotic scoliosis of the thoracolumbar spine. Marked dextrorotatory scoliosis due to unequal asymmetrical disc degeneration on the left side of the upper lumbar discs.

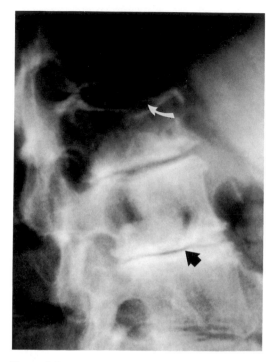

Figure 2.5. A vacuum osteochondrosis of the L2-L3 disc is noted (*arrow*). This represents the culmination of probably decades of degeneration. A compression defect of the superior L1 vertebral body is noted (*curved arrow*).

TRIPLE JOINT COMPLEX AND INSTABILITY

Figures 2.1 through 2.18 represent examples of disturbed kinematics of the functional spinal unit (Fig. 2.19), which is defined as the ligaments, apophyseal joints, and disc joining two adjacent vertebrae (1). The intervertebral disc anteriorly and the two apophyseal joints posteriorly comprise the triple joint complex. It can be noted in all of the above cases that alteration in one structure of the triple joint complex or the functional spinal unit leads to disturbed kinematics and pain.

Instability of the Spinal Unit

The change most often the result of dysfunction of the triple joint complex is termed instability. Instability is defined as the loss of the ability of the spine, under physiological loads, to maintain relationships between vertebrae in such a way that there is neither initial damage nor subsequent irritation to the spinal cord or nerve roots and, in addition, there is no development of incapacitating deformity or pain due to structural changes (2).

From Figures 2.1 through 2.18, we can see that instability may be introduced by facet asymmetry, disc injury, developmental and acquired scoliosis, degenerative disc disease, congenital anomalies, and pathological states.

Instability of a lumbar segment exists when it has abnormal movement, whether such motion be aberrant hypermobility or hypomobility. It may be pain-producing or below the level of pain production. Farfan (3) defines clinical instability as that symptomatic condition in which, in the absence of new injury, a physiological load induces abnormally large deformations at the intervertebral joint. He further describes two types of mechanical intervertebral joint failure: those due to axial compression and those due to axial torsion. Of these two types of injury, only torsional injury is considered to lead to instability, since both the

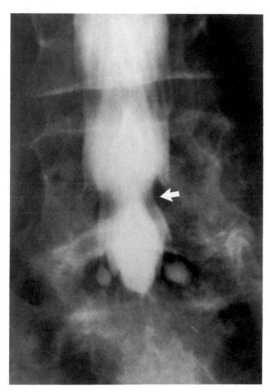

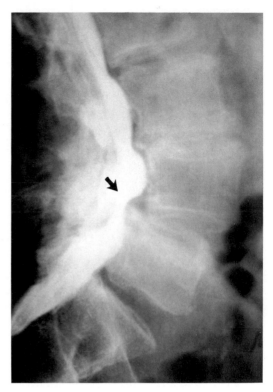

Figure 2.6. Myelogram showing stenotic narrowing (*arrow*) of the dye-filled subarachnoid space at L4-L5 level due to degenerative spondylolisthesis of L4 on L5 as shown in Figure 2.7.

Figure 2.7. Lateral view of the patient in Figure 2.6 shows the degenerative spondylolisthesis of L4 and the accompanying stenosis of the cauda equina (*arrow*).

annulus fibrosus and the facet joints fail simultaneously, rendering the joint unable to resist a repeated torsion until healing has occurred, with scar tissue formation. Compression injuries, on the other hand, damage only the end plate of the vertebra, leaving the functional spinal unit its capacity to support the superimposed weight with the annulus, facet joint, and vertebral body.

Examples of Instability of the Intervertebral Disc

Figures 2.20 and 2.21 show the instability of the intervertebral disc in true pars interarticularis fracture spondylolisthesis. Figure 2.20 shows the anterolisthesis of the fifth lumbar body on the sacrum, and the almost total return to normal alignment on vertical traction is seen in Figure 2.21.

Figure 2.22 shows the neutral standing position of a degenerative spondylolisthesis slippage;

the marked further unstable slippage in flexion is shown in Figure 2.23.

Both of these examples indicate that there has been disc damage and instability, allowing this translation of one spinal unit upon the other.

LATERAL FLEXION DISC MECHANICS IN RADIOGRAPHIC STUDY OF THE LUMBAR SPINE AND PELVIS

The biomechanics of the lumbar spine and pelvis are well shown radiographically by use of the dynamic lateral bending study. Without it, one of the most important tools of diagnosis of lumbar mechanics is lost. Weitz (4) revealed the accuracy of lateral bending studies by comparing his findings to those of myelography and surgery. He found that, of 46 patients, 12 had normal bending studies, and of these, six had midline disc protrusions and two had stenosis. Of the 34 patients with abnormal bending studies, 28 had disc pro-

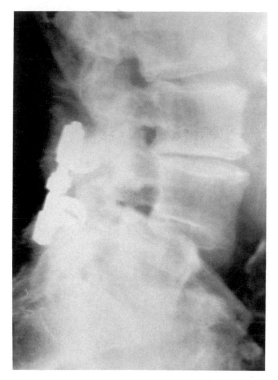

Figure 2.8. Lateral view shows surgical stabilization of the degenerative spondylolisthesis.

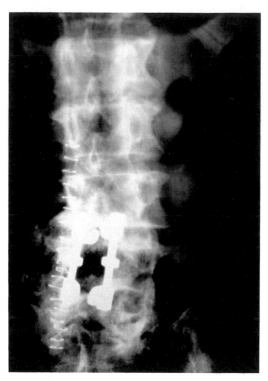

Figure 2.9. Anteroposterior view of patient in Figure 2.8 showing surgical stabilization of the degenerative spondylolisthesis.

trusions confirmed at both myelography and surgery. Two of the 34 had abnormal bending studies that were confirmed at surgery despite negative myelography. Both patients had lateral disc protrusions, with normal bending away from the protrusion and impaired bending toward the protrusion. There was no instance of a patient with an ipsilateral list and a negative myelogram.

Bending Study Accuracy

Van Damme et al. (5) compared the relative efficacy of clinical examination, electromyography, plain film radiography, myelography, and lumbar phlebography in the diagnosis of low back pain and sciatica. They found that *the bending studies had diagnostic reliability equal to that of myelography* and lumbar phlebography.

In 1942, Duncan and Haen stated that the postural attitude assumed by a patient with a disc protrusion was such as to avoid further compression of the disc: "This posture entails a list of the spine away from the side of the lesion and since the mass is extruding posteriorly, an attitude of

forward flexion is assumed" (6). They took films of the patient in lateral flexion to each side and in flexion and extension and found that, "in the majority of our cases, these films have demonstrated a lack of spinal mobility localized to the involved joint" (6). They also found that, in patients with laterally placed herniation, the myelograms were consistently found to be normal. (Author's note: We know that lateral discs can be so far lateral as not to contact the dye-filled subarachnoid space, thus giving a false negative myelogram—one reason for the 30 to 40% inaccuracy of myelography.) They also took postoperative bending films, which showed that once the sequestrum had been removed from the involved joint there was immediate restoration of joint mobility.

In 1948, Falconer et al. (7), in a study of 25 patients with ipsilateral list and 17 with contralateral list, with the summit medial or lateral to the nerve root in both subgroups, discussed the importance of list in lumbar disc disease. They found that scoliosis was due to spasm designed to exert the least possible "strain" on the surround-

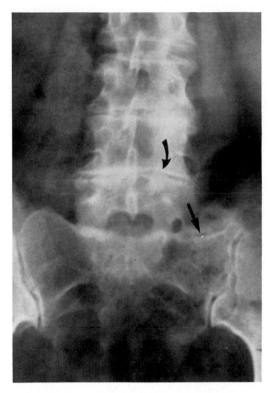

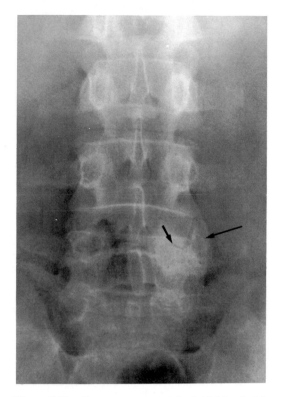

Figure 2.10. Transitional L5 vertebra with left pseudosacralization (*straight arrow*) and degeneration of the L4-L5 disc above (*curved arrow*) (Bertolotti's syndrome).

Figure 2.11. Facet asymmetry at the L4-L5 level with hyperplasia of the right superior L5 facet (*long arrow*) and a facet lamina pseudoarthrosis formed by the inferior facet of L4 in contact with the lamina of L5 (*short arrow*).

ing structures, but they were unable to correlate the direction of the curvature with the side of the symptoms. One year later, Hadley (8) noted that in certain patients with nerve root pressure, the foramen is not allowed to become smaller on lateral flexion toward the affected side, although normal wedging may take place at this level when the patient bends to the opposite direction.

Schalimtzek (9) and Hasner et al. (10) performed motion studies for diagnosis of herniated discs. Hasner et al. discovered that if lateral bending is inhibited, either the normal angulation between vertebral bodies may be less pronounced, or a state of parallelism may be noted. They (9, 10) also found that the vertebral bodies may even be divergent from each other on the side where the lateral bending takes place.

Breig (11) states that the patient's posture in an acute back disorder represents a compromise between the need to minimize tension in the dura and the root and the need to reduce the bulge of the prolapsed disc. He believes that it is not un-

common to see a patient with a flattened lumbar region flex the spine forward to minimize the herniation and ipsilaterally to relieve tension on the root, such as occurs in a patient with an axillary herniation (author's note: a medial disc).

Controversy Regarding Lateral Flexion Accuracy

Porter and Miller (12) do not find lateral flexion as diagnostic as other authors and state that, in a study of 100 patients with trunk list and back pain, they found a total of 49 that fulfilled the criterion of a symptomatic lumbar disc lesion, and 20 of these required surgical excision of the disc. The side of the list was not related to the side of the sciatica or to the topographic position of the disc in relation to the nerve root. Twice as many patients listed to the left as to the right, and there was some evidence that the side of the list may be related to hand or leg dominance.

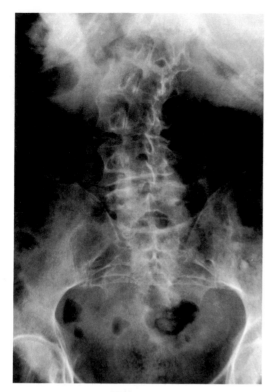

Figure 2.12. Levorotatory scoliosis is seen on this posteroanterior x-ray.

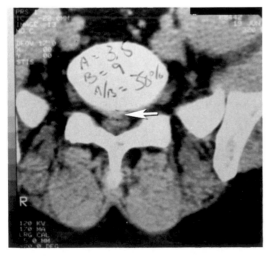

Figure 2.13. *Arrow* points to a disc protrusion occupying 38% of the sagittal diameter of the vertebral canal diameter. CT scan was performed when the patient was in pain.

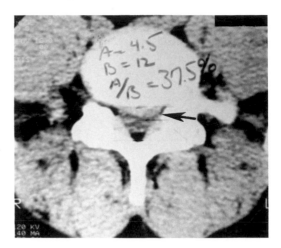

Figure 2.14. Comparison with Figure 2.13 shows reduction of the disc protrusion to be negligible while the patient is pain-free (*arrow*).

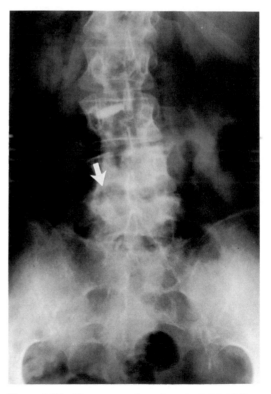

Figure 2.15. Facetectomy (*arrow*) on the left L4-L5 articulation for removal of an extreme lateral disc prolapse has resulted in left lateral flexion subluxation and degenerative changes of the intervertebral disc on the left. (Case courtesy of David Taylor, D.C., Joliet, Illinois.)

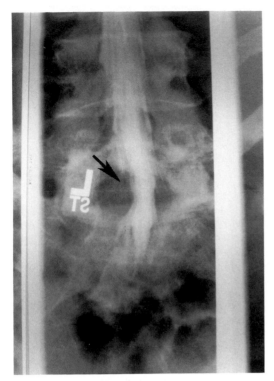

Figure 2.16. Myelographic filling defect (*arrow*) due to L5-S1 intervertebral disc protrusion.

Finneson (13) has demonstrated both ipsilateral and contralateral listing caused by the relationship of the protrusion to the nerve root.

Nachemson believes that "the information obtained from ordinary x-rays is . . . mostly irrelevant" (14). Weitz, therefore, states, "It is with this impetus that we urge lateral bending (dynamic) x-ray studies rather than static films in patients clinically suspected of having lumbar disc herniations" (4).

RADIOGRAPHIC STUDIES

Lateral bending studies are performed to determine aberrant lateral flexion of a functional spinal unit in relation to its adjacent segments. These studies are most beneficial in determining subluxation, as in hypomobility of the static subluxation accompanying intervertebral disc protrusion. For study of the L4-L5 level, routine anteroposterior (AP) views in lateral flexion are adequate, but for study of the L5-S1 level, the tilt view must be used because the sacral angle and lumbar lordosis make viewing of the lateral flexion of L5 on the sacrum impossible.

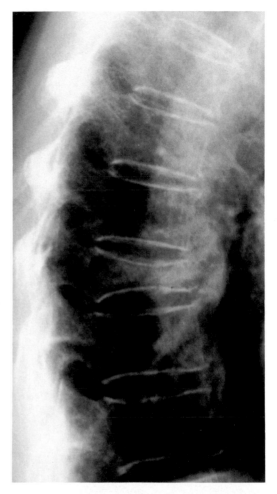

Figure 2.17. Compression fracture with flexion deformity of the T8 vertebral body.

For the tilt view, take the lateral lumbar view as shown in Figure 2.24. Next, draw the sacral promontory line and measure the angle made by this line with the horizontal. Then tilt the x-ray tube to match this angle (Fig. 2.25), with the center ray 1.5 inches inferior to the intercrestal line centered to the midline. In addition to the neutral posteroanterior (PA) view, the lateral bending studies are performed by having the patient slide his hand down his thigh while keeping his feet flat on the floor directly beneath the hip joints and keeping his knees straight (Fig. 2.26). These studies may be performed with the patient either sitting or standing, depending on the doctor's preference, and provide information on the following:

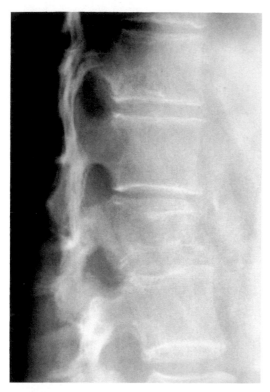

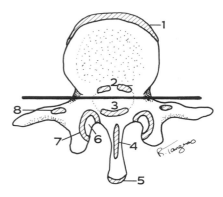

Figure 2.19. The schematic anatomical representation of a lumbar spinal segment. *1,* Anterior longitudinal ligament; *2,* posterior longitudinal ligament; *3,* ligamentum flavum; *4,* interspinous ligament; *5,* supraspinous ligament; *6,* facet joint; *7,* facet capsule; *8,* intertransverse ligament.

Figure 2.18. Pathological fracture of the T12 vertebral body.

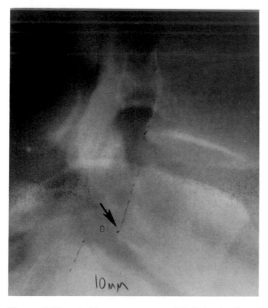

Figure 2.20. A 10-mm true spondylolisthesis slip of L5 on the sacrum is seen (*arrow*) in a weight-bearing film.

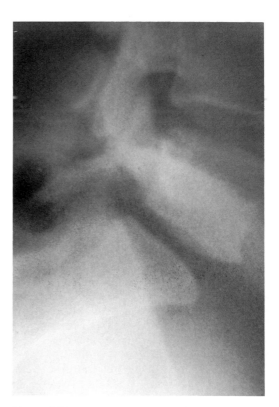

Figure 2.21. Vertical distraction of the Figure 2.20 spondylolisthetic slip shows complete reduction.

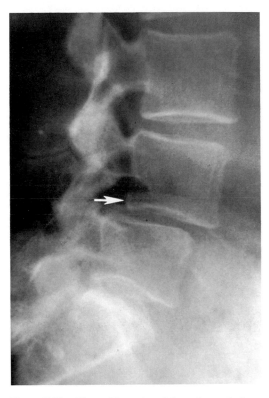

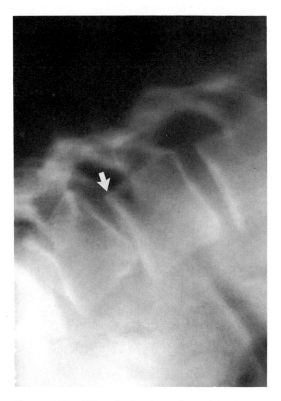

Figure 2.22. Neutral lateral upright radiograph shows approximately 15% slippage of L4 on L5 (*arrow*) with an intact partes interarticularis but a degenerative pseudospondylolisthesis.

Figure 2.23. When flexion is performed by the patient shown in Figure 2.22, marked instability is shown as L4 further translates on L5 to approximately 30% slippage (*arrow*).

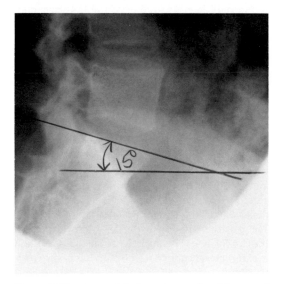

Figure 2.24. An upright lateral spot view. The sacral angle measured 15°.

1. Fixation (hypomobile) subluxation due to either disc protrusion or facet incongruity;
2. Relief of disc or facet lesions following manipulation, as normal physiological mobility returns.

Figure 2.27 is an illustration of lateral bending antalgic postures and their effect on the medial and the lateral discs.

Figures 2.28 through 2.30 are the roentgenographic studies that correlate with the schematic representations in Figure 2.27 of the disc protrusion causing nerve root compression. They are lateral bending studies of the L5-S1 level in a patient with pain down the right first sacral dematome, and they provide clinical evidence of a right lateral fifth lumbar disc protrusion. Figure 2.28 is the PA neutral view. Note the left lateral flexion subluxation of L5 on the sacrum and the tropism at L5-S1, with the right facets being sagittal and the left facets being obliquely coronal in

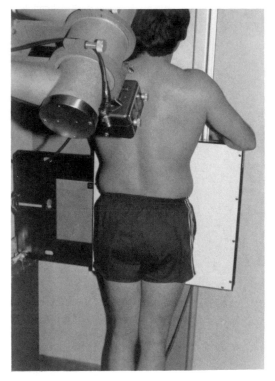

Figure 2.25. Tube tilted to match sacral angle and centered to L5-S1 level.

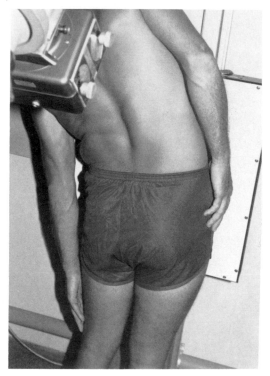

Figure 2.26. Lateral flexion is performed by having the patient slide his hand down his thigh while bending laterally.

their planes of articulation. Dye from prior myelography can be seen in the dural root sleeve.

Figure 2.29 is the left lateral bending study. Note spinous process deviation to the left. Figure 2.30 is the right lateral bending study and shows failure of right lateral movement of L5 on the sacrum. L5 is a hypomobile fixation subluxation, as evidenced by failure of lateral flexion or spinous process motion beyond the midline, which occurs in lateral disc protrusion.

Howe (personal communication, 1980) has said that the disc lesion is an area of hypomobility on the cineradiography study. Movement occurs above or below the disc lesion subluxation, but the disc is a hypomobile segment.

Figures 2.31 and 2.32 demonstrate the mechanics of the antalgic leans shown in Figures 2.28, 2.29 and 2.30.

Figures 2.33, 2.34, and 2.35 are studies of a patient with right medial disc protrusion at L5-S1. Figure 2.33 is the neutral PA view of the L5-S1 interspace in this patient with pain down the right first sacral dermatome. Note the right lateral flexion of L5 on the sacrum and the tropism

present, with the L5-S1 left facets being sagittal and the right facets being coronal. Figure 2.34 shows right lateral bending of the lumbar spine. Note a Lovett-positive scoliosis. Figure 2.35 shows attempted left lateral bending of the lumbar spine with failure of lateral flexion of L5 on the sacrum and with hypomobility of the segments above to laterally flex left. This subluxation pattern is quite compatible with the motion studies observed during physical examination.

Figure 2.36 is a schematic representation of the antalgia in the patient in Figures 2.33, 2.34, and 2.35.

White and Panjabi (2) state that lateral bending produced 2° to 3° of motion at L5-S1, and Tanz (15) has found that lateral bending produces 7° to 8° of motion at L4-L5 and L3-L4. The greater mobility at the L4-L5 level than at the L5-S1 level would help to account for the greater lateral subluxation occurring in disc protrusions.

Figures 2.37, 2.38 and 2.39 are studies of an L4-L5 left medial disc protrusion. Figure 2.37 is

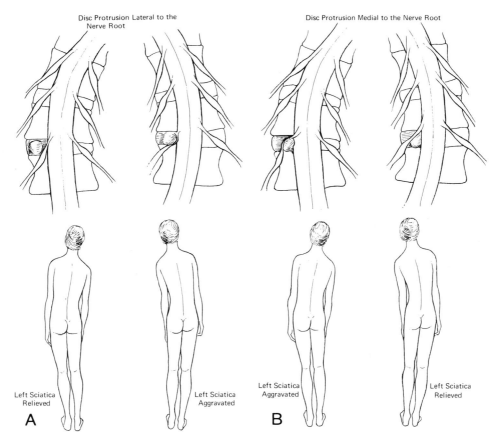

Figure 2.27. Relief or aggravation of pain with lateral flexion may indicate whether the disc protrusion is lateral or medial to the nerve root. (Reproduced with permission from Finneson BE. *Low Back Pain*. Philadelphia, JB Lippincott, 1973, p 302.)

the neutral PA view of L4-L5 and shows L4 in left lateral flexion subluxation on L5. The patient has left L5 dermatome pain indicative of a left L4-L5 medial disc lesion. Figure 2.38 is the left lateral bending study of the lumbar spine, with good lateral bending shown above L4-L5. Figure 2.39 is the right lateral bending study and shows failure of lateral flexion of L4 on L5. This is a fixation hypomobile discogenic subluxation. Note the motion of the lumbar levels above L4-L5 to the right.

Figures 2.40, 2.41, and 2.42, respectively, are schematic representations of antalgia in the patient in Figures 2.37, 2.38, and 2.39.

Lovett Reverse Scoliosis

Figure 2.43 is a standing AP lumbopelvic view of a patient who has had two myelograms for persis-

tent low back and right leg first sacral dermatome pain. This x-ray, if read alone, might be interpreted as being relatively erect, with no spinal unit subluxation patterns. There is tropism at L5-S1, with the right facet being sagittal and the left facet being coronal.

Figure 2.44 reveals normal lateral bending to the left. The spinous processes deviate to the concavity on the left and the bodies on the right.

Figure 2.45, however, is most informative; without it, misinterpretation of this spine would have occurred. In this right lateral flexion study, a Lovett reverse curve is shown. The spinous processes deviate to the convexity on the left, and the bodies deviate to the concavity on the right. There is some right lateral flexion of L4 on L5, of L3 on L4, and of L2 on L3, but there is also marked inferiority of the right hemipelvis on right lateral bending.

122 patients with surgically confirmed pathology consisting of either herniated lumbar disc, spinal stenosis, or both, were given preoperative metrizamide myelography and computerized myelography. When each myelogram and CT scan was read blindly by a neuroradiologist who knew nothing of the patient's surgical pathology, clinical examination, or results of the other preoperative tests, myelography was found to be more accurate than computed tomography in the diagnosis of herniated lumbar disc (83% vs. 72%). In the diagnosis of spinal stenosis, myelography was slightly more accurate than computed tomography (93% vs. 89%). Based on this study, which was said to be the largest surgically confirmed case study ever done, Bell et al. concluded that metrizamide myelography is more accurate than computed tomography in the diagnosis of both herniated lumbar disc and spinal stenosis and remains the diagnostic study of choice for these conditions. Furthermore, metrizamide myelography gives the added advantage of visualizing the thoracolumbar junction and thus affords the opportunity to diagnose occult spinal tumors.

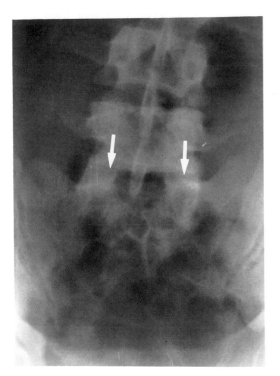

Figure 2.33. Neutral posteroanterior view of L5-S1. Note right lateral flexion of L5 on the sacrum (*arrow*). Tropism can be seen at L5-S1.

Accuracy of X-ray Interpretation by Various Professionals

Phillips (26) reported that spinal radiographs, whether interpreted by medical or chiropractic radiologists, have minimal value in predicting the presence or absence of low back complaints and, in particular, have no value in epidemiological studies.

Deyo et al. (27) had two skeletal radiologists independently interpret lumbar spine studies from 100 walk-in patients with low back pain. Intraobserver variability was assessed by having each perform duplicate readings on a random sample of films 1 month later. Each reader used a standardized form to record 43 data items for each examination, including the presence or absence of 17 specific abnormalities. Intraobserver agreement was generally better than interobserver agreement, but still only moderate. For patients with clinically low risk of systemic disease, the predictive value of a "positive" x-ray is low, and observer disagreements lower it further, constituting another reason to avoid radiography for low-risk patients.

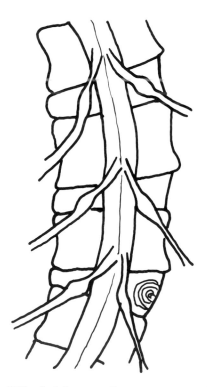

Figure 2.32. Left lean to relieve pressure caused by disc protrusion lateral to nerve root.

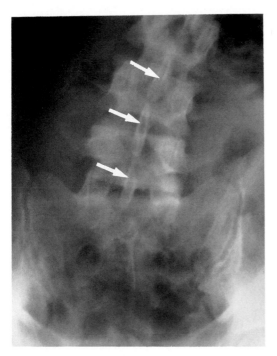

Figure 2.34. Right lateral flexion view showing Lovett-positive curve with spinous deviation into the concavity of the curve (*arrows*).

Discography

Another imaging modality not widely used, but increasingly discussed due to its tremendous ability to reveal the internal derangement of the nucleus pulposus and annulus fibrosus, is discography. It has been stated to be more reliable than CT scanning in assessment of disc integrity (28).

Discography coupled with CT scanning was found to be a useful diagnostic adjunctive procedure (29) in the assessment of 22 patients with continued, undiagnosed symptoms of low back and sciatic pain for an average of 14 months. The patients studied had had prior negative evaluations, including electromyography (EMG), CT scanning, and/or metrizamide myelography. Three-level, posterolateral, extradural discography was performed on the side opposite the sciatica. One to six hours after discography, CT scanning was performed on all injected discs; 91% demonstrated abnormal discograms at one or more levels. CT imaging demonstrated contrast tracking to the periphery of the disc in 82%. Discography reproduced the patient's symptoms in 77%. The direction of contrast tracking seen on scanning correlated with clinical symptoms in

73% and with symptoms at discography in 82%. CT scanning was thought to be a useful adjunct to lumbar discography in patients with prior negative evaluations.

The benefits of discography were described in 500 patients with negative or inconclusive iophendylate myelograms (30). Discography remains the ideal complementary examination to demonstrate normal or diseased disc morphology, and its findings were confirmed during surgery in 97.8% of explored discs. Discography is also a valuable clinical test, since the injection may reproduce the patient's symptoms. Its observations were decisive in the surgeon's decision whether or not to explore a disc: 97.3% of patients submitted to laminectomy had an abnormal discogram, and 73% of these patients experienced reproduction of clinical symptoms during the procedure. Myelography is superior to discography in demonstrating sequestered fragments, pachymeningitis, and spinal stenosis, but it was nevertheless not helpful in 56% of the pa-

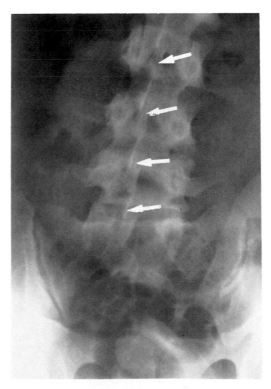

Figure 2.35. Left lateral flexion view showing Lovett failure curve with failure of the lumbar bodies to flex left and the spinous processes rotating left (*arrows*).

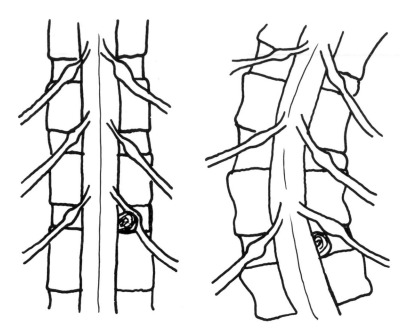

Figure 2.36. Schematic of L5 right medial disc protrusion in relation to the right S1 nerve root. The patient leans right to move the nerve root away from the disc; i.e., the patient leans into the side of the pain (*right side*) to relieve the pressure from an L5 disc protrusion medial to the S1 nerve root.

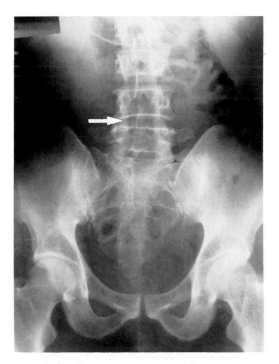

Figure 2.37. Posteroanterior view of the lumbar spine shows left lateral subluxation of L4 on L5 (*arrow*).

tients with these conditions, in whom the diagnoses were made in the operating room.

Extraforaminal disc herniation was found to be best identified by discography (31). Atypical disc herniation, especially extraforaminal disc herniation (EFDH), is apt to be overlooked, because myelography and peridurography can give false positive and false negative findings. Eleven cases of EFDH were confirmed by operative treatment. This number is a very small percentage of the total, but if these cases had not been diagnosed correctly, the results of surgery would have been poor. Selective lumbosacral radiculography and nerve root block techniques are very useful in determining the nerve root involved. Discography is an excellent diagnostic technique for finding the relationship between the nerve root and hernia mass. Extraforaminal disc herniation must be kept in mind as a cause of lumbar radiculopathy.

Magnetic Resonance Imaging

Powell et al. (32) reported on 302 women aged 16 to 80 without symptoms of spinal disease who had their lumbar intervertebral discs examined by magnetic resonance imaging (MRI). The prevalence of one or more degenerated discs increased linearly with age, but disc degeneration was already present in over one-third of the women aged 21 to 40 years; these young women may prove to be at special risk of disc prolapse later in life. The high prevalence of symptomless disc degeneration must be taken into account when MRI is used for assessment of spinal symptoms.

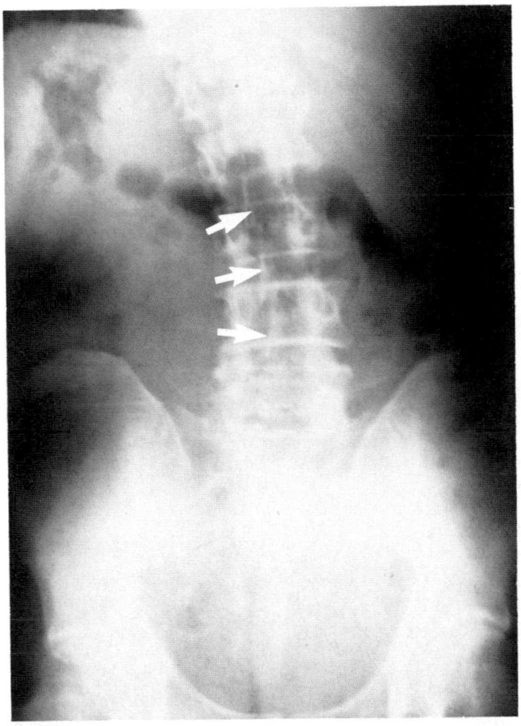

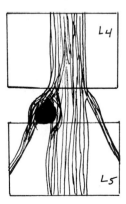

Figure 2.38. Left lateral flexion view showing normal lateral flexion mechanics. All segments have spinous process rotation into the concave side (Lovett-positive motion) (*arrows*).

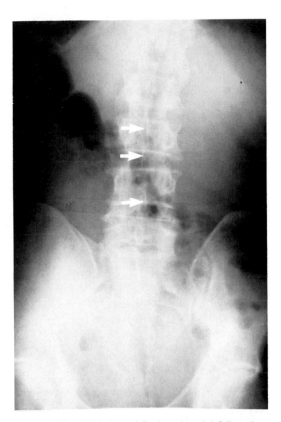

Figure 2.39. Right lateral flexion view. L4 fails to laterally flex right on L5. The spinous processes do not rotate right (Lovett motion failure) (*arrows*).

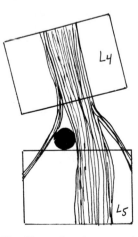

Figure 2.40. Illustration demonstrating how standing erect pulls the L5 nerve root into the L4 medial disc protrusion.

Figure 2.41. Illustration demonstrating how left lateral bending pulls L5 nerve root away from the L4 medial disc protrusion and relieves pain.

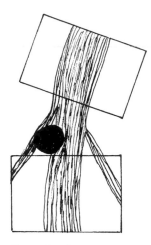

Figure 2.42. Illustration demonstrating how right lateral bending pulls the L5 nerve root into the left L4 medial disc protrusion and aggravates pain.

Gibson et al. (33) found a consistent pattern of gradual loss of signal from the nucleus pulposus, culminating in a complete loss of nuclear signal in all cases after chemonucleolysis. The time required for this change to occur varied between 6 and 18 weeks. Transitory minor end-plate changes were present in five patients, probably representing a mild chemical discitis.

Technically adequate MRI examinations are equivalent to CT and myelography in the diagnosis of lumbar canal stenosis and herniated disc disease. CT and MRI can be complementary studies, and surface coil MRI can be viewed as an alternative to myelography (34).

A study (35) showed that healthy intervertebral disc behavior on loading depends greatly on water content: that is, the high water content of the nucleus in early life (85 to 95%) is the most important factor in resistance to compression. On the other hand, the water content is determined by the major macromolecular components of the disc. These major components are collagen I and II, and the proteoglycan matrix. The nucleus of young discs contains 65% of its dry matter weight as proteoglycan, whereas the corresponding figure for the annulus is only 20%. The collagen ratios are reversed. It seems likely that the proteoglycan matrix is responsible for the hydrodynamic properties of the nucleus, even

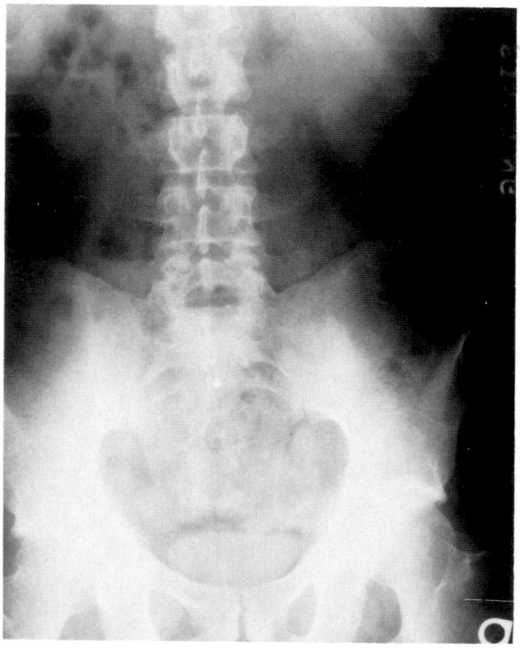

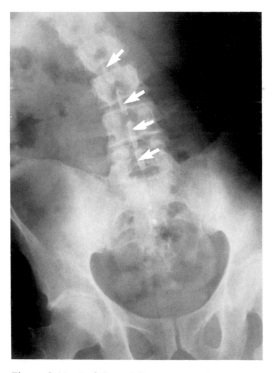

Figure 2.44. Left lateral flexion view of the patient seen in Figure 2.43. Normal Lovett-positive motion is shown with spinous processes rotated to the concave side (*arrows* on spinous processes).

Figure 2.43. Posteroanterior neutral view of the lumbar spine which appears quite free of lateral curvature.

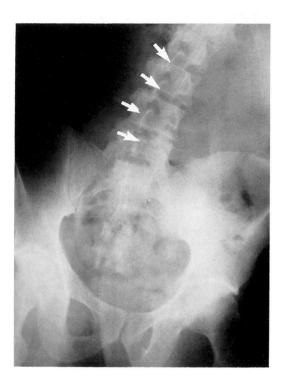

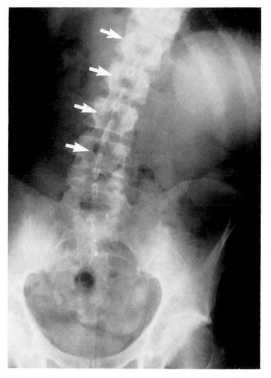

Figure 2.45. Right lateral flexion of the patient shown in Figure 2.44. Abnormal lateral movement with spinous process deviation to the convex side (Lovett negative) is shown (*arrows*). The right hemipelvis drops markedly.

Figure 2.46. Repeat view of the patient seen in Figure 2.45 following 2 weeks of Cox flexion distraction manipulation. The right hemipelvis is level now. The spinous processes rotate to the midline instead of the convexity (*arrows*).

though it is also known from recent works that collagen II, which has a high concentration in the nucleus, may absorb a higher percentage of water than does collagen I.

Initial results suggest that MRI is a particularly suitable way to follow the changes in the state of water in intervertebral discs.

Role of Myelography in Disc Lesion Diagnosis

Authorities have expressed opposing opinions on the use of myelography. Day (20) says that there is need for improvement in the diagnosis and treatment of the lumbar disc disease. Furthermore, he states that the diagnosis can be made on the basis of history and physical examination alone. He believes that myelography has grave shortcomings, since it provides indirect evidence by the indentations of the Pantopaque (iophendylate) column. Myelography is reliable only when herniations contact this column. Day advocates use of the dis-

cogram in preference to use of the myelogram. Rothman and Simeone (17), however, dislike use of the discogram.

Semmes (21) states that the clinical findings and history are more reliable than myelograms because nearly one-third of myelograms are uncertain or misleading. He explains that the myelogram is too frequently used for diagnosis and as an indication for surgical treatment. It is wholly unnecessary in the diagnosis of the average patient requiring surgery for a ruptured disc, and is hardly justifiable in cases not requiring surgery. He used myelograms in less than 3% of his last 350 surgeries.

In their article concerning lumbar spondylolisthesis with ruptured disc, Scoville and Corkill (22) say that seven of 17 patients with spondylolisthesis and ruptured disc had negative myelograms.

Abdullah et al. (23), in their article on extreme lateral lumbar disc herniation, state that this type of disc herniation is outside the anatomical boundary of the spinal canal and cannot be demonstrated by myelography. The classic clinical manifestations of an extreme lateral lumbar disc lesion are necessary for the diagnosis, and discography often proves helpful. According to Abdullah et al., whenever neurological findings suggest upper lumbar nerve root compression, the chances are four to one that an extreme lateral disc herniation is responsible. Categorically stated, a systematic diagnostic approach to the disc lesion, up to but excluding the use of myelographic exploration, can yield an excellent diagnostic impression about the level and type of disc lesion in relationship to the nerve root it compresses.

Myelographic Dye Suitability

In myelography, a study comparing iohexol and iopamidol showed comparable radiographic quality, with iopamidol being slightly better tolerated (36).

Comparison of the dyes used in myelography was performed by means of a double-blind study (37) that compared metrizamide with the new iodinated water-soluble nonionic contrast medium, iopamidol, for conventional and CT lumbosacral myelography. Both contrast agents were used in 30 patients, and were equivalent in terms of image quality and clinical accuracy. Headaches and nausea were less severe using iopamidol. The most striking difference was found in adverse neurobehavioral reactions and associated electroencephalographic abnormalities, which were noted in 17% of the metrizamide group but were not seen with the use of iopamidol. Iopamidol appears to be superior to metrizamide for intrathecal applications.

Outpatient myelography was studied over a 2-year period in 92 outpatients who underwent lumbar myelography using iopamidol (38). The incidence and severity of adverse reactions associated with myelography in these cases were compared with those in 116 patients who underwent iopamidol myelography as inpatients. The hospitalized patients received 10 ml, and the outpatients 8 or 10 ml, of contrast medium. The severity of complications was graded as very mild, mild, moderate, or severe. The complication rate was 37% in the hospitalized patients and 40% in the outpatients. Adverse reactions, mostly in the form of headache, were very mild in approximately two-thirds of cases in each group, and moderate or severe in 15% of the inpatients and 24% of the outpatients presenting complications. The incidence of moderate or severe reactions was lower in the outpatients receiving 8 ml of contrast medium than in those given 10 ml of iopamidol. Lumbar myelography performed on an outpatient basis is a safe procedure. The outpatient regimen considerably reduces the cost of myelography and indirectly increases the availability of beds in orthopedic and neurological units.

MRI, CT, Discography, or Myelography in Disc Hydration State

Troisier (39) states that it is a well-known fact that both surgery and chemonucleolysis can cure a patient suffering from root pain due to a prolapsed intervertebral disc. However, the failure rate after intradiscal injection of chymopapain remains important. Analysis of unsuccessful chemonucleolysis shows that about two-thirds of failures are due to a remaining discal fragment. Only discography, not CT scan or myelography, can demonstrate invasion of the prolapsed area. A large, well-filled protruding area characterizes a "good" image; when this is present, there is a 76% incidence good results. Likewise, lateralization of the pain response (in the buttock or the affected limb) is correlated with a 42% success rate and a 13% failure rate. A combination of good images and lateralized pain, seen in 24.8% of the cases, correlates with a 97.5% incidence of good results. Therefore, discography should be a factor in the decision between surgery and chemonucleolysis and should be considered as a preoperative examination.

Hickey et al. (40) state that a loss of water from the nucleus during aging was demonstrated by a reduction and change in the distribution of the M values for an 82-year-old disc, as compared with a 16-year-old disc. Values of T1 and T2 indicated that there was a difference in the chemical environment of water molecules in the nucleus pulposus and annulus fibrosus; the extent of this difference was much greater for younger than for older discs. High-resolution MR images from discs of living subjects showed almost as much detail as those from experimental specimens, but in the latter, the laminated structure of the annulus was resolved.

Evaluation of CT against myelography was reported by Kornberg et al. (41), with six patients with abnormal myelograms found to have evidence of a herniated nucleus pulposus at the L5-S1 level on CT scan. Their conclusion was that the sensitivity of CT in diagnosing a herniated nucleus pulposus is greater than that of myelography if images in the exact plane of the disc can be obtained.

MRI and CT Differential Diagnosis of Disc Herniation from Postoperative Scarring

Firooznia et al. (42) stated that computerized tomography of the lumbar spine, without and with intravenous administration of contrast medium, was performed in 113 consecutive patients who had previously had spine surgery for disc herniation and had persistent or recurrent symptoms. Fifty-two patients underwent surgical reexploration. It was possible to make the diagnosis of normal postoperative status, disc herniation, or scarring in 31 (60%) of the 52 patients with the use of CT scans without intravenous contrast enhancement. CT with intravenous contrast enhancement was useful in 12 of the remaining patients (23%). Enhancement of the margins of a herniated disc occurred in 37 (71%) of the patients. There was near-homogenous enhancement of postoperative scarring in 34 (65%) of the patients. Intravenous contrast medium was particularly helpful when disc herniation and scarring were both present, by delineating the margins of a herniated disc and enhancing the entire substance of the scar. In symptomatic postoperative patients, CT of the lumbar spine without intravenous contrast medium should be performed initially. If a definitive diagnosis is not established, CT with intravenous contrast enhancement should be considered.

Another study (43) shows that differentiation between recurrent herniation of the nucleus pulposus (RHNP) and postoperative epidural fibrosis (scar) is difficult on both clinical and radiological grounds, including myelography and CT. In this setting, it is likely that MRI, or to a lesser degree CT with contrast enhancement (CT/C), will provide a more definitive diagnosis than conventional CT.

Weiss et al. (44) studied 65 patients with recurrent radicular complaints after operation for lumbar disc herniation with CT examination before and after intravenous contrast application (volume, 1.5 to 2.0 ml/kg of body weight; flow rate, 0.35 ml/s). Postsurgical hypertrophic scar tissue showed definite contrast enhancement, whereas disc herniation remained unenhanced. Intravenous contrast application is recommended in patients previously operated upon for disc herniation. Accuracy was reported at 67%. The dye used was angiografin.

Mikhael et al. (45) studied 10 normal adult volunteers, 75 patients with low back pain and/or lumbar radiculopathy, 16 patients following chymopapain treatment, 14 patients with recurrent symptoms following disc surgery, and two patients with distal cord compression with scanning on a Fonar 3000 permanent magnet scanner. Of all the patients, 98 had additional CT scans of the lumbar spine and 82 had myelography. Lumbar MRI and CT scans were both diagnostic in cases of herniated and extruded discs. MRI scan showed more information concerning the degenerative state of the intervertebral discs. It was relatively more accurate in detecting small bulging and herniated discs without ruptured annulus and in determining the relation of the migrated fragments of the extruded discs to both the back of the vertebrae and the thecal sac. Moreover, lumbar MRI matched the clinical response of disc disease to chymopapain treatment more than lumbar CT scan. In addition, the MRI studies differentiated more accurately between postoperative epidural fibrotic changes and recurrent herniated and/or extruded disc, and detected laterally herniated lumbar discs. Myelography was the diagnostic study in cases of arachnoiditis.

The use of the contrast agent gadolinium diethylenetriaminepentaacetic acid/dimeglumine (Gd-DTPA) prior to MRI (and also CT) allows the scar to be enhanced with the contrast dye, whereas the disc material is not so enhanced. Hueftle (46) describes a Gd-DTPA contrast-enhanced MRI to differentiate epidural fibrosis scarring from recurrent disc protrusion, and states that failed back surgery syndrome has been seen in 10 to 40% of patients who undergo back surgery and that it is characterized by intractable pain and varying degrees of functional incapacitation. The differentiation of fibrosis from disc protrusion is important because the result of reoperation for epidural fibrosis is not generally good as in recurrent disc protrusion.

Pre- and postcontrast MRI images were done on 30 cases of failed back surgery syndrome. Seventeen patients had surgical and pathological correlation of the MRI findings at 19 disc levels. The precontrast studies had a sensitivity, specificity, and accuracy of 100%, 71%, and 89%, respectively. The enhanced MRI studies correctly depicted the character of abnormal epidural soft tissue in 17 patients at all 19 levels. Scar showed heterogeneous enhancement on the early T1-weighted spin-echo images obtained within 10 minutes after contrast material administration. Herniated disc did not show significant enhancement on the early studies but showed variable degrees of enhancement on delayed images in nine of 12 cases. Results showed that precontrast and early postcontrast T1-weighted spin-echo studies are highly accurate in separating epidural fibrosis from herniated disc. Hueftle (46) speculates that this may be the premier procedure for accurate differentiation of fibrosis and disc tissue.

Value of Attenuation Numbers for Identifying Anatomical Structures

Helms et al. (47) report normal CT attenuation values for various structures in the lumbar spine which were obtained on several CT scanners. The wide range of normal values makes using absolute CT numbers unreliable. The utility and pitfalls of using attenuation numbers in the spine are discussed, and several examples are illustrated. CT numbers used as absolute values can be misleading; used as relative values for comparison with other structures, however, they can be quite valuable.

The following tissues were sampled: thecal sac at L3, L4, L5, and S1 levels; ligamentum flavum; epidural fat; normal disc material (bulging annulus and herniated nucleus pulposus); nerve roots; and dorsal root ganglia.

One of the most useful aspects of computed tomography is its ability to distinguish subtle tissue density differences. The density of a herniated disc has been shown to be greater than the density of the thecal sac.

There are reports that refute the above findings strongly, and for the purposes of this text I will only state that, regardless of the imaging modality, careful clinical correlation with the imaging findings is needed to arrive at the diagnosis. This is even more necessary with the advent of MRI, which so commonly shows us numerous disc protrusions, making it mandatory to utilize clinical findings. I previously quoted Semmes

(21), who stated that the clinical examination and findings are more reliable than the myelogram. I agree heavily with this comment.

Clinical Findings Must Be Correlated with Imaging Diagnoses

CASE PRESENTATION

The case presented here is a good example of numerous imaging modalities being performed on a patient, with differing clinical diagnoses from each modality. This patient suffered from low back and left leg pain, for which she had been treated by a general practitioner with nonsteroidal antiinflammatory drugs. He referred her to a neurosurgeon, who performed an epidural steroid injection with no relief.

The patient then had MRI performed, which revealed an L4-L5 disc bulging, which was interpreted as being more than an annular bulge (Fig. 2.47). It was felt to be more prominent on the right than on the left, and the T2 surface coil studies demonstrated a diminished signal intensity from the L4-L5 disc. The impression from the MRI was degenerative disc disease at the L4-L5 level with annular bulging of the disc.

A myelogram was then performed, as seen in Figures 2.48 and 2.49. It was negative.

A CT scan, seen in Figure 2.50, was negative for any disc pathology or stenosis of the vertebral canal.

Plain x-rays, shown in Figures 2.51 and 2.52, reveal good disc spaces with no evidence of degenerative disc disease. Lateral flexion studies (Fig. 2.53 and 2.54) reveal failure of spinous process rotation to the left concavity on left lateral flexion motion. This correlates with a lateral left disc protrusion impression. The reader is urged to study lateral bending studies described earlier in this chapter.

The aforementioned imaging studies left the surgeon, and our clinic as well, when the patient came to us, with a mixed diagnostic impression. Here was a patient with low back and fifth lumbar dermatome pain, whose myelogram and CT were negative while the MRI revealed evidence of some degeneration and bulging of the L4-L5 disc.

Our approach in this case was to do a complete examination, with neurological and orthopedic workup. These revealed that the straight leg raises were negative; there were +2 deep reflexes of the ankle, knee, and hamstrings; and there was no motor weakness. The circulation of the lower extremities was normal. The patient had no pain on coughing, sneezing, or straining to move the bowel.

Treatment of this case was then administered, consist-

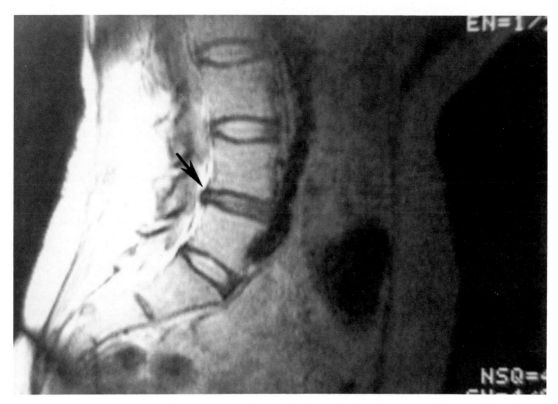

Figure 2.47. MRI showing an L4-L5 disc protrusion (*arrow*) and a diminished signal intensity at L4-L5 compared to the other disc levels. This represents degenerative disc disease with annular protrusion at the L4-L5 disc level.

ing of flexion distraction manipulation, physiological therapeutics, low back wellness school, and a home exercise program. The patient was relieved of her symptoms.

In our opinion, this patient might well have first been treated with conservative care, and then, if adequate (50%) relief was not shown after 3 to 4 weeks of such care, the more sophisticated imaging procedures might have been performed.

RELIABILITY OF CLINICAL EXAMINATION IN DIAGNOSIS OF LUMBAR DISC HERNIATION WITHOUT IMAGING MODALITIES

What about the ability of the clinical examination to diagnose the level of disc lesion? Let's look at some factual data on this question. Hakelius (48) reported a 63% correlation between clinical neurological signs and operatively proven pathology. Similar data were reported by Hirsch (49), who reported a 55% correlation between neurological signs and the presence of a herniated lumbar

disc. *They found that the presence of a positive straight leg raising sign in addition to positive neurological signs produced the correct diagnosis in 86% of their patients. When a positive myelogram, however, was correlated with the positive neurological examination and positive straight leg raising sign, the accuracy increased to 95%.*

Consider that chiropractic physicians in private practice, often not privileged to have the sophistication of hospital-based imaging instruments such as CT, MRI, or myelography, rely greatly on their own capabilities in clinical, orthopedic, and neurological examination to diagnose their patients. Now chiropractors and their patients can appreciate the extensive training given in undergraduate school in the performance of excellent spinal and clinical examinations. The future will dictate that the careful clinical correlative diagnosis will become more important as imaging modalities such as MRI show us greater disc changes and numerous disc protrusions while being incapable of identifying the offending level. The chiropractic physician may expect 86% accu-

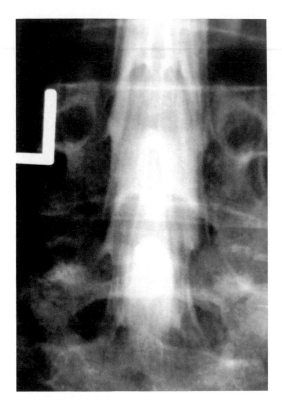

Figure 2.48. The myelogram of the patient seen in Figure 2.47 is negative in the posteroanterior study.

curate than myelography alone, both in predicting the presence or absence of nerve root involvement and in distinguishing disc prolapse from bony entrapment. Provided the clinical criteria were clearly defined, patients with three or more of the four criteria were usually found to have a disc prolapse, while bony entrapment could frequently be identified with one or two criteria. It is concluded that in practice, although lumbar disc prolapse is well recognized, clinical assessment and diagnostic criteria need to be defined more clearly to match increasingly sophisticated radiology.

The predominant symptom in both was root pain, with or without paresthesia (51). In bony entrapment, this was sometimes related to walking; that is, the key feature was reproduction of root pain on walking. Most disc prolapses produced root irritation signs, and features of nerve irritation were usually more marked than those of nerve compression. In contrast, bony entrapment frequently produced root compression signs with only minor root irritation and surprisingly free straight leg raising.

All surgeons agree in principle that diagnosis and decisions to operate should be based on clinical criteria and that radiological investigations should be used to complement and not replace clinical judgment (51).

racy in the correct diagnosis with a carefully performed clinical examination.

Hirsch (49) reported 93% accuracy in diagnosing disc lesions with clinical and myelographic correlation; however, Firooznia et al. (50) reported the same accuracy for CT scanning in 89 surgically confirmed cases. Of 12 instances of disagreement, two were due to incorrect interpretations, five were in previously operated patients, three in spondylolisthesis, and two in spinal stenosis.

Clinical Diagnostic Criteria Compared to Myelography

Morris et al. (51) performed a prospective study of 185 patients undergoing first-time lumbar surgery, comparing how accurately clinical criteria and water-soluble myelography predicted the operative findings. Clinical diagnostic criteria of *(a) nerve root pain, (b) root irritation signs,* and *(c) neurological signs of root compression* supplemented by *(d) myelography* were shown to be much more ac-

Sensory Examination Findings and Their Diagnostic Accuracy

Weise et al. (52) studied the significance of sensory changes determined by pinprick and light touch in individuals with a herniated lumbar disc. They found that right-left differences in Semmes-Weinstein pressure thresholds of more than 15 mg/mm^2 enabled them to localize disc lesions to a specific root in 100% of the patients, and differences in vibratory thresholds of more than 3.5 μm localized the correct level in 88% of cases. Light touch and pinprick testing could not duplicate these good results and only resulted in correct identification of the nerve root involved in 50% of patients. The correct dermatome tested was confirmed by patient criteria prior to the sensory examination by having a positive straight leg raising sign, motor or reflex asymmetry, a single nerve root dermatome involvement, and a positive CT scan or myelogram.

Schofferman et al. (53) feels that pain in the lower extremity may prove to be useful diagnostically. The exact distribution of pain is elicited, as

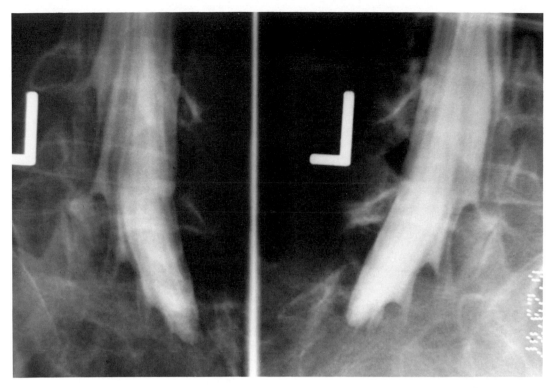

Figure 2.49. The oblique views also are negative for cauda equina or nerve root compression by disc protrusion.

well as the quality of pain, to separate referred pain from radicular pain. Leg pain in the absence of neurological deficiency is referred pain, while pain with neurological deficit is radicular. However, in early radicular pain, the neurological deficit may not yet be present. True positive nerve root tension signs suggest radicular pain, even in the absence of frank neurological deficit. Referred pain shares the same distribution as the innervation of the affected zygapophyseal joints. Pain arising from the facet joints of L4-L5 or L5-S1 will be felt in the posterior thigh and occasionally in the medial or lateral calf, and back pain is usually greater than leg pain. Numbness or tingling may accompany this pain. *Posterior joint pain (facet, ligament, annulus) occasionally, but rarely, extends beyond the calf and into the foot.* Radicular pain is caused by nerve root irritation, inflammation, or compression. The predominant and more severe pain is usually felt in the thigh and is present in the posterior lateral calf, extending to the toes. Dermatomal radiation may not be exact, and much overlap exists. However, certain patterns are characteristic: L3 pain involves the groin and anterior medial thigh; L4 pain involves the ante-

rior thigh and medial calf, as well as the gluteal area; L5 pain involves the lateral thigh as well as the lateral and possibly medial calf, and the great toe; S1 nerve involvement is felt in the posterior thigh, posterior calf, and lateral aspect of the foot and heel.

White (54) states that annular disc tears, by means of nociceptor nerve endings in the annulus fibrosus, cause pain referral to the low back, buttock, sacroiliac region, and lower extremity even in the absence of neural compression.

Comparison of Clinical and Imaging Modalities

The correlation of standard diagnostic studies in the diagnosis of disc herniation was studied in 100 patients by Schoedinger (55). One hundred patients with surgically proven ruptured lumbar discs were studied in terms of their diagnostic workup. Four studies—electromyogram, CT scan, myelogram, and epidural venogram—were evaluated independently and in combination. No one study was consistently abnormal; however, epidural venography was diagnostic in 74% of

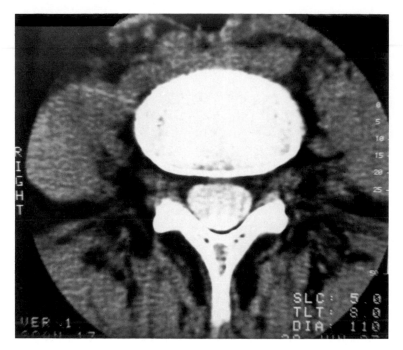

Figure 2.50. The CT scan of this patient is negative.

cases. CT scanning and electromyographic examination, when used in combination, were found to be reliable in confirming the diagnosis of lumbar disc rupture in 84% of cases. In no instance were all preoperative diagnostic studies normal when a diagnosis of herniated nucleus pulposus was proven surgically. It seems, therefore, that *a detailed history and physical examination* in combination with a positive result in at least one of the diagnostic studies appears sufficient to establish the diagnosis of lumbar disc rupture.

Localization of Lumbar Disc Herniation by Symptoms and Signs

Kortelainen et al. (56) reported that neurological symptoms and signs in patients with sciatica were studied prospectively and compared with myelographic and operative findings in 403 cases with lumbar disc herniation, with special reference to accuracy of the clinically diagnosed level. Neurological symptoms and signs of involvement of a single root were present in 239 cases, and of two roots in 154 cases in L4-L5 and L5-S1 herniations. Pain projection into the fifth lumbar distribution was a very important symptom for clinical

identification of the fifth lumbar root involvement and gave a level of diagnostic accuracy comparable to myelography, while pain projection into the first sacral distribution was less reliable, especially in cases with signs of two roots. The neurological picture of high herniations was completely unreliable. Lumbar myelography or computed tomography is recommended as a routine preoperative study.

Pain in the fifth lumbar area was due to an L4-L5 disc herniation in 80% of cases, and pain in the S1 area was due to a disc lesion at L5-S1 in 63% of cases and to an L4-L5 rupture in 34%.

The straight leg raising test was usually positive in all levels of herniation (94%). However, it was strongly positive (positive under 30°) more frequently in herniations of the lower discs. The sign was bilaterally positive in 41% of cases.

The Achilles reflex was the most generally affected neurological sign (52%). It was pathological in all levels of herniation, though more so in L5-S1 disc ruptures (56).

Weakness of extension of the great toe (45%) was almost as common as the pathological Achilles reflex. Sensory defects were associated with 38% of the disc ruptures. They were most common in the area of the first sacral root and were caused by L5-S1 disc herniation in 61% of the

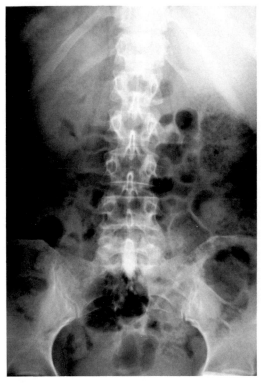

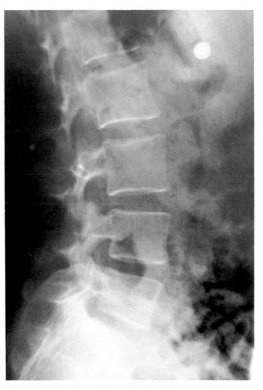

Figure 2.51. The lumbar spine in anteroposterior projection is not remarkable for lateral flexion or rotatory subluxation.

Figure 2.52. Lateral projection shows no degenerative disc disease and good sagittal curvature.

cases and by L4-L5 disc rupture in the rest. Sensory changes in the area of the fifth nerve root were less common and were due to L4-L5 disc lesions in 80% and to L5-S1 disc rupture in 20% of the cases.

Pain projection to L5 alone with associated S1 signs, usually a pathological Achilles reflex, was 75% correct in diagnosis of the L4-L5 level disc rupture. Pain in the L5 area with extensor hallucis weakness was 92% accurate despite concomitant S1 findings.

Extensor hallucis weakness and sensory defect in the L5 area were 100% reliable in level diagnosis of fourth disc herniation despite accompanying pain projection to the first sacral area in all cases and a pathological Achilles reflex in some instances. A pathological Achilles reflex and sensory defect in the S1 area, on the other hand, had no level diagnostic significance in the presence of pain projection to the L5 area.

The cough impulse test (74%) and Lasègue's sign (94%) were the most frequently positive clinical signs, as has been reported previously.

Projected pain could be localized according to the distribution of the lumbar and the first sacral roots in 93% of the disc ruptures.

The Achilles reflex is of multiple root origin, and affection of any root may cause reflex disturbance. In this study, the reflex was pathological both in the fourth disc (37%) and fifth disc (71%) lesions.

Extensor hallucis weakness was due to fifth lumbar disc rupture in about 70% of the cases, and was associated with either pain projection or sensory defect of the fifth nerve root even if signs of the first sacral nerve root were present.

Disc herniations with signs of two roots were more often fourth disc lesions. Clinical level diagnosis was more accurate in fourth than in fifth lumbar disc ruptures, with pain projection as the leading sign. This seems to be due to true double root compression rather than to variations in innervation, that is, fourth disc herniation more often compresses the first sacral root than the fifth disc lesion compresses the fifth lumbar root (56).

In conclusion, Kortelainen (56) stated that segmentally localized pain projection is very im-

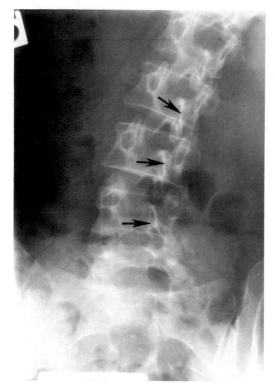

Figure 2.53. Right lateral flexion shows the spinous processes to rotate to the concavity on the right (*arrow*) representing a Lovett positive, or normal, vertebral rotation into the side of lateral flexion.

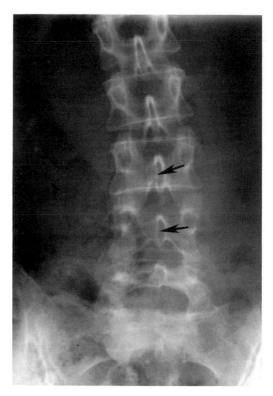

Figure 2.54. Left lateral flexion shows that the spinous processes at the L3-L4 levels do not rotate into the left concavity of the curve (*arrows*), representing a Lovett failure rotation. Contrast this rotation of the spinous processes into the convexity of the curve with the rotation of the spinous processes into the concavity, as seen in Figure 2.53. Failure of rotation by the spinous processes into the concavity, as well as failure of lateral flexion of the vertebral bodies into the side of lateral flexion, occurs in patients with disc protrusions.

portant in clinical level diagnosis of lumbar disc herniation. In cases with signs of a single root, additional motor, reflex, or sensory disturbances of the appropriate root raise the level of diagnostic accuracy to that of myelography. In the presence of the signs of two roots, pain projection to the fifth lumbar area still usually refers to fourth disc rupture, but multiple signs of first sacral root dysfunction are essential for the correct level diagnosis of the fifth disc herniation. The differences in reliability of level diagnosis are mainly due to more frequent double root compression in fourth lumbar disc ruptures.

Clinical diagnosis is not completely reliable in lower lumbar herniations, even in cases with signs of a single root, and it is practically impossible in high herniations. Cases with evident root compression and normal or indeterminate myelography should be checked by CT before proceeding to surgery to avoid unnecessary explorations (56).

REFERRED PAIN SYNDROMES TO THE LOWER EXTREMITY

A retrospective study of 1293 cases of low back pain treated over a 12-year period revealed that sacroiliac joint syndrome and posterior joint syndromes were the most common referred pain syndromes, whereas herniated nucleus pulposus and lateral spinal stenosis were the most common nerve root compression lesions (57). Referred pain syndromes occurred nearly twice as often as nerve root compression syndromes and frequently mimicked their clinical presentation. Combined lesions occurred in 33.5% of cases. Lateral spinal stenosis and herniated nucleus pulposus coexisted in 17.7%. In 30% of the cases of spondylolisthesis, the radiographic findings were incidental and the source of pain was the sacroiliac joint. Distinguishing radicular from referred pain, recognizing coexisting lesions, and correlating diagnostic imaging with the overall clinical presentation facilitates formulation of a rational plan of therapy (57).

NEUROANATOMY AND ITS ROLE IN DIAGNOSING DISC HERNIATION

Let's discuss the anatomy of the lumbosacral plexus and other plexi of the lumbar spine and pelvis. Dietemann et al. (58) state that the main nerves of the pelvis and lower limbs arise from the lumbar and sacral plexi. Understanding of the neurological findings related to paravertebral and pelvic pathology requires complete and accurate knowledge of the anatomy of these regions. The lumbar plexus is formed by anastomosis of the ventral rami of the four first lumbar nerves. The lumbar plexus lies within the posterior portion of the psoas muscle.

Iliohypogastric and Ilioinguinal Nerves

The iliohypogastric and ilioinguinal nerves arise from the first lumbar nerve. The iliohypogastric nerve is distributed to the skin of the upper lateral part of the buttock (lateral branch) and the skin of the pubis, and also has muscular branches to the abdominal wall. The ilioinguinal nerve extends to the upper and medial regions of the thigh and, in men and boys, to the skin of the penis and scrotum; in girls and women, it extends to the skin of the pubis and the labium majus.

Genitofemoral Nerve

The genitofemoral nerve arises from the first and second lumbar nerves. It has a genital branch, which supplies the cremaster, the skin of the scrotum in boys and men, or the skin of the mons pubis and labium majus in females, and a femoral branch, which supplies the skin of the upper part of the femoral triangle.

Lateral Cutaneous Nerve

The lateral cutaneous nerve of the thigh arises from the second and third lumbar nerves, supplying the skin on the lateral aspect of the thigh and the lateral aspect of the buttock.

Femoral Nerve

The femoral nerve is the largest terminal branch and arises from the dorsal branches of the ventral rami of the second, third, and fourth lumbar nerves. The femoral nerve supplies the skin of the anterior aspect of the thigh and of the medial border of the leg, the quadriceps of the thigh and sartorius, and the iliac muscles.

Obturator Nerve

The obturator nerve arises from the ventral branches of the ventral rami of the second, third, and fourth lumbar nerves.

Sciatic Nerve

The sciatic nerve is the continuation of the sacral plexus. It is the largest nerve in the body, measuring 2 cm across at its origin. It leaves the pelvic cavity through the greater sciatic foramen, below the piriformis muscle, and passes behind the sacrospinal ligament at its insertion on the ischial spine, then running downward between the greater trochanter of the femur outside and the tuberosity of the ischium inside; at this level, the nerve is located in front of the greatest gluteal muscle and behind the obturator internal and gemellus muscles, and the quadratus femoris muscle.

The sciatic nerve supplies the skin of the posterior and lateral border of the leg and foot and also the muscles of the leg and foot and the posterior muscles of the thigh.

Pudendal Nerve

The pudendal nerve derives from the second, third, and fourth sacral nerves and is the most important branch of the plexus. It supplies the skin of the perineum, scrotum, and penis (or labium majus and clitoris); branches are also distributed to the external anal sphincter, to the skin around the anus, to the muscles of the perineum, and to the pelvic viscera (58).

Scrotal Pain in Disc Compression of S2 and S3 Nerve Roots

Scrotal pain is described anatomically by White and Leslie (59), who present a 20-year-old man who had consulted his general practitioner 15 months earlier because of continuous right scrotal pain. A consultant urologist excluded testicular disease and referred him to a pain clinic, but an ilioinguinal and genitofemoral nerve block did not relieve the pain. The pain was found to be reproduced by straight leg raising, so an orthopedic opinion was sought.

The pain was exacerbated by leaning forward, coughing, or moving suddenly. The patient's lumbar lordosis was slightly flattened, and there was no forward flexion of the lumbar spine. Straight leg raising was limited to 20° on the right by severe scrotal pain. There were no objective neurological signs.

At operation, an intervertebral disc protrusion was found to be impinging on the first sacral nerve root on the right. The disc was incised, and a good decompression was achieved. The pain relief was immediate and permanent.

The posterior two-thirds of the scrotum is innervated by the second and third sacral nerves. Central disc lesions may compress the lower sacral roots, but no such compression was demonstrated in this case. An upper lumbar disc lesion is a rare cause of scrotal pain, and in such cases there may be no restriction of straight leg raising. The distribution of pain did not seem to be related to the level of the disc protrusion, yet decompression of the first sacral nerve root relieved the symptoms. Perhaps the anomaly of bone segmentation, besides predisposing to disc degeneration, was associated with an anomaly of nerve root segmentation. This case emphasizes the value of examination of the lumbar spine in cases of unexplained scrotal pain (59).

Summary of Low Back and Leg Pain Production

Nachemson (60), in a discussion of the role of the disc in low back and leg pain, concludes:

1. Disc hernia is usually preceded by one or more attacks of low back pain.

2. Following intradiscal injection of either hypertonic saline or contrast media, it is often possible, in patients with complaints of pain as well as in normal subjects, to artificially cause the same type of pain as that which occurs from disc degeneration.

3. Investigations have been performed in which thin nylon threads were surgically fastened to various structures in and around the nerve root. Three to four weeks after surgery, these structures were irritated by pulling on the threads, but pain resembling that which the patient had experienced previously could be registered only from the outer part of the annulus and the nerve root.

4. Pathoanatomically radiating ruptures are known to occur in the posterior part of the annulus, reaching out toward the areas in which naked nerve endings are located. Such single ruptures in the lumbar discs are first manifested in people about 25 years old, the same age at which the low back pain syndrome becomes clinically important. Various theories on how these ruptures elicit pain exist.

5. Of all the structures that theoretically could be involved in the pain process, only the disc shows changes that could account for the anatomical changes at such an early age. Such changes in other structures in the region generally show up much later in life, and then only secondary to severe disc degeneration.

6. Although a late sign, disc degeneration is noted on radiographs of patients between 50 and 60 years old and has been seen significantly more often in those who have had back pain than in those who have not.

The facet joints have been demonstrated to show histological signs of arthritis very late in life and always secondary to degenerative changes in the discs.

Findings of Various Authorities on Nerve Supply to the Disc

When this author was in undergraduate school, we were taught that the disc had no nerve supply, and most technique applications in manipulation were done with this idea in mind. With the knowledge of the sensitivity of the annulus fibrosus and even the nucleus, as described by some, we have a much better understanding of pain etiology in the low back and have modified our manipulative treatments, as discussed in Chapter 12 "Care of the Intervertebral Disc." This change in manipulative approach is to avoid irritation of the pain-sensitive annular fibers of the disc by the application of rotatory motion. Such rotation seems to be strongly associated with the onset of severe low back pain and should therefore be avoided in the acutely damaged disc patient. Let's review the nerve supply of the disc according to various authorities:

1. Bernini and Simeone (61) state that the sinuvertebral nerve supplies the posterior longitudinal ligament, annulus fibrosus, and neurovascular contents of the epidural space.

2. Nachemson (60) found that the outer annulus and nerve root were the most pain-sensitive and reproduced the patient's presurgical symptoms when stimulated 3 to 4 weeks postsurgically.

3. Farfan (62) points out that there is increasing evidence that there are unmyelinated nerve endings, usually associated with pain reception, in the posterior annulus and even penetrating the nucleus. The posterior longitudinal ligament is well innervated.

4. Helfet and Gruebel-Lee (63) have shown that when a radial tear penetrates the outer annulus, there is an attempt at healing by ingrowth of granulation tissue. Naked endings of the sinuvertebral nerve have been identified in this granulation tissue. These may be pain receptors, which would explain discogenic pain in the absence of herniation.

5. Bogduk (64) says that the sinuvertebral nerve supplies the annulus fibrosus and the posterior longitudinal ligament. It runs up and down two segments, supplying the annulus and posterior longitudinal ligament above and below.

6. Tsukada (65) and Shinohara (66) claim that nerve fibers exist not only in the posterior longitudinal ligament but also in the nucleus and notochord. Malinsky (67) and Hirsch et al. (68) observed that nerve fibers penetrated into the outer layers of the disc. Tsukada (65) and Shinohara (66) found nerve endings in granulation tissue within the inner layers of the annulus and in the nucleus of some degenerated discs. In another article, Yoshizawa et al. (68) found profuse free nerve terminals in the outer half of the annulus but no such terminals in the nucleus.

7. Sunderland (69), at the National Institute of Neurological and Communicative Disorders and Stroke (NINCDS) Conference, 1975, stated that the recurrent meningeal nerve supplies the dura, intervertebral disc, and associated structures.

8. Edgar and Ghadially (70) say that the sinuvertebral nerve divides into ascending, descending, and transverse branches adjacent to the posterior longitudinal ligament. Lazorthes (71) states that this nerve supplies the neural laminae, the intervertebral disc at the adjacent levels, the posterior longitudinal ligament, the internal vertebral plexus, the epidural tissue, and the dura mater. Concerning the tissues supplied by this nerve, however, there is still disagreement; some authorities do not believe that there is such a wide distribution. Tsukada (65) and Shinohara (66) found that the outer annulus is innervated in a normal disc but that fine nerve fibers accompany granulation tissue present in a degenerated disc. In one instance, fine fibers were observed in the nucleus. Most of these were naked nerve endings and probably mediated pain sensation. Edgar and Ghadially (70) found that sinuvertebral nerves supply the anterior dura. In spinal stenosis, therefore, irritation of the sinuvertebral nerve may be the mechanism of claudication pain.

Well-Substantiated Neurological Facts

In discussing the lumbar intervertebral disc syndrome, Bogduk (64) states that there are four elements of the nervous system which may be involved in the production of this syndrome: the lumbosacral nerve roots, the spinal nerves, the dorsal rami, and the sinuvertebral nerves. The nerve root is usually irritated because of its being stretched over a protruding or prolapsed disc. The irritation of the spinal nerve may result from arthrosis of the zygapophyseal joints, ligamentum flavum hypertrophy, osteophytes, intervertebral disc protrusion, subluxation, spondylolisthesis, infection, tumor, fracture, Paget's disease, or ankylosing spondylitis. The dorsal rami (which supply the zygapophyseal joints, the erector spinae muscles and their related fascia and skin, the periosteum of the vertebral arches, the multifidus muscles, the interspinous ligament, and the interspinous muscles) are irritated by articular facet arthrosis, subluxation, sacroiliac joint arthrosis, spinous process impingement, strain of the sacral joints, hyperlordosis, scoliosis, myositis, muscle spasm, and reactions secondary to sclerosis or arthrosis of the articular facets. The sinuvertebral nerve, also known as the recurrent meningeal nerve, supplies the posterior longitudinal ligament as well as the annulus fibrosus of the disc. A descending branch runs caudally for a maximum of two segments, supplying the annulus fibrosus and the posterior longitudinal ligament. An ascending branch may also behave similarly. Any lesion of the annulus or posterior longitudinal ligament is capable of setting up pain impulses in the sinuvertebral nerve.

Two basic causes of low back pain are internal

derangements of the intervertebral disc and irritation of the zygapophyseal articulation. The ontogeny of low back pain concerns two structures: the disc and facet. Debate continues as to which is the initial lesion and which is a secondary or compensatory change. After study, this author believes that the initial change takes place in the intervertebral disc, which later affects the articular facet. Vernon-Roberts and Pirie (72) state that a direct relationship exists between the degree of disc degeneration, the marginal osteophyte formation on vertebral bodies, and the apophyseal joint change, which suggests that disc degeneration is the primary event leading to the clinical condition of degenerative spondylosis.

INTERVERTEBRAL DISC BIOMECHANICS—NORMAL AND ABERRANT

In people between the ages of 30 and 40 years, the nucleus has a water content of 80% (73). Puschel (74) says that this fluid content decreases with age. DePukey (75) found that the average person is 1% shorter in height at the end of the day than on first arising in the morning. He also found that a person in the first decade of life is 2% shorter at bedtime, and a person in the eighth decade of life is 0.5% shorter. This difference he attributes to decreasing water content in the disc which occurs with advancing age.

Hendry (76) believes that the hydrodynamics of the disc result from the gel structure of the nucleus pulposus, enabling it to absorb nine times its volume of water. No chemical bond influences this water content, as it can be mechanically expressed under pressure; thus, there is the decrease of 1% average height from weight bearing in a day.

The nucleus pulposus occupies about half the disc surface area and bears the vertical load, while the annulus bears the tangential load (77). Because of nuclear degeneration, shift in stress and weight-bearing forces occurs. Bradford and Spurling state that the ratio of the anterior to posterior weight-bearing forces of the body is 15:1; therefore, lifting 100 lb with the arms extended places a total pressure of 1500 lb on the nucleus pulposus. Even more revealing is the finding of Morris et al. (78) that a 170-lb man lifting 200 lbs exerts a force of 2071 lb on the L5-S1 disc space.

Discography is performed by the injection of contrast material into the nucleus, which normally will accept approximately 1 cc of solution. If the injection duplicates the patient's symptoms, disc protrusion, irritating the annulus and/or nerve root, is signified. Figure 2.55 reveals normal and abnormal nuclear appearances on discography.

Gresham and Miller (79) carried out postmortem discography on 63 fresh autopsy specimens; the patients who came to autopsy ranged in age from 14 to 80 years and had relatively asymptomatic backs. The results of this study are presented in Table 2.1.

Abnormalities in the disc reduce its capacity to aid in supporting torsional loads of the spine by about 40% (77).

Degeneration of the intervertebral disc and subsequent changes in adjacent vertebrae and ligaments are termed *spondylosis*. Fissuring of the annulus fibrosus occurs posteriorly, usually where the common ligament is least strong (80). Finneson (77) describes two disc changes following injury (Fig. 2.56): disc herniation (or protrusion) and spondylosis. He notes that in less than 20% of patients with annular tears or fissures, a large fragment of nucleus bulges forth to compress a nerve root, producing classic disc symptoms. Usually, however, the annulus never completely tears and contains the nucleus within its boundary with only slight protrusion.

Table 2.1.
Results of Postmortem Discography from a Study by Gresham and Miller (Total Autopsies, 60)[a]

Group	Age range (years)	Findings
I	14–34	90% normal discs
		10% degenerated discs
II	35–45	25% normal discs
III	46–59	25% normal discs at L3-L4
		0% normal discs at L5-S1
IV	60 and over	5% normal discs
		0% normal at L5-S1
		2% normal at L4-L5[b]
		3% normal at L3-L4[c]

[a]Data from Gresham JL, Miller R: Evaluation of the lumbar spine by diskography. *Orthop Clin* 67:29, 1969.
[b]One autopsy in 60.
[c]Two autopsies in 60.

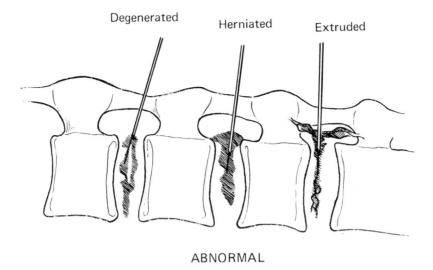

Figure 2.55. Some abnormal discogram configurations. (Reproduced with permission from Finneson BE: *Low Back Pain,* ed 2. Philadelphia, JB Lippincott, 1980, p 104.)

Finneson goes on to say that fibrosis of the annulus fibrosus occurs as the annulus loses its sponginess and elasticity. The disc space thins, with sclerosis of the cartilaginous end plates and new bone formation around the periphery of the contiguous vertebral surfaces occurring. The altered mechanics place stress on the posterior diarthrodial joints, causing them to lose their normal nuclear fulcrum for movement. With the loss of disc space, the plane of articulation of the

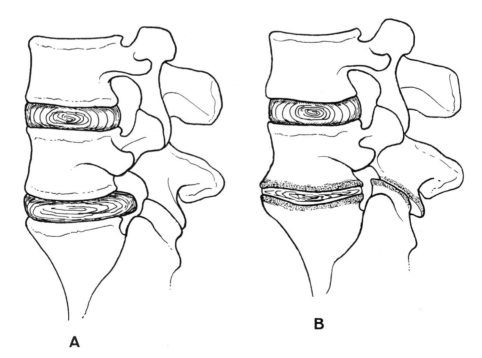

Figure 2.56. **A**, Herniation of the nucleus pulposus. **B**, Spondylosis. (Reproduced with permission from Finneson BE: *Low Back Pain,* ed 2. Philadelphia, JB Lippincott, 1980, p 437.)

facet surfaces is no longer congruous. This stress results in degenerative arthritis of the articular surfaces. Complete fibrous ankylosis of the disc and articular surfaces is possible.

Definitions and Illustrations of Disc Protrusion and Prolapse

Two terms are used to describe disc degenerative change allowing nuclear herniation. They are *contained disc* and *noncontained disc*. They refer to the state of the annulus fibrosus, that is, whether it is intact and restraining the nucleus pulposus, termed a contained disc; or whether it has completely radially torn to allow the nuclear material to sequester or free-fragment into the vertebral canal.

Disc protrusion (Fig. 2.57) is an extension of nuclear material through the annulus into the spinal canal with no loss of continuity of extruded material. Protrusion and herniation are synonymous.

Disc prolapse (Fig. 2.58) occurs when the extruded material loses continuity with the existing

nuclear material and forms a free fragment in the spinal canal. Disc prolapse is the most common indication for disc surgery.

Protrusion of disc material (Fig. 2.59) exists when the bulging nuclear material is contiguous with the remaining nucleus pulposus, and the annulus fibrosus is stretched, thinned, and under pressure. Epstein (81) notes that the pressure within the nucleus pulposus is 30 psi and mentions that Nachemson and Morris found that this pressure is 30% less in the standing position than in the sitting position and is 50% less in the reclining position than in the sitting position. Keep in mind, also, that cerebrospinal fluid pressure is 100 to 200 mm of water in the recumbent posture and 400 mm in the sitting posture (82). It is important, therefore, that the patient with a protruding disc avoid sitting.

Disc prolapse (Fig. 2.60), as stated earlier, exists when the extruded nuclear material loses continuity with the existing nuclear material and forms a free fragment within the spinal canal.

Figure 2.61 illustrates that a disc may protrude either lateral to a nerve root, medial to a

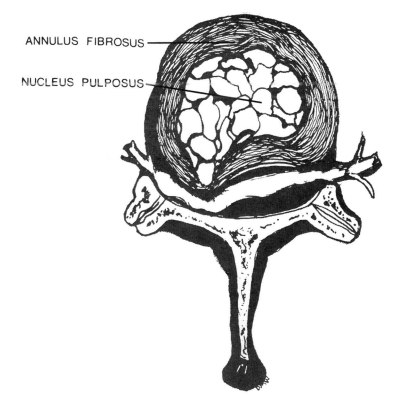

Figure 2.57. Nuclear protrusion. The annulus fibrosus is still intact although weakened with nuclear bulge.

ANNULUS FIBROSUS

NUCLEUS PULPOSUS

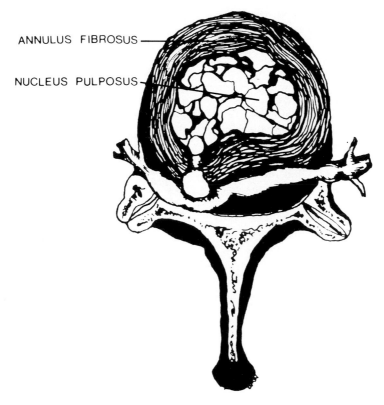

Figure 2.58. Nuclear prolapse. The annulus fibrosus is completely torn, allowing nuclear escape into the posterior vertebral canal as a free fragment.

nerve root, under a nerve root, or in a central position. When the disc protrudes lateral to the nerve root, the patient assumes an antalgic lean away from the side of the disc lesion (Fig. 2.62). When the disc protrudes medial to the nerve root, the patient assumes an antalgic lean into the side of disc lesion or pain (Fig. 2.63). With a central disc lesion, the patient assumes a flexed posture of the lumbar spine with or without lean to either side. With protrusion under the nerve root, the patient may assume no lean.

The dermatome chart (Fig. 2.64) reveals innervation of the sensory nerves of the lower extremity. Ninety percent or more of lumbar disc lesions occur at either the L4-L5 or L5-S1 disc level. The L4-L5 disc usually compresses the fifth lumbar nerve root, resulting in pain sensations down the lower extremity in the fifth lumbar nerve root innervation. The L5-S1 disc usually compresses the first sacral nerve root, resulting in pain distribution down the first sacral dermatome of the lower extremity. Lecuire et al. (83) found that of 641 patients with disc lesion, 307 showed

definite S1 dermatome patterns, 267 showed definite L5 dermatome patterns, and 67 showed mixed patterns, Sixty percent of these patients had an antalgic lean. A single disc lesion was noted in 562 patients, with 47% occurring at L5-S1, 39% occurring at L4-L5, and 2% occurring at L3-L4. Myelograms were performed on 238 of the 641 patients prior to surgery. Knowledge of specific innervation of the nerve root is important in deciding which disc is involved. By ascertaining the antalgic posture, the clinician may determine whether the problem is a medial, a central, or a lateral disc protrusion.

Therefore, there are two facts of primary importance in the evaluation of a patient: the side of sciatic pain distribution, and the side of antalgic inclination; i.e., whether the patient leans toward or away from the side of pain (Fig. 2.65).

The author finds that the level of disc involvement usually is the site of vertebral rotational and lateral flexion changes; this level may be observed on visual examination of the patient's spine. Often it is noted only on x-ray examination; x-ray studies can be made with the patient in both a recumbent and a standing position, since no difference is noted in these disc cases. The site of lateral flexion and rotation change may be quite noticeable or only very slightly discernible on radiographs; therefore, close correlation with the history and clinical examination is needed to pinpoint the site of disc protrusion. In other cases, the x-ray finding is quite striking regarding the amount of flexion and rotational change that results in a sciatic scoliosis. Some cases of disc prolapse requiring surgery, however, often reveal minimal change in functional spinal unit relationships. An interesting observation is that sciatic scoliosis often appears as a Lovett failure or as reverse scoliosis; i.e., there is a failure of body rotation or a rotation to the convexity of the scoliosis by the vertebral bodies instead of toward the side of concavity. Another point to remember is that a false negative is sometimes reported on myelography when a laterally protruded disc lies too far lateral to the subarachnoid space to impress upon it. Compilation of these findings delineates the nerve root and disc involved.

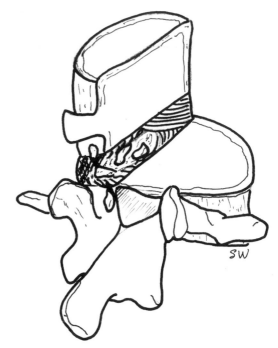

Figure 2.60. In nuclear prolapse, the annulus completely tears, allowing escape of free fragments of nuclear material into the vertebral canal or extremely laterally into the intervertebral foramen.

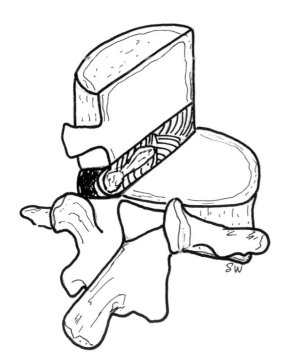

Figure 2.59. In nuclear protrusion, the annular fibers are containing the bulging nuclear material.

Nerve Root Origin from Cauda Equina

A discussion of the normal anatomical relationship of the nerve root origin from the dural sac and its ultimate exit via its intervertebral foramen is in order before proceeding. The adult spinal cord ends at the level of L1-L2 at the conus medullaris, continuing caudally as the filum terminale to attach at the back of the coccyx. The filum terminale is encased in dura mater to the level of S2. At each vertebral level, a pair of nerve roots leave the dural sac, with each enclosed by dural nerve root sleeves. In the lumbar spine, these nerve roots pass directly downward, forming the caude equina surrounding the filum terminale, until their eventual exit from each respective intervertebral foramen. The origin of the nerve root from the dural sac (cauda equina) is about one segment above the exit from its intervertebral foramen (IVF). The nerve root runs down laterally to the IVF from which it exists. Specifically, the fourth lumbar root exits the dural sac at the level of the third lumbar disc to exit the IVF one vertebra below; the fifth lumbar nerve root exits the dural sac at the level of the fourth lumbar disc to exit the IVF one vertebral segment below; the first sacral root exits the dural sac at the fifth lumbar disc level, passing down to the first sacral IVF; and the second sacral nerve root lies medial to S1, originating at the lower border of the fifth lumbar disc.

From Figure 2.66, it can be seen that the L4 nerve root can be compressed at its origin and course by the protrusion of the third lumbar disc, that the L5 nerve root can be compressed by the fourth lumbar disc, and that the S1 and S2 nerve roots can be compressed by the fifth disc protrusion.

Intradiscal Pressure Changes

Pressure changes within the nucleus pulposus as they relate to postural and physiological stresses are shown in Figures 2.67, 2.68 and 2.69.

From Figures 2.67 and 2.68, it can be noted that Déjérine triad and sitting raise the intradiscal pressure six times higher than does recumbency.

Changes in the Intervertebral Disc

Turek (84) states that the annulus fibrosus begins to show concentric cracking and cavitation in children as young as age 15. This dehydration and cracking of the annulus may progress silently for many years, with the nucleus bulging through these cracks, causing the annulus to be thinned and weakened at its periphery. Relatively little force may cause the annulus to tear, allowing the nucleus to burst forth. Ritchie and Fahrni (85) mention that an ingrowth of vascular tissue takes place through the end plates, from the cancellous bone of the vertebral body into the nucleus pulposus. The fluid content of the nucleus decreases with increasing age until approximately 70% of the nucleus is fluid in a person at age 77, as compared with 88% in a newborn. This degeneration of the disc is accompanied by remodeling of the vertebral bodies. Herniation of the nucleus into the vertebral end plate at the site of vascular proliferation is termed Schmorl's node. The rupturing of the nuclear material anteriorly and laterally results in periosteal proliferation or osteophyte formation.

This thinning of the intervertebral disc is accompanied by changes in the facet articulations as well. The facet joints lose their spacing as their articular cartilage shows degenerative changes because of the stress encountered by disc degeneration. The facets lose their gliding motion of one upon another, and the synovium undergoes hypertrophic proliferation, typically known as osteoarthrosis. This former condition, involving the loss of intervertebral disc height and the accompanying osteophytic and subchondral sclerotis changes, has been termed discogenic spondylosis. The latter condition, involving facet arthrosis, is consequently termed discogenic spondyloarthrosis. The changes of the two articular facets and the disc (triple joint complex) are outlined in Figure 2.70.

Clinical Picture of Disc Degeneration

Yong-Hing and Kirkaldy-Willis (86) describe three clinical stages in the natural history of spinal degeneration.

1. Stage of Dysfunction. In the beginning there is little demonstrable pathology. Patient finds are subtle or absent, and conservative care is highly successful. Lumbago and rotatory strain are commonly diagnosed.

2. Stage of Instability. Abnormal movement of the motion segment of instability exists. Patient complaints are more severe, and objective findings are present. Conservative care is used and sometimes surgery.

3. Stage of Stabilization. Severe degenerative changes of the disc and facets reduce motion, and improvement may be experienced. Stenosis is now very probable.

Nachemson's (60) findings agree with the above second and third stages; he says that histological signs of arthritis have been demonstrated in the facet joints very late in life and always secondary to degenerative change in the disc.

It should be remembered that both the disc and the articular facet are capable of producing low back pain. It is interesting to study the work of Lora and Long (87), who were able to trace scleratogenous pain when various facet levels of the lumbar spine were irritated. L5-S1 facet stimulation resulted in referred pain to the coccyx, hip, posterior thigh, groin, inguinal ligament, and perineum; L4-L5 facet stimulation resulted in pain to the coccyx, posterior hip, and thigh and was less intense than that following irritation of the L5-S1 facets. L3-L4 facet stimulation resulted

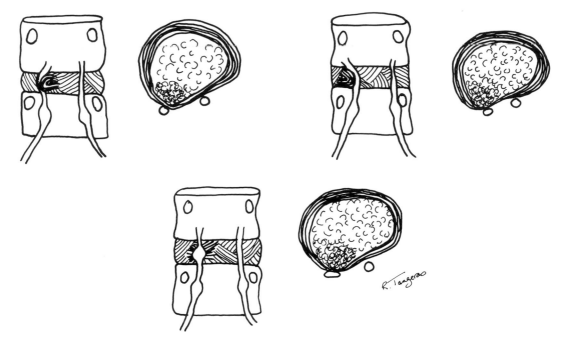

Figure 2.61. Nerve root displacement by disc protrusion. *Upper left,* Medial disc displaces nerve laterally. *Upper right,* Lateral disc displaces nerve root medially. *Lower center,* Disc lies directly under nerve root, stretching it.

in pain radiating upward into the thoracic area, flank, and anterior thigh. Irritation of the articular facets at T12, L1, L2, and L3 produced no leg or coccyx sensation.

Arns et al. (88) states that the first stage of disc lesion begins with protrusion of the nucleus pulposus into the outer rings of the annulus fibrosus, resulting in low back pain. This lesion is characterized by local pain that is increased by coughing and sneezing, paravertebral muscle spasm, and antalgia of the lumbar spine. Neurological symptoms are not present. The next stage involves penetration of the nucleus pulposus into the outer rings of the annular fibers, producing pressure on the spinal nerve roots which creates radiating pain down the leg. Neurological signs are now present.

Farfan (62) has defined three stages of disc disease:

1. Annular bulge (protrusion);
2. Facet arthrosis as the disc thins and extrudes;
3. Stenosis if stages 1 and 2 are severe, with tautening of nerve root.

Discal thinning allows the pedicles of the superior vertebra to lower, thus compressing the nerve roots as they course toward the intervertebral foramen for emergence (89, 90). Figure 2.71 shows the normal pedicle-nerve root relationship, and Figure 2.72 shows the relationship between the narrowed disc and the pedicle compression of the nerve root. Thus, another reason can be seen for the constant back and sciatic pain before and after a surgical procedure. The reader should note, also, the effect of short, thickened pedicles in conjunction with disc thinning, further narrowing the vertebral canal.

DISCUSSION OF PHYSIOLOGICAL AND ABNORMAL LUMBAR MOTIONS

Centrode Locations in Lumbar Kinematics

To start the discussion of lumbar mechanics, let's begin with axis motion study. The path traced by the instantaneous axis of rotation of the intervertebral disc, termed its *centrode,* was studied in varying stages of degeneration of the disc. The centrodes of normal discs were compared with the degenerative state in 47 cadaveric spines, 22 of which were also evaluated with axial loading. The normal disc centrode fell within the posterior

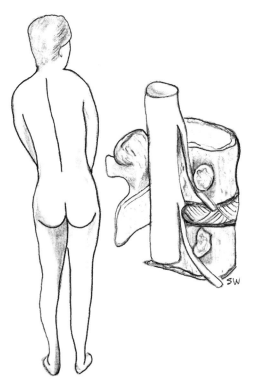

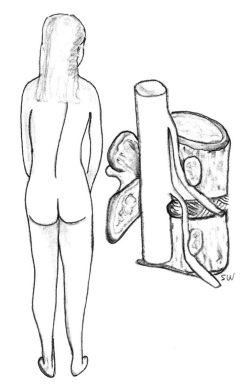

Figure 2.62. Sciatic scoliosis in a patient with a right lateral disc protrusion.

Figure 2.63. Sciatic scoliosis in a patient with right medial disc protrusion.

half of the disc space (Fig. 2.73) and averaged 21 mm in length in 10 specimens. In the earliest stages of degeneration, the centrode lengths increased significantly (average, 116 mm) (Fig. 2.74). In specimens with moderate disc degeneration, the centrode also migrated inferiorly into the L5 vertebra (Fig. 2.75 through 2.78). Axial loading did not appear to influence the centrode lengths or position. This technique detected 94% of unstable spines, as compared with flexion and extension radiographs, which detected 25% of unstable spines by excessive mobility (90a).

From the above centrode location changes in discal degeneration, one can see that the concept that the nucleus pulposus moves within the annular restraints as a marble, or that it can be moved about under manipulation as such, should be met with skepticism. The nuclear material seems to move out of its confines through radial annular tears in an amoeboid or pseudopodia-like fashion, and its return to the interstices of the annular disc fibers must be through this same rent or tear. The escape of nuclear fluid through

the tear in the annular fibers is similar to the formation of a vascular aneurysm.

The nucleus pulposus is located centrally within the posterior compartment of the disc at the juncture of the central and posterior thirds. It contains various mucopolysaccharides in the form of glucosaminoglycan, which has the ability to imbibe fluids to nine times its own volume. The nucleus fills 40% to 50% of the total disc area, and because of imbibition of fluids, it takes on a stiffness within its cells called turgor. At a person's birth, the water content of a disc is 70% to 90%; the content decreases with increase in the age of the person. The intradiscal pressures drop with loss of fluid; thus, disc herniation occurs most often when the person is between 20 and 50 years old and the intradiscal pressures are their greatest.

The annulus fibrosus contains the nucleus pulposus by concentric laminated bands of fibrous tissue which gradually form at the boundary of the nucleus without a sharp area of differentiation (Fig. 2.79). Sharpey's fibers attach

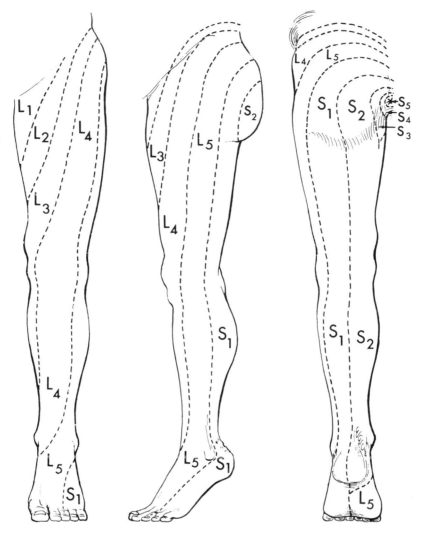

Figure 2.64. Dermatome chart of lower extremity.

the annular fibers to the end plates in the inner area and to the osseous tissue in the periphery.

Rotation Mechanics of the Lumbar Spine

Rotation of the lumbar spine is precluded by the action of the facet processes aligned across the path of rotation, blocking the movement. The knowledge that rotation occurs invites an explanation. While the effective rotation contributed by each lumbar segment in the total vertebral movement is small, it adds up to a real capability, often acknowledged only when a patient experiences its loss. Rotation primary spin is expected to occur about a center of motion dominated by the disc until the opposing facet makes contact and resists further movement across the facet plane. In the presence of further torque, one expects a migration of the center of motion to occur toward the resisting facet and, using this as a fulcrum, a pseudo-spin would tend to occur as a result of lateral shear or displacement of the disc (Fig. 2.80) (90b).

Rotation is felt to be a complex motion facilitated by the effective shape of the articular surface of the disc, an arcuate motion that occurs across the disc and is associated with swing in both the lateral and anteroposterior planes. The

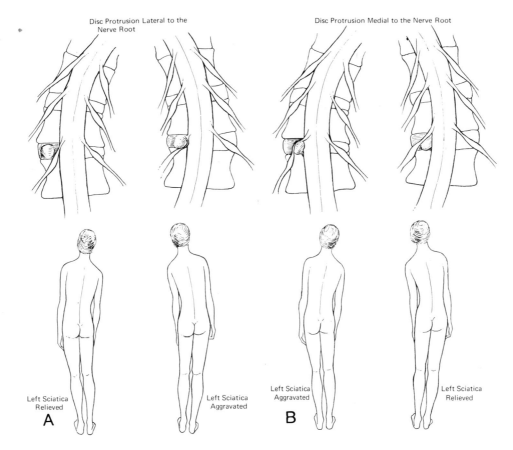

Figure 2.65. Relief or aggravation of pain with lateral flexion may indicate whether the disc protrusion is lateral or medial to the nerve root. (Reproduced with permission from Finneson BE: *Low Back Pain*, ed 2. Philadelphia, JB Lippincott, 1980, p 302.)

intervertebral disc is the primary articulation in the vertebral column, comprising a joint with about three degrees of freedom. This allows both spin about a mechanical axis and swing of the mechanical axis in two mutually independent directions, for example, in the anteroposterior and lateral planes (Fig. 2.81) (90b).

The posterior complex and, in particular, the architecture of the posterior facet joints, act as a control mechanism not only to restrict the motion of the primary articulation but also to control the motion to satisfy the anatomical requirements for motion of the segment while retaining segment strength and stability.

A centrode, rather than a single point, indicates that the articular surface has a varying curvature, and one would expect the disc to articulate as if it were a flat, ovoid diarthrosis, as shown schematically in Figure 2.82.

The disc has a potential for three degrees of freedom. Lateral flexion is accompanied by rotation in a monodal movement. The posterior elements of the motion segment cause rotatory movement during both flexion and lateral flexion, as shown in Figure 2.83.

Summary of Lumbar Mechanics

The bony parts and soft tissues of a cross section of the lumbar spine can be divided into anterior and posterior elements. The dividing line is just behind the vertebral body, with the body, the disc, and the anterior and posterior longitudinal ligaments lying anteriorly. The neural arch with its processes, the intervertebral (apophyseal or facet) joints, and the different ligaments attached to the bony elements lie posteriorly. The back muscles are distributed mainly lateral and poste-

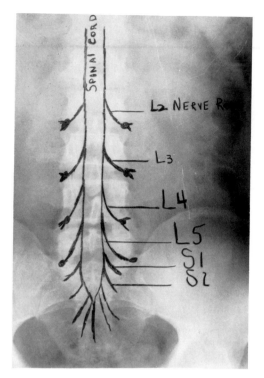

Figure 2.66. Schematic overlay of exiting cauda equina nerve roots in relation to the vertebral column and disc level.

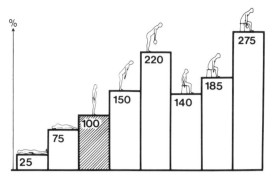

Figure 2.67. Relative change in pressure (or load) in the third lumbar disc in various positions in living subjects. (Reproduced with permission from Nachemson AL: The lumbar spine, an orthopaedic challenge. *Spine* 1(1):61, 1976.)

rior to the neural arch, but there are also anterolateral muscles (91).

The division is not merely anatomical but has a functional (mechanical) purpose. The anterior elements provide the major support of the column and absorb various impacts; the posterior struc-

tures control patterns of motion. Together they protect the dural content, which is surrounded by the neural arch.

Being synovial in nature, these joints undergo degenerative changes as age progresses. These changes are usually secondary to degeneration of the disc and, therefore, occur later in life. It is obvious that the decrease of intervertebral disc height accompanying degeneration has an effect on the apophyseal joints in stress distribution. It becomes germane, therefore, to postulate on the importance of mechanical factors in degenerative changes. The importance of mechanical factors to these changes is also indicated by the fact that severe osteoarthritis of the apophyseal joints is common in the presence of scoliosis, kyphosis,

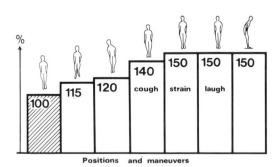

Figure 2.68. Relative change in pressure (or load) in the third lumbar disc in various maneuvers in living subjects. (Reproduced with permission from Nachemson AL: The lumbar spine, an orthopaedic challenge. *Spine* 1(1):61, 1976.)

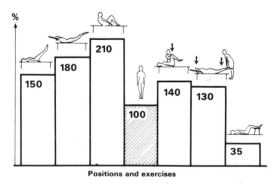

Figure 2.69. Relative change in pressure (or load) in the third lumbar disc in various muscle-strengthening exercises in living subjects. (Reproduced with permission from Nachemson AL: The lumbar spine, an orthopaedic challenge. *Spine* 1(1):61, 1976.)

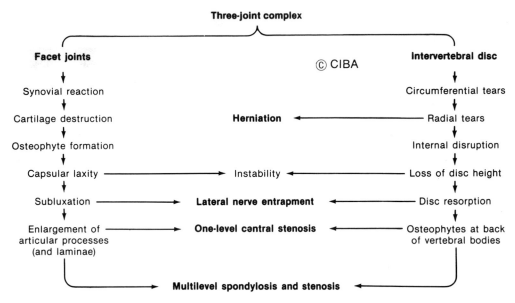

Figure 2.70. Pathogenesis of the nerve root entrapment syndrome. (Reproduced with permission from Keim HA, Kirkaldy-Willis WH: Clinical symposia. *Ciba Found Symp* 32(6):89, 1980. CIBA Pharmaceutical Company, Division of CIBA-GEIGY Corporation. All rights reserved.)

block vertebrae, spondylolisthesis, and vertebral body collapse.

Normal function of the apophyseal joints is important in stabilizing the motion segment and controlling its movement. The discs and ligaments are thus protected. Loads applied to the lumbar spine are normally shared between the joints and discs. This load sharing can be influenced by the type of loading, the geometry of the motion segment, and the stiffness of the participating structures (91).

Miller et al. (92) have reported on the manner in which the intervertebral disc and the posterior elements share loads placed on the lumbar mo-

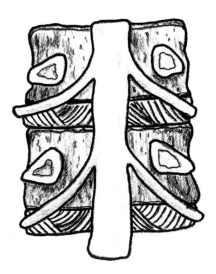

Figure 2.71. Normal pedicle to nerve root distance.

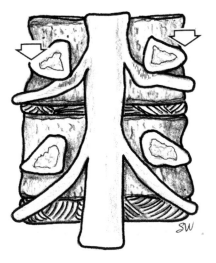

Figure 2.72. Tethering of the nerve root as the pedicle settles down upon it and as the disc space narrows or hyperextension subluxation of the superior vertebral arch occurs.

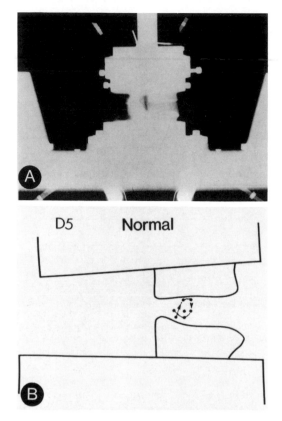

Figure 2.73. Normal spine: **A,** radiograph; **B** centrode. (Reproduced with permission from Seligman JV, Gertzbein SD, Tile M, Kapasouri A: Computer analysis of spinal segment rotation in degenerative disc disease with and without axial loading. *Spine* 9(6):569, 1984.)

tion segment. For their report they made use of a two-dimensional biomechanical model to examine this load sharing. The model incorporated two rigid bodies to represent the vertebrae and six elastic springs to represent the tissues of the intervertebral disc and the posterior elements. Compression loads were resisted almost totally by the model intervertebral disc, but both the intervertebral disc and the posterior elements contributed substantially to resisting anteroposterior shear and flexion-extension loads. Motion segment morphology was a major determinant of load sharing in the model disc response to anteroposterior shear.

Both the intervertebral disc and the apophyseal (facet) joints of low lumbar motion segments are suspected sources of low back pain. When a low back disorder occurs, pain is aggravated by some physical activities but not by others. Different physical activities impose different loads on

both the disc and the facets; perhaps pain aggravation is related to those loading patterns. Hence, it is important to know how much of a load imposed on a motion segment is distributed to the intervertebral disc, how much is distributed to the apophyseal joints, and what the determinants of that distribution are.

Range of Internal Loads

Provided that facets were present, a shear force applied to the motion segment was resisted primarily by a combination of intervertebral disc shear and facet compression or tension. The portion of the overall shear resistance contributed by disc shear versus that contributed by facet tension compression depended little on how far posterior to the disc the facets were but depended very much on their superior-inferior location. When the facets were low, almost all of that resistance was provided by shearing of the intervertebral disc. When the facets were high, each mechanism contributed substantially to the total resistance. Thus, in response to a large anteroposterior shear force, both the intervertebral disc and the facet joints can be loaded lightly to moderately, or they can be loaded heavily. Which circumstance occurs seems to depend primarily on the location of the facets relative to the disc in the superior-inferior direction (92).

Facet inclination angle did not seem critical to motion segment response. When the facets were tilted 20° from the frontal plane, the facets were compressed 300 N at most in response to the 2500-N compression force. When the facets were tilted only 5°, they were compressed 120 N at most. That is, *facet inclination angle had only a modest effect on compression response.* In response to the 500-N shear force, changing the superior-inferior location of the facets by 2 cm caused about three times the change in load sharing between disc shear and facet inclination of 15° (92).

Conclusions

The findings (92) suggest that when loads typical of those experienced in vivo are applied to a lumbar motion segment, the following occur:

1. The apophyseal joints are not loaded heavily by compression or flexion-extension loads but can be heavily loaded by anteroposterior shear loads.

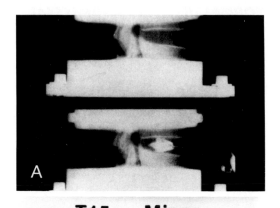

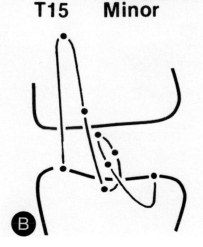

Figure 2.74. Minor degenerative disc disease: **A,** radiograph and discogram; **B,** centrode. (Reproduced with permission from Seligman JV, Gertzbein SD, Tile M, Kapasouri A: Computer analysis of spinal segment motion in degenerative disc disease with and without axial loading. *Spine* 9(6):569, 1984.)

cause small fractures in this region and can be responsible for episodes of back pain. The diagnosis of these fractures is usually missed.

Under compressive load, the highest compressive strains were recorded near the bases of the pedicles and deep surfaces of the pars interarticularis (93).

Experiments were carried out on cadaveric lumbar spines to determine the mechanical function of the apophyseal joints (94). It was found that in lordotic postures the apophyseal joints resist most of the intervertebral shear force and share in resisting the intervertebral compressive force. Apophyseal joints prevent excessive movement from damaging the discs. The posterior an-

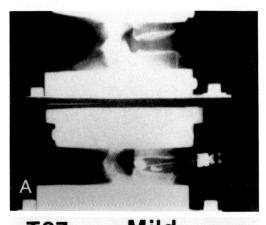

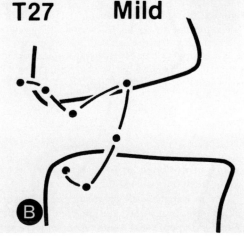

2. Resistance developed by the apophyseal joints is not very effective in relieving loads on the intervertebral disc when the motion segment is compressed. It can be effective in relieving the disc, however, when the segment is flexed, extended, or anteroposteriorly sheared.

3. In response to anteroposterior shear loads, the location of the facet joints relative to that of the intervertebral disc in the superior-inferior direction is a major determinant of what loads each structure will bear.

Pathological, experimental, and clinical studies indicate that excessive strain concentration may occur in the posterior elements of the spine and be increased by extension. These strains may

Figure 2.75. Mild degenerative disc disease: **A,** radiograph and discogram; **B,** centrode. (Reproduced with permission from Seligman JV, Gertzbein SD, Tile M, Kapasouri A: Computer analysis of spinal segment motion in degenerative disc disease with and without axial loading. *Spine* 9(6):570, 1984.)

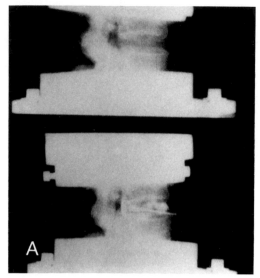

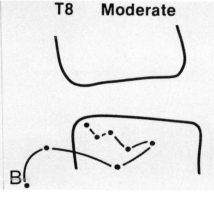

Figure 2.76. Moderate degenerative disc disease: **A**, radiograph and discogram; **B**, centrode. (Reproduced with permission from Seligman JV, Gertzbein SD, Tile M, Kapasouri A: Computer analysis of spinal segment motion in degenerative disc disease with and without axial loading. *Spine* 9(6):570, 1984.)

NORMAL DISC AND APOPHYSEAL JOINT ANATOMY AND PHYSIOLOGY

Normal Kinematics of the Lumbar Spine

Structural physiology begins with an understanding of normal spinal mechanics. Studies have been done to measure the ranges of active flexion and extension, axial rotation, and lateral bending in the lumbar spines of normal volunteers in vivo, and to assess the relation between the primary and accompanying movements in the other planes (95).

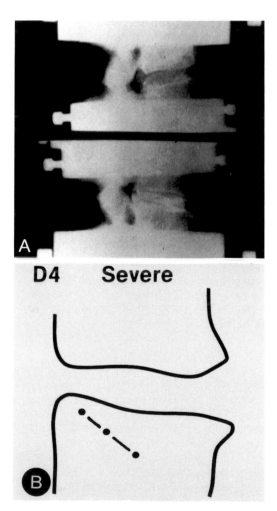

Figure 2.77. Severe degenerative disc disease: **A**, radiograph and discogram; **B**, centrode. (Reproduced with permission from Seligman JV, Gertzbein SD, Tile M, Kapasouri A: Computer analysis of spinal segment motion in degenerative disc disease with and without axial loading. *Spine* 9(6):571, 1984.)

nulus is protected in torsion by the facet surfaces and in flexion by the capsular ligaments.

Recent experiments performed on cadaveric spines have determined the mechanical properties of the apophyseal joints when they are subjected to loading regimes calculated to simulate movements and postures in life. This experimental evidence has been collated to give a concise account of the mechanical function of the apophyseal joints and to indicate under what circumstances they might sustain damage.

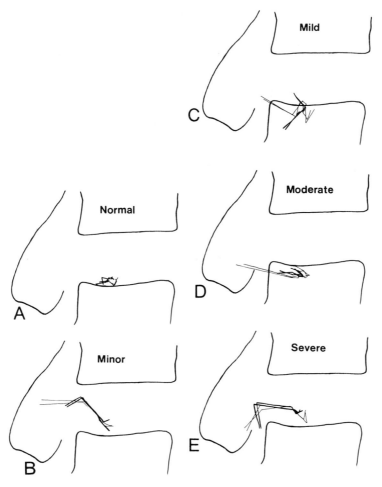

Figure 2.78. Axial loading. Thick lines represent centrodes from unloaded runs. Thin lines represent centrodes from axial-loaded runs (70 lb). On each figure all four centrodes are from the same spine. **A**, Normal spine; **B**, minor spine; **C**, mild spine; **D**, moderate spine; **E**, severe spine. The terms minor, mild, moderate, and severe refer to the degenerative state of the disc. (Reproduced with permission from Seligman JV, Gertzbein SD, Tile M, Kapasouri A: Computer analysis of spinal segment motion in degenerative disc disease with and without axial loading. *Spine* 9(6): 572, 1984.)

The movements of flexion and extension of the L5-S1 level were larger than at the other levels. On inspection, it was apparent that some subjects flexed more than they extended at L5-S1, while the others extended more than they flexed. L5-S1 does not demonstrate a consistent range of motion patterns, although the total range of flexion plus extension remains similar.

Lateral bending at L4-L5 is markedly limited compared to the upper three lumbar levels.

During voluntary flexion and extension, there is found little accompanying rotation or lateral flexion. In axial rotation, there is a consistent pattern of accompanying lateral flexion. At the upper three lumbar levels, axial rotation is accompanied by lateral flexion in the opposite direction. That is, if the voluntary axial rotation is to the right, the accompanying lateral bend is to the left, and vice versa. At L5-S1, if lateral bending occurs, it is always in the same direction as the axial rotation (95).

The magnitude of accompanying axial rotation during lateral bending suggests that the lumbar spine is also twisted to its limit in the opposite direction during this maneuver. In voluntary axial rotation, the accompanying lateral bends were generally one-half to two-thirds of the full range seen in voluntary lateral bending.

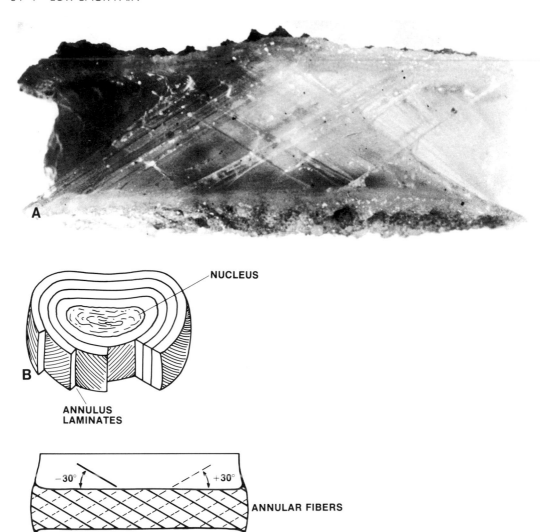

Figure 2.79. Intervertebral disc. **A**, A photograph of a disc clearly shows the annular fibers and their orientation. **B**, The disc consists of a nucleus pulposus surrounded by the annulus, which is made of concentric-laminated bands of annular fibers. In any two adjacent bands, the fibers are oriented in opposite directions. **C**, The fibers are oriented at about ±30° with respect to the placement of the disc. (Photograph courtesy of Dr. Leon Kazarian.) (Reproduced with permission from White AA, Panjabi MM: *Clinical Biomechanics of the Spine*. Philadelphia, JB Lippincott, 1978, p 3.)

The L4-L5 level is a transition point for coupled axial rotation and lateral bending. Since L4-L5 also has the largest degree of flexion and extension in the lumbar spine, it is felt that this joint experiences higher stresses than the other lumbar levels and gives a mechanical reason for L4-L5 to have the highest incidence of intervertebral joint pathology.

Ten degrees of lateral bending occurs in the upper three lumbar levels, while there is significantly less movement—6° and 3°—at the L4-L5 and L5-S1 levels, respectively.

In flexion and extension, accompanying axial rotation of 2° or more and lateral bending of 3° or more occur rarely, and any larger amount of rotation should be considered abnormal (95).

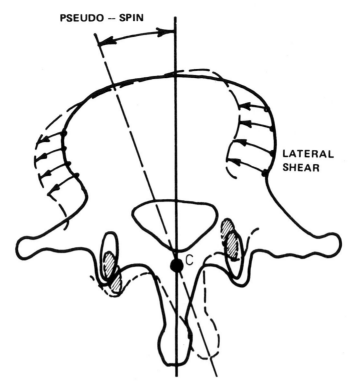

Figure 2.80. "Accessory rotation" due to lateral disc shear. (Reproduced with permission from Scull ER: Joint biomechanics and therapy: contribution or confusion? In Glasgow EF, Twomey LT, Scull ER, Kleynhans AM, Idczak RM (eds): *Aspects of Manipulative Therapy.* New York, Churchill Livingstone, 1985, pp 9–12.)

Weight-Bearing Changes in the Disc

The disc bears vertical axis weight and distributes it tangentially to the annular fibers. The disc also bears tensile stresses at the annular fibers during rotation motion. The nucleus bears the vertical load and the annular fibers bear the tangential load in a normal disc. Degeneration causes redistribution of the loading mechanism, with the annular fibers bearing most of the vertical load.

On compression loading, the cartilaginous end plate is most susceptible to fracture, allowing rupture of nuclear material into the cancellous bone (Schmorl's nodes). The vertebral body (Fig. 2.84) is next most susceptible to fracture. There is an audible crack as the body gives way, occurring at compression loads of 1,000 to 1,700 lb in young specimens and at as little as 300 lb in older specimens. With the annulus intact, the disc will not compress without vertebral compression. (77).

Virgin (96) also observed that even if postero-lateral incisions were made in the annulus fibrosus all the way to the nucleus and then loaded in compression, there would still be very little change in the elastic properties of the annulus and definitely no disc herniation.

Rotational Changes in the Disc

In the lumbar spine, the axis of rotation is between the articular facets in the arch of the vertebra, with the annular fibers resisting the axial shearing stresses (Fig. 2.85). On flexion and extension, the axis of rotation passes close to or within the nucleus pulposus, so that for the most part the nucleus pulposus can be considered the center of motion in a sagittal plane.

Gregersen and Lucas (97) studied axial rotation of the spine while the trunk was rotated from side to side. Approximately 74° of rotation occurred between T1 and T12, and the average cumulative rotation from the sacrum to T1 was 102°. Very little rotation occurred in the lumbar spine, as compared with that in the thoracic

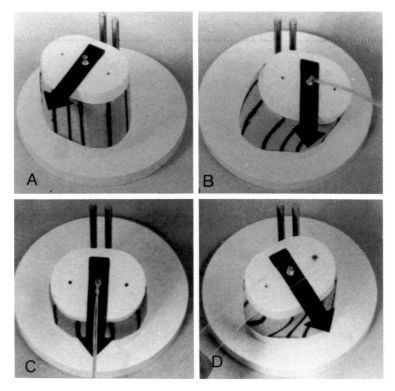

Figure 2.81. Three degrees of freedom of the isolated IV disc. **A**, Model of the isolated disc without posterior elements; **B**, lateral swing; **C**, anterior/posterior swing; **D**, rotation or spin. (Reproduced with permission from Scull ER: Joint biomechanics and therapy: contribution or confusion? In Glasgow EF, Twomey LT, Scull ER, Kleynhans AM, Idczak RM (eds): *Aspects of Manipulative Therapy.* New York, Churchill Livingstone, 1985, pp 9–12.)

spine; again, this is a reflection of the orientation of the facet joints. Measurements of rotation obtained during walking indicated the following (77):

1. The pelvis and the lumbar spine rotate as a functional unit.
2. In the lower thoracic spine, rotation diminishes gradually up to T7.
3. T7 represents the area of transition from vertebral rotation in the direction of the pelvis to rotation in the opposite direction, that of the shoulder girdle.
4. The amount of rotation in the upper thoracic spine increases gradually from T7 to T1.

Lumsden and Morris (98) measured axial rotation at the lumbosacral level in vivo and found that approximately 6° of rotation occurred at this level during maximum rotation. Approximately 1.5° of rotation occurred during normal walking. They also found that rotation at L5-S1 was not measurably affected by asymmetrically oriented facets (tropism); it has always been associated with flexion of L5 on the sacrum.

White and Panjabi (2) state that the disc annulus supports two types of stress—the normal or perpendicular and the shearing or parallel. Shear stresses are larger in magnitude, and there is no provision for resisting shear stress in the way that annular fibers resist normal perpendicular stresses by the alternating annular layers. Thus, the risk of disc failure is greater with tensile loading than with compression loading.

When a disc is subjected to torsion, there are shear stresses in the horizontal as well as the axial plane. The magnitude of these stresses varies in direct proportion to the distance from the axis of rotation (Fig. 2.86). The stresses at 45° and 60° to the horizontal are shown in Figure 2.86. Shear stresses that are perpendicular to the fibers' direction may produce disc failure.

The application to proper lifting (Fig. 2.87) can be considered with the above tensile stress failures.

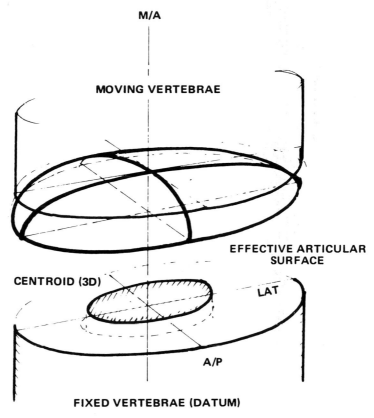

Figure 2.82. The effective articulation of the intervertebral disc. (Reproduced with permission from Scull ER: Joint biomechanics and therapy: contribution or confusion? In Glasgow EF, Twomey LT, Scull ER, Kleynhans AM, Idczak RM (eds): *Aspects of Manipulative Therapy.* New York, Churchill Livingstone, 1985, pp 9–12.)

Disc Resistance to Force

RESISTANCE TO INTERVERTEBRAL SHEAR FORCE

Adams and Hutton (98a) report that when an intervertebral joint is loaded in shear (Fig. 2.88A), the apophyseal joint surfaces resist about one-third of the shear force, while the disc resists the remaining two-thirds. However, this passive resistance to shear is complicated by two features. First, when an intervertebral disc alone is subjected to sustained shear, it readily creeps forward. In an intact joint, this readiness to creep would manifest as stress relaxation, thus placing an increasing burden on the apophyseal joint surfaces until, in the limit, they would resist all of the intervertebral shear force. Second, the muscle slips attached to the posterior part of the neural arch brace it by pulling downward. This prevents any backward bending and brings the facets more

firmly together. This means that, in the intact joint, the intervertebral disc is subjected only to pure compression and that the intervertebral shear force is resisted by the apophyseal joints, producing a high interfacet force.

RESISTANCE TO INTERVERTEBRAL COMPRESSIVE FORCE (98a)

The absence of a flattened articular surface in the transverse plane at the base of the articular facets quite clearly suggests that apophyseal joints are not designed to resist intervertebral compressive force. Experiments confirm that, provided the lumbar spine is slightly flattened (as occurs in erect sitting or heavy lifting), all the intervertebral compressive force is resisted by the disc. However, when lordotic postures, such as erect standing, are held for long periods, the facet tips do make contact with the laminae of the subadjacent vertebra and bear about one-sixth of the compressive force (Fig. 2.88**B**).

The contact may well be of clinical significance, since it will result in high stresses on the tips of the facet and, possibly, nipping of the joint capsules (Fig. 2.89). Perhaps this is why standing for long periods can produce a dull ache in the small of the back that is relieved by sitting or by using some device, such as a bar rail, to induce slight flexion of the lumbar spine. Disc narrowing results in as much as 70% of the intervertebral compressive force being transmitted across the apophyseal joints.

With increasing extension of an intervertebral joint, the compression force transmitted across the apophyseal joints increases, and it is likely that the extension movements are limited by this bony contact. Thus it is possible that hyperextension movements could cause backward bending of the neural arch, eventually resulting in spondylolysis, but again only as a fatigue fracture.

RESISTANCE TO TORSION

The apophyseal joints are oriented to resist rotation and protect the soft tissues from the effects of torsion (98a).

RESISTANCE TO FLEXION

The capsular ligaments of the apophyseal joint play the dominant role in resisting flexion of an intervertebral joint. In full flexion, as determined by the elastic limit of the supraspinous and interspinous ligaments, they provide 39% of the joint's resistance. The balance is made up by the disc (29%), the supraspinous and interspinous ligaments (19%), and the ligamentum flavum (13%) (98a).

Effects of Posture on the Lumbar Spine

Current ideas on what constitutes "good posture" are rather vague. The usual advice, possibly based on esthetic and military traditions, is to "sit up straight" and "don't slouch." Paradoxically, sitting up straight is taken to mean sitting with a lumbar lordosis and not allowing the lumbar spine to flex and flatten its curve (99).

As far as the lumbar spine is concerned, there is no reliable evidence that sitting up straight is, in fact, beneficial. On the contrary, population studies have shown that lumbar disc degeneration is rare among people who habitually sit or squat in postures that flatten the lumbar spine. Such postures are instinctively assumed by children and by many adults. If these natural preferences are to be discouraged and advice given on posture, then such advice should be founded on scientific evidence.

POSTURE AND THE LOADING OF THE APOPHYSEAL JOINTS (99)

These joints stabilize the spine and protect the discs from both excessive flexion and axial rotation. They also play a major role in resisting shear and compressive forces, although this varies considerably with posture.

In the erect posture, the apophyseal joints resist most of the shear force acting on the spine, as well as about 16% of the compressive force. The resulting stress between the articular surfaces is concentrated in the lower margins of the joint. If the disc is unusually narrow and degenerate, the facets may come into close apposition and may then resist up to 70% of the compressive force on the spine.

In the flexed posture, the apophyseal joints resist the shear force but now play no part in resisting the intervertebral compressive force. The stress between the articular surfaces is lower than in the erect posture and is concentrated in the middle and upper parts of the joint. In the flexed posture there is no extraarticular impingement.

POSTURE AND THE LOADING OF THE INTERVERTEBRAL DISC (99)

The intervertebral discs and vertebral bodies comprise the main weight-bearing column of the lumbar spine. Posture affects the way this column resists the loads applied to it but has little effect on the magnitude of these loads.

Under load, an unwedged disc tends to behave as a hydrostatic body exerting a uniform compressive stress on the vertebral end plates. By wedging a disc, we complicate this slightly: young nondegenerate discs remain hydrostatic, but mature and degenerate discs sustain pressure gradients. This means that when a mature disc is wedged in the erect posture, the highest compressive stresses are transmitted through the posterior annulus and the lowest through the anterior annulus. Similarly, in flexed postures the highest compressive stresses are transmitted

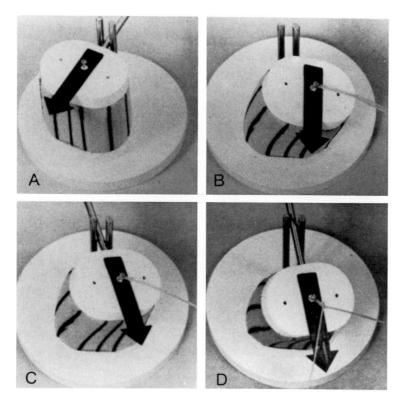

Figure 2.83. Motion of the IV disc with posterior coupling. **A**, Model of the disc with posterior coupling; **B**, lateral chordal swing without coupling; **C**, lateral chordal swing and adjunct rotation initiated by posterior coupling; **D**, combined lateral and A/P swing movement with posterior coupling. (Reproduced with permission from Scull ER: Joint biomechanics and therapy: contribution or confusion? In Glasgow EF, Twomey LT, Scull ER, Kleynhans AM, Idczak RM (eds): *Aspects of Manipulative Therapy*. New York, Churchill Livingstone, 1985, pp 9–12.)

through the anterior annulus and the lowest through the posterior annulus (99).

Fluid flow is caused by pressure changes on the disc. High pressure causes fluid to be expelled from the disc, while low pressure (lying down, for example) allows the proteoglycans in the disc to suck in fluid from surrounding tissue. Flexed postures increase this fluid exchange because they cause more fluid to be expelled from the disc than do erect postures.

FLEXION EFFECTS ON THE FACET AND DISC

The advantages and disadvantages of flexing the lumbar spine are summarized here. Let us first consider the advantages (99).

Reducing the high stresses that can be found on the tips of the facet joints may well be significant. In a lordotic posture, the stress between the facet surfaces can exceed the peak levels found in the articular cartilage of the hip and knee and may be responsible for the very high incidence of osteoarthritis in these joints.

Advantages of flexion:
  Reduced stresses at the apophyseal joints;
  Reduced compressive stress on the posterior annulus;
  Improved transport of disc metabolites;
  High compressive strength of the spine.
Disadvantages of flexion:
  Increased compressive stress on the anterior annulus;
  Increased hydrostatic pressure in the nucleus at low load levels.

How Do Discs Absorb Compressive Loads?

Discs absorb shock by squeezing fluid out of the nucleus and/or by allowing the fibers of the outer

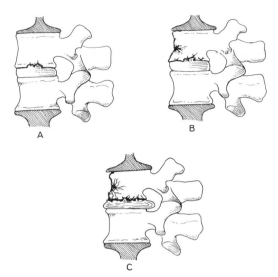

Figure 2.84. **A**, The cartilaginous end plates are most susceptible to spinal compression. **B**, The vertebral body is the second most susceptible unit of the spine. **C**, The normal nucleus pulposus and annulus fibrosus are least susceptible to pressure. (Reproduced with permission from Finneson BE: *Low Back Pain*, ed 2. Philadelphia, JB Lippincott, 1980, p 39.)

shell to stretch. Studies of disc fibers suggest that they have only limited elasticity and can only stretch to 1.04 times their initial length before suffering irreparable damage. When the disc is compressed, for instance when we lift a heavy object or jump from a great height and land on our feet, this limited elasticity does not present a major problem. Indeed, when we are standing upright, the disc fibers can take 10 times as much compression as can the vertebrae themselves, so a

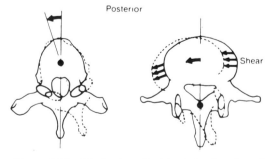

Figure 2.85. Mechanism of axial rotation in a thoracic (*left*) and a lumbar (*right*) vertebra. (Reproduced with permission from Finneson BE: *Low Back Pain*, ed 2. Philadelphia, JB Lippincott, 1980, p 34.)

very heavy load will crush bones before it ruptures a disc.

Disc fibers are less able to cope with torsion than with compression because with torsion the stress concentrates at points of maximum curvature. Because the disc shell is made of layers of fibers which lie obliquely to each other in a crisscross pattern, torsion tends to shear one layer from another, further weakening the total structure. As a result, we stand a much greater risk of damaging our discs when we try to lift an object and twist our body around at the same time.

Sitting and Its Effects on the Intervertebral Disc

The intradiscal pressure within the nucleus pulposus is lowest when the patient is recumbent and is highest when the patient is sitting in a flexed position. Nachemson (60) has measured the relative pressure within the third lumbar disc of people in various positions and has found that these pressures range between 25 and 275 as the person moves from the recumbent to the sitting flexed posture.

Fahrni (100) states that he studied a jungle population in India who squat rather than sit and sleep on the ground rather than in beds. These people had no concept of posture principles whatsoever but had a zero incidence of back pain. Furthermore, x-rays of the lumbar spine in 450 of these people of ages 15 to 44 years showed no incidence of disc narrowing. Thus, sitting is to be avoided in treatment of low back pain, especially with intradiscal involvement.

Fromelt et al. (101) found that bending, twisting, and lifting were the most common causes of low back pain and disc injury. The effect of rotational instability on the lateral recess is shown in Figure 2.90.

Osmotic Principles of the Disc

The human intervertebral disc acts as an osmotic system. Water, salt, and other low-molecular-weight substances penetrate the cartilage plates and annulus fibrosus. The content of water, sodium, potassium, and ashes in different regions of 69 human lumbar intervertebral discs was examined before and after being loaded with certain weights. Under load, the disc loses water (annulus, 11%; nucleus, 8%) and gains sodium and potassium. The higher concentration of elec-

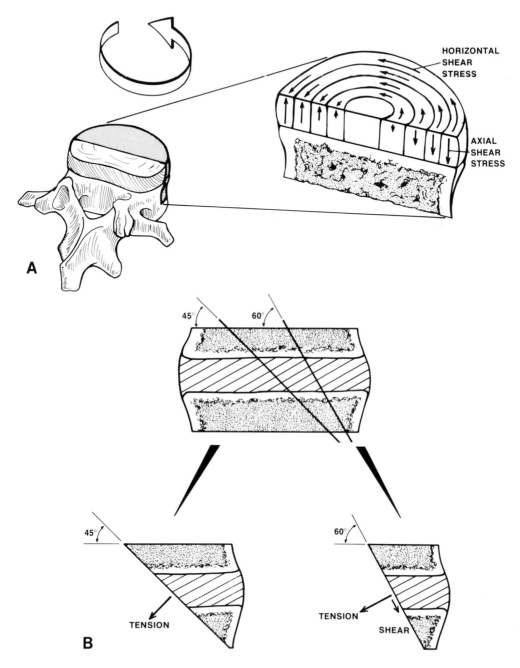

Figure 2.86. Disc stresses with torsion. **A**, Application of a torsional load to the disc produces shear stresses in the disc. These are in the horizontal plane as well as in the axial plane, and both are always of equal magnitude. They vary, however, at different points in the disc in proportion to the distance from the instantaneous axis of rotation. **B**, At 45° to the disc plane, the stresses are normal (i.e., there are no shear stresses). At 60° to the disc plane, perpendicular to the annular fibers, however, both types of stresses are present, normal as well as shear. The normal stresses are efficiently taken up by the annular fibers. (Reproduced with permission from White AA, Panjabi MM: *Clinical Biomechanics of the Spine.* Philadelphia, JB Lippincott, 1978, p 16.)

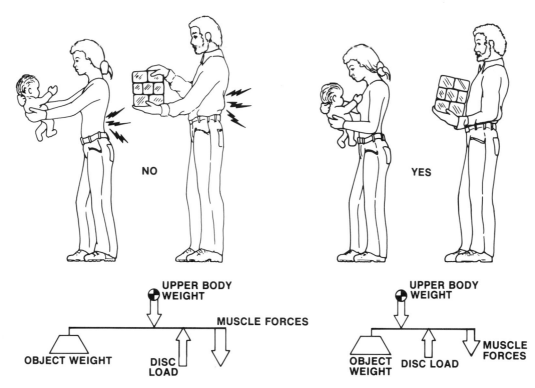

NO

YES

UPPER BODY WEIGHT

MUSCLE FORCES

OBJECT WEIGHT

DISC LOAD

UPPER BODY WEIGHT

OBJECT WEIGHT

DISC LOAD

MUSCLE FORCES

Figure 2.87. Diagram of the ergonomics of proper lifting. The load on the discs is a combined result of the object weight, the upper body weight, the back muscle forces, and their respective lever arms to the disc center. On the *left*, the object is farther away from the disc center, compared to the object on the *right*. The lever balances at the *bottom* show that smaller muscle forces and disc loads are obtained when the object is carried nearer to the disc. (Reproduced with permission from White AA, Panjabi MM: *Clinical Biomechanics of the Spine.* Philadelphia, JB Lippincott, 1978, p 331.)

trolytes in the disc after a long period of loading increases its osmotic absorption force and enables the disc to hold back the remaining water, even against a considerable pressure. After reduction of pressure, water is quickly reabsorbed, and the disc gains height and volume. The pumping mechanism maintains the nutritional and biomechanical function of the intervertebral disc (102).

Suspension Effects on the Lumbar Spine

Roentgenological investigation of the lumbar spine was done in the standing and suspended position in 100 healthy adult male volunteers. Spinal and external morphology were studied. The aim of this work was to identify correlations between the modifications of shape and size of the suspended lumbar spine and external morphol-

ogy. Such correlations were sought to establish a functional approach to anthropometry. This study demonstrated that the suspended position led to lengthening of the spine in 70% of the sub-

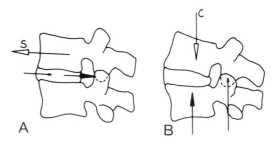

A   **B**

Figure 2.88. The apophyseal joint and the intervertebral disc share in resisting shear *(S)* and compression *(C)*. (Reproduced with permission from Adams MA, Hutton WC: The mechanical function of the lumbar apophyseal joints. *Spine* 8(3):328, 1983.)

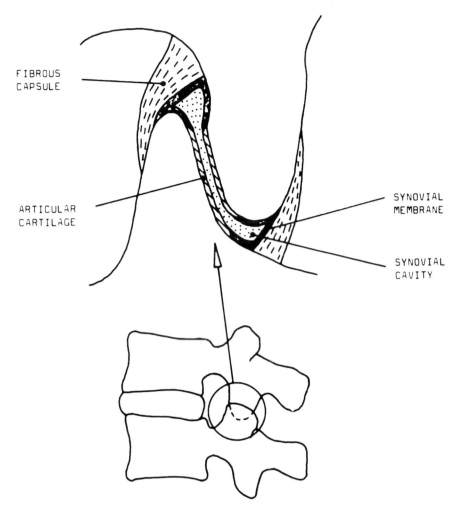

Figure 2.89. An apophyseal joint cut through in the sagittal plane. (Reproduced with permission from Adams MA, Hutton WC: The mechanical function of the lumbar apophyseal joints. *Spine* 8(3):328, 1983.)

jects examined, shortening of the spine in 22%, and mainly straightening of the spine in 8% (103).

The phenomenon of elongation of the lumbar spine when the body is placed in the suspended position is dependent upon tonic muscle activity. Shortening of the lumbar spine in the suspended position was seen in apparently longitypic and thin subjects. This somatotype has been linked to "tonic" temperament. Straightening of the lumbar spine without lengthening under the effect of suspension was observed in subjects with relatively high body weight and accentuated lumbar curvature.

In 70% of the subjects studied, increased size of the intervertebral spaces was seen when the body was placed in the suspended position, i.e.,

by a traction force of approximately 40 to 50% of body weight. The results may have practical applications in the use of therapeutic traction. Indeed, in this respect our results underline the need to obtain muscle relaxation and show that mild traction may be effective. Furthermore, elimination of lordosis is not proof of the efficacy of traction on the intervertebral discs. Longitypic subjects may be more resistant to traction compared to other somatotypes (103).

ANATOMICAL AND DEMOGRAPHIC FACTORS IN LOW BACK PAIN

Three hundred twenty-one males, ages 18 to 55, had standardized tests to determine height,

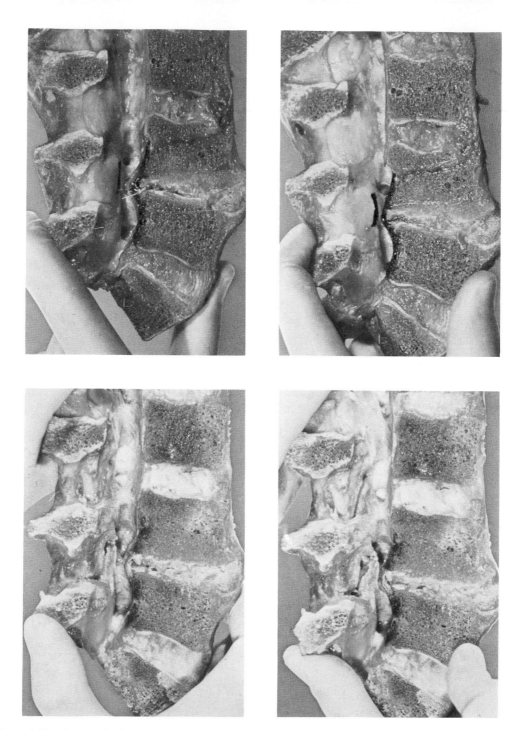

Figure 2.90. Longitudinal section of the lumbar spine. The posterior joint and disc at L3-L4 are normal. Those at L4-L5 show marked degenerative changes with rotational instability. *Top left*, Before rotation. The *black line* on the *left* is placed over the front of the superior articular process. Note the size of the lateral recess. *Top right*, Same specimen. The spinous process of L5 has been rotated out of the picture (toward the viewer). This rotation displaces the superior articular process forward with narrowing of the lateral recess. *Bottom left*, Same as *top left*, with the lateral extension of the ligamentum flavum removed. Note the marked degeneration of the posterior joint and disc and the size of the lateral recess. *Bottom right*, Same as *top right*, with the lateral extension of the ligamentum flavum removed. The spinous process of L5 has again been rotated as in *top right*. The posterior joint surfaces are separated. The lateral recess is narrowed by forward displacement of the superior articular process. (Reproduced with permission from Yong-Hing K, Reilly J, and Kirkaldy-Willis WH: The ligamentum flavum. *Spine* 1(4):232, 1976.)

weight, Davenport index, leg length inequality, determination of flexion and extension torques, flexion/extension balance, range of motion, straight leg raising, and lumbar lordosis. A total of 106 (33.0%) had never experienced low back symptoms; 144 (44.9%) had or were having moderate low back pain (LBP); and 71 (22.1%) had or were having severe low back symptoms. These three subgroups showed no significant differences in height, weight, Davenport index, lumbar lordosis, or leg length inequalities. LBP patients had less flexor and extensor strength and were flexor-overpowered, had diminished range of motion for spinal extension and axial rotation ($P=0.003$, $P=0.0005$), and had diminished straight leg raising capacity ($P=0.004$). A multivariate correlation matrix demonstrated no typical pattern of associated abnormalities except that a diminished spinal range of motion in one plane was associated with the anticipated diminishment in all other planes of motion, and often with greater restrictions of straight leg raising tests (104).

Men with a height of 180 cm or more showed a relative low back pain risk of 2.3 (95% confidence limits, 1.4 to 3.9), and women with a height of 170 cm or more showed a relative risk of 3.7 (1.6 to 8.6), compared with those who were more than 10 cm shorter (1.0). In men, but not in women, increased body mass index proved to be an independent risk factor for herniated lumbar disc, whereas the thickness of triceps skinfold had no predictive significance. Height and heavy body mass may be important contributors to the herniation of lumbar intervertebral discs (105).

Measurements made from plain lumbar radiographs were used to compare the size and shape of the lumbar vertebral canals between various categories of occupation and work load among 77 men and 118 women with a history of low back pain. The mean anteroposterior foraminal diameters proved to be wider in female farm workers than in other women, especially in the vertebra 1.3 (17.1 vs. 15.4 mm). However, the men who did heavy manual work had smaller anteroposterior foraminal diameters than the men whose work involved less physical labor (difference at L5, 9.4 vs. 10.8 mm). Female farm workers were found to have shorter interarticular distances than females in other occupational groups. In the men who reported working in stooped postures or who reported lifting and carrying heavy objects at work, the interarticular distances were wider than in men who had no such exposures (106).

Correlation of Age, Weight, Height, and Body Curve to Low Back Pain

Correlations of age, height, weight, lordosis, and kyphosis with noninvasive spinal mobility measurements were studied in 301 men and 175 women, aged 35 to 55 years, who suffered from chronic or recurrent low back pain. Correlations of the different spinal movements with the degree of LBP were analyzed, with corrections for these relationships. Age had significant indirect correlations with most of the mobility measurements, but the effect of height was minor. Weight had considerable negative correlations with the mobility measurements, except lateral flexion. Lordosis and kyphosis had significant relationships with mobility in the sagittal and frontal planes. Thoracolumbar mobility had higher correlations with LBP than mobility of the lumbar spine. Thoracal spinal mobility alone also correlated with LBP. Lateral flexion and rotation, except for rotation in women, had stronger relationships than forward flexion and extension with LBP (107).

Of all 30-, 40-, 50-, and 60-year-old inhabitants of Glostrup, a suburb of Copenhagen, 82% (449 men and 479 women) participated in a general health survey, which included a thorough physical examination relating to the lower back. The examination consisted of anthropometric measurements, flexibility/elasticity measurements of the back and hamstrings, and tests for trunk muscle strength and endurance. *The main findings were that good isometric endurance of the back muscles may prevent first-time occurrence of LBT (low back trouble) in men and that men with hypermobile backs are more liable to contract LBT.* Recurrence or persistence of LBT was correlated primarily with the interval since last LBT episode: the more LBT, the shorter the intervals had been. Weak trunk muscles and reduced flexibility/elasticity of the back and hamstrings were found as residual signs in particular, among those with recurrence or persistence of LBT in the follow-up year (108).

In all, 28.9% of the sample (29.8% of the men and 27.9% of the women) had leg length discrepancies equal to or greater than 1 cm. The leg length discrepancy showed no significant predictive power for first-time occurrence of LBT in the follow-up year or for recurrence or persistence of

LBT, but when tested in relation to whether that subject ever had LBT prior to the initial examination, the group with prior LBT was found to contain significantly more participants with unequal leg length than the group with no prior LBT (x^2=9.19, df=1, P=0.0025). Of those with LBT, 46% (264 of 569) had unequal leg length. This figure was of the same magnitude in all eight sex/age groups. Neither the magnitude of the inequality nor whether the right or left side was shortest was found to provide any additional information regarding LBT (108).

Children's Incidence of Low Back Disc Herniation

Herniated discs in children and adolescents can be extremely disabling and difficult to diagnose because of the paucity of neurological abnormalities and the consequent suspicions of hysteria.

One percent of patients operated upon for discal herniation are between 10 and 20 years of age. Spinal fusion should be considered when discal herniation is complicated by the presence of transitional vertebrae and spordylolisthesis, which because of instability contribute to the persistence of back pain (109).

One study reported on twenty-five teenage children with herniated lumbar intervertebral discs with accompanying structural anomalies (109). Three had transitional vertebrae; 11 had spinal stenosis confirmed at surgery; one had tropism; and one had spondylolysis.

The unusual frequency of transitional vertebrae dominates all of the cases reviewed. When associated with hyperlordosis, which also seriously compromises the mechanical efficiency of the spine, the result is often residual back pain and disability.

The true incidence of lumbar disc herniation in children is unknown. In white patients, the percentage varies from 0.8% in Rugtveit's series to 3.8% in the group reviewed by O'Connell. In Japan, the frequency is unusually high, from 7.8% to 22.3%, possibly related to earlier ages of employment (109).

Disc Annular Fiber Damage and Pain Production

This author remembers that Charles Ray, M.D., at the Challenge of the Lumbar Spine in 1985, referred to the annular fibers of the disc as resembling the plies of a tire. When damaged by loss of elasticity, pain begins. He felt that metabolic disturbance of collagen is a cause of low back pain and that torsion caused instability of the annulus fibrosus.

Discs of 25 specimens of human lumbar motion segments were subjected to an internal division of the annulus fibrosus, sparing only a peripheral layer 1 mm thick. Thus an attempt was made to simulate an internal disruption of the annulus caused by a traumatic episode or a degenerative process. The disc bulge that developed at the site of the injury was observed under axial compression fracture and after intradiscal injection. Under 1000-N load, the bulge amounted to less than 0.5 mm; typically, it increased to less than 1.0 mm after fracture. An extrusion of disc material at the site of the annulus injury was never observed. The results suggest that a radial division of the annulus is not sufficient to produce a clinically relevant disc herniation; further prerequisites are a fragmentation of the disc material and a separation from the end plates (110).

Annular tears can, by nociceptor nerve endings in the annulus fibrosus, cause pain referral to the low back, buttock, sacroiliac region, and lower extremity even in the absence of neural compression (54).

Correlation of Low Back Pain with Specific Conditions

In the classic low back syndrome commonly referred to as "muscle spasms" or "a strained back," the pain usually comes from the disc. The classic history is of someone who has had some vague intermittent discomfort but is able to carry on normal activities. Then one day he bends over to pick something up, he feels something snap, and over the next several hours he develops an acute low back problem, with or without leg radiation. If there is no sciatica—no leg radiation—it is most likely that there is a weak annulus fibrosus, usually at the L4-L5 or the L5-S1 interspace. The patient probably is getting microscopic tears in that weakened annulus, which will cause acute episodes of back pain. It may not be a disc herniation, just a disc bulge, which causes the acute onset of pain and which subsides quite rapidly (111).

Facet Syndromes

Most facet joint problems are secondary to degenerative disc disease. The overall syndrome begins with disc problems. There is a weakening in the annulus, with or without true herniation of the disc, and there is settling of the disc; the facet joints are therefore under more strain because of the instability that has occurred. They may or may not be subluxed, depending on how narrow the disc space is, and then they will develop osteoarthritic changes secondary to the disc disease, but the original problem is a problem with the discs.

Does subluxation of the facet produce pain in itself? Absolutely (111). Facet pain, first of all, is pain from a joint. Therefore, one of the major symptoms is stiffness. If patients have stiffness after rest, such as when waking up in the morning or after riding long distances in an automobile or a plane, which improves if they get up and move around, and if, on physical examination, leaning to the side reproduces achy stiffness, then it is felt that the facet joint is the source of the problem.

Innervation of the Zygapophyseal Joint

In a study of lower zygapophyseal facet joints, nerves have been demonstrated in the synovial folds by means of a silver impregnation method. The diameter of the nerves ranged from 0.6 to 12 μm; the number of fibers per nerve ranged from 1 to 5. They generally run a course separate from blood vessels, indicating that they are afferent nerves that probably have a nociceptive function. This finding may be relevant to low back pain (112).

The fibrous capsule of the zygapophyseal joints is well innervated (112). It is less certain whether the ligamentum flavum, which forms the ventral portion of the joint capsule, is innervated. A small number of free neural structures described as nerve endings have been found. The question of innervation of the synovial membrane is even more contentious. According to Mooney and Robertson (113), the zygapophyseal joint synovial membrane contains a rich nerve supply, but their claim is not supported by histological evidence. Hadley (114) and Wyke (personal communication, 1983) did not find nerves in the synovial folds of the zygapophyseal joints. Indeed, Wyke (115) emphasized that there are no receptor nerve endings of any kind in the synovial

tissue or in the intraarticular menisci in these joints in mature individuals (112).

It is reasonable to assume from most studies, although controversial, that all human zygapophyseal joint synovial folds are innervated.

Entrapment of intraarticular synovial inclusions that protrude between moving parts of zygapophyseal joints has been implicated as a cause of low back pain (115a, 115b). Therefore, the demonstration of nerves, unrelated to blood vessels, in the synovial folds and joint inclusions has potential clinical significance in relation to low back pain (112).

Spondylolisthesis

Patients with this condition usually present in the late teenage years or early 20s with a history of back pain that may sound very similar to a disc herniation. They may have chronic back discomfort and leg pain caused by root compression in the region of the spondylolisthesis.

Also, patients with symptomatic spondylolisthesis usually have tight hamstring muscles, and if the slippage is great enough, one can palpate a step-off in the back that is due to the prominence of one of the spinous processes (111).

If someone who is 40 years old has had recent onset of back pain, and the radiographs demonstrate spondylolisthesis, chances are that the pain is due not to the spondylolisthesis but, rather, to a disc problem.

Spinal Stenosis

The typical patient with spinal stenosis is someone in his 50s or 60s or older who has had chronic back discomfort through the years, suggesting a chronic degenerative disc problem; who subsequently develops degenerative changes in the facet joints, frequently with a mild degenerative scoliosis as well; and who then subluxes one of the vertebrae forward at the joint level. This usually occurs at L4, in contrast to the spondylolytic spondylolisthesis in teenagers, which is almost always at L5. Patients with degenerative spondylolisthesis caused by facet joint problems will experience the symptoms of spinal stenosis, with a certain amount of back discomfort, but their major complaint will be that their legs do not work any more. They cannot walk very far. They develop a heaviness, a sensation of vague paresthesia, in the lower extremities, usually unassociated with any cramping to suggest vascular claudication. This type of leg discomfort, leg weakness, is almost always relieved by sitting down. The classic story is of a woman who goes shopping. She can walk into one store and then has to come out into the mall and sit down because her legs just will not carry her any farther. Radiographs in such a person will frequently show degenerative spondylolisthesis of L4. Plain films will frequently give the answer, but the CT scan is the best way of determining the exact amount of stenosis (111).

CASE PRESENTATION OF DEGENERATIVE SPONDYLOLISTHESIS STENOSIS

A 67-year-old white female was seen in our office with a chief complaint of low back pain and radiating pain into the right leg to the great toe. This patient had had back surgery two times, 11 years and 2 years previously, both times for pain down the left L5 nerve root to the great toe. This time the pain was in the right L5 nerve root.

Examination of this patient revealed her vital signs to be within normal limits. She had night pain, and walking aggravated her leg pain. Her Déjérine triad was negative. The ranges of motion were 80° flexion, 5° extension, 10° lateral bending, and 20° bilateral rotation. Her straight leg raising signs were bilaterally positive at 50°, creating leg pain. Motor evaluation revealed weakness on dorsiflexion of the right foot and great toe. The left ankle jerk was decreased, and the right ankle jerk was +2. There was hypesthesia of the right L5 and S1 dermatomes to pinwheel examination.

X-ray examination (Figs. 2.91 and 2.92) taken in AP and lateral views reveals evidence of decompressive laminectomies at the L4 and L5 levels and a 25% anterior slippage of the L4 vertebral body on L5. The L5-S1 disc reveals an extreme degenerative change. An oblique view (Fig. 2.93) reveals the outline of the lamina from the decompressive laminectomy performed in the past. Figures 2.94 and 2.95 are flexion and extension studies of the lumbar spine which reveal 5 mm of anterior translation of L4 on L5 in flexion and 3 mm on extension. This exceeds the normally seen 3 mm, which would be considered within normal motion at a given functional spinal unit level.

The impression of this case is as follows:

1. Pseudospondylolisthesis of L4 on L5, a 25% slippage;
2. Discogenic spondyloarthrosis L5-S1;
3. Unstable L4-L5 disc as evidenced by flexion and extension study;

4. Decompressive laminectomies at the L4-L5 segments.

Treatment of this case consisted of gentle flexion distraction manipulation over a small flexion roll under the abdomen. The patient was placed on knee-chest exercises and abdominal strengthening exercises, and attended low back wellness school to learn how to use the spine in daily living with minimal irritation. We told the patient that 50% relief of her symptoms would be an excellent clinical result, and anything over that would be a clinical bonus. We told her that 100% relief of this back problem is not feasible unless perhaps some surgical maneuver could be developed to provide it. We found that, within a 4-week period of care, this patient had attained 50% subjective relief. That relief consisted primarily of alleviation of the leg pain. She continued to have low back pain that was relieved by lying down and was aggravated in the upright posture.

We felt that this was a most interesting case of a postsurgical spine that developed instability at the L4-L5 level. The question arises as to whether or not the decompression of the L4 laminae diminished the ability of the L4 vertebra to resist the spondylolisthesis movement.

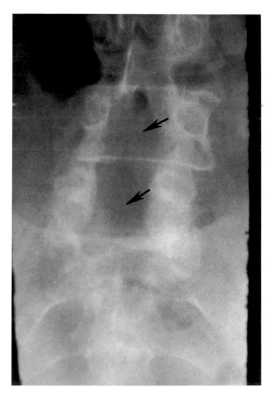

Figure 2.91. Anteroposterior lumbar spine x-ray reveals decompressive laminectomy (*arrows*) at the L4 and L5 levels.

ABNORMAL DISC AND APOPHYSEAL JOINT ANATOMY AND PHYSIOLOGY

The horizontal curvatures of the posterior surfaces of the lumbar vertebral bodies have been quantitatively evaluated by means of a simple measuring device (Fig. 2.96). The measurements were done near the superior and inferior vertebral margins. A horizontal concavity was always found in L1-L3; in L5 a posterior convexity was prevalent; and L4 occupied an intermediate position (Fig. 2.97). The degree of concavity of the posterior vertebral bodies is important in the evolution of lumbar canal stenosis (116).

Degenerative Disc Changes

One hundred thirty-nine discs from cadaveric lumbar spines were injected with a mixture of radiopaque fluid and dye. Discograms were taken, and the discs were then sectioned in the sagittal plane. Examination of the sections revealed that injected fluid did not at first mix with the disc ma-

trix but pushed it aside to form pools of injected fluid. The location of these pools, and hence the appearance of a discogram, depended on the stage of degeneration of the disc (117).

Then the stage of degeneration was used to explain the distribution of injected fluid, and hence the appearance of the discogram (Table 2.2).

1. Cottonball. The radiopaque shadow appears to be contained within the nucleus and is of uniform density. The shape is not necessarily round or centrally located.

These discs showed no signs of degeneration. The annulus was white and unfissured, and in noninjected specimens the nucleus was a soft white amorphous gel that contained no fissures or fibrous lumps.

2. Lobular. The radiopaque shadow appears to be contained within the nucleus and has a lobular appearance, being denser near the end plates and less dense or absent in the center. Typical shapes resemble a hamburger or horseshoe. The lobes can overlap to give the superficial appearance of a cottonball, but the lobular nature is revealed by the variation in density. Occasionally only one lobe is filled on injection.

These were typical mature discs with the nu-

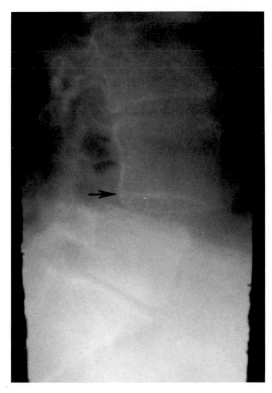

Figure 2.92. L4 (*arrow*) is 25% slipped anteriorly on L5 as a degenerative spondylolisthesis.

Table 2.2.
The Five Types of Discogram and the Stages of Disc Degeneration They Represent[a]

Discogram Type		Stage of Disc Degeneration
1. 1Cottonball		No signs of degeneration. Soft white amorphous nucleus
2. Lobular		Mature disc with nucleus starting to coalesce into fibrous lumps
3. Irregular		Degenerated disc with fissures and clefts in the nucleus and inner annulus
4. Fissured		Degenerated disc with radial fissure leading to the outer edge of the annulus
5. Ruptured		Disc has a complete radial fissure that allows injected fluid to escape. Can be in any state of degeneration

[a]Reproduced with permission from Adams MA, Dolan P, Hutton WC: The stages of disc degeneration as revealed by discograms. *J Bone Joint Surg* 68B:37, 1986.

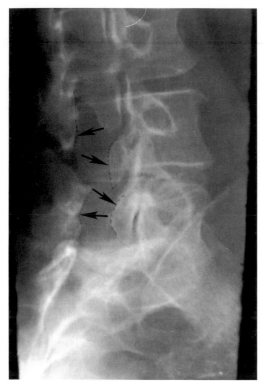

Figure 2.93. The *arrows* point to the surgically removed laminar outlines on oblique view.

limit (usually 1 to 3 ml) to the volume of fluid that can be injected.

These discs were usually degenerated, being fibrous and often discolored and narrowed. There were always one or more radial fissures in the annulus, and these usually led to the posterior or posterolateral border of the disc. The fissure occurred either in the midplane of the disc or near one end plate. The posterior annulus often bulged beyond the edge of the vertebral bodies.

5. Ruptured. The discogram shows contrast material extending to the outer edge of the annulus and escaping from the disc entirely. There may be a large quantity of contrast material within the disc space, or most may escape on injection. There is no limit to the volume of fluid that can be injected (117).

These discs come in all stages of degeneration, but there is always a complete radial fissure, usually in the posterior annulus.

cleus starting to coalesce into fibrous lumps, separated from the annulus and cartilage end plates (and occasionally from each other) by softer material.

3. Irregular. The radiopaque shadow has an irregular shape and appears to penetrate into the inner annulus.

These discs showed distinct signs of degeneration, with a fibrous nucleus and clefts and small fissures in the nucleus and inner annulus. There was poor differentiation between nucleus and annulus. The injected fluid formed pools around the fibrous lumps of nucleus and in the fissures in the inner annulus. There was little mixing with the matrix. Injection into isolated pieces of disc was generally easy in all locations except the outer annulus.

4. Fissured. The discogram shows the radiopaque shadow reaching to the outer edge of the annulus (perhaps beyond the edge of the vertebral body), but no contrast material escapes from the disc through the annulus. There is a definite

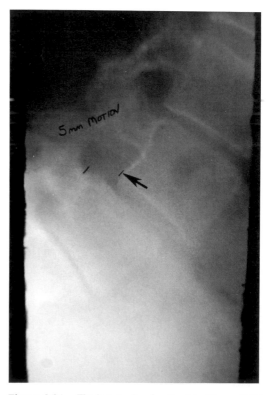

Figure 2.94. Flexion study of patient in Figure 2.92 shows 5 mm of anterior translation (*arrow*) of L4 on L5 compared to neutral lateral upright study.

Intervertebral Osteochondrosis

Intervertebral osteochondrosis is a common degenerative process involving the nucleus pulposus. With advancing age, dehydration and desiccation of the intervertebral disc, particularly the nucleus pulposus, are observed. These changes begin in the 2nd or 3rd decade of life and become prominent in middle-aged and elderly individuals. The nucleus appears friable and loses the elastic quality it possessed in youth. It becomes yellow or yellow-brown in color, and the onion-skin appearance of the nucleus pulposus changes, with the development of cracks or crevices within its substances. The cracks produce an abnormal space into which surrounding gas, principally carbon dioxide and nitrogen, collects. The gas produces a radiolucency on radiographs or CT, an occurrence that is called a "vacuum" phenomen. (Fig. 2.98**A** and **B**). The radiolucent collections are initially circular or oval, and they later elongate in a linear fashion, extending into the annulus fibrosus. This vacuum phenomenon differs from a radiolucent collection at the mar-

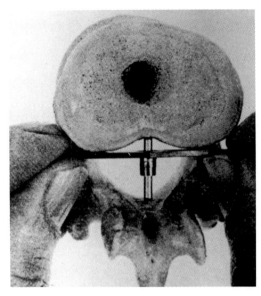

Figure 2.96. The measuring instrument in use at the superior vertebral border. The protruding part of the movable rod of the instrument was after the measuring determined by a magnifying monocular with a built-in scale, allowing estimation in tenths of a millimeter. (Reproduced with permission from Larsen JL: The posterior surface of the lumbar vertebral bodies. Part 2. *Spine* 10(10):901, 903, 1985.)

gin of the intervertebral disc, which may accompany a different process, spondylosis deformans; and from radiolucent collections within the vertebral bodies (vacuum vertebral body), which may accompany ischemic necrosis of bone. A discal vacuum phenomenon generally excludes the presence of infection (118).

As the process of intervertebral osteochondrosis progresses, the intervertebral disc diminishes in height, the annular fibers bulge, and the cartilaginous end plates degenerate and fracture. Adjacent trabeculae in the subchondral regions of the vertebral bodies thicken. Radiographically, at this stage, disc space loss and body sclerosis of peridiscal areas of the vertebral body are seen. The sclerosis is generally well defined. The discovertebral junction is usually sharply marginated, differing from the ill-defined margin that accompanies infection. An associated finding is a radiolucent focus within the vertebral body, representing the site of a cartilaginous node (Schmorls' node) that is caused by intervertebral herniation of a portion of the disc through the degenerating cartilaginous end plate.

Pathological and radiographic features of in-

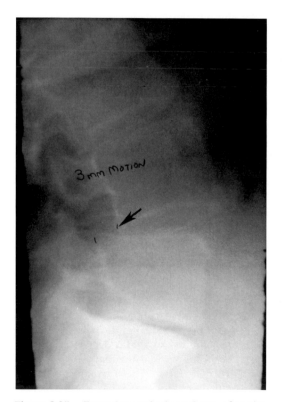

Figure 2.95. Extension study shows 3 mm of motion of L4 on L5 (*arrow*) compared to neutral posture.

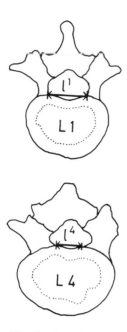

Figure 2.97. The drawing shows typical horizontal curvatures at L1 and L4, demonstrating the longer stretch of the horizontal upper (HU) in the upper than in the lower lumbar spine. (Reproduced with permission from Larsen JL: The posterior surface of the lumbar vertebral bodies. Part 2. *Spine* 10(10):901, 903, 1985.)

tervertebral osteochondrosis are most prominent in the lower lumbar region and are observed in men more commonly than in women.

With breakdown in Sharpey's fibers, the propulsive force of the nucleus pulposus leads to anterior and lateral displacement of the annulus fibrosus. The displacement produces elevation of the anterior longitudinal ligament and traction at the site of attachment of the ligament to the vertebral body. This site is several millimeters from the discovertebral junction. The osteophytes resulting from the abnormal ligamentous traction course first in a horizontal direction before turning in a vertical one. Eventually, the osseous excrescences may bridge the intervertebral disc (118).

CAUSE OF NITROGEN GAS FORMATION IN OSTEOCHONDROSIS VACUUM CHANGE

Gas-containing cleft-like spaces in the intervertebral disc indicate, in most instances, a process of cartilage degeneration. The crevices formed in

the degenerated disc cartilage become low-pressure spaces that attract gases from surrounding interstitial fluid. The chemical analysis of these gas collections in the disc space shows a 90 to 92% concentration of nitrogen. This is understandable considering diffusion gradients, solubility coefficients, and partial pressures of nitrogen, oxygen, and carbon dioxide. Nitrogen, a metabolically inert gas, is the dominant element trapped in any low-pressure space created in degenerated disc cartilage, distracted synovial joints, or aseptic necrosis of bone. Similarly, when a vertebra undergoes collapse secondary to ischemic necrosis, the volume of bone is reduced, and cleft-like spaces are formed. There is low pressure in these spaces, especially when hyperextension of the spine distracts the apposing surfaces of the cleft. Thus, the vacuum sign may become accentuated or appear only when the spine is in hyperextension (119).

Corticosteroid-Induced Aseptic Necrosis of Bone

The relationship between aseptic necrosis of bone and long-term corticosteroid treatment is well established. In patients with chronic corticosteroid treatment, it is well established. In patients with chronic corticosteroid therapy, biopsy-proven aseptic necrosis of bone has been reported in vertebrae exhibiting the vacuum sign (119).

Criteria for Determining the Level of Disc Involvement

MacGibbon and Farfan (120) give criteria for determining the level of disc degeneration by markings on a plain film study of the lumbar spine (Fig. 2.99). Basically, they state that when the intercrestal line passes through the upper half of the fourth lumbar vertebral body and when the transverse processes of L5 are well developed, the L4-L5 disc degenerates first. If the intercrestal line passes through the body of L5 and L5 has short transverse processes, the L5-S1 disc degenerates first. The higher the intercrestal line, the greater the risk of L4-L5 degeneration; and the lower the intercrestal line, the greater the risk of L5-S1 degeneration. They further state that, if it is assumed that discs are injured and degenerate solely because of torsional strains, the high intercrestal line and long transverse processes

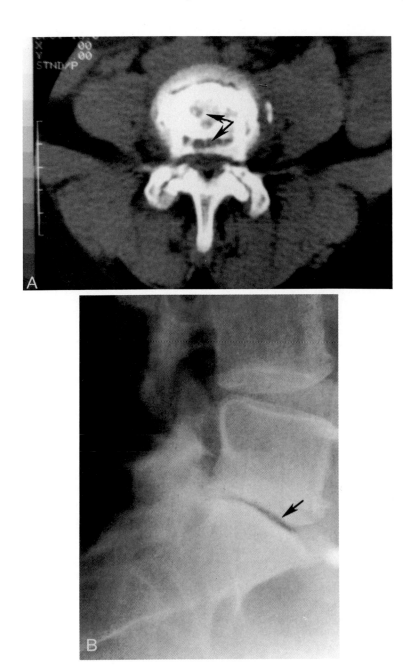

Figure 2.98. Osteochondrosis of the disc with vacuum phenomenon (*arrows*) as shown: **A**, on CT scan, and **B**, on plain x-ray.

become antitorsional devices, protecting the L5-S1 discs and indicating the likelihood of degeneration at L4-L5. Similarly, the low intercrestal line and small transverse processes, providing no protection against torsion, indicate the likelihood of degeneration at either the L4-L5 or the L5-S1 disc. We would, therefore, expect a high odds ratio for L4-L5 disc degeneration in the protected spines and a more equal odds ratio when there is no protection.

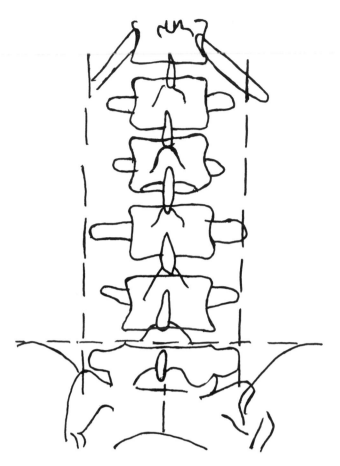

Figure 2.99. Intercrestal and transverse process lines drawn for determining probable level of disc degeneration.

The criteria for probable L4-L5 degeneration are:

1. A high intercrestal line passing through the upper half of L4;
2. Long transverse processes on L5;
3. Rudimentary rib;
4. Transitional vertebra.

The criteria for L5-S1 degeneration are:

1. An intercrestal line passing through the body of L5;
2. Short transverse processes on L5;
3. No rudimentary rib;
4. No transitional vertebra.

Surgical fusion has an effect similar to that of the intercrestal lines described by MacGibbon and Farfan. Fusion places the mobility at the segment above the fusion and can cause disc de-

generation at that level. The following case demonstrates this.

CASE PRESENTATION

The patient was hospitalized for low back and left sciatic pain. A spinal fusion was carried out from the third lumbar vertebra through the second sacral vertebra, involving a graft along the transverse and spinous processes.

The patient lived in low back pain and leg pain discomfort for 2 years. She then sought chiropractic care. Examination revealed that the patient had left leg fifth lumbar dermatome sciatica and left fourth lumbar medial disc protrusion.

Figure 2.100 reveals that at the L2-L3 intervertebral disc space there is a right lateral flexion subluxation of L2 on L3 with marked discogenic spondyloarthrosis present. Normally, 75% of the motion of the lumbar spine occurs at L5-S1, and as that disc degenerates, the

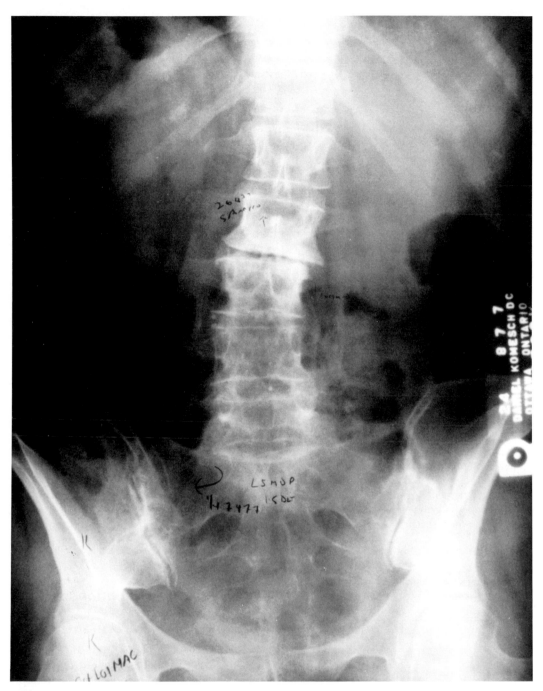

Figure 2.100. Right lateral flexion subluxation of L2 on L3 and advanced discogenic spondyloarthrosis of L2-L3. L2-L3 cannot perform all the movements that normally occur at the lower lumbar levels and degenerates severely following lumbar fusion.

motion moves progressively upward, so typically L4-L5 will be the next disc to degenerate. In this patient with attempted fusion from L3 through the sacrum, the point of maximum mobility was changed to L2-L3. The resultant degenerative change, therefore, occurred at the L2-L3 intervertebral disc joint, which was never intended to tolerate such hypermobility. This patient has to be splinted with back support to prevent future pain when lifting, bending, or twisting.

Age Incidence of Lumbar Disc Protrusion

In the study of surgical data on 6565 disc protrusions/herniations, a localization at the L4-L5 level was found in 3361 cases (51%), while the number at the L5-S1 level amounted to 2749 (42%). After adding disc pathology at the levels L5-L6, L6-S1, and S1-S2 to the group of L5-S1, the total number is increased to 2819 (43%). Above L4 the incidence is remarkably lower, showing a progressive decrease in the cranial direction. The preponderance of the L4-L5 localization corresponds with the overall frequency of 51% based on various studies, with abundant case material, in the literature (121).

In order to study the correlation between age and localization, the 6565 cases of disc protrusion/herniation are classified according to decade of life at the time of surgery. The highest overall frequency is found in the 5th decade (33%). In the 4th decade, the percentage is somewhat lower (28%), while it is remarkably less in the others. This is especially the case in patients 10 to 19 years of age, and in those who are older than 60 years.

In Table 2.3, the percentages of the respective localizations per decade are shown. It will be clear from the two first columns (L1-L2-L3 and L3-L4) that a percentage increase of cases occurs while the patients grow older (121). A more stable situation is demonstrated by the third column

Table 2.3.
Distribution of Protruded/Herniated Lumbar Discs above L3, at L3-L4, at L4-L5, and at L5-S1 per Decade (%)[a]

Age	L1-L2-L3	L3-L4	L4-L5	L5-S1
20	—	2.4	50.0	45.2
21–30	0.4	3.6	45.0	48.2
31–40	—	3.7	48.7	46.8
41–50	0.2	3.8	52.1	43.2
51–60	2.0	10.4	54.9	31.7
61–70	3.2	13.0	57.8	25.3
71–80	4.3	26.1	52.2	13.1

[a]Reproduced with permission from Luyendijk W: The localization of protruded lumbar discs in advancing age. *Acta Neurochir* 85:168–171, 1987.

(L4-L5), while the last column (L5-S1) shows a gradual decrease that becomes considerable after the age of 50 years.

The outcome of all this demonstrates quite clearly that, overall, protruded/herniated discs in older people usually are located at a higher level than in younger patients. This is a confirmation of what was previously postulated in the literature.

Regardless of the level, L5-S1 shows a steep decrease in the incidence after the age of 40 years.

It is tempting to correlate this phenomenon with a progressive fibrosis of the intervertebral discs occurring predominantly and primarily at the caudal levels. As can be expected, the final fibrosis of the intervertebral disc will prevent the formation of a protrusion (121).

Meaning of Lumbar Lordosis

Two lordotic angles were measured on roentgenograms of 973 adults in a prospective and retrospective review. The majority of the films were taken because of lumbar complaints. The mean lumbosacral (LS) angle (L2-sacrum) was 45.05°± 0.85°. The mean lumbolumbar (LL) angle (L2-L5) was 29.96°±0.74°. Only minor differences were found between a standardized (prospective) and a nonstandardized (retrospective) group. There was a statistically significant difference between men and women with both LS and LL angles, but no racial differences were observed. A "routine" supine lateral lumbar spine roentgenogram is a very accurate means of measuring lordotic angles. A lordotic angle of less than 23° defines hypolordosis, and more than 68°, hyperlordosis (122).

Radiographic Evaluation of Lumbosacral Lordosis— Recumbent versus Upright

In adults, the radiographic evaluation of vertebral slippage and lumbosacral lordosis is equally reliable in the recumbent and standing positions (123).

Lordosis in Low Back Pain Patients

No differences in the variation of the lordosis were found when spinal x-rays from men who denied any earlier back pain history were compared with those of men who claimed prior low back injury or chronic low back disability. This suggested that the shape of the lumbar lordosis as noted on survey x-ray techniques is not important for the occurrence of either acute or chronic low back pain. Thus, comments by physicians about minor variations in the amount of lumbar lordosis on plane views of the lumbar spine should be disregarded (124).

Two groups, of 150 people each, were analyzed. They were between the ages of 35 and 40 and had been engaged in heavy work all their lives. One group was under treatment for low back pain, and the other group denied any history of low back pain at any time in their lives. The main points that were found in this study were the following: There was no statistical difference in the anatomical variants seen on x-ray in both groups. The measurements for lordosis and lumbosacral angle were distributed similarly in both groups. There was no correlation between the anatomical variants that presumably gave rise to some degree of mechanical insufficiency and the degrees of degenerative disc changes that were observed. The only correlation that was noted was a correlation between disc degeneration and age (125).

Effects of Lumbar Spine Musculature

The musculature of the lumbar spine is of primary importance in the control of the efficiency of the spinal mechanism. The system of loading, which results in observable physiological response, maintains the compressive load at virtually 90° at the bisector of the disc for all weights and all angles of forward flexion (126).

The abdominal mechanism involves the posterior ligamentous system, comprising the midline ligaments, the lumbodorsal fascia, the facet capsular ligaments, the ligamentum flavum, and the posterior longitudinal ligament. The abdominal muscles and the lumbodorsal fascia contribute significantly to the balancing of the external moments.

The lumbodorsal fascia is attached to the spinous processes in the midline. The lateral margin of the fascia is attached to the ribs above and to the pelvis below. In its mid portions, the lateral margin of the fascia is continuous with the insertion of the transversus abdominis (TA) and the internal oblique (IO) muscles.

It is not clear what mechanism(s) is (are) contributing to the restraining of the fascia edges. Because the TA and the IO are attached to the edges of the fascia, it is attractive to assume that these muscles do restrain its edges. Hence these muscles must fire in order to maintain the fascia width (126).

In the lift sequence, the lumbodorsal fascia requires the muscle fibers attached to the fascia to stay in the same plane as the fascia if maximum efficiency is to be achieved. This cannot be done unless the abdominal cavity is pressurized to a level sufficient to ensure the proper shape and to support the hoop tension generated by the contracting muscles. This is the primary reason for the existence of the intraabdominal pressure (IAP). Once the abdominal cavity is pressurized, it follows that the pelvic floor and the diaphragm will spread apart unless there is a force that will maintain their relative spatial position. The rectus abdominis does not generate any movement on the spine. It simply counterbalances the action of the IAP on the two end caps of the abdominal cavity.

The system of loading can be deduced from the magnitude and direction of forces calculated at the intervertebral joint. Of first interest is the role of the nucleus pulposus. The entire lift is accomplished in 0.3 second, with maximum stress being applied in probably the first 0.1 second of the lift. This is to be compared with recordings of intradiscal pressure done by Nachemson (60) using equipment with a 500-hertz band. The intradiscal pressure rise achieved its maximum approximately 1 second after the load was applied. These recordings show clearly that the intradiscal pressure remains constant during the application of the load and then slowly rises to a maximum in about 3 seconds.

It must be noted that the component of shear due to the external forces is significant. The posterior ligamentous system and the extensors almost balance this external shear, leaving a small remainder component to be absorbed by the disc and the facets. Hence it is apparent that the disc probably sees no shear, and the facets see little if any shear. It must also be appreciated that because muscles and ligaments have different moments and shear contribution, they must function together if the resultant shear at the intervertebral joint is to be minimal.

Flexion at the intervertebral joint is brought

about by applying the load anterior or posterior to some point that may be considered as the neutral point. The eccentricity of the applied load must, however, remain within the confines of the disc annulus (126).

In conclusion, first, the abdominal mechanism utilizing intraabdominal pressure has been described and quantified. Second, simulations show that the lumbodorsal fascia, under control of the abdominal muscles, contributes to reduce the stress at the intervertebral joint. Third, the musculature of the lumbar spine is of primary importance in the control of the efficiency of the spinal mechanism. *Finally, the system of loading that results in observable physiological response maintains the compressive load at virtually 90° at the bisector of the disc for all weights and all angles of forward flexion* (126).

TRUNK STRENGTH DURING LIFTING

Twenty male workers with 2- to 18-year histories (median, 5.5 years) of low back pain went through strength tests of trunk flexion and extension and a series of standardized lifts. The IAP and the electromyographic activity of the oblique abdominal muscles and the erector spinae muscles were recorded. The results were compared with those in 20 healthy men exposed to similar loads at work and at leisure:

1. The low back patients had reduced abdominal muscle strength (-25%) compared with the healthy controls.
2. The IAP during lifting was the same in the two groups despite the difference in abdominal muscle strength.
3. The trunk extension strength was the same in the two groups.
4. The oblique abdominal muscles were only moderately activated during lifting (5 to 15% of maximum activity with 25 kg) both in low back patients and in healthy controls.
5. The erector spinae muscle was strongly activated during lifting (40 to 60% of maximum activity with 25 kg) both in low back patients and in healthy controls.
6. During backlifting, the duration of erector spinae activity varied. Back patients had extended activity compared with the healthy controls. Stiffness seemed to affect the duration of activity in both groups.
7. The oblique abdominal muscles seem to be of no decisive importance to the IAP (127).

Strength and endurance measures were obtained with patients stabilized in the upright sitting position. Both trunk flexors and extensors were evaluated.

Statistically significant differences were found in isometric extension strength, endurance, and extension/flexion strength ratio. No significant strength difference was found between the normal and the organic patient groups (128).

MULTIFIDUS MUSCLE

Dissection studies revealed that the fibers of the lumbar multifidus are divided by distinct cleavage planes into five bands. Each band arises from a lumbar spinous process and is innervated unisegmentally. The lumbar multifidus is therefore composed of five myotomes arranged such that the fibers that move a particular segment are innervated by the nerve of that segment (129).

With aging, the multifidus adopts an increasingly postural role as slow fibers predominate. Correspondingly, the muscle is less adapted to carrying out rapid phasic movements (130).

A technique for recording electromyographic (EMG) activity from specific lumbar segments of multifidus has been developed based on recent morphological studies.

In a study, bilateral EMG recordings of the lower four lumbar segments of multifidus were obtained during various movements of the trunk in the prone, standing, and sitting positions in a group of 17 normal subjects. The possibility of independent activity of the various segments of the muscle has been studied. Patterns of muscular activity during various movements of the trunk were described. A possible clinical application of the technique of specific lumbar segment EMG of multifidus has also been discussed (131).

MULTIFIDI AS ROTATOR MUSCLES OF THE LUMBAR SEGMENTS

From an analysis of the attachments of the various muscles, it could be discerned that all the lumbar back muscles act to increase the compressive load on the lumbar spine and tend to accentuate the lumbar lordosis. The action of the multifidus is at right angles to the spinous processes, so this muscle can act only as a posterior sagittal rotator of lumbar vertebrae. In addition to acting as posterior sagittal rotators, the lumbar fibers of the longissimus and iliocostalis muscles exert a significant component of their action in the horizontal plane, particularly at lower lumbar levels, and so are disposed to resist ventral translation of lower lumbar vertebrae (spondylolisthesis). These are the only muscles in the back that control ventral displacement of the lumbar vertebrae during flexion and reverse ventral displacement during extension. This action is ignored in current models of lumbar spine stability but must be considered as a factor that assists the ligaments and bony factors that prevent ventral displacement of lumbar vertebrae during flexion of the vertebral column (132).

CHEMISTRY OF THE INTERVERTEBRAL DISC AND APOPHYSEAL JOINT ARTICULATIONS

Since the major functions of the intervertebral disc appear to be mechanical, and since the overall mechanical properties of the annulus fibrosus as an organ and as a tissue are likely to be a function of the molecular chemistry and organization of its major structural component, collagen, one would expect, on general biological grounds and on a broad interpretation of Wolff's law applied at the molecular level, that there should be distinct differences in this component of the annulus fibrosus as a function of annulus geometry. One would expect portions of the annulus subjected to very different kinds and distributions of internal stresses and strains to reflect these structural differences by appropriate changes in the chemistry, interaction properties, and organization of collagen, the major structural component of the annulus fibrosus (133).

In support of this point of view, one may cite the following:

1. There is a significant overall increase in type I collagen in annuli fibrosi with increasing age;
2. Type I collagen increases principally in the outer lamellae of the posterior quadrant; and
3. The cells of the annulus fibrosus above a degenerative disc synthesize type I collagen almost exclusively. Thus, the synthesis of increased amounts of type I collagen, and the resorption of type II collagen and its replacement by type I collagen, may be directly and causally related to the eventual mechanical and biological failure of the annulus and of the intervertebral disc as a whole (133).

Nutritional Flow into Cartilage

The role of joint movement in the nutrition of adult cartilage has been well established. Exercise of the joint appears to increase the penetration of cartilage by nutrients from the synovial fluid. Maroudas et al. suggest that the squeezing of synovial fluid into and out of the cartilage surface produced by cyclical compression of cartilage is not a major factor but that the increased flow of nutrients from synovial fluid into cartilage is due more to the agitation of the fluid film on the cartilage surface during exercise. This would indicate that the nutrition of articular cartilage could be maintained by passive movement without concomitant loading of the joint surfaces (134).

All Discs Show Degeneration, Not Just One

Fifteen lumbar spines were collected postmortem (135). The intervertebral discs were assigned morphological grades and were analyzed for water, collagen, and proteoglycan.

In general, if any disc in a lumbar spine is degenerate, all discs in the spine will have a low proteoglycan concentration regardless of their morphological grade, suggesting that degeneration usually occurs only in spines in which all discs have a low proteoglycan concentration. Loss of proteoglycan from all discs would be associated with loss of water, with consequent narrowing of the disc spaces and excessive movement of the entire spinal segment (135).

Age Incidence of Disc Degeneration

Measurements of disc thickness, shape, and degeneration were recorded from 204 postmortem lumbar spines. The "true average disc height" increased with age as the discs "sank" into the vertebrae. These results add information to previous studies that indicate that the loss of transverse trabeculae of lumbar vertebrae is primarily responsible for the change in shape of both vertebrae and discs in the elderly. While the incidence of disc degeneration does increase in old age, the majority of the discs examined did not show evidence of any such change (136).

Collagen Changes by Enzyme Action

The collagenolytic enzyme systems in the normal and prolapsed human intervertebral discs have been studied. Normal discs obtained postmortem contained a novel collagenase with specificity toward type II collagen and gelatin but with little or no activity against type I collagen.

In summary, in the prolapsed disc there is a change in the normal pattern of collagenolytic enzymes. Instead of being directed against type II collagen, they are directed against type I collagen and elastin. It remains possible that this is a consequence of disc prolapse, but equally this alteration in enzyme pattern may be the precipitating factor in prolapse. This latter hypothesis will be further tested in animal experimentation (137).

Concepts of Pain Production by Damaged Disc Tissue

The concept that the intervertebral disc is per se biochemically active after injury has not yet been widely accepted in clinical practice. Crock (138) states:

1. The capillaries related to the vertebral endplate cartilage drain via a subarticular collecting vein system into the internal vertebral venous plexus or directly into veins of the marrow spaces in the spongiosa of the vertebral body.

2. Trauma to an intervertebral disc, inflicted by heavy lifting or by the high-speed application of force of short duration, may damage disc components, resulting in the production of irritant substances that may drain either into the spinal canal, irritating nerves, or into the vertebral body, thus setting up an autoimmune reaction.

3. The following clinical syndrome may then develop: *(a)* intractable back pain with aggravation of pain and loss of spinal motion with any physical exercise; *(b)* leg pain; *(c)* loss of energy; *(d)* marked weight loss; *(e)* profound depression.

4. Patients with this syndrome will be found to have: *(a)* normal plain roentgenograms of the spine; *(b)* normal myelograms; *(c)* normal CT scans of the spine; *(d)* usually normal blood examination; *(e)* normal neurological findings on clinical examination.

5. If this syndrome is present, *(a)* the patients will have abnormal discograms; *(b)* pain will be reproduced by as small a volume as 0.3 ml of dye, due to hypersensitivity of the pain fibers within the disc substance; *(c)* the final volume of dye accepted will be in excess of normal; *(d)* the discographic patterns on x-ray films will be abnormal.

This hypothesis suggests that in certain individuals, especially after trauma, a syndrome develops resulting from the production of chemical substances by the damaged disc tissues (138).

Disc degeneration is characterized histologically by loss of tissue in the nucleus, increasing thickness of the collagen fibers, and the occurrence of fissures both in the center and in the periphery of the disc. Insufficient diffusion into the disc has been said to account for premature disc degeneration.

In a study of the pH of discs of patients operated upon for lumbar rhizopathy, a marked decrease of pH was noted in some discs. These cases also showed an abundance of connective tissue scarring around the nerve roots.

A number of mechanisms could have caused this increase in hydrogen ion concentration, but a separate study demonstrated that the main factor was probably an increased concentration of lactic acid, the concentration of which was found to be directly correlated with the hydrogen ion concentration of the nucleus.

Thus, this study suggests that two nutritional routes are open for the intervertebral disc: *(a)* diffusion through the central portion of the end plate from marrow space cartilage contacts, and *(b)* diffusion through the annulus fibrosus from the surrounding vessels (139).

Does the Disc Have Circulation?

The imbibition of fluids into the nucleus pulposus has always interested this author, as it relates to the possible nutritional advantages of supplying minerals and glucosaminoglycan orally to patients with disc degeneration in an attempt to reverse the degenerative process. An exciting factor was shown by Eismont et al. (140) when they found penetration of antibiotics into the nucleus pulposus following an 8-hour course of intramuscular antibiotic injections.

Immunological Implications of Lumbar Disc Disease

Naylor et al. (141) state that a hypothesis to explain the chemical process of disc prolapse would include the initial change as a disturbance of the normal protein-polysaccharide synthesis-depolymerization equilibrium in favor of increased or unbalanced depolymerization, with the changes in the proteoglycan metabolism being associated with an increased fluid content and, thus, increased intradisc tension. This could then produce an episode of disc nuclear herniation. Five acid glycerophosphatases have been isolated from disc material. These lysosomal enzymes can be shown to degrade the intervertebral disc. Of these five acid glycerophosphatases isolated in normal nuclei, two have the same activity during prolapse, one has a lower activity, and the others have some deficiencies. The studies of Naylor et al. suggest that lysosomal enzymes present in the nucleus pulposus of the prolapsed intervertebral disc are capable of degrading the protein-polysaccharide complexes.

Elves et al. (142) studied 12 patients with prolapsed intervertebral discs. All patients had discectomy performed. Eight of these patients had protrusion, and four had sequestration or prolapse with free fragmentation of the disc. Three of the four patients with prolapse showed an immune response to their own disc material. None of those with protrusion gave a positive immune reaction.

Naylor et al. (141) found a significant enhancement of IgM and IgG in patients with lumbar disc prolapse. They suggest that either a nonspecific antigen process or stimulation of an antibody humoral system is the factor in the development of disc prolapse. Gertzbein (143) states that there is evidence for an autoimmune mechanism in the degeneration of the lumbar disc.

It was Falconer (as discussed in Ref. 141) who originally stated that, on myelography, defects could still be observed in patients whose low back and leg pain had been completely relieved. Thus, there is evidence to support the claim that the pain from disc prolapse is caused by chemical irritation as well as mechanical irritation of nerve roots. Once the degradation products of prolapse are dissipated, the relief of symptoms may be imminent.

Direct chemical analysis, x-ray crystallography, and electron microscopy have shown that disc degeneration shows a fall in the total sulfate, both keratin and chondroitin, although no pH change occurs. In disc herniation, there is a fall in total proteoglycan level, chiefly chondroitin sulfate, and probably in keratosulfate fractions.

The chemical explanation of disc prolapse expressed here is that initially there is a disturbance of the normal protein-polysaccharide synthesis which is associated with an increased fluid content and intradiscal pressure that produces the damage to the annulus, with repeated episodes producing advanced degeneration of the disc. *What creates these changes? The lysosomal enzymes of arthritis and rheumatoid arthritis are similar and may produce the disc changes of herniation.* Ruptured discs have been shown to release *acid phosphatase,* which degrades the protein-polysaccharide complexes of the intervertebral disc (141).

Bobechko and Hirsch (as discussed in Ref. 141) showed that the intervertebral disc could act as an antigen, with the common antigenic determinant located in the region of the glycosaminoglycan to the protein core.

IgM, IgG, and IgA have been isolated in the serum of patients with prolapse and not in the serum of normal healthy people (143). It is primarily IgG and IgM that are elevated in patients with lumbar disc prolapse.

A reaction between IgM and the protein polysaccharide complex has been shown to produce *amyloid* similar to that found in the amyloid-containing tissues of patients with rheumatoid arthritis (141).

Many believe that chronic degeneration of the disc is an autoimmune disease with antibodies directed at components of the nucleus pulposus which normally are shielded from the circulation and the reticuloendothelial system. A highly significant increase of serum IgM was reported in patients with proven Schmorl's nodes, narrowed disc spaces, or neurological signs of disc damage, compared with age-matched controls (144) (Fig. 2.101).

Chemical Irritation of a Nerve Root as a Pain Producer

DISC PROLAPSE AS CHEMICAL IRRITANT OF NERVE ROOT

For more than a decade, orthopedic surgeons have considered the likelihood of chemical irritation of the nerve root in association with disc prolapse as the cause of the very acute pain following injury. This view has arisen from the frequent finding at operation of a swollen, inflamed nerve root without bone pressure. The chemical content of the nerve root lists glycoprotein as a constituent. Previously, it was shown that the carbohydrate capsule of the pneumococcus liberates histamine and other H substances from per-

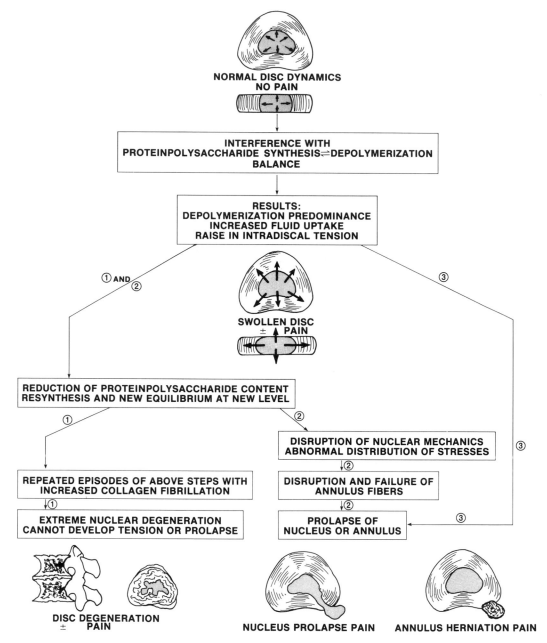

NORMAL DISC DYNAMICS
NO PAIN

INTERFERENCE WITH
PROTEINPOLYSACCHARIDE SYNTHESIS⇌DEPOLYMERIZATION
BALANCE

RESULTS:
DEPOLYMERIZATION PREDOMINANCE
INCREASED FLUID UPTAKE
RAISE IN INTRADISCAL TENSION

① AND ②   ③

SWOLLEN DISC
± ↑ PAIN

REDUCTION OF PROTEINPOLYSACCHARIDE CONTENT
RESYNTHESIS AND NEW EQUILIBRIUM AT NEW LEVEL

①   ②

DISRUPTION OF NUCLEAR MECHANICS
ABNORMAL DISTRIBUTION OF STRESSES   ③

REPEATED EPISODES OF ABOVE STEPS WITH   **DISRUPTION AND FAILURE OF**
INCREASED COLLAGEN FIBRILLATION   **ANNULUS FIBERS**

EXTREME NUCLEAR DEGENERATION   **PROLAPSE OF**
CANNOT DEVELOP TENSION OR PROLAPSE   **NUCLEUS OR ANNULUS**   ③

DISC DEGENERATION
± PAIN   **NUCLEUS PROLAPSE PAIN**   **ANNULUS HERNIATION PAIN**

Figure 2.101. This flow diagram explains the biomechanical hypothesis of the basic mechanisms of spine pain, disc prolapse, and disc degeneration. A number of mechanical factors mentioned in this chapter probably play a large role in the clinical presentation and outcome of these various biochemical phenomena. (Reproduced with permission from White AA, Panjabi MM: *Clinical Biomechanics of the Spine.* Philadelphia, JB Lippincott, 1978, p 291.)

fused organs much in the same way as venom. Direct tests of the nucleus pulposus pharmacologically show the presence of 1 to 4 μg of histamine per gram, but no tryptamine and no slow-reacting substance or kinin. Extract of the glycoprotein from human nucleus pulposus releases considerable quantities of histamines, edema fluid, protein, and another amine with four times the mobility of histamine from the isolated perfused lung of the guinea pig. The acute pain in disc lesion is due to local irritation of the nerve root producing edema and release of protein and H substances at the site of disc injury. Relief of pain by cortisone accords with these findings, since cortisone inhibits the peripheral response to II substances (145).

Disc Annular Irritation as Source of Low Back Pain

Anatomical studies have demonstrated the presence of nociceptive nerve endings in the annulus fibrosus of the lumbar intervertebral disc. Annular tears can, therefore, cause pain referral of purely discogenic origin into the low back, buttock, sacroiliac region, and lower extremity even in the absence of neural compression. Neural compression caused by an annular tear that has progressed to become a protruded disc is an obvious source of pain. Disc protrusion without neural compression can precipitate an inflammatory response with secondary radiculitis, raising the possibility of chemically induced inflammatory neural pain (146).

The lumbar zygapophyseal joints, i.e., facet joints, are well innervated and thus are potent potential pain generators. Facet arthropathy can cause low back pain as well as referral of pain into the buttock and lower extremity.

Basic anatomy and pathophysiology of lumbar nerve injury reveal that the motor (i.e., ventral) nerve root and sensory (i.e., dorsal) nerve root pass dorsal and lateral to the intervertebral disc.

EFFECTS OF SMOKING ON DISC CIRCULATION AND LOW BACK PAIN INCIDENCE

To open this discussion, I would like to cite an interesting study (147) on lung cancer incidence in smoking. Although it does not deal with low back pain, it is an important issue. In the study, the available epidemiological studies of lung cancer and exposure to other people's tobacco smoke (exposure was assessed by whether or not a person classified as a nonsmoker lived with a smoker) were identified and the results combined. There were 10 case-control studies and three prospective studies. Overall, there was a highly significant 35% increase in the risk of lung cancer among nonsmokers living with smokers compared with

nonsmokers living with nonsmokers (relative risk, 1.35; 95% confidence interval, 1.19 to 1.54). The increase in risk among nonsmokers living with smokers compared with a completely unexposed group was thus estimated as 53% (relative risk of 1.53).

This analysis, and the fact that nonsmokers breathe environmental tobacco smoke, which contains carcinogens, into their lungs, and that the generally accepted view is that there is no safe threshold for the effect of carcinogens, leads to the conclusion that breathing other people's tobacco smoke is a cause of lung cancer. About one-third of the cases of lung cancer in nonsmokers who live with smokers, and about one-quarter of the cases in nonsmokers in general, may be attributed to such exposure (147).

It is often thought by physicians that veterans have a much higher prevalence of smoking than the general population. To test this perception, all patient charts on the medical and surgical wards of the Denver Veterans Administration Hospital were reviewed on August 24, 1986, for reported smoking habits.

Nearly twice as many inpatients (50.7%; 74 of 146) as outpatients (27.0%; 126 of 466) were current smokers ($p < 0.001$, X^2). The age-adjusted smoking rate among inpatients (63.5%) was almost double the national rate (33%), while there was no significant difference between the outpatient rate (35.6%) ($p > 0.10$, Poisson) and the national rate.

There is indeed a high prevalence of smoking and smoking-related diseases among VA hospital inpatients. In contrast, outpatient veterans smoke at a rate similar to the national average (148).

Smoking Reduces Discal Circulation by 50%

Particularly in the case of large human discs in which the balance between nutrient utilization and supply is precarious, any loss in blood utilization and supply is precarious, and any loss in blood vessel contact or reduction in blood flow at the periphery of the disc could lead to nutritional deficiencies and build-up of waste products (149).

In an experimental study, the influence of cigarette smoke on nutrition of the intervertebral disc was investigated.

The animals used (six dogs and eight pigs)

were anesthetized, intubated, and kept ventilated in a respirator. An additional pumping system was attached to the respirator so that the smoke could be administered. During the testing time, blood gases and intradiscal oxygen tension were measured continuously. After the smoking period, radioactive isotopes (sulphate and methyl glucose) were introduced intravenously. The animals were sacrificed at various times after the infusion, and their spines were quickly excised and analyzed.

A smoking period of 3 hours reduced the transport efficiency to about 50%. The effect of smoke decreased when the exposure ceased. The concentration gradients were close to normal after 2 hours of "recovery."

These findings demonstrate that cigarette smoke significantly affects the circulatory system outside the intervertebral disc. The most pronounced effect was the reduction in solute exchange capacity. When there is reduction of the transport of substrate, which is necessary for the cells in order to fulfill the prevailing energy demands in the tissue, the inevitable consequence over a longer period of time will be deficient nutrition (149).

Smoking and Exercise Incidence in Low Back Pain

We compared the exercise and smoking habits of 576 patients suffering low back and leg pain with those of 50 persons who stated that they were asymptomatic. Thirty-three percent of low back and leg pain sufferers smoked, as compared to 14% of those without pain. Concerning exercise, 47% of low back or leg pain sufferers, as compared to 86% of nonsufferers, exercised regularly. Specifics as to the amount of smoking (by packs of cigarettes, amount of pipe tobacco, or number of cigars smoked daily) were given in this paper, as well as the number of times weekly a person exercised and for how long. A higher percentage of persons not suffering from low back or leg pain exercise regularly, more frequently, and longer at each session than those who suffer from these pains. Likewise, a higher percentage of those without low back and leg pain did not smoke, as compared to those who did have low back or leg pain. These statistics would indicate that there is less low back and leg pain in those who exercise regularly and avoid smoking (150).

Further factors concerning low back pain are of interest. Cigarette smoking was associated with an increased risk of prolapsed disc (151). A person's risk of prolapsed disc was increased by about 20% for each 10 cigarettes smoked per day, on the avearsge, during the past year.

Patients with severe low back pain were more likely to be cigarette smokers and had a greater tobacco consumption, as measured by both the number of cigarettes smoked per day and the number of years of exposure (152). Fifty-three percent of 288 men with severe low back pain smoked, while only 39.6% of 368 men without pain smoked, and 43.8% of 565 men with moderate low back pain smoked.

In a retrospective study, smoking was identified as being significantly associated with medically reported episodes of low back pain. Svensson (153) and Svensson and Andersson (154) identified a similar association in Swedish industrial workers, and they speculated that coughing leading to increased intradiscal pressure was the mechanism responsible for this relationship. A Danish study (155) supported this idea by identifying coughing and chronic bronchitis, but not smoking, as important in the etiology of low back complaints.

Frymoyer et al. (156) indicated that smoking and coughing were related to low back pain but that coughing alone was insufficient to account for the difference in back complaints in subjects who smoked. It might be that smokers have emotional, recreational, or occupational differences, although multivariate analysis of a retrospective and epidemiological survey did not confirm that speculation. The nicotine equivalent of one cigarette, when injected into a dog, may cause a reduction in the blood flow in the vertebral body. It is believed conceivable that decreased diffusion of nutrients into the disc by such alteration of blood flow could adversely affect discal metabolism and render the disc more susceptible to mechanical deformities (157).

Other studies have suggested that smoking and/or coughing is a risk factor for prolapsed lumbar disc (155, 158) and for back pain in general. In fact, it now seems that spinal disorders can be added to the rather long list of diseases associated with cigarette smoking. The mechanisms for the association with smoking are not entirely clear. One plausible mechanism is that smoking brings about coughing, which in turn puts more pressure on discs. In one study (152), the association of coughing with prolapsed lumbar disc was negligible. While this might suggest the existence of some other mechanism for the effect of smoking on intervertebral discs, the tendency of smokers to deny that they cough may also contribute to the lack of association with coughing. Smoking was identified as significantly associated with low back pain episodes reported by Frymoyer et al. (152), Svensson (153), and Svensson and Andersson (154). Svensson and colleague (153, 154) studied 940 Swedish men aged 40 to 47 years in a random sample as to low back pain in relation to other diseases. Included was the prevalence of smoking as one of nine variables correlated to low back pain. Smoking habits were evaluated in the following manner: those who had a daily consumption of 1 g of tobacco or who had stopped smoking within 3 months before the interview were considered to be smokers; persons who had never smoked or who had previously smoked continuously for less than 1 month were considered nonsmokers; and the remaining were regarded as ex-smokers. One cigarette was considered equivalent to 1 g of tobacco, and a cheroot 2 g. Four categories were used: 1 to 4, 5 to 14, 15 to 24, and 25 or more grams per day, respectively.

Of all men investigated, 42.5% were smokers, 23.2% were ex-smokers, and 34.2% were nonsmokers. Twenty-seven percent of the men had a daily consumption of more than 15 g of tobacco. The median value of the duration of the smoking habit among the smokers was 25 years. Productive cough was found in 21.1% of the men and breathlessness on exertion in 16.6%.

Svensson and colleague (153, 154) found that the proportion of smokers among the men with low back pain was larger than among the controls, and that the association between low back pain and smoking persisted in the analysis. This interesting finding was also reported by Frymoyer et al. (156). In recent years, a positive correlation between smoking and diminished mineral content of bone has been identified (159, 160). Microfractures of the trabeculae in the lumbar vertebral bodies caused by osteoporosis are a possible cause of low back pain (161). Further investigations will perhaps clarify the connection between smoking and low back pain.

Frymoyer et al. (156) analyzed the records of 3920 patients and found that 11% of males and 9.5% of females reported an episode of low back pain during a 3 year interval. The low back pain sufferers were more likely to be cigarette smokers, particularly when smoking was accompanied by a chronic cough. In 203 men aged 18 to 55 years with low back pain, 33% were smokers, while only 13.6% of 1649 men without low back pain were smokers ($p < 0.001$). Of 196 women aged 18 to 55 years with low back pain, 26% smoked, whereas of 1872 women without low back pain, on 12.1% smoked ($p < 0.001$).

Frymoyer et al. (156) believed this to be an unexpected association between low back pain and smoking. They speculated that smoking might influence low back pain by one of three possible mechanisms. First, smokers might possibly be constitutionally or emotionally selected in a biased fashion for the low back complaint. Although smoking was related to anxiety and depression, this was found in preliminary analysis to be uniform throughout the male and female populations with and without low back pain. Hence there does not appear to be a specific selective bias for low back pain patients who smoke and also have other psychological risk factors to a greater extent than the population at large. Second, smoking might produce significant hormonal and/or other alterations that increase the low back pain. Third, smoking might produce other problems that lead to a greater incidence of low back pain. Those patients who had low back pain had a greater reported incidence of chronic cough, and this suggests the possibility that mechanical stresses induced by coughing may be relevant to the low back complaint. The extent to which chronic coughing and smoking are related to this population is currently under study. Biering-Sorenson (162) identified coughing, but not smoking, as important in the etiology of low back complaints.

SHORT-LEG BIOMECHANICS AND BASIC CORRECTION

The possible association between pelvic obliquity and low back pain was investigated in low back pain patients and a control population (163).

The clinical importance of leg length inequality depends on the degree of the inequality and its relationship with a number of conditions and problems:

1. A possible correlation between the resultant pelvic obliquity and any degenerative changes in the lumbar spine such as arthrosis, spondylosis, etc.;
2. A possible association with low back pain;
3. A correlation with hip joint degenerative changes;

4. A correlation with knee joint degenerative changes—"long leg arthropathy";
5. Psychological difficulties associated with the esthetic consequences of the postural deformity.

However, the vast majority of patients with leg length inequality of 1 cm or more have no known etiology for this inequality, which arises during normal growth without any apparent pathology.

Radiographic asymmetric structural changes in the lumbar spine, which appear to be correlated with pelvic obliquity and the consequent postural lumbar scoliosis, were described in two groups of nonacute low back pain patients: those with a leg length difference of greater than 9 mm, and those with no leg length difference (0 to 3 mm). With leg length inequality, concavities in the end plates of lumbar vertebral bodies, wedging of the fifth lumbar vertebra, and traction spurs appear (164).

Disc Protrusion on Long-Leg Side

In 700 patients, aged 14 to 89 years, with chronic low back pain, the incidence of leg length inequality (LLI) was two to five times that observed in the sympton-free control group. In a series of 228 cases of sciatica, the pain radiated to the longer leg in 78%. In 241 cases, the chronic unilateral hip pain symptoms and arthrotic changes were located on the long-leg side. In 73% of 180 cases with chronic unilateral knee symptoms and arthroses, the symptoms were found on the short-leg side (165).

These observations may logically be interpreted by the biomechanical effects of LLI on the musculoskeletal system. Pelvic tilt caused by LLI is generally compensated with a functional scoliosis convex to the short-leg side. During bending of lumbar motion segments, the discs are compressed on the concave side of the curve and put a tensile load on the opposite side. On the compression side, the disc bulges. In case of LLI, the disc bulges in the posterolateral direction toward the spinal nerve root on the long-leg side. The lateral bending of the lumbar motion segment is always coupled with an axial rotation, so that the posterior elements tend to rotate toward the concavity of the curve. These complicated bending and torsional loads on lower intervertebral joints, ligaments, and especially on discs may be etiological factors for low back symptoms associated with LLI (165).

Hip Osteodegenerative Arthritis on Long-Leg Side

Present knowledge of hip biomechanics supports the contention that the stresses imposed on the hip on the side of the longer leg are greater than normal; those on the short side are comparably reduced. Indirect measurements by various authors have demonstrated greater stress on the hip if the pelvis is adducted, a persistent and chronic condition of the hip joint on the side of a long leg. Furthermore, the pressure on the acetabulum will be displaced laterally in those circumstances. The consistent pattern of degeneration in unilateral superolateral osteoarthritis of the hip is what would be expected if the consequences of leg length disparity were as described. Leg length inequality may be a major contributing factor in the development of unilateral degenerative disease of the hip of this type (166).

Gauging Leg Length Inequality

A useful way to estimate leg length disparity clinically employs the same postural considerations outlined in the discussion of x-ray methodology. The patient stands with the feet parallel and about 7 inches apart. The examiner sits behind the patient. The patient should stand erect and look forward, not downwards. The knees must be straight and the pelvis centered over the feet. If significant leg length disparity exists, three observations will be made: (a) the upper lateral thigh on the long side will protrude; (b) scoliosis will be apparent; (c) the examiner's hands placed on top of the iliac crests will rest at different heights. All three of these findings should be present if the estimation of disparity is to be trusted.

The next step is to place, under the foot of the presumed short side, a block of an appropriate thickness (e.g., 1/4 inch, 3/8 inch, 1/2 inch) and to repeat the observations. The thighs should now be symmetrical, the spine straight, and the hands level.

The final step, and one that should not be omitted, is to place the same block under the presumed longer leg. The three observations originally made should now be exaggerated. Unless these simple checks confirm the initial observations, the reliability of the estimate of leg length disparity is in doubt. The size of the block necessary to bring the pelvis to an appropriate level is an indication of the amount of disparity (166).

Short-Leg Incidence and Correction

This author (J.M.C.) (167) found that 11% of 576 low back cases had a leg length discrepancy of more than 6 mm after maximum correction of the patient's mechanical faults had been performed and maximum improvement attained. In that study, 6 mm was the minimal shortness of one femoral head that was corrected. Up to 9 mm difference, a heel lift was inserted. Over 10 mm difference, the entire lift was placed on the heel and 5 mm less under the sole of the shoe. Also, if desire for vanity purposes, up to 9 mm could be placed inside the shoe and the remainder of a lift over 9 mm placed under the heel and sole.

Correction of Leg Length Disparity in This Author's Clinic

To outline the treatment protocol used in our clinic to correct leg length disparities, a study will be summarized which examined visual leg length insufficiency detection and correction as compared with established radiographic procedures on 41 consecutive patients.

Cailliet (168) uses visual correction with three points of reference to determine short leg and its correction: (a) iliac crest levelness; (b) vertical appraisal of the spine from the sacral base (the spine should be perpendicular to the sacral base); and (c) levelness of the posterosuperior iliac spine (PSIS) dimples. Lifts of varying thickness are placed under the foot of the short leg in both leg length corrective procedures.

Cailliet's study (168) found that the visual method of measurement did not differ significantly from the x-ray method of measurement for leg length insufficiency. This allowed us to level the iliac crests on the short-leg side and low hemipelvis in comparison to the opposite side by placing lifts under the short extremity. We then took an x-ray through the femoral heads with the patient standing to confirm that the heads were now indeed level. In 75% of the cases of short leg, the buildup seen visually to level the pelvic iliac crests was the amount needed on x-ray to correct for the insufficiency. This allowed us to minimize radiation to the patient by having only to take one x-ray to confirm levelness of the femoral heads. In the other 25% of cases, we had to add to or subtract from the buildup until we found correction.

PROCEDURE TO LEVEL THE ILIAC CRESTS FOR SHORT-LEG CORRECTION

The patient is examined standing barefoot with both legs fully extended at the same distance apart as the femoral heads. First, at arms length, the doctor places one index finger on each iliac crest and evaluates the horizontal level of the pelvis. It is desirable for the crests to be level. If they are not, a short leg may be present, and there may be a need for correction. Secondly, the "dimples" noted in most people in the region of the sacroiliac joints can be "lined up" by eye and furnish another estimate of pelvic level. It is also desirable to have the dimples horizontal. We found that, except in obese or very thin patients, the dimples were easily visualized. The third phase of visual evaluation involves observation of the lumbar spine in its vertical position related to the base of the sacrum. The spinous processes of the vertebrae are usually prominent and can be seen in the groove created by the erector spinae muscle groups. The desired position of the spine is at a right angle to the sacral base. If an oblique vertical position is noted, either the spine is curved or the sacral base is not level. A short leg may curve the spine or tilt the sacral base. These observations were used as indicators of discrepancy.

If these three clinical methods of determining pelvic obliquity indicated any leg length discrepancy, correction was performed. Boards of predetermined and marked thickness were placed under the foot of the short leg until the pelvis became horizontal as gauged by the three methods described above. The board thickness required to achieve a level pelvis is the shortness of the leg corrected. Board thickness was either 3, 6, 12, 18, or 25 mm (Fig. 2.102).

Following the visual determination and correction of the pelvic inferiority, radiographic short-leg study was performed with the patient barefoot in an upright position. Focal film distance was 40 inches, with the central ray centered anterior-to-posterior at the height of the femoral heads. (In accordance with Chamberlain's view (169), the patient's feet must be directly under the femoral heads in order to prevent distortion (167). Giles and Taylor (170) note that the x-ray tube must be at the height of the femoral heads to avoid artificially inducing differences due to the divergent ray (171).) The radiological technician was not informed of the visual correction previously recorded. When the film was viewed, a

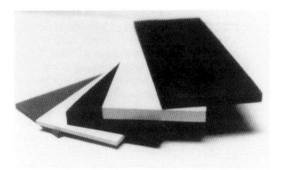

Figure 2.102. Lifts used in corrective procedures. (Reproduced with permission from Aspegren DD, Cox JM, Trier KK: Short leg correction: a clinical trial of radiographic vs. non-radiographic procedures, *Journal of Manipulative and Physiological Therapeutics,* vol 10, issue 5, pp 233–237, ©by the National College of Chiropractic, 1987.)

horizontal line was drawn perpendicular to the vertical side of the film across the top of the highest femoral head (Fig. 2.103). The same boards used to level the pelvis previously were used to build up the short leg and level the femoral heads

(Fig. 2.104). The board was placed under the entire sole on the side of the low femoral head. A second x-ray was taken to confirm the proper height requried for correction (Fig. 2.105).

RESULTS

The overall results of the study show that, in 13 of 41 cases, visual determination was as accurate as radiographic appraisal. A second group of 13 cases were correct within 3 mm when compared to the x-ray standard. Six were off by 6 mm, and eight by 9 mm. One patient was corrected and found to be 12 mm off when compared to the standing x-ray films.

In reviewing the results, it was generally found that the difference between visual and x-ray measurements for leg length insufficiency and musculoskeletal disorders is minimal. Table 2.4 demonstrates that the mean x-ray measurement is 4.73 mm. Ranges and standard deviations are also equal.

Furthermore, in testing for a significant difference between visual and x-ray measures (Table 2.5), it is found that the Z score is 0.128, which is

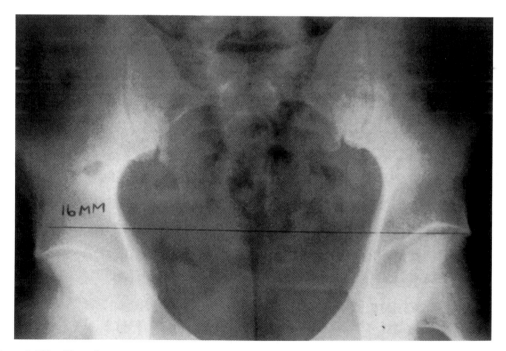

Figure 2.103. X-ray demonstrating 16-mm difference in femoral head height. (Reproduced with permission from Aspegren DD, Cox JM, Trier KK: Short leg correction: a clinical trial of radiographic vs. non-radiographic procedures, *Journal of Manipulative and Physiological Therapeutics,* vol 10, issue 5, pp 233–237, ©by the National College of Chiropractic, 1987.)

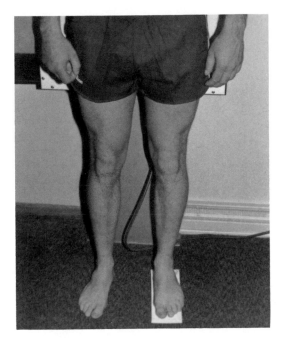

Figure 2.104. Photograph of patient being radiographed with short leg build-up in place.

not significant at the $P = 0.05$ level. Therefore, the null hypothesis stands, which says that there is no difference between the two types of measurements.

Technically, x-ray measurement is considered most accurate. Table 2.6 shows that 15 of the visual measurements equal the x-ray measurement, while 14 are less than and 12 are greater than the x-ray measurement. There is a significant relationship between visual and x-ray measures. The η^2 further shows that the relationship is very strong (0.885).

Table 2.4.
Description of Visual and X-ray Measurements[a]

Concept	Mean[b]	Range[b]	SD[b]	η
Visual	4.88	0–19	5.28	41
X-ray	4.73	0–19	5.03	41

[a]Reproduced with permission from Aspegren DD, Cox JM, Trier KK: Short leg correction: a clinical trial of radiographic vs. non-radiographic procedures, *Journal of Manipulative and Physiological Therapeutics*, vol 10, issue 5, pp 233–237, © by the National College of Chiropractic, 1987.
[b]Measurements are all reported in millimeters.

Table 2.5.
Is There a Difference between Visual and X-ray Measurements?[a]

Concept	Mean	SD	Z[b]
Visual	4.88	5.28	0.128
X-ray	4.73	5.03	

[a]Reproduced with permission from Aspegren DD, Cox JM, Trier KK: Short leg correction: a clinical trial of radiographic vs. non-radiographic procedures, *Journal of Manipulative and Physiological Therapeutics*, vol 10, issue 5, pp 233–237, © by the National College of Chiropractic, 1987.
[b]Note: The Z score is not significant at the $P = 0.05$ level.

This study found that the visual method of measurement did not differ significantly from the x-ray method of measurement for leg length insufficiency. Furthermore, it was found that, when comparing those cases in which the visual measurement was less than the x-ray measurement and those in which the visual measurement was greater, there was a significant relationship between visual and x-ray measurements. The η^2 demonstrates that there is a very strong relationship between visual and x-ray methods of measurement.

Table 2.6.
Is There a Difference between Those Visual Scores That Are Less Than and Those That Are Greater Than X-ray Measurement?[a]

Visual scores equal to x-ray = 15
Visual scores less than x-ray = 14
Visual scores greater than x-ray = 12

	ANOVA Analysis			
Dependent variable:	X-ray measurement			
Independent variables:	Sum SQ	DF	F	SIG
Visual	797.55	4	54.9	0
Groups	325.70	2	44.8	0
Between groups (explained)	893.80	8	30.8	0
Within groups (error)	116.25	32		
Total	1010.05	40		

[a]Reproduced with permission from Aspegren DD, Cox JM, Trier KK: Short leg correction: a clinical trial of radiographic vs. non-radiographic procedures, *Journal of Manipulative and Physiological Therapeutics*, vol 10, issue 5, pp 233–237, © by the National College of Chiropractic, 1987.
[b]To determine strength of relationship: Eta (η^2) = 0.885.

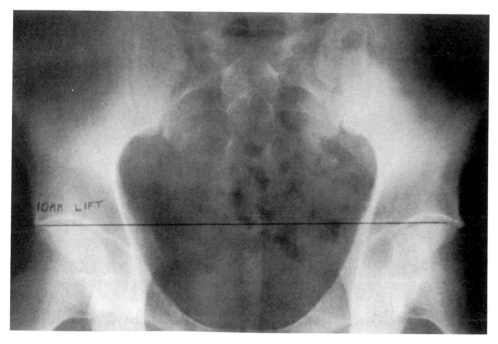

Figure 2.105. Same patient as in Figure 2.103, only requiring 10 mm to level the femoral heads. (Reproduced with permission from Aspergren DD, Cox JM, Frier KK: Short leg correction: a clinical trial of radiographic vs. non-radiographic procedures, *Journal of Manipulative and Physiological Therapeutics,* vol 10, issue 5, pp 233–237, © by the National College of Chiropractic, 1987.)

LUMBAR SPINE MOTION DYNAMICS AND ABERRANCIES

A nonlinear three-dimensional finite element program (Fig. 2.106) has been used to analyze the response of a lumbar L2-L3 motion segment subjected to axial torque alone and combined with compression. Torsion is primarily resisted by the articular facets that are in contact and by the disc annulus. The ligaments play an insignificant role in this respect. For the intact segment, with an increase in torque, the axis of rotation shifts posteriorly in the disc so that under maximum torque it is located posterior to the disc itself (Fig. 2.107). Loss of disc pressure increases this posterior shift, whereas removal of the facets decreases it. Torque, by itself, cannot cause the failure of disc fibers but can enhance the vulnerability of those fibers located at the posterolateral and posterior locations when the torque acts in combination with other types of loading, such as flexion. The most vulnerable element of the segment in torque is the posterior bony structure (172).

Further analysis by the L2-L3 three-dimensional study showed (173):

1. The motion segment exhibits stiffening effects with increasing sagittal plane moments. It is found to be stiffer in extension than in flexion. The segmental stiffness reduces slightly in flexion with the loss of disc pressure and considerably in extension with the removal of the facets.

2. In contrast to the case under flexion moment, when relatively high intradiscal pressures are generated, under extension moment negative pressures (suction type) of low magnitude are predicted.

3. The presence of large intradiscal pressure resists the inward bulge of the inner annulus layers. However, when the disc loses its pressure, the inner annulus layers at the anterior region bulge inward markedly under flexion moment.

4. Comparison of the predicted stresses and strains in the various segmental materials with their reported ultimate values leads to the following conclusions: (*a*) Ligaments: Only the vulnerability of the interspinous ligament to rupture at its medial site can be concluded. (*b*) Annulus ground substance: Large tensile radial strains are computed to occur at anterior and posterior locations under flexion and extension mo-

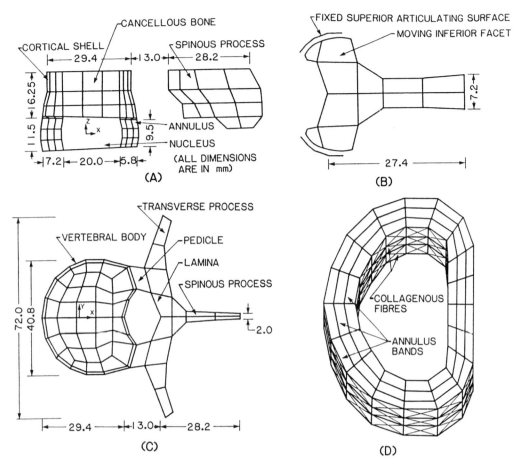

Figure 2.106. Finite element grid of the motion segment. **A,** Sagittal cross-section; **B,** horizontal section of the posterior bony elements at $z = 5$ mm; **C,** horizontal cross section at $z = 22$ mm; **D,** annulus layers and fiber orientation. Measurement of z is done at the sagittal cross-section at the top level of the upper vertebral body as a function of axial torque. (Reproduced with permission from Shirazi-Adl A, Ahmed AM, Shrivastava SC: Mechanical response of a lumbar motion segment in axial torque alone and combined with compression. *Spine* 11(9):915–924, 1986.)

ments, respectively. Such strains may cause circumferential clefts between the annulus layers, the frequency of occurrence of which is reported to increase with age. Large tensile axial strains are also predicted, which may correspond with the observation of horizontal splits in the annulus parallel to the end plates (173). (*c*) Annulus collagenous fibers: The maximum fiber strains are computed to be larger in flexion than in extension and occur posterolaterally in the innermost annulus layer of a normal disc. Loss of disc pressure reduces these strains. The fact that the magnitude of the maximum fiber strain is larger than the fibers' reported elastic limit and that the maximum strains occur at the posterolateral fibers in

the normal disc suggests that hyperflexion in combination with other types of loading might induce failure of these fibers commonly seen in conjunction with disc prolapse (173).

Mechanical Factors in Lumbar Motion

In cadaver studies, sustained lordosis produced abnormal loading of apophyseal joints. Forward bending wedged the discs, rendering them vulnerable to fatigue injuries (174). Excessive flexion at some spinal levels caused posterior ligament damage, and a strong contraction of the

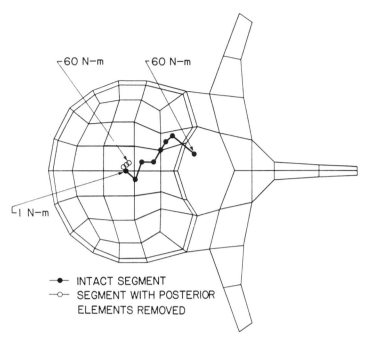

⌐60 N–m   ⌐60 N–m

⌐1 N–m

—●— INTACT SEGMENT
—○— SEGMENT WITH POSTERIOR
      ELEMENTS REMOVED

Figure 2.107. Predicted change in the location of the axis of rotation with increasing torque (1 N-m to 60 N-m) at the top level of the upper vertebral body. (Reproduced with permission from Shirazi-Adl A, Ahmed AM, Shrivastava SC: Mechanical response of a lumbar motion segment in axial torque alone and combined with compression. *Spine* 11(9):915–924, 1986.)

back muscles then caused prolapse of the intervertebral disc.

The center of rotation for flexion was just anterior to the center of the disc. The average forward bending force necessary to damage an intervertebral joint in flexion was 4938 N (1097.3 lb). Most resistance came from the disc and capsular ligaments. The supraspinous and interspinous ligaments were slack for the few degrees of flexion but were the first structures to sustain damage at the limit of the physiological range, which averaged 8.4° of flexion. Data on the tensile properties of the apophyseal joint capsule ligaments were used to predict that these ligaments would be damaged after 11.6° of flexion on the average.

The center of rotation for axial rotation was poorly defined but was usually located in the posterior annulus or neural arch. Nearly all of the resistance to torsion came from the disc and the facet surfaces in compression, with the percentage from each depending on the location of the center of rotation. On compression, the apophyseal joints of nondegenerated discs sustained damage after only 1° to 3° of rotation, and those in degenerated discs sustained damage after 7° of rotation. Resistance for isolated discs to torque was found to be smooth and reproducible for at least 10°. The authors of these cadaver studies (174) believe that the *disc was not damaged by rotation, since they found that the disc was capable of 10° of rotation.* They also believe that the facet would fracture before the disc would tear. They point out that *flattening or slight flexion of the lumbar curve unloads the facets and compresses the disc which would not be damaged, as is the facet.* They believe that *lordosis is the cause of pain and degeneration of the facets.* Full flexion can distort the lamellae of the disc, giving rise to radial fissures in the annulus which can produce pain and protrusion of the nucleus. Therefore, according to them the order of damage in heavy lifting injuries is:

1. Damage to the supraspinous and interspinous ligaments;
2. Damage to the capsular ligaments of the apophyseal joints;
3. Prolapse of the disc occurring with muscular contraction and hyperflexion of the lumbar spine.

The combination of a degenerated annulus and a turgid nucleus is the most vulnerable to injury. *A slightly protruding nucleus can cause bleeding of the posterior longitudinal ligament that can cause pain.*

The term *functional spinal unit* (FSU) replaces the term *motion segment.* Posner et al. (175) defined the FSU as being the ligament, apophyseal joints, and disc joining two adjacent vertebrae. Posner et al. attempted to determine the stability and instability of the lumbar FSU. Seven lumbar spines and sacra were removed from cadavers within 6 hours of death; the spines were subjected to flexion and extension experiment. In flexion, intertransverse and posterior longitudinal ligaments and the disc failed, with the end plates pulling off the vertebral bodies. In extension, the intertransverse ligament again failed, whereas the apophyseal capsule and the ligamentum flavum pulled off their attachments to the bone.

Effects of Flexion and Extension on the Lumbar Structures

The effects of flexion (Fig. 2.108) on the lumbar spine are:

1. Decrease in the intraspinal protrusion of the lumbar intervertebral disc;
2. Slight increase in the length of the anterior wall of the spinal canal;
3. Significant increase in the length of the posterior wall of the spinal canal;
4. Stretching and a decreased bulge of the yellow ligaments within the spinal canal;
5. Stretching and a decreased cross-sectional area of nerve roots;
6. An overall general increase in spinal canal volume and decreased nerve root bulk.

The effects of extension (Fig. 2.109) are:

1. Bulging of the intervertebral discs into the spinal canal;
2. Slight decrease in the anterior canal length;
3. Moderate decrease in the posterior canal length;
4. Enfolding and protrusion of the yellow ligaments into the spinal canal;
5. Relaxation and an increase in the cross-sectional diameter of the nerve roots;
6. An overall decrease in the volume of the lumbar spinal canal and an increased nerve root bulk.

For these reasons, patients seek flexion for relief of back pain, and this is the premise on which the use of flexion distraction manipulation for correction of disc protrusion is based.

EFFECTS OF FLEXION AND EXTENSION ON THE LUMBAR CANAL

Breig (as discussed in Ref. 176) has shown that extension of the lumbar spine causes protrusion of the intervertebral disc with dorsal displacement of the cauda equina roots. On myelography, Ehni and Weinstein (176) showed that extension produces total block and flexion permits the contrast medium to pass through the blocked area. Reaching overhead or bending backward causes the common complaint of painful paresthesia or numbness in both legs (177).

Dyck et al. (177) showed that extension pro-

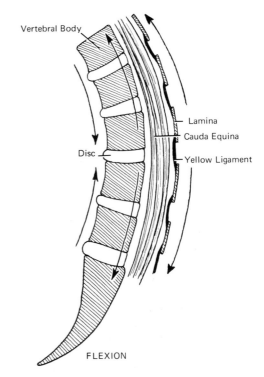

Figure 2.108. Increased spinal canal volume and decreased nerve root (cauda equina) bulk with flexion. (Reproduced with permission from Finneson BE: *Low Back Pain,* ed 2. Philadelphia, JB Lippincott, 1980, p 432.)

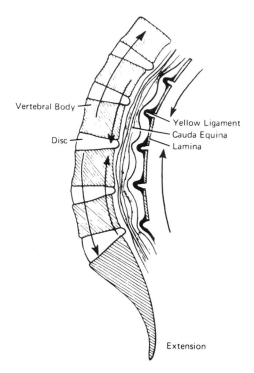

Vertebral Body

Yellow Ligament
Cauda Equina
Lamina

Disc

Extension

Figure 2.109. Decreased spinal canal volume and increased nerve root bulk with extension. (Reproduced with permission from Finneson BE: *Low Back Pain*, ed 2. Philadelphia, JB Lippincott, 1980, p 432.)

motes lumbar stenosis and forward flexion reduces it.

Raney (178) performed a series of myelograms that showed that with flexion of the lumbar spine, the posterior bulge of the posterior annulus and posterior longitudinal ligament disappeared as the anterior margin of the vertebral bodies approached each other and the posterior margins separated. The myelographic column became flat, and the dural sac closely approximated the back of the posterior longitudinal ligament and annulus. Even though the force propelling the disc posteriorly is increased by flexion, the tightening of the posterior annulus and posterior longitudinal ligament in flexion improves the barrier to a greater extent, with the net effect being reduction of the posterior protrusion. In prolapse, this relief has not been found. Therefore, the flexed position obliterates the disc bulge and relieves the irritated nerve root in the bulging disc.

Pilling (179), who performed myelography on patients in the upright position, showed that a protrusion is reduced in the flexion position because the posterior longitudinal ligament and annulus are stretched and the disc spaces are widened posteriorly. A prolapse would not show such reduction.

With epidurography, Matthews and Yates (180) showed that with distraction of 120 lb, there is reduction of a disc protrusion.

Extension causes the ligamentum flavum, the disc, and the posterior longitudinal ligament to narrow the sagittal diameter of the vertebral canal, whereas flexion reverses this (181).

McNeil et al. (182) demonstrated the extensor muscles to be the weakest in the low back. We, therefore, exercise them after the patient has had relief of his low back and leg pain.

White and Panjabi (2) showed that with bending of the spine, the disc bulges on the concave side of the curve and collapses on the convex side of the curve. In flexion, the disc protrudes anteriorly and depresses posteriorly.

Finneson (77) showed disc protrusion on extension and reduction on flexion (Figs. 2.108 and 2.109).

EFFECTS OF FLEXION AND EXTENSION ON THE SPINE

Cadaveric lumbar motion segments (consisting of two vertebrae and the intervening disc and ligaments) were loaded to simulate forward bending movements in life, and the flexion angle at the elastic limit was measured (183). These flexion angles were then compared with flexion angles obtained from x-rays of healthy volunteers in the erect standing and fully flexed positions. The comparison showed that, when people adopt the static, fully flexed posture, the osteoligamentous lumbar spine is flexed about 10° short of its elastic limit.

The results imply that the lumbar spine is normally well protected by the back muscles in the relaxed, fully flexed posture. Special mechanisms must be identified to explain forward bending injuries.

For a typical motion segment, a 2° reduction in flexion means a 50% reduction in the resistance to bending moment, and hence a 50% reduction in the bending stresses in the posterior annulus and intervertebral ligaments. At the limit of the range of flexion, the osteoligamentous spine resists a bending moment equal to about 50% of that exerted by the upper body in forward bending. This means that at the more moderate angles of flexion found in life, only about 5% (i.e., 50% of 50%) of the upper body's forward bending moment will be resisted by the spine; the rest will be resisted by the lumbodorsal fascia, back muscles, etc. Therefore, it appears that there is little chance of damaging the lumbar spine in the static toe-touching posture (183).

For flexion/extension mode, more mobility exists at the L4-L5 level than at L1-L2. For lateral bending mode, more mobility is observed at the L1-L2 level than at the L4-L5 level (184).

EFFECTS OF FLEXION AND EXTENSION ON DURAL SAC DURING MYELOGRAPHY

Penning and Wilmink (185) performed measurements on 40 lateral lumbar myelograms in flexion and extension with the object of analyzing changes in position and shape of the dural sac in spinal movements. There proved to be an anterior displacement of the entire lumbar dural sac in lumbar extension, most likely caused by shortening and thickening of the flaval ligaments. In addition, the anterior dural surface was indented at the L3-L4 and L4-L5 interspaces by posterior bulging of the discs in extension. This encroachment was partially compensated by dual bulging into areas with a rich and compressible venous plexus behind the vertebral bodies and the L5-S1 disc. While the patterns of dural movements showed individual variations, these trends were found in all diagnostic and anatomical subgroups. One subgroup (with root involvement at L4-L5) showed marked dorsal encroachment upon the dural sac in extension at the same level.

In distinction to these posture-dependent changes in cross-sectional area of the spinal canal, Breig (186) has stressed the influence of flexion-extension movements upon longitudinal spinal dimensions. In spinal flexion, there is marked elongation of the spinal canal with concomitant stretching of the dural sac and nerve root fibers. This is thought to have a bearing on the production of nerve root symptoms in cases with disc herniation (185).

MODERATE FLEXION FINDS LUMBAR SPINE STRONGEST

Accurate measurement of lumbar spine curvature is important because the curvature affects the stresses acting on the apophyseal joints and

intervertebral discs. In moderate flexion, the lumbar spine is at its strongest; in full flexion, the discs are vulnerable to fatigue damage, and in hyperflexion, the intervertebral ligaments can be sprained and the discs can prolapse suddenly. Therefore, in order to evaluate the risks of a job involving bending and lifting, it is necessary to measure how much the lumbar curve is flexed in each bending movement (187).

Forty-one cadaveric lumbar intervertebral joints from 18 spines were flexed and fatigue-loaded to simulate a vigorous day's activity. The joints were then bisected and the discs examined. Twenty-three out of 41 of the discs showed distortions in the lamellae of the annulus fibrosus and, in a few of these, complete radial fissures were found in the posterior annulus (188).

FLEXED POSTURES IMPROVE TRANSPORT OF METABOLITES

A study (190) compared postures that flatten (that is, flex) the lumbar spine with those that preserve the lumbar lordosis. Flexed postures have several advantages: flexion improves the transport of metabolites in the intervertebral discs, reduces the stresses on the apophyseal joints and on the posterior half of the annulus fibrosus, and gives the spine a high compressive strength. Flexion also has disadvantages: it increases the stress on the anterior annulus and increases the hydrostatic pressure in the nucleus pulposus at low load levels.

The disadvantages are not of much significance, and we conclude that it is mechanically and nutritionally advantageous to flatten the lumbar spine when sitting and when lifting heavy weights (190).

FLEXION OCCURRENCE AT PELVIS VERSUS LOW BACK

In normal subjects, lumbar motion accounts for 63% of gross flexion, with 37% due to pelvic motion in the range up to about 90° of flexion. Low back pain subjects exhibit less gross motion than normal subjects (54%), with the ratio of lumbar flexion to gross flexion decreased from 63% to 43%. Range-of-motion exercising can significantly increase functional pain-free range both in lumbar (71%) and pelvic (39%) motion over a 3-week period (191).

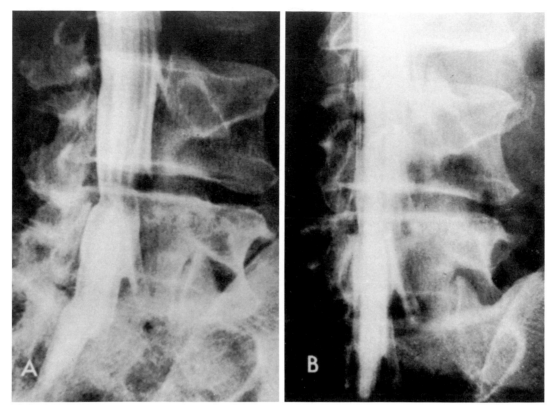

Figure 2.110. Effects of lumbar flexion-extension movements upon root involvement. **A,** Water-soluble lumbar myelogram, RPO projection, showing compression of the emerging left L5 root in extension (*left*), with swelling of nerve root and cutoff of root sheath filling. Note also dorsal indentation in dural sac at same level. **B,** Flexion view (*right*) shows that compression of L5 root and dural sac has been relieved. Right L5 root (not illustrated) showed similar posture-dependent involvement. (Reproduced with permission from Penning L, Wilmink JT: Posture-dependent bilateral compression of L4 or L5 nerve roots in facet hypertrophy. *Spine* 12(5):489, 1987.)

EFFECTS OF FLEXION AND EXTENSION ON THE SPINAL CANAL

Myelographic studies show that flexion opens the anterolateral angles of the spinal canal, creating relief of the nerve roots. Conversely, extension closes the anterolateral angles, causing bilateral root involvement, as evidenced by the conventional myelogram in extension (Fig. 2.110). In extension, nerve root involvement signs are maximal, while in flexion they tend to disappear (192, 193). This seems to indicate some posture-dependent narrowing of the spinal canal rather than disc herniation as the cause of the problem. Facet hypertrophy, both of the facet and its covering ligaments, has long been felt to be a possible factor in narrowing of the spinal canal (194, 195), but difficult to prove in plain radiography of the lumbar spine. Penning and Wilmink (196)

were able to show the presence of facet hypertrophy, sometimes in combination with an abnormally bulging but not necessarily herniated disc.

In 12 patients with myelographic evidence of bilateral root involvement at the L3-L4 or L4-L5 levels, postmyelographic CT studies were performed in flexion and extension. They showed concentric narrowing of the spinal canal in extension, and widening with relief of nerve root involvement in flexion (Fig. 2.111). This could be attributed to the presence of marked degenerative hypertrophy of the facet joints, narrowing the available space for dural sac and emerging root sleeves. In extension of the lumbar spine, bulging of the disc toward the hypertrophic facets causes a pincers mechanism at the anterolateral angles of the spinal canal, with the risk of bilateral root compression. This mechanism is enhanced in these cases by marked dorsal indentation of the dural sac because of anterior move-

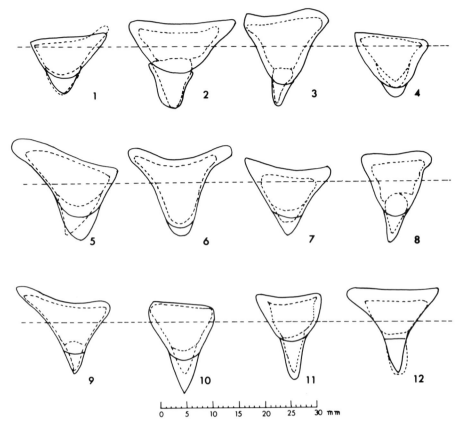

Figure 2.111. Drawings of dural sac and dorsal fat pad outlines in flexion and extension in the 12 patients. Drawings are made by tracing the outlines of dural sac and dorsal fat pad from maximally (4X) enlarged CT slices. *Solid lines* = outlines in flexion. *Broken lines* = outlines in extension. The *horizontal line* represents the interfacet line. (Reproduced with permission from Penning L, Wilmink JT: Posture-dependent bilateral compression of L4 or L5 nerve roots in facet hypertrophy. *Spine* 12(5):495, 1987.)

ment of the dorsal fat pad in extension. The authors of the study believe that the radiologically described mechanism forms the anatomical basis of neurogenic claudication and posture-dependent sciatica (196).

The closing of the anterolateral angles can be explained by bulging of the disc in extension, as shown in Figure 2.112. This bulging, described by Knuttson (197), in 1942, among others, is a physiological phenomenon caused by the approximation of the dorsal parts of the vertebral end plates. Thus, no disc pathology is needed to explain the narrowing or complete occlusion of the anterolateral angles of the spinal canal in facet hypertrophy. This facet hypertrophy may reduce the distance between disc and facet to such a

degree that normal disc bulging in extension is sufficient to close the lateral recesses. In the majority of the patients, the dorsal surface of the disc had a symmetric appearance. It is possible that, in some of these instances, disc bulging in extension was pathologically increased due to disc degeneration and subsequent approximation of adjoining vertebrae, but this was impossible to measure. More marked asymmetry was noted in a minority of patients, indicating that disc pathology (abnormal bulging, disc prolapse) in these cases might have played an additional role. Hypertrophy of the flaval ligaments has also been mentioned as a cause of additional narrowing of the spinal canal but, like abnormal disc bulging, this is difficult to quantify (196).

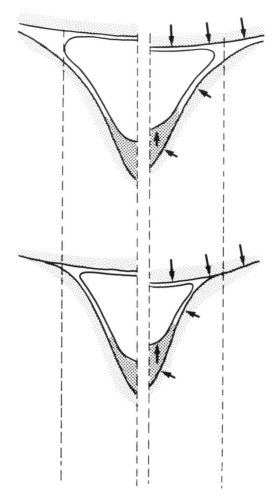

Figure 2.112. Effects of flexion-extension in normal canal (*above*) and in individual with facet hypertrophy (FH) (*below*). *Left*, Flexion; *right*, extension. In normal canal, extension causes reduction of cross-sectional area available for dural sac through combined bulging of disk, flaval ligaments and retrodural fat pad, without endangering available space for dural sac and emerging nerve roots. In individual with FH, loss of reserve space, already present in flexion, enhances narrowing of spinal canal and lateral recesses in extension, and pinching effect upon dural sac and emerging nerve roots. (Reproduced with permission from Penning L, Wilmink JT: Posture-dependent bilateral compression of L4 or L5 nerve roots in facet hypertrophy. *Spine* 12(5):496, 1987.)

FAT PAD CHANGES DURING MOTION

An additional mechanism contributing to root compression in extension is the anterior movement of the dorsal fat pad. In previous studies, it has been noted that in patients with bilateral root involvement at L4-L5, marked dorsal indentation of the dural sac in extension takes place. That the dorsal indentation of the dural sac is related to anterior motion of the dorsal fat pad came as a surprise because it had always been presumed that the flaval ligaments would cause the dorsal indentation, as is the case in spondylotic myelopathy in the cervical spine (198). However, the examples (Figs. 2.113 and 2.114*B* and *D*) show that when lumbar lordosis increases and the laminae approach one another, the fat pad, which cannot be compressed but, being semiliquid, is easily deformed, decreases in its longitudinal dimension and as a result thickens in the transverse plane. Being bordered dorsolaterally by flaval ligaments, the fat pad can expand only in an anterior direction at the expense of the dural sac. This forward

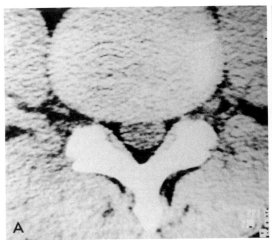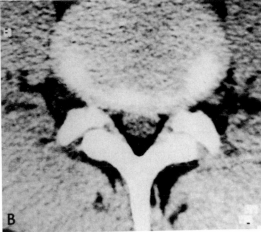

Figure 2.113. Flexion-extension CT in normal individual. Note increase in depth of black epidural fat from **A**, lumbar flexion to **B**, extension, at the expense of the dural sac. Combination of fat thickening and disc bulging, both physiological, cause reduction of cross-sectional area of dural sac amounting, in this example, to approximately 30%. (Reproduced with permission from Penning L, Wilmink JT: Posture-dependent bilateral compression of L4 or L5 nerve roots in facet hypertrophy. *Spine* 12(5):497, 1987.)

expansion of the dorsal fat pad is enhanced by some thickening of the flaval ligaments in extension. This thickening by shortening was previously described in a cadaver study by Knuttson (197). In almost all patients, transverse flattening and sometimes some anterior displacement of the entire fat pad due to flaval thickening in extension, probably in combination with slight anterior movement of the lamina with respect to the disc, are seen. The effect of the anterior movement of the dorsal fat pad in extension is anterior displacement of the dural sac with increased presentation of the emerging root sleeves to the pincers mechanism at the anterolateral angles (196).

Measurements were performed on 40 lateral lumbar myelograms in flexion and extension with the object of analyzing changes in position and shape of the dural sac in spinal movements. There proved to be an anterior displacement of the entire lumbar dural sac in lumbar extension, most likely caused by shortening and thickening of the flaval ligaments. In addition, the anterior dural surface was indented at the L3-L4 and L4-L5 interspaces by posterior bulging of the discs in extension. This encroachment was partially compensated by dural bulging into areas with a rich and compressible venous plexus: behind the vertebral bodies and the L5-S1 disc. While these patterns of dural movements showed individual variations, these trends were found in all diagnos-

tic and anatomical subgroups. In spinal flexion, there is marked elongation of the spinal canal with concomitant stretching of the dural sac and nerve root fibers (185).

Velocity of Motion May Be a Factor in Back Pain

Trunk mobility, as defined by trunk angle, has long been considered an acceptable means to evaluate the degree of impairment in patients with low back pain. However, biomechanically, there is reason to believe that patients with low back pain may exhibit significant sensitivity to trunk velocity of motion as well as angular mobility factors. Thus, it is suggested that trunk velocity be used as a quantitative measure of low back disorder and that it be used as a means to monitor the rehabilitative progress of patients with low back pain (199).

Effect of Spinal Fusion on Adjacent Segment Motion

The effects of spinal fusion on the fused segments and the adjacent, unfused segments play a significant role in the clinical effectiveness of spinal fusion for low back pain with or without sciatica. Much of the information on this important subject is derived from clinical impressions. All types

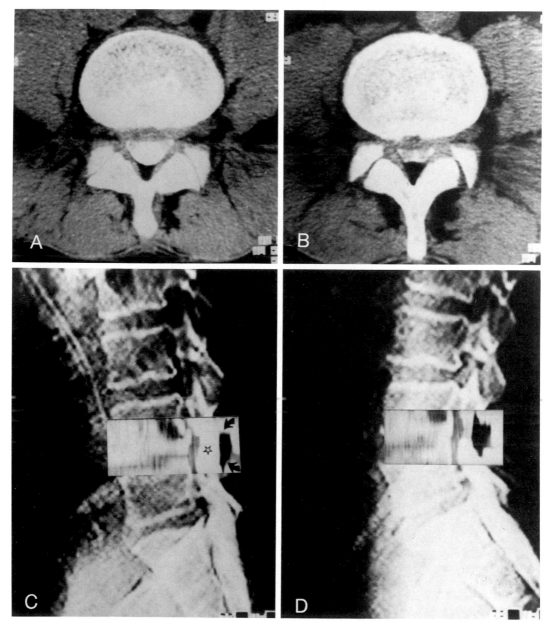

Figure 2.114. Flexion-extension CT. Transverse sections (**A, B**) and lateral views (**C, D**) are shown. Lateral views are composed of scanograms with midsagittal reformats of CT sections superimposed at L4-L5 (*insets*). Note marked anterior expansion of dorsal fat pad (*between arrows*) from flexion (**A, C**) to extension (**B, D**), indenting posterior surface of dural sac (*asterisks*) due to thickening of flaval ligaments and approximation of laminae. Note narrow lateral angle, in flexion (**A**), formed by disc surface and flaval ligaments. Thickening of flaval ligaments and increased disc bulging in extension (**B**) causes "pincers mechanism," pinching ventrolateral angles of dural sac and emerging L5 roots. (Reproduced with permission from Penning L, Wilmink JT: Posture-dependent bilateral compression of L4 or L5 nerve roots in facet hypertrophy. *Spine* 12(5):498, 1987.)

of fusion resulted in increased bending and axial stiffness. All types of fusion demonstrated stabilizing effects on the fusion and produced increased stress on the adjacent, unfused segments, especially the facet joints (200).

Resistance of Ligamentous and Bony Elements

RESISTANCE TO FLEXION

The capsular ligaments of the apophyseal joints play the dominant role in resisting flexion of an intervertebral joint. In full flexion, as determined by the elastic limit of the supraspinous and interspinous ligaments, the capsular ligaments provide 39% of the joint's resistance. The balance is made up by the disc (29%), the supraspinous and interspinous ligaments (19%), and the ligamentum flavum (13%) (94).

In hyperflexion, the supraspinous and interspinous ligaments are damaged first, followed by the capsular ligaments and then the disc. Bending forward and to one side, however, could damage the capsular ligaments first because the component of lateral flexion would produce extra stretching of the capsule away from the side of bending while not affecting the supraspinous and interspinous ligaments which lie on the axis of lateral bending.

In flexion, as in torsion, the apophyseal joints protect the intervertebral disc. Once the posterior spinal ligaments have been sprained in hyperflexion, the wedged disc is able to prolapse into the neural canal if subjected to a high compressive force.

DISC CHANGES AFFECT MOVEMENT MORE THAN FACET CHANGES

The influence of the posterior vertebral ligamentous and bony elements on the sagittal range of motion of the lumbar spine has been investigated by observing the effects of sectioning ligaments and pedicles in 17 cadavers of both sexes with an age range from 14 to 78 years. The investigation showed that the apophyseal joints provide a greater restraint to flexion and extension movements than do the lumbar ligaments. It also showed that the age changes that most severely affect movement in elderly persons occur in the intervertebral discs rather than in the posterior elements (201).

RESISTANCE TO INTERVERTEBRAL SHEAR FORCES

When an intervertebral joint is loaded in shear, the apophyseal joint surfaces resist about one-third of the shear force, while the disc resists the remaining two-thirds (94). This passive resistance to shear is complicated by two features, however. First, when an intervertebral disc alone is subjected to sustained shear, it readily creeps forward. In an intact joint, this readiness to creep would manifest itself as stress relaxation, thus placing an increasing burden on the apophyseal joint surfaces until they resist all of the intervertebral shear force. Second, the muscle slips attached to the posterior part of the neural arch brace it by pulling downward. This prevents any backward bending and brings the facets more firmly together. This means that, in the intact joint, the intervertebral disc is subjected only to pure compression and that the intervertebral shear force is resisted by the apophyseal joints, producing a high interfacet force.

RESISTANCE TO INTERVERTEBRAL COMPRESSIVE FORCE

The absence of a flattened articular surface in the transverse plane at the base of the articular facets clearly suggests that apophyseal joints are not designed to resist intervertebral compressive force. Experiments confirm that, provided the lumbar spine is slightly flattened (as occurs in erect sitting or heavy lifting), all the intervertebral compressive force is resisted by the disc. When lordotic postures such as erect standing are held for long periods, however, the facet tips do make contact with the laminae of the subadjacent vertebra and bear about one-sixth of the compressive force (94).

This contact may well be of clinical significance, since it will result in high stresses on the tips of the facets, and possibly, nipping of the joint capsules. Perhaps this is the reason standing for long periods can produce a dull ache in the small of the back which is relieved by sitting or by using some device, such as a bar rail, to induce slight flexion of the lumbar spine. Disc narrowing results in as much as 70% of the intervertebral compressive force being transmitted across the apophyseal joints. Three such specimens tested exhibited gross degenerative changes in the apophyseal joints (94).

With increasing extension of an intervertebral

joint, the compressive force transmitted across the apophyseal joints increases, and it is likely that the extension movements are limited by this bony contact. Thus, it is possible that hyperextension movements could cause backward bending of the neural arch, eventually resulting in spondylolysis, but again only as a fatigue fracture.

RESISTANCE TO TORSION

Axial rotation of the lumbar spine takes place about a center of rotation in the posterior disc or neural canal. (If axial rotation of the lumbar spine were to occur about some axis posterior to the apophyseal joints, it would be most strongly resisted by the fibers of the anterior annulus fibrosus, since the posterior annulus would be nearer to the center of rotation.) The apophyseal joints are oriented to resist such rotations and protect the soft tissues from the effects of torsion.

Forced axial rotation could occur from a fall on one shoulder or from activities involving high angular momentum, such as discus throwing. Awkward bending (i.e., forward and to one side) is often mistakenly thought to involve significant axial rotation of the lumbar spine. Unlike axial rotation, awkward bending is limited by soft tissues and can lead to ligamentous damage and disc prolapse (94).

For normal intervertebral discs to fail completely, they must be rotated to angles of 22.6° on the average, although microscopic damage will occur at angles somewhat less than this. The margin of safety must be quite high in the lower lumbar spine, however, when we consider that because of the orientation of the facets the T12-L1 discs can be safely rotated about 5° to each side.

CONCLUSION

The function of the lumbar apophyseal joints is to allow limited movement between vertebrae and to protect the discs from shear forces, excessive flexion, and axial rotation. They are not well suited to resist intervertebral compressive forces and are usually protected by the discs. The ligaments of the apophyseal joints are most likely to be damaged in bending forward and to one side. The capsule could be a source of pain in sustained lordotic postures (94).

Rotational Effects on Lumbar Structures

EFFECTS OF ROTATION ON THE INTERVERTEBRAL DISC

Farfan (202) proved that torsional stresses of a magnitude encountered in daily living play a major role in initiating lumbar disc degeneration. He found that, in compression loading of the lumbar spine, the nucleus pulposus was the last structure to fracture, with the vertebral body fracturing by compression before the disc would so yield. When experiments were devised to test the effects of rotation on the lumbar spine, the normal range of axial rotation at the lumbosacral joint was less than 9°.

The annulus fibrosus may be subdivided into a peripheral portion of thick, firmly attached, well-formed laminations and an inner, softer, less well structured portion surrounding the nucleus pulposus. When the disc is subjected to torsion, the resulting damage is found in the outermost layers of the disc but does not involve the longitudinal ligaments and possibly not the most superficial annular laminae. The inner portions of the annulus remain undisturbed. There is increasing evidence that there are unmyelinated nerve endings (usually associated with pain reception) distributed throughout the posterior annulus and even penetrating the nucleus (62).

Measurement of the degree of rotation occurring at the lumbosacral joint has been as high as 9° but is usually 5° or less (62). During walking, minimum rotation occurs between vertebrae; walking at 3.65 mph results in a total rotation of 11° between T1 and the sacrum with 0.2° to 0.6° of this occurring at the lumbosacral joint. The lumbosacral joint can be rotated 3° to 13° during twisting to one side.

TORQUE ROTATION CURVES

Rotation was applied to fresh human lumbar spine specimens at the rate of 3.6°/min. This corresponds to the rate of rotation applied during walking at 3.5 mph (62). The following changes took place at various degrees of rotation:

1. 0° to 3°. During this phase, there was little increase of torque with increasing rotation.

2. 3° to 12°. In this second portion of the curve, a major torque was proportional to the applied rotation. During this phase, much tissue was expressed from the specimen. The fluid seemed to come from the vertebral body bone surfaces adjacent to the disc.

3. 12° to 20°. In this portion of the curve, there was little increase of torque with increase of applied rotation. During this phase, the curve showed numerous small dips just prior to failure. These small indentations in the recordings were often accompanied by sharp cracking noises emanating from the specimen. Nothing was observed at the specimen's surface to explain these sounds.

The torque rotational curves were similar for intact whole joints, for the isolated disc, and for facet joint preparations. *"The normal range of rotation in the human lumbosacral joint probably is limited to less than 5°. Our experiments suggest that the range may even be 3° or less"* (62) (emphasis added). The average torque at failure for intact whole intervertebral joints with normal discs was found to be 750 to 900 inch-lb, nearly twice as high as that for joints with degenerated discs. The average angle of rotation at failure for whole joints with normal discs was 22.6°, while for degenerated discs it was 14.3°. The resistance of the normal disc to this torque is approximately 300 inch-lb, while that of a degenerated disc is about 200 inch-lb. The posterior apophyseal joints also provide resistance to rotation, totaling about 250 inch-lb.

Morris (as discussed in Ref. 97) states that the average cumulative rotation from the sacrum to the first thoracic vertebra is 102°, with 74° of this rotation occurring between the first and the 12th thoracic vertebra. The rotation at the lumbosacral level in vivo is approximately 6°. Figure 2.115 shows the rotational damage to the intervertebral joints at various degrees of rotation.

Farfan (62) believes that it is possible to state with some certainty that the first pathological changes that occur in the disc occur in the annulus. These take the form of small circumferential separations between the lamellae of the annulus, which have been recorded in children as young as age 10 (85, 203). He states that it is impossible to

say whether the process of intervertebral joint degeneration begins in the disc, end plate, or neural arch complex. The changes may occur simultaneously in all three locations. The incidence of disc degeneration is highest at L5-S1, next highest at L4-L5, and third highest at L3-L4.

ROTATION NOT FOUND IN THE LOW LUMBAR SPINE

Maigne (204) states that facet orientation at the lumbar spine permits only flexion and extension. The thoracic spine, by virtue of its facet facings, should have a high degree of mobility, especially in rotation. *"No rotation is possible in the lumbar spine by virtue of the facet orientation and form"* (emphasis added). Therefore, the highest degree of rotation and lateral flexion must take place at the level of the thoracolumbar spine.

Helfet and Gruebel-Lee (63), in discussing the instability of the lumbar spine with regard to range of motion, point out that rotation injuries affect primarily the intervertebral disc itself.

UPRIGHT VERSUS RECUMBENT ROTATION OF THE LUMBAR SPINE

CASE PRESENTATION

This case is of a 23-year-old white woman who had a history of low back pain but no leg pain. At the time this x-ray study was done, she was being treated only for left shoulder pain; her low back was totally asymptomatic.

Consequently, we performed rotation studies on the spine in order to determine any differences in rotation from the standing to the recumbent non-weight-bearing rotational posture.

The anteroposterior view (Fig. 2.116) reveals that this patient has tropism at L5-S1, with the right facet being sagittal and the left being coronal. The hip and sacroiliac joints are adequate. The lateral view (Fig. 2.117) reveals a moderate increased lumbar lordosis. The disc spaces are normal.

Figures 2.118 and 2.119 were taken with the patient in

	NORMAL DISC	DEGENERATED DISC
Average angle of rotation at failure	22.6°	14.3°
Resistance to torque	300 in-lb.	200 in-lb.

Figure 2.115. Annular fiber failure in rotation.

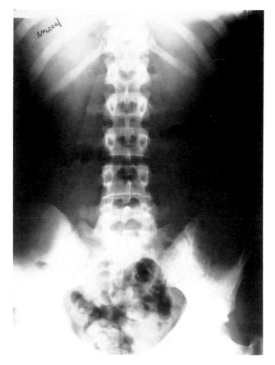

Figure 2.116. Neutral anteroposterior view. Tropism is present at L5-S1.

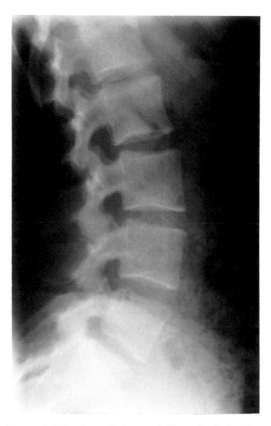

Figure 2.117. Lateral view—mild hyperlordosis. The disc spaces are normal.

the standing weight-bearing posture. Figure 2.118 reveals left rotation, and Figure 2.119 reveals right rotation. There is lateral flexion of L4 and L5 with actual Lovett reverse rotation of the spinous process at L4 on left lateral flexion and with minimal Lovett positive rotation on right rotation. Normally, the spinous process would deviate to the concave side; instead, it deviates to the left, to the convex side, and this is called a Lovett reverse curve. This may indicate a minimal rotatory capability at L4; there is no rotation at the L5 level.

Figures 2.120 and 2.121 are, respectively, right and left lateral rotation studies of the lumbar spine with the patient in the recumbent position. These films were taken with the patient rotating to each side while in the recumbent position and being supported with foam padding in the thoracic spine as maximum rotation is attained. The purpose of this study is to see whether there is any difference between the muscular contractions causing rotatory change when the patient is in a recumbent position and those causing change when the patient is in a weight-bearing position. As you can see, there is actually no discernible rotation with the patient in the recumbent posture.

This author interprets this to mean that rotation, if possible, is greatest when the patient is in the upright posture. This might also make sense if one considers that most back injuries occur during flexion in the upright

posture, with either lifting or rotating in combination motion.

COMPARISON OF LATERAL FLEXION AND ROTATION OF THE LUMBAR SPINE

CASE PRESENTATION

This case is of a 34-year-old white woman with low back and left lower extremity pain. She has had numerous episodes of low back pain in the past few years but has had leg pain for only the past 2 weeks.

The rotation movement of the lumbar spine is studied by comparison with lateral flexion movement. Figures 2.122, 2.123 and 2.124 are neutral and lateral bending films showing normal motion. Figures 2.125 and 2.126 reveal a sacral angle of 33° and a lumbar lordosis of 50°. Figure 2.127 shows no stenosis present. Figure 2.128 is a posteroanterior tilt view of the same patient as in Figure 2.122.

Figures 2.129 and 2.130 are, respectively, left and right rotation studies made by having the patient rotate at the

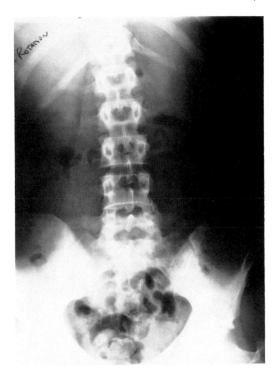

Figure 2.118. Left rotation of the lumbar spine in upright posture.

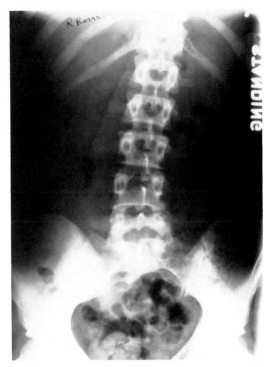

Figure 2.119. Right rotation of the lumbar spine in the upright posture.

waist while holding the pelvis fixed on the bucky. Note that L5 does not rotate measurably and L4 bends laterally but that rotation is no greater than the lateral bendings reveal. There is definite increased rotatory movement of the upper lumbar vertebral bodies, coupled with lateral flexion.

ROTATIONAL AND LATERAL FLEXION CAPABILITIES OF THE LUMBAR SPINE

A three-dimensional radiographic technique was used to investigate the ranges of active axial rotation and lateral bending plus the accompanying rotations in places other than those of the primary voluntary movements in two groups of normal male volunteers. There was approximately 2° of axial rotation at each intervertebral joint, with L3-L4 and L4-L5 being slightly more mobile. Lateral bending of approximately 10° occurred at the upper three levels, while there was significantly less movement, 6° and 3° at L4-L5 and L5-S1, respectively. In the upper lumbar spine, axial rotation to the right was accompanied by lateral bending to the left, and vice versa. At L5-S1, axial rotation and lateral bending generally accompa-

nied each other in the same direction, while L4-L5 was a transitional level (205).

TORSIONAL VERSUS COMPRESSIVE DISC INJURY

The effect of cyclic torsional loads on the behavior of intact lumbar intervertebral joints was investigated. Failure locations occurred in such diverse regions as end plates, facets, laminae, capsular ligaments, and so forth. All specimens exhibited a synovial fluid discharge from the apophyseal joint capsule sometime during testing. Posttest examinations of all the cartilage surfaces showed fibrillation, whether or not the intervertebral joint failed (206).

Cyclic torsional fatigue loads produce undesirable effects: (a) leakage of synovial fluid at the apophyseal joints; (b) fibrillation of the facet cartilage surface (Table 2.7); and (c) fracture of various elements of the vertebra. The "failures" lead to weakening and improper functioning of apophyseal joints and disc. In the absence of synovial fluid, the apophyseal joint may exhibit more bony contact and higher friction. Under chronic in

Table 2.7.
Failures Observed in Specimens Tested at Constant Torque Levels (Mode II)[a,b]

Number of Failures	Type of Failure Observed		Number of Specimens Failed at Torque (N-m)				Total
			11.3	22.6	33.9	45.2	
1	Vertebral body	Superior	1	0	1	1	3
(VC)		Inferior	1	2	1	0	4 = 7
2	Facets cracks	Unilateral	1	0	2	2	5
(FC)		Bilateral	0	1	1	1	3 = 8
3	Torn capsules	Unilateral	0	0	2	1	3
(TC)		Bilateral	1	3	0	1	5 = 8
4	Annulus in tears		0	3	0	2	5
(TA)							
5	Lamina crack	Unilateral					
(LC)		Bilateral	1	1	3	0	5
	2 + 3		1	1	2	2	6
	1 + 3		1	2	1	0	4
	1 + 4		0	2	0	0	2
	2 + 4		0	1	0	1	2
	3 + 4		0	2	0	2	4
	1 + 2 + 3		1	1	1	0	3
	2 + 3 + 4		0	2	0	2	4
	1 + 3 + 4		0	2	0	0	2
	1 + 2 + 4		0	1	0	0	1
	1 + 2 + 3 + 4 + 5		1	1	3	0	5

[a]Reproduced with permission from Liu YK, Goel VK, Dejong A, Njus G, Nishiyama K, Buckwalter J: Torsional fatigue of the lumbar vertebral joints. *Spine* 10(10):899, 1985.
[b]The fibrillation of facet articular cartilage and a discharge of fluid from apophyseal joints were observed in all the specimens regardless of whether the specimens failed or not.

vivo loading, the rate of damage may exceed the rate of repair by the cellular mechanisms of the body. Prolonged exposure to cyclic torsional loads producing more than ±1.5° of angular displacement per segment is detrimental to elements of the lumbar spine. Since these elements contain nociceptors, their disturbance may lead to low back pain (206).

Fifteen discs were studied in pure compression, flexion and extension, axial rotation, and shear. The largest strains were in torsion (207).

During axial rotation, the oblique fibers, running counter to the direction of movement, are stretched, while the intermediate fibers with opposite orientation are relaxed. The tension reaches a maximum in the central fibers of the annulus, which are the most oblique. The nucleus is therefore strongly compressed, and the *internal pressure rises in proportion to the angle of rotation* (208).

Kapandji records that Cailliet states: "It has been shown by myelography that there is posterior protrusion of the intervertebral disc from hyperextension" (208).

Cailliet speaks of the "concept that rotary trauma in later life causes rupture of the outer annular fibers." He goes on to say, "Gradually the outward intradiscal pressure causes radial tears to occur in the disc.

"Compressive forces applied directly to the functional unit will cause vertebral body compression before any disc disruption of the intact disc. Rotational forces, however, place torque upon the annular fibers which become disrupted, and the intradiscal nuclear pressure is no longer contained."[a]

Regarding disc herniation, Cailliet and Kapandji (208) agree on the effect of microtrauma: Cailliet states, according to Kapandji, "The strain or repeated stresses have frequently occurred prior to the acute onset and have set the stage for the ultimate herniation. By setting the stage is meant the weakening of the annulus fibrosus which diminishes the elastic recoil against a stress. A minimal stress applied on the disc that is contained within a weakened defective annulus may cause the nuclear material to herniate."[b]

---

[a] From Kapandji I: The physiology of the joints (Letter to the Editor). *J Orthop Sports Phys Therapy* 3(November):40: 1986.
[b] From Kapandji I: The physiology of the joints (Letter to the Editor). *J Orthop Sports Phys Therapy* 3(November):40, 1986.

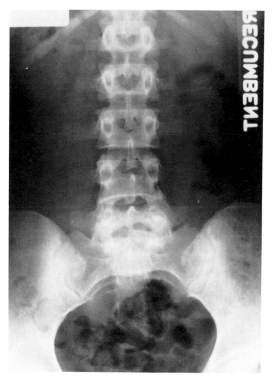

Figure 2.120. Right rotation of the lumbar spine in the recumbent supine position.

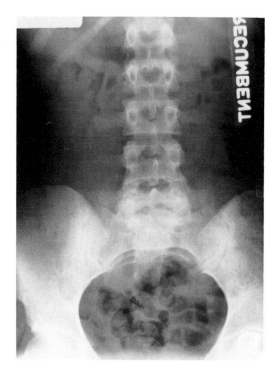

Figure 2.121. Left rotation of the lumbar spine in the recumbent supine position.

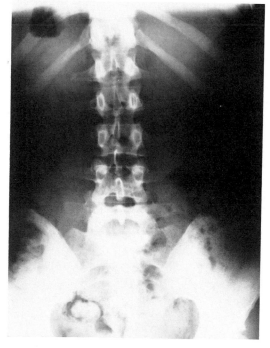

Figure 2.122. Neutral anteroposterior view of the lumbar spine and pelvis.

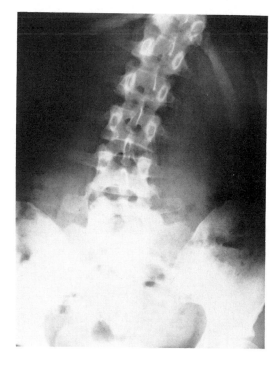

Figure 2.123. Right lateral flexion.

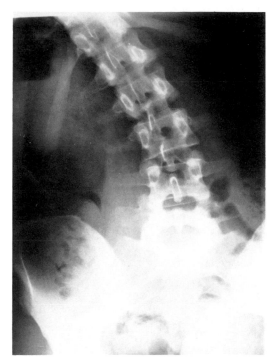

Figure 2.124. Left lateral flexion.

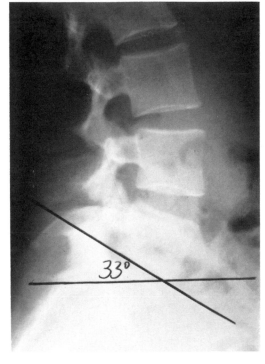

Figure 2.125. Sacral angle measurement.

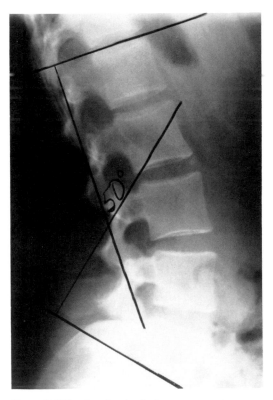

Figure 2.126. Lumbar lordosis measurement.

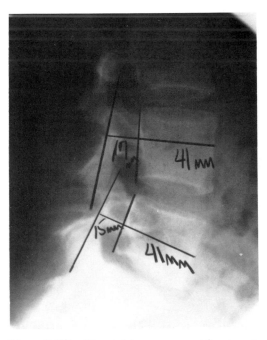

Figure 2.127. Eisenstein's measurement for stenosis.

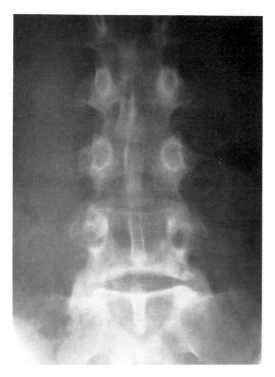

Figure 2.128. Posteroanterior tilt view of L5-S1. Note the centered position of the spinous processes.

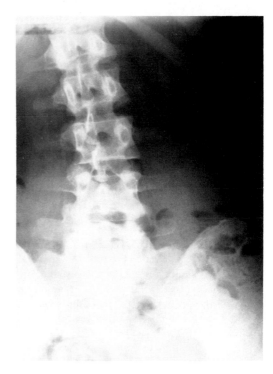

Figure 2.129. Left lumbar spine rotation in the upright posture.

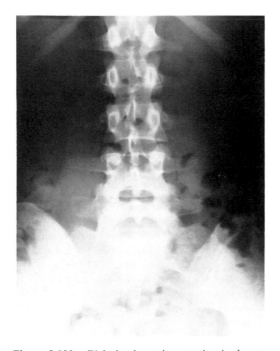

Figure 2.130. Right lumbar spine rotation in the upright posture.

The most harmful motions appear to be rotations, since these produce both compression and shear. The patient should be counseled to reduce such activities as shoveling and lifting, as well as recreational activities such as handball, squash, tennis, cycling, and gardening (209).

ANNULUS FIBROSUS DAMAGE BY ROTATION ON CONCAVE SIDE OF CURVE

Lindblom, Percy, and others (210) have reported that the injection of saline solution or of some other solution into the appropriate disc space may reproduce the symptoms of some patients who are suffering from low back and sciatic pain. However, if Novocain is injected into these same discs, the pain is eliminated. Similarly, Feffer, as reported by Lindblom, has reported that the injection of the hormone hydrocortisone into the appropriate disc space has relieved symptoms in a substantial proportion of patients in whom rupture and actual protrusion or extrusion of a disc fragment had not occurred (210).

Under axial compression, failure occurred

due to fracture of one of the vertebral end plates and collapse of the underlying vertebral body.

In these tests, failure of the annulus fibrosus occurred only as the result of extremely rapid cyclic bending combined with mild axial compression.

NUCLEUS PULPOSUS MIGRATES TO THE CONCAVE SIDE OF CURVE

It is commonly stated that the nucleus pulposus is the structure by which stresses are distributed uniformly to the annulus fibrosus and cartilaginous plates. It is furthermore stated in the literature that the nucleus pulposus moves toward the convex side of the curve when the spine bends to either side or forward and backward. The behavior of two specimens subjected to combined axial loading and bending in this investigation did not seem consistent with this concept. The annulus invariably bulged on the concave side, apparently as the result of compression between the opposing vertebral surfaces (211).

In order to study the effect of increased pressure on the intervertebral disc, rats' tails were tied up and fixed in the shape of a U. It was found that degeneration and even rupture of the annulus fibrosus occurred on the concave side of the tails while the convex side remained normal (210).

The intervertebral disc herniations causing low back and sciatic pain are predominantly situated on the concavity of the curvature. The location of intervertebral disc herniation is different in men and women: the fifth lumbar intervertebral disc is more often affected in women than in men (210).

Disc or Facet as the Etiology of Back Pain

Vernon-Roberts and Pirie (72) state that there is a direct relationship between the degree of disc degeneration, marginal osteophyte formation on vertebral bodies, and apophyseal joint changes, which suggests that disc degeneration is the primary event leading to the clinical condition of degenerative spondylosis. They also state that they have evidence that enables them to speculate on the role of prolapse in disc degeneration and in the genesis of osteoarthrosis of the apophyseal joints.

Nachemson (60) found that arthrosis of the articular facets was always secondary to disc degeneration.

Thus, it is strongly implied that internal de-rangement of the intervertebral disc, namely, the nucleus pulposus, begins the aberrant mobility of the lumbar spine. The degenerative changes occurring thereafter in the disc spread posteriorly into the arch of the vertebra. We know that both the disc and the facet are pain-producing entities and that specific attention must be given to both of these structures in the treatment of low back pain. Furthermore, it also seems most likely that a combination of surgery and manipulation may be the answer for many people: that is, surgery for the disc prolapse and manipulation for the altered motoricity of the articular facet.

The effects of rotation have been well summarized by Eagle (212), who states that the main cause of severe long-lasting back pain is the damaged intervertebral disc, and once a disc is damaged there is nothing a surgeon can do to repair it. Nor are discs able to repair themselves. Therefore, if we are to prevent back pain, it would be useful to know how much stress the disc fibers can withstand before they give way.

Eagle (212) quotes the work of Hukins and Hickey (213) of Manchester University, who state that the most hazardous maneuvers to the low back are bending and twisting. They won the 1979 Volvo Bioengineering Award for their paper proving that annular failure and tearing are caused by torsion and forward bending, causing nuclear protrusion and low back pain. They found that the maximum rotation that will not damage the annular fibers at L5-S1 is $3°$.

Miller (214) states that during the lifting of a weight of 200 lb, the disc carries an average of 91% of the load and the facet joint carries no more than 12%. Low facet joints put more weight on the disc than do high facet joints. *The facets carry very little weight on compression but accept large loads on bending.* The amount of load on the facets is 50% on flexion and extension and 30% on torsion.

An in vitro experimental study was carried out to measure the induced loading on human lumbar facets due to varying amounts of compressive axial load (215). Testing was done on the L2-L3 and L4-L5 spinal motion segments obtained from cadavers at autopsy. The compressive loading was applied with the spinal specimens first in a neutral position and then in an extended position. In particular, this study demonstrated that the absolute facet loads remain relatively constant with increasing segmental compressive loads such that the facet load expressed as a percentage of the load applied to the segment decreases with increasing axial loads. It also demonstrated that with increasing loads in extension the contact area moves cranially at L2-L3 and caudally at L4-L5. Furthermore, it indicated that after a facetectomy the load on the remaining facet is reduced substantially, although peak pressure increases. Finally, this study demonstrated that there is a substantial difference in facet loadings between the L2-L3 and the L4-L5 segments.

A comparison of segments at L2-L3 and L4-L5 at different axial loads in the neutral position shows that the facets at L2-L3 generally take more load than those at L4-L5. The same trend is also observed during extension. Furthermore, the normal load on the facets is always higher in extension than in the neutral position. This holds true for both the L2-L3 and L4-L5 levels.

Observations based on these data indicate:

1. The average peak pressure for all axial compressive loads is higher in extension than in the neutral position at both the L2-L3 and the L4-L5 levels.
2. The peak pressure is generally higher at the L2-L3 level than at the L4-L5 level in both the neutral and the extended positions.

The facet pressure rather than the facet load, therefore, may be playing a significant role in the degenerative changes of facets.

Contrary to expectations, a unilateral facetectomy causes a significant reduction in the load borne by the remaining facet in both the neutral and the extended positions. This may be explained by the fact that since the facet load on the left side is eliminated by performing a unilateral facetectomy, equilibrium is substantially altered. The superior vertebral body is now free to drift away from the inferior body, thus reducing positive contact at the remaining facets. This phenomenon again reinforces the above observation that pressure rather than load is the precipitating factor in facet degeneration.

A second unexpected phenomenon observed in this study is that in many cases the contact decreases with increasing loads.

Do Facets Irritate the Nerve Roots to Cause Sciatica?

Mooney and Robertson (113) injected local anesthetic into the facet joints of 100 consecutive patients with "disc syndrome." One-fifth had long-term relief and one-third had partial relief of lumbago and sciatica. Carrera (216) succeeded in providing some relief to seven of 20 patients by injection. Dory (217) found that the articular capsule nearly always burst during arthrography, and the path of leaking medium provided a possible explanation of how steroids relieve pain on injection. It might be that the injected anesthetic or steroid directly affects the nerve root and can give partial or temporary relief.

VULNERABILITY OF NERVE ROOTS TO COMPRESSION DEFECTS

The dorsal nerve roots have a larger diameter than the ventral nerve roots, which some feel may explain the greater susceptibility of the sensory axons to compressive forces. The S1 nerve roots are approximately 170 mm long, while the L1 nerve roots are 60 mm long. The nerve roots as well as the spinal nerves are composed of axons that have arisen within the substance of the spinal cord and course to their final destination in the periphery. These axons may exceed 100 cm in length (146).

Spinal nerve roots lack the connective tissue protection that sheaths peripheral nerves. This sheathing has considerable mechanical strength and possesses properties to form a barrier to diffusion of certain molecules. The spinal nerve roots, therefore, are at a disadvantage mechanically and possibly biochemically. The nerve roots are surrounded by cerebrospinal fluid, however, and this, together with the dura, does give the spinal nerve roots an element of mechanical protection. The dura of a spinal nerve root appears to be continuous with the epineurium of the peripheral nerve.

It must be kept in mind that the nerve root complex must be extraordinarily mobile. Nerve roots must change length depending on the degree of flexion, extension, lateral bending, and rotation of the lumbar spine. Lumbar nerve roots limited in motion by fibrosis of either intraspinal or extraspinal origin will create traction upon the nerve root complex, causing ischemia and secondary neural dysfunction. This fact must also be kept in mind during the rehabilitation process. Flexibility exercises must be designed to maintain nerve root mobility.

Intraneural blood flow is markedly affected when the nerve is stretched about 8% over the original length. Complete cessation of all intraneural blood flow is seen at 15% elongation.

The dorsal root ganglion, because of its fibrous capsule as well as its rich vascular supply, may, indeed, be more susceptible to changes in intraneural blood flow as well as to the development of secondary intraneural edema with consequent fibrotic change. This may explain sensory symptoms even in the absence of evidence of sensory loss on gross neurological examination (146).

Weight-Bearing Stresses on the Disc and Facet

Changes in body height have been used as a measure of summarizing disc compression due to creep. Under controlled circumstances, changes in body height can be used as a measure of the load on the spine. This can be of great value in ergonomic evaluations of workplaces, equipment, and tasks. There are, however, many factors influencing the shrinkage as a response to a certain load, which have to be controlled. The duration of the load is one obvious example. Also, age and individual factors, the time of day, hours of sleep, getting up time, and previous loads are other influences.

An interesting fact is the quick recovery when the spine is unloaded (218).

The in vitro static load displacement characteristics of the intact and injured human lumbar intervertebral joint have been investigated in a loading apparatus that allows entirely unconstrained relative motion between the joint members. The spatial relative displacement produced by a given load, with and without preloads, was measured. The significant observations are summarized as follows (219):

1. Joint flexibilities measured by raising the initial intradiscal pressure show that: (a) For force loads, the joint is most flexible in anterior shear and least flexible in axial compression; the flexibility in anterior shear is an order of magnitude greater than in compression. The flexibilities in posterior shear and lateral bending are one-half and one-third of that in anterior shear, respectively. (b) For torque loads, the joint is most flexible in flexion. The flexibility in extension is around 60% of that in flexion, while in lateral bending it is approximately an average of those in flexion and extension. The joint is least flexible in axial torque, the flexibility being less than 30% of that in flexion.

2. The load displacement results of the two sequential sectioning series of experiments show that: (a) In the load range considered in the experiment, the disc is by far the major load-bearing element in lateral and anterior shears, axial compression, and flexion. In lateral shear and axial compression, at higher displacements, the facets may transmit part of the load through the joint. Also, with increased displacement, the facet capsules (in anterior shear) and the facet capsules and the posterior ligaments (in flexion) are likely to be important. (b) The facets play a major load-bearing role in posterior shear and axial torque (219).

FACET STIFFNESS UNDER LOADING

Three-dimensional load deformation data were obtained for intact posterior elements and isolated facet joint capsules of five lumbar motion segments. Considerable variability was observed among specimens.

The load deformation data showed that, in response to 30.2=N loads applied in anterior, posterior, or lateral shear, or in tension or compression, the mean displacements of the inferior facet joint centers of the superior vertebral body ranged from 0.5 to 1.8 mm (220).

Disc versus Facet Weight-Bearing Proportion

Results of study of six lumbar segments revealed that the normal facets carried 3 to 25% of the weight-bearing load. If the facet joint was arthritic, the load could be as high as 47%. The transmission of compressive facet load occurs through contact of the tip of the inferior facet with the pars of the vertebra below. The data also show that an overloaded facet joint will cause rearward rotation of the inferior facet, resulting in the stretching of the joint capsule. The finite element model predicted an increase in facet load due to a decrease in disc height. The following hypothesis is proposed: Excessive facet loads stretch the joint capsule and can be a cause for low back pain (223).

The disc carries an average of 91% of the load in lifting 200 lb, and the facet joint carries no more than 12%. Low facet joints put more weight on the disc, while high facet joints put less weight on the disc. *The facets carry very little weight in compression but accept large amounts in bending* (214).

ARTICULAR FACETS CARRY MORE WEIGHT THAN KNEE JOINTS

The pedicle-facet complex normally carries only 20% of the vertical pressure applied at the interspace (224). This constitutes 10 times the weight per square inch applied to the knee joints (225). As the disc loses turgor and resilience, its ability to resist compressive forces and to maintain normal intervertebral separation and alignment fails. This throws an additional burden on the facet articulations and may accelerate the changes of degenerative arthrosis (226).

A comparison of segments L2-L3 and L4-L5 at different axial loads in neutral mode shows that the facets at L2-L3 generally take more load than those at L4-L5.

The same trend is also observed for the extension mode at both the L2-L3 and L4-L5 levels. Furthermore, in extension the normal load at the facets is always higher than in the neutral mode. This holds for both the L2-L3 and L4-L5 levels.

This indicates that the facet pressure rather than the facet load may be playing a significant role in the degenerative changes of facets (215).

Effect of Degenerative Disc Disease on Weight Bearing

The intervertebral disc is considered to be one of the structures of major importance in painful conditions of the spine. An injury to the disc can affect overall spinal mechanics—both the behavior of the disc itself, and that of other spinal structures. For example, it can lead to altered sharing of the load between the disc and the apophyseal joints.

The two load-bearing components of the disc are *(a)* the nucleus, in the central region, which is surrounded by *(b)* the annulus fibrosus, consisting of fibrous tissue in concentric laminated bands. The nucleus is generally under compressive stress, while the annular layers, especially the outer layers, carry tensile stresses. The stresses in the two components balance each other as well as the load carried by the disc. A disturbance in any one component of the disc, such as a decrease in the water content of the nucleus or an injury to the annulus, may be thought to affect the mechanical behavior of the other component as well as that of the disc as a whole (227).

The stages of injury to the functional spinal unit are:

1. Asymmetric disc injury at one FSU;
2. Disturbed kinematics of FSUs above and below injury;
3. Asymmetric movements at facet joints;
4. Unequal sharing of facet loads;
5. High load on one facet joint;
6. Cartilage degeneration, and/or facet atrophy and narrowing of IVF (227).

STAGES OF DISC PROLAPSE

Fifty-two cadaveric lumbar motion segments were subjected to fatigue loading in compression and bending to determine if the intervertebral discs could prolapse in a gradual manner (Fig. 2.131). Prior to testing, the nucleus pulposus of each disc was stained with a small quantity of blue dye and radiopaque solution. This enabled the progress of any gradual prolapse to be monitored by direct observation and by discogram. Six discs developed a gradual prolapse during the testing period. The injury starts with the lamellae of the annulus being distorted to form radial fissures; then, nuclear pulp is extruded from the disc and leaks into the spinal canal. The discs most commonly affected were from the lower lumbar spine of young cadavers. Tests on 10 older discs with preexisting ruptures showed that such discs are stable and do not leak nuclear pulp (228).

Cadaveric lumbar spine specimens of "motion segments," each including two vertebrae and the linking disc and facet joints, were compressed. The pressure across the facet joints was measured using interposed pressure-recording paper. This was repeated for 12 pairs of facet joints at four angles of posture and with three different disc heights. The results showed that pressure between the facets increased significantly with narrowing of the disc space and with increasing angles of extension (Table 2.8). Extraarticular impingement was found to be caused, or worsened, by disc space narrowing. Increased pressure or impingement may be a source of pain in patients with reduced disc spaces (229).

Nerve Root Compression Changes in Disc Degeneration

An instrumented probe mounted on the anterior surface of the lumbar spine over an excised lumbar intervertebral disc was used to simulate a disc protrusion in 12 fresh cadavers. The contact force between probe and nerve root was mea-

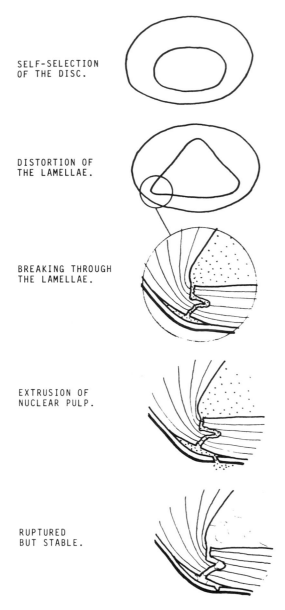

SELF-SELECTION
OF THE DISC.

DISTORTION OF
THE LAMELLAE.

BREAKING THROUGH
THE LAMELLAE.

EXTRUSION OF
NUCLEAR PULP.

RUPTURED
BUT STABLE.

Figure 2.131. The five stages of gradual disc prolapse. (Reproduced with permission from Adams MA, Hutton WC: Gradual disc prolapse. *Spine* 10(6):530, 1985.)

Table 2.8.
Average Peak Pressures of 24 Joints

Posture	Peak Pressure (kg/cm^2)	Disc Height	Peak Pressure (kg/cm^2)
Flexion 4°	56.8	Unaltered	51.6
Neutral	63.9	Loss of 1 mm	70.1
Extension			
4°	72.8	Loss of 4 mm	83.3
6°	79.4		

both proximal and distal to the intervertebral disc appears to play an important role in this regard.

Narrowing the disc space significantly decreased the force on the nerve root for a given probe protrusion (230).

Pain Production in the Facet with Disc Degeneration

Disc space narrowing causes a marked increase in peak pressure between opposed facets in the zygapophyseal joints, and it is known that there is an association between osteoarthrosis of the zygapophyseal joints and osteophytic lipping of vertebral bodies. However, osteoarthrosis of the zygapophyseal joints need not always occur at the same level as intervertebral disc degeneration (231). Harrison et al. (232) found vascular profusion accompanying degenerative changes in the hip joint. According to Arnoldi (233), intraosseous hypertension may be a factor of importance in the pathomechanics of certain types of low back pain, and it is well known that pain of vascular origin is a recognized clinical phenomenon. Giles and Taylor's (234) study describes vascularization of a zygapophyseal articular cartilage in minor osteoarthrosis (Fig. 2.132 and 2.133). This vascularization presupposes innervations of these blood vessels by vasomotor nerves.

A survey of the literature concerning osteoarthrosis of the zygapophyseal joints of the lumbar spine has not revealed a previous description of an extensive vascular supply to cartilage showing minor osteoarthrosis, as has been demonstrated in this study. The vascular supply shown in this study may well be indicative of an attempt at cartilage repair, and this repair need not be limited to the periphery of the joint. The presence of this vascularization may indicate that low back pain of vascular origin could be experienced by patients with minor osteoarthrosis (234).

sured as a function of two independent variables: probe protrusion depth and disc space height.

The force produced by the probe on the nerve root progressively increased as the probe was advanced against the nerve root due to the tension produced in the nerve root. The anatomical fixation of the nerve root within the neural canal

Degenerative Changes of Vertebral Plates

Degenerative change at the end plate of the discovertebral joint was studied in the elderly adult by correlating the histological and radiographic findings. Undecalcified ground sections were made from 21 autopsied lumbar spines that demonstrated no evidence of disease except age-related osteoporosis. Histological examination (Figs. 2.134–2.138) showed that the cartilaginous end plates were degenerated to various extents and were replaced by subchondral bone proliferation (endochondral bone formation) in the direction of the joint space. In advanced cases, this histological finding was reflected in radiographs as a subchondral sclerotic zone protruding toward the disc space. The degree of end-plate change was positively correlated with disc space narrowing and the vacuum phenomenon (degeneration of the nucleus pulposus), but not with osteoporosis and vertebral compression. Anatomically and functionally, this may be the most common form of degeneration at the discovertebral joint end plate. Further study will be necessary to clarify the process (235).

Treatment Effects on Disc and Facet Articulations

EPIDURAL STEROID INJECTION

Epidural anesthetics and steroids have been widely used for more than 20 years in the treatment of low back pain and pseudo-radicular or radicular pain.

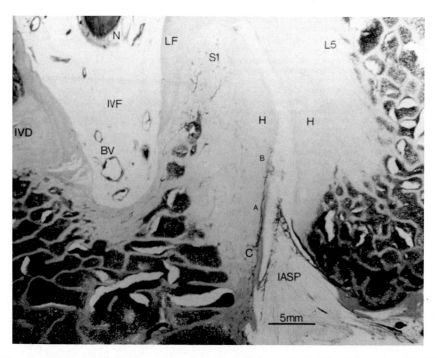

Figure 2.132. A sagittally cut histological section from the medial one-third of the right zygapophyseal joint of a cadaver. Note the blood vessel extending from the subchondral bone of the superior articular process of the sacrum into the articular cartilage which shows minor osteoarthrosis. Note that this sagittal section reveals the anatomy of the inferomedial intraarticular synovial inclusion that projects into the wide opening of the inferior joint recess. The intraarticular synovial inclusion is a highly vascular adipose structure with a synovial membrane lining. *BV*, blood vessels; *C*, capillary—parts A and B; *H*, hyaline articular cartilage; *IASP*, intraarticular synovial inclusion; *IVD*, intervertebral disc at the lumbo-sacral joint; *IVF*, intervertebral foramen; *LF*, ligamentum flavum; *L5*, inferior articular process of the fifth lumbar vertebra; *N*, nerve; *S1*, superior articular process of the first sacral segment. (Reproduced with permission from Giles LGF, Taylor JR: Osteoarthrosis in human cadaveric lumbo-sacral zygapophyseal joints, *Journal of Manipulative and Physiological Therapeutics*, vol 8, issue 4, pp 241–242, ©by the National College of Chiropractic, 1985.)

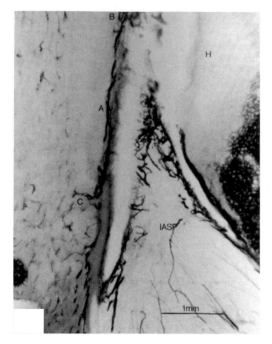

Figure 2.133. This figure represents magnification of the blood vessel shown in Figure 2.132. *C*, capillary—parts A and B; *H*, hyaline articular cartilage; *IASP*, intraarticular synovial protrusion. (Reproduced with permission from Giles LGF, Taylor JR: Osteoarthrosis in human cadaveric lumbo-sacral zygapophyseal joints, *Journal of Manipulative and Physiological Therapeutics*, vol 8, issue 4, pp 241–242, ©by the National College of Chiropractic, 1985.)

Seven women and nine men, aged 27 to 59 years (mean, 45 years) with lumbar pain and sciatica had epidural blocks once with 80 mg of methylprednisolone acetate and lidocaine in individual doses. By means of a visual analogue scale, 10 of these patients (62%) reported relief of half the pain the following day. One month later, only seven patients (43%) reported relief of one-third of the pain. Only one patient benefited ultimately (after 6 months). In the remaining patients, complaints were unaffected by the epidural injection (236).

This author has found this procedure of very limited benefit to low back pain patients.

Posture Effects on Lumbar Spine

A series of experiments showing how posture affects the lumbar spine is reviewed. Postures that flatten (that is, flex) the lumbar spine are compared with those that preserve the lumbar lordosis. Flexed postures have several advantages: flexion improves the transport of metabolites in the intervertebral discs, reduces the stresses on the apophyseal joints and on the posterior half of the annulus fibrosus, and gives the spine a high compressive strength. Flexion also has disadvantages: it increases the stress on the anterior annulus and increases the hydrostatic pressure in the nucleus pulposus at low load levels.

The disadvantages are not of much significance, and we conclude that it is mechanically and nutritionally advantageous to flatten the lumbar spine when sitting and when lifting heavy weights (237).

On the basis of posture, humans can be divided into squatters and non-squatters. A comparative study of the two groups follows:

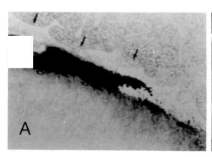
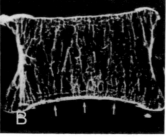
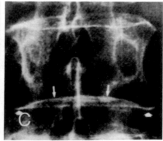

Figure 2.134. Inferior surface of L3 in a 75-year-old man. **A**, Histological section (undecalcified, Villaneuva bone staining, original magnification × 10). Cartilaginous end plate is sufficiently retained (*open arrows*). Note small protrusion of subchondral bone (*arrowhead*). **B**, Low-kilovoltage contact radiograph. **C**, Clinical radiograph. Appearance of the bone end plate (*thin arrows*) and epiphyseal ring (*thick arrows*) is almost normal. (Reproduced with permission from Aoki J, et al.: End plate of the discovertebral joint: degenerative change in the elderly adult. *Radiology* 164(2): 412, 1987.)

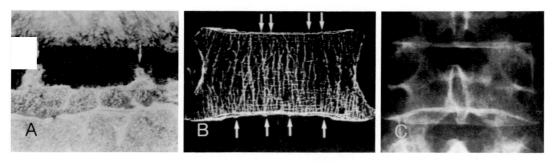

Figure 2.135. Superior surface of L4 in an 82-year-old man. **A, B,** Small projections of subchondral bone into the cartilaginous end plate can be observed (*arrows*). **C,** Radiograph shows completely normal appearance of the end plate. (Reproduced with permission from Aoki J, et al.: End plate of the discovertebral joint: degenerative change in the elderly adult. *Radiology* 164(2):412, 1987.)

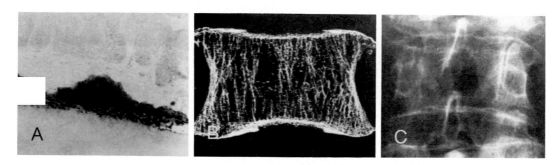

Figure 2.136. Inferior surface of L4 in a 72-year-old woman. **A,** Cartilaginous end plate is replaced by subchondral bone proliferation. Border between the cartilaginous end plate and fibrous cartilage is flat, whereas the cartilage-bone border is undulatory. **B,** Newly formed subchondral bone makes a thin sclerotic zone. **C,** Radiograph fails to reflect the histological finding, because the direction of x-ray is not appropriate. (Reproduced with permission from Aoki J, et al.: End plate of the discovertebral joint: degenerative change in the elderly adult. *Radiology* 164(2):413, 1987.)

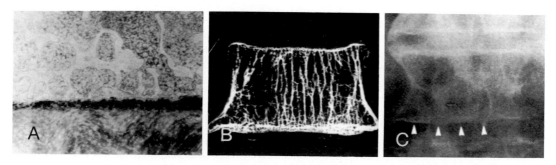

Figure 2.137. Inferior surface of L1 in an 82-year-old woman. **A,** Thickness of the cartilaginous end plate is markedly reduced. **B,** Newly formed subchondral trabeculae are fine and intimate, forming a protrusive thin sclerotic zone. **C,** Radiograph reflects the histological changes well (*arrowheads*). (Reproduced with permission from Aoki J, et al.: End plate of the discovertebral joint: degenerative change in the elderly adult. *Radiology* 164(2):413, 1987.)

1. On the basis of radiographic studies, the incidence of degenerative change in the intervertebral disc in primitive squatting populations is considerably less than that found in civilized peoples.

2. The suggestion is made that lordosis is implicated in the pathogenesis of degeneration, but further studies are required (237a).

Intraabdominal Pressure Effects on Spinal Unloading

The ability of a partial or full Valsalva maneuver (voluntary pressurization of the intraabdominal cavity) to unload the spine was investigated in four subjects. During the performance of five isometric tasks, intraabdominal and intradiscal pressures and surface myoelectric activities in three lumbar trunk muscle groups were measured. The tasks were carried out without voluntary pressurization of the intraabdominal cavity and then when the subjects performed partial and full Valsalva maneuvers. A biomechanical model analysis of each task was made to help interpret the experimental measurements. Intraabdominal pressure was found not to be an indicator of spine load in these experiments. The Valsalva maneuvers did raise intraabdominal pressure, but in four of the five tasks it increased rather than decreased lumbar spine compression (238).

Apophyseal Joint Resistance to Compression

Cadaveric lumbar intervertebral joints were loaded to simulate the erect standing posture (lordosis) and the erect sitting posture (slightly flexed). The results show that, after the intervertebral disc has been reduced in height by a period of sustained loading, the apophyseal joints resist about 16% of the intervertebral compressive forces in the erect standing posture, whereas in the erect sitting posture they resist none. The implications of this in relationship to degenerative changes and to low backache are discussed below.

Compression forces of up to 11 times the superincumbent body weight can be imposed on the lumbar spine by daily activities.

If the aim is to reduce the compressive forces on the disc, some degree of lordosis is needed. This posture, however, in addition to loading the apophyseal joints, places high compressive loads on the posterior annulus, which is the focus of degenerative changes. It has indeed been suggested that our Western lordotic posture promotes intervertebral disc degeneration. Slight flexion, on the other hand, has the advantage of relieving both the apophyseal joints and the posterior annulus of compressive force (239).

Routine daily activities seldom impose large loads on the spine in shear, bending, or torsion. In bending and torsion, in particular, it usually falls to the trunk muscles rather than the motion segments to balance moments. This occurs because few physical activities require lumbar motion segments to flex, extend, bend laterally, or twist more than a few degrees. Few physical activities involve significant motions in shear. In response to only small motions, the motion segments can develop only small moment and shear resistances (240).

Trunk Length in Low Back Pain

Of 446 pupils aged 13 to 17 years, 115 were found to have a history of back pain. These pupils tended to have decreased lower limb joint mobility and increased trunk length compared to pupils without back pain. In 77 pupils whose site of back pain was identified, 38 had pain associated with the lumbar spine. These pupils had an increased trunk length, while those with thoracolumbar or thoracic pain did not. Back pain was more common in those who avoided sports (241).

Diurnal Stress Variations on Lumbar Spine

Forward bending movements subject the lumbar spine to higher bending stresses in the early morning compared with later in the day. The increase is about 300% for the discs and 80% for the ligaments of the neural arch. It is concluded that lumbar discs and ligaments are at greater risk of injury in the early morning (242).

TROPISM

In the literature on the subject of normal facings of the lumbar articular facets, there is a variance of opinion. Some investigators believe that sagittal facings are normal, whereas others believe that coronal facings are normal. In our clinical study (243) of patients with vertebral disc lesions, we recorded which facet findings were involved at all lumbar levels. We believe that this is the first

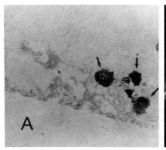
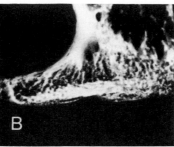
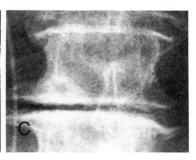

Figure 2.138. Inferior surface of L1 in a 75-year-old woman. **A,** Cartilaginous end plate is completely lost, and the surface of subchondral bone is crushed. Small herniated cartilaginous nodes can be observed (*arrows*). **B,** Texture of end-plate zone is different from that of triangular area of thickened preexisting trabeculae. **C,** Both triangular sclerotic-area and protrusive subchondral sclerotic zone can be observed on the radiograph. (Reproduced with permission from Aoki J, et al.: End plate of the discovertebral joint: degenerative change in the elderly adult. *Radiology* 164(2):413, 1987.)

controlled study documented in the chiropractic and, perhaps, the medical literature concerning which facet facings are involved in lumbar disc lesions. It must be stressed that these findings are based on x-rays of patients with disc protrusion or prolapse.

Tropism (from the Greek word *trope*, a turning) refers to an anomaly of articular formation in which the two articular facings are not the same; i.e., instead of both being sagittal or both coronal, each side assumes a different facing, as shown in Figure 2.139.

From Tables 2.9 and 2.10, it can be inferred that sagittal facet facings are typical in the upper lumbar spine, whereas coronal facet findings are typical in the lower lumbar spine. In 18 of 56 cases of disc lesion (32%), anomalies of articular tropism were present. The most difficult cases to treat were those involving the sagittal facet facings at the level of discal protrusion or prolapse, especially when a medial disc was involved.

The directional plane of articulation of the facets allows for specific movement. Sagittal facets flex and extend, while coronal facets bend laterally. The combining of these two directional opposing forces places excessive stress on the annular fibers of the intervertebral disc (IVD), which tear in nuclear protrusion. The axis of rotation of a lumbar vertebral unit is between the articular facets, with the body rotating forward of this axis (77). Therefore, the altered motoricity of a sagittal and coronal combination creates stress on both the disc and articular facets in all motions of the lumbar spine.

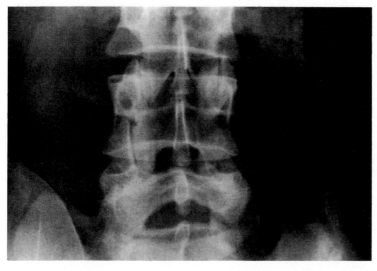

Figure 2.139. X-ray study reveals tropism of the articular facets, with the right L4-L5 facet facings being coronal and the left being sagittal. Note that the facet facings at L5-S1 are bilaterally coronal.

Table 2.9.
Percentage of Facet Facings in 56 Cases of Lumbar Disc Lesion, by Location and Position

	L1-L2		L2-L3		L3-L4		L4-L5		L5-S1	
	Right	Left	Right	Left	Right	Left	Right	Left	Right	Left
Sagittal	74	72	55	64	47	43	29	29	7	5
Coronal	23	26	40	34	41	53	64	65	91	95
Semisagittal	3	2	5	2	12	4	7	6	2	

Table 2.10.
Average Percentage of Facet Facings at Each Level in 56 Cases of Lumbar Disc Lesion

	L1-L2	L2-L3	L3-L4	L4-L5	L5-S1
Sagittal	73	59.5	45	29	6
Coronal	24.5	37	47	64.5	93
Semisagittal	2.5	3.5	8	6.5	1

Facet tropism, therefore, creates stress on the lumbar spine during motion. In this situation, rotation takes on added importance, since it places maximum stress on the annular fibers, which must tear in order for the nucleus pulposus to protrude, creating the typical disc syndrome with sciatica.

According to Farfan et al. (202), the IVD is capable of great compressive loads. They also believe that Schmorl and Beadle were inaccurate when they stated that the compressive load was the mechanical basis of disc degeneration.

By application of torsional loading to 90 IVD joints (proven normal by discogram) from 66 necropsy specimens, the amount of rotation needed to cause failure of the normal disc was determined to be 22.6°; in cases of degenerated disc, the angle of failure was 14.3°. Degenerated discs show a consistently smaller torsional angle of failure. Farfan et al. concluded that the IVD is injured by rotation within a small normal range of movement and that disc protrusion is a manifestation of annular tearing by torsional injury.

According to Cailliet (168), 75% of lumbar flexion occurs at the lumbosacral articulation. He further states that the shearing stress of the fifth lumbar vertebra on the sacrum increases proportionately to the anterior angulation of the sacrum. We have applied these ideas on stress to our knowledge of the facet articular plane and believe that the coronal facet facing at L5-S1 al-

lows greater stability than does the sagittal facet facing at L5-S1.

We believe, therefore, that the following conclusions are justified.

1. Sagittal facet articulation facings are normal for the upper lumbar spine, and coronal facet articulation facings are normal for the lower lumbar spine.

2. Even with the lesser number of sagittal facings in the lower lumbar spine, tropism at the level of disc lesion occurred in 32% of the cases; therefore, there is a prominence of disc lesions in cases of sagittal facings and of tropism.

3. Rotation is the most damaging motion of the low back, resulting in tearing of the lumbar disc annular fibers which allows for nuclear protrusion.

4. Sagittal facets or anomalies of tropism create additional stress on the spine during rotation. Rotation in this situation may be much less than normal before annular disc fibers tear.

5. Patients with anomalous facet facings are at high risk for developing a disc lesion on rotation.

6. In one of every five patients, there is an asymmetrical orientation of the articular facets of the spine at a single level and abnormal spinal motion; these patients, therefore, are predisposed to develop low back and sciatic pain syndromes (226).

7. In patients with articular tropism, the joints rotate toward the side of the more oblique facet (244). Figures 2.140 and 2.141 reveal how tropism changes the force distribution and applies additional torsion to the disc. Furthermore, tropism may predispose to degenerative arthrosis at these facets.

Finally, articular tropism or asymmetry of the articular facets can lead to the manifestation of lumbar instability as joint rotation. This rotation occurs toward the side of the more oblique facet and can place additional stress on the annulus fibrosus of the intervertebral disc and capsular ligaments of the apophyseal joints.

Because the posterior elements maintain stability of the spine, they play an important role in the triple joint complex of the facets and disc. Tropism occurs most commonly in the two lowest lumbar levels (245, 246). Keep in mind that these are synovial joints, and shearing forces place compression on facet surfaces. This compression is greater in less obliquely facing facets. Less oblique facets have greater interfacet forces, predisposing them to degenerative forces.

Arthrosis of the facets is rare in patients under 30 and is found progressively more frequently and is more severe as these patients age (247).

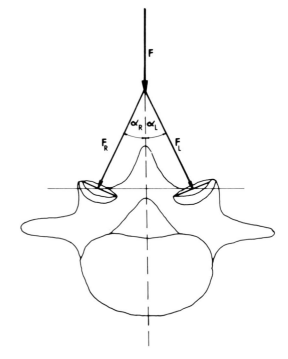

Figure 2.140. Forces (F) acting on symmetrically oriented superior articular facets. (Reproduced with permission from Cyron BM, Hutton WC: Articular tropism. *Spine* 5(2):170, 1980.)

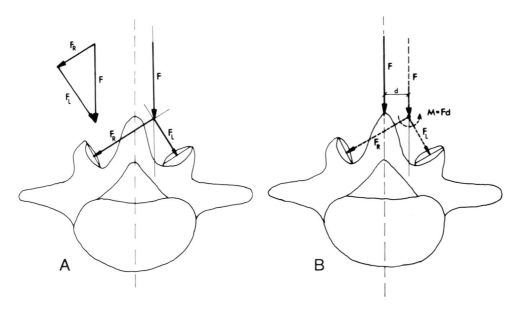

Figure 2.141. Forces (F) acting on asymmetrically oriented superior articular facets. **A,** The force F acts at the point of concurrency and is distributed unevenly to the articular facets. **B,** The force is offset from the point of concurrency, and additional torsion is applied to the joint. (Reproduced with permission from Cyron BM, Hutton WC: Articular tropism. *Spine* 5(2):171, 1980.)

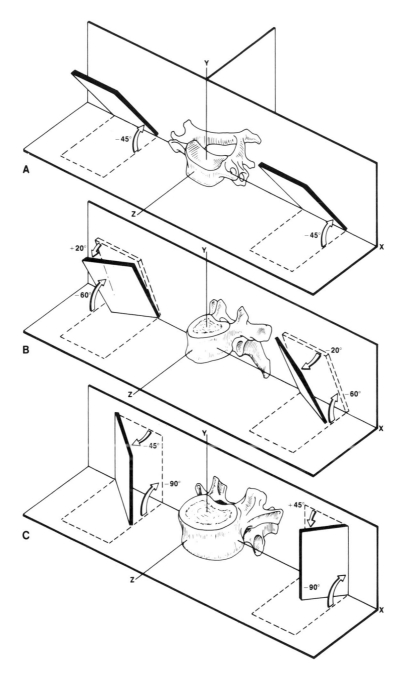

Figure 2.142. Orientation of the facet joints. A graphical representation of the facet joint inclinations in various regions of the spine is obtained by rotating two cards lying in the horizontal plane through two consecutive angles, i.e., *x*-axis rotation followed by *y*-axis rotation. Typical values for the two angles for the three regions of the spine follow. **A**, Cervical spine: −45° followed by 0°. **B**, Thoracic spine: −60° followed by +20° for right facet rotation, or −20° for left facet rotation. **C**, Lumbar spine: −90° and −45° for right facet rotation or +45° for the left facet rotation. (These are only rough estimates.) There are variations within the regions of the spine and between different individuals. (Reproduced with permission from White AA, Panjabi MM: *Clinical Biomechanics of the Spine*. Philadelphia, JB Lippincott, 1978, p 22.)

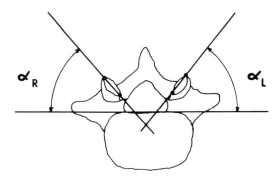

Figure 2.143. Measurement of facet orientation. (Reproduced with permission from Cyron BM, Hutton WC: Articular tropism. *Spine* 5(2):170, 1980.)

Also, intervertebral arthritis is more common at L3-L4 and L4-L5 than at L5-S1, where the facets are less obliquely faced. Badgley (245) reports that arthritis of the facets is more common in cases of tropism and lesions of articular capsules, granular ossification, calcification, and adhesions

of the meningeal covering of the nerve root adjacent to it.

The normal plane of articulation of the lower lumbar facets (Fig. 2.142) is 45° to the body sagittal or coronal planes (2). The inferior facets are convex, whereas the superior facets are concave.

Figure 2.143 shows the normal 45° angle of inclination (244). Figure 2.140 shows that the vector forces are equally balanced on the two facets in the case of a symmetrically oriented articular facet, whereas Figure 2.141 shows that the forces shift to the side of the more obliquely faced facet in the case of tropism. It is on the side of the more obliquely faced facet that the posterolateral annular fibers tear.

Thoracolumbar Facet Orientation

The disc degeneration in the thoracolumbar junctional region (T10-L1) of 37 male cadaveric spines was recorded with the use of discography. From 24 of these spines, the facet joint orientation and degenerative findings of the facet, costo-

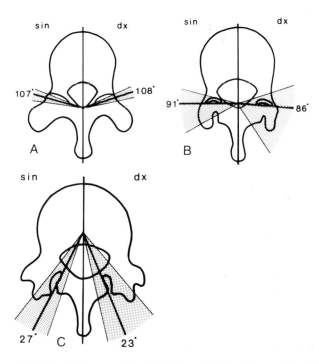

Figure 2.144. Median and 10th and 9th percentiles (*shaded area*) of facet joint angles of 24 cadaveric spines at **A**, T10-T11, **B**, T11-T12, and **C**, T12-L1. At T10-T11, facet orientation was always nearly frontal. At T11-T12, the facet angles showed widest variation. At T12-L1, facet orientation was usually of lumbar type, i.e., nearly sagittal. (Reproduced with permission from Malmivaara A, Videman T, Kuosma E, Troup JDG: Facet joint orientation, facet and costovertebral joint osteoarthrosis, disc degeneration, vertebral body osteophytosis, and Schmorl's nodes in the thoracolumbar junctional region of cadaveric spines. *Spine* 12(5):460, 461, 1987.)

vertebral joints, vertebral bodies (osteophytosis) and discs, and Schmorl's nodes were recorded directly from bones. At T11-T12, the most common site for the transitional zone between thoracic and lumbar facet type, there was a marked variation in the orientation of facets (Fig. 2.144). The occurrence of degenerative findings and Schmorl's nodes at the three levels in the region differed (Figs. 2.145–2.147). At T10-T11, disc degeneration, vertebral body osteophytosis, and Schmorl's nodes were most common (anterior degeneration). At T12-L1, facet and costovertebral joint degeneration were dominant (posterior degeneration). At T11-T12, disc degeneration, vertebral body osteophytosis, Schmorl's nodes, and facet and costovertebral joint degeneration all occurred (anterior and posterior degeneration). The results point to a pathoanatomical association between degenerative changes and facet orientation (248).

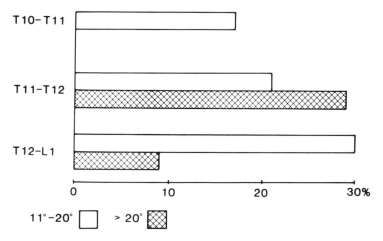

Figure 2.145. Asymmetry of the facet joints at different levels of the thoracolumbar junctional region (T10-L1) of 24 cadaveric spines. Asymmetry of >20° was most common at T11-T12. (Reproduced with permission from Malmivaara A, Videman T, Kuosma E, Troup JDG: Facet joint orientation, facet and costovertebral joint osteoarthrosis, disc degeneration, vertebral body osteophytosis, and Schmorl's nodes in the thoracolumbar junctional region of cadaveric spines. *Spine* 12(5):460, 461, 1987.)

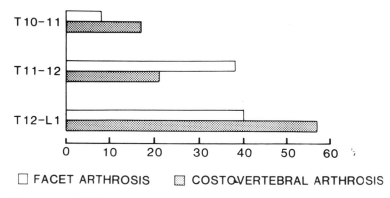

Figure 2.146. Percentages of slight to severe facet joint and costovertebral joint osteoarthrosis (posterior degeneration) at different levels of the T-L region (T10-L1) in 24 cadaveric spines. Assessments from bone specimens. Posterior degeneration was most common at T12-L1. (Reproduced with permission from Malmivaara A, Videman T, Kuosma E, Troup JDG: Facet joint orientation, facet and costovertebral joint osteoarthrosis, disc degeneration, vertebral body osteophytosis, and Schmorl's nodes in the thoracolumbar junctional region of cadaveric spines. *Spine* 12(5):460, 461, 1987.)

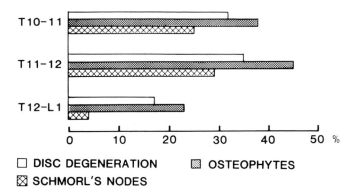

Figure 2.147. Percentages of moderate to severe general disc degeneration, vertebral body osteophytosis, and Schmorl's nodes (anterior degeneration) at different levels of the T-L region (T10-L1) in 24 cadaveric spines (disc degeneration in 37). Anterior degeneration was least common at T12-L1. (Reproduced with permission from Malmivaara A, Videman T, Kuosma E, Troup JDG: Facet joint orientation, facet and costovertebral joint osteoarthrosis, disc degeneration, vertebral body osteophytosis, and Schmorl's nodes in the thoracolumbar junctional region of cadaveric spines. *Spine* 12(5):460, 461, 1987.)

Facet Facings in Upper Compared to Lower Lumbar Spine

The relationship between the angulation of the facet joints and that of the caudad parts of the corresponding laminae in the transverse plane was investigated with CT at the vertebral levels L3-L4, L4-L5, and L5-S1 (Fig. 2.148). At the level of L3-L4, both the facet joints and the caudad portions of the laminae tend toward a sagittal orientation, while at L5-S1, the orientation is more toward the frontal plane. At the level of L4-L5, they occupy an intermediate position. A highly significant correlation between the orientation of these structures is demonstrated. The caudad parts of the laminae may be considered buttresses for the inferior articular processes of the same vertebra (249).

Sagittal Facets Promote Disc Prolapse

In the synergistic complex formed by the intervertebral disc and posterior articular processes, the latter play a significant role in protecting the disc and blocking forward movement of the spine. This role is of special importance at the level of the lumbosacral interface, whose inclination contributes to increasing the shearing forces acting on the disc. The orientation of the lumbosacral articular processes modifies the distribution of the mechanical stress acting at their level.

The relationship between the orientation of the articular processes and the stress transmitted to the disc was studied by computed tomography (31 subjects without disc prolapse, 35 subjects with disc prolapse, 110 operative reports). Sagittal orientation of the facet joints, which is consistently more pronounced on the right side, seems to promote the occurrence of disc prolapse at the lumbosacral level (250).

Controversy Exists over Facet Symmetry in Disc Degeneration

No useful correlations were found between facet asymmetry and asymmetry of the canal, or canal rotation, or degenerative change. Coronally oriented facets withstand shear but do not resist rotation. There was no greater incidence of degenerative change in vertebrae with coronally oriented facets. The role of asymmetric apophyseal joints was discussed by Farfan (202). In this study, however, no correlation between the degree of facet asymmetry and the size of the vertebral osteophytes was found.

If facet asymmetry predisposed an individual to rotational displacement, either it is not necessarily associated with degenerative change, or it is so infrequent an occurrence that it was not detected in this series of specimens (251).

Radiographs of the lumbar spine frequently demonstrate asymmetry of posterior articular facets, but this is asymptomatic in patients with

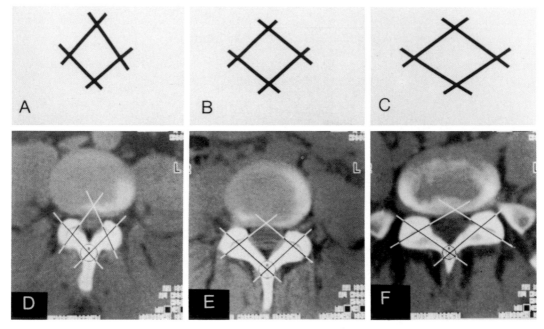

Figure 2.148. **A, B, C**, Quadrangles composed of the mean values for transverse interfacet-joint and interlaminar angles at L3-L4, L4-L5, and L5-S1, respectively. **D, E, F**, CT scans of each of the three levels show the formation of the quadrangles. They represent individual values, not the mean values shown in **A**, **B**, and **C**. (Reproduced with permission from Van Schaik JPJ, Herbiest H, Van Schaik FDJ: The orientation of laminae and facet joints in the lower lumbar spine. *Spine* 10(1):63, 1985.)

good abdominal and lumbar muscles when the anomaly is only of a moderate degree. It can, however, cause rotatory instability of the subjacent vertebra, leading to lumbago. It is then frequently associated with osteoarticular complications affecting the posterior arch, this being a logical consequence of a sequence of changes which can be explained by simple mechanical factors (252).

Determining Tropism by Plain Film versus CT Study

A study by this author (253) found the accuracy of defining tropism on plain x-ray study of 20 patients to have been 27% by one interpreter and 50% by another. CT was the accurate diagnostic modality against which plain x-ray study was compared.

Tropism is a common anomaly, with an occurrence of 17 to 31% in several large series (249, 254, 255, 256). Tropism is reported in higher incidence in patients with clinically and surgically proven disc herniations as opposed to a lower incidence in persons without back complaints

(257). It is a biomechanical factor of importance to the manipulative physician. Plain x-ray has limited accuracy in diagnosing facet articular plane, while CT is the best modality for viewing the entire contour of the zygapophyseal joints.

CONCLUSION

At the conclusion of this lengthy chapter, I wish to state that my intention has been to cover pertinent research in lumbar spine biomechanics which will positively influence the daily regimens of care administered by practitioners of chiropractic or allopathic medicine. The principles presented in this chapter formulate the diagnostic and therapeutic discussions in the remainder of the text.

References

1. Posner I, White AA, Edwards WT, Hayes WC: A biomechanical analysis of the clinical stability of the lumbar and lumbosacral spine. *Spine* 7(4): 374–389, 1982.
2. White AA, Panjabi MM: *Clinical Biomechanics of*

the Spine. Philadelphia, JB Lippincott, 1978, pp 15, 22, 55.

3. Farfan HF, Gracovetsky S: The nature of instability. *Spine* 9(7):714–719.

4. Weitz EM: The lateral bending spine. *Spine* 6(4): 388–397, 1981.

5. Van Damme W, Hessels G, Verhelst M, Van Laer L, Van Es I: Relative efficacy of clinical examination, electromyography, plain film radiography, myelography and lumbar phlebography in the diagnosis of low back pain and sciatica. *Neuroradiology* 18:109–118, 1979.

6. Duncan W, Haen TI: A new approach to the diagnosis of herniation of the intervertebral disc. *Surg Gynecol Obstet* 75:257–267, 1942.

7. Falconer MA, McGeorge M, Begg AC: Surgery of lumbar intervertebral disc protrusion: study of principles and results based upon 100 consecutive cases submitted to operation. *Br J Surg* 1: 225–249, 1948.

8. Hadley LA: Construction of the intervertebral foramen—a cause of nerve root pressure. *JAMA* 140:473–475, 1949.

9. Schalimtzek M: Functional roentgen exam of degenerated and normal intervertebral discs of the lumbar spine. *Acta Radiol [Suppl] (Stockh)* 116: 300–306, 1954.

10. Hasner E, Schalimtzek M, Snorrason E: Roentgenographic examination of function of lumbar spine. *Acta Radiol [Diagn] (Stockh)* 37:141–149, 1952.

11. Breig A: *Adverse Mechanical Tension in the Central Nervous System.* New York, John Wiley & Sons, 1978.

12. Porter RW, Miller CG: Back pain and trunk list. *Spine* 11(6):596, 1986.

13. Finneson BE: *Low Back Pain.* Philadelphia, JB Lippincott, 1973.

14. Nachemson AL: The lumbar spine, an orthopaedic challenge. *Spine* 1(1):59–69, 1976.

15. Tanz SS: Motion of the lumbar spine, a roentgenographic study. *Am J Roentgenol Radium Ther Nucl Med* 69:399–412, 1953.

16. Rees WS: Slipped disc syndrome. *Med J Aust* 2: 948, 1973.

17. Rothman RH, Simeone FA: *The Spine.* Philadelphia, WB Saunders, 1975, vol 2, pp 444, 468.

18. Feffer H: How to prevent back pain. *US News World Rep* (April):47–48, 1975.

19. Cyriax J: *Textbook of Orthopedic Medicine,* ed 5, vol 1, *Diagnosis of Soft Tissue Lesions.* Baltimore, Williams & Wilkins, 1969, pp 389–397.

20. Day PL: Early interim and long term observations on chemonucleolysis in 876 patients with special comments on the lateral approach. *Clin Orthop* 99:63–69, 1974.

21. Semmes RE: *Ruptures of the Lumbar Intervertebral Disc.* Springfield, IL., Charles C Thomas, 1964, pp 17–18.

22. Scoville WB, Corkill G: Lumbar spondylolisthesis with ruptured disc. *J Neurosurg* 40:530, 1974.

23. Abdullah AF, Ditto EW, Byrd EW, Williams R: Extreme lateral disc herniations, clinical syndrome and special problems of diagnosis. *J Neurosurg* 41: 229–233, 1974.

24. Weisel SW, Tsourmas N, Feffer H.L, Citrin CM, Patronas N: A study of computer-assisted tomography. I. The incidence of positive CAT scans in an asymptomatic group of patients. *Spine* 9(6): 549–551, 1985.

25. Bell GR, Rothman RH, Booth RE, Cuckler JM, Garfin S, Herkowitz H, Simeone FA, Dolinskas C, Han SS: A study of computer-assisted tomography. II. Comparison of metrizamide myelography and computed tomography in the diagnosis of herniated lumbar disc and spinal stenosis. *Spine* 9(6):552–556, 1985.

26. Phillips RB, Frymoyer JW, MacPherson BV, Newburg AH: Low back pain: a radiographic enigma. *J Manipulative Physiol Ther* 9:3, 183, 1986.

27. Deyo RA, McNiesh LM, Cone RO: Observer variability in the interpretation of lumbar spine radiographs. *Clin Res* 33(2):A228, 1985.

28. Graham CE: A prospective comparative study of lumbar discography versus CT scanning in the assessment of the integrity of 270 lumbar discs. *J Bone Joint Surg* 69B, 1987.

29. McCutcheon ME, Thompson WC: CT scanning of lumbar discography: a useful diagnostic adjunct. *Spine* 11(3):257–259, 1986.

30. Milette PC, Melanson D: A reappraisal of lumbar discography. *J Can Assoc Radiol* 33(September): 176–182, 1982.

31. Kurobane Y, Takaahashi T, Tajima T, Yamakawa H, Sakamoto T, Sawaumi A, Kikuchi I: Extraforaminal disc herniation. *Spine* 11(3): 260–268, 1986.

32. Powell MC, Szypryt P, Wilson M, Symonds EM, Worthington BS: Prevalence of lumbar disc degeneration observed by magnetic resonance in symptomless women,. *Lancet* (December): 1366–1367, 1986.

33. Gibson MJ, Buckley J, Mawhinney RR, Mulholland RC, Worthington BS: The changes in the intervertebral disc after chemonucleolysis demonstrated by magnetic resonance imaging. *Proceedings of the British Institute of Radiology* 59(704):808, 1986.

34. Modic MT, Masaryk T, Boumphrey F, Goormastic M, Bell G: Lumbar herniated disc disease and canal stenosis: prospective evaluation by surface coil MR, CT, and myelography. *AJR* 7(4):709–717, 1986.

35. Bobest M, Furo I, Rompa K, Pocsik I, Kuncz A: ¹h Nuclear magnetic resonance study of intervertebral discs: preliminary report. *Spine* 11(7): 709–711, 1986.

36. Hoe J, Tan L: A comparison of iohexol and

iopamidol for lumbar myelography. *Clin Radiol* 37:505, 1986.

37. Drayer BP: A double blind clinical trial of iopamidol versus metrizamide for lumbosacral myelography. *J Neurosurg* 58(April):531–537, 1983.

38. Postacchinia F, Massobrio M: Outpatient lumbar myelography: analysis of complications after myelography comparing outpatients with inpatients. *Spine* 10(6):567–570, 1985.

39. Troisier O, Cypel D: Discography: an element of decision. *Clin Orthop* 206:70–78, 1986.

40. Hickey D, Aspden R, Hukins D, Jenkins J, Sherwood I: Analysis of magnetic resonance images from normal and degenerate lumbar intervertebral discs. *Spine* 11(7):702, 1986.

41. Kornberg M, Usner MC, Rechtine GR, Dupuy TE: Computed Tomography in the diagnosis of a herniated disc at the L5-S1 level. *Spine* 9(4):433–436, 1984.

42. Firooznia H, Kricheff I, Rafii M, Golimbu C: Lumbar spine after surgery: examination with intravenous contrast-enhanced CT. *Radiology* 163(1):221, 1987.

43. Sotiropoulos S, Chafetz N, Genant HK, Winkler M: Assessment of the post-operative lumbar spine: distinction between post-operative fibrosis and recurrent disc herniation—I.V. contrast enhanced CT vs. MRI. *Invest Radiol* 21(9):15, 1986.

44. Weiss T, Treisch J, Kazner E, Kohler D, Collmann H, Claussen C: CT of the postoperative lumbar spine: the value of intravenous contrast. *Neuroradiology* 28:241–245, 1986.

45. Mikhael MA, Ciric I, Kudrna JC, Hindo WA: Recognition of lumbar disc disease with magnetic resonance imaging. *Comput Radiol* 9(4):213–222, 1985.

46. Hueftle MG: Lumbar spine: postoperative MR imaging with Gd-DTPA. *Radiology* 167(3):817, 1988.

47. Helms CA, Vogler JB, Wall SD: CT attenuation numbers in the lumbar spine and their ability in diagnosing disc disease. *Comput Radiol* 9(5):291–297, 1985.

48. Hakelius A: Prognosis in sciatica. *Acta Orthop Scand* 129(Suppl):1–76, 1970.

49. Hirsch C: Efficiency of surgery in low back disorders. *J Bone Joint Surg* 47A:991, 1965.

50. Firooznia H, Benjamin V, Kricheff I, Rafii M, Golimbu C: CT of lumbar spine disc herniation: correlation with surgical findings. *AJR* 142 (March):587–592, 1984.

51. Morris EW, Paola MD, Vallance R, Waddell G: Diagnosis and decision making in lumbar disc prolapse and nerve entrapment. *Spine* 11(5):436–439.

52. Weise MD, Garfin SR, Gelberman RH, Katz MM, Thorne RP: Lower extremity sensibility testing in patients with herniated lumbar intervertebral discs. *J Bone Joint Surg* 67(8):1219–1224, 1985.

53. Schofferman J, Zucherman J: History and physical examination. *Spine: State of the Art Reviews* 1(1):14, 1986.

54. White A: Failed back surgical syndrome. *Spine: State of the Art Reviews* 1(1):149–159, 1986.

55. Schoedinger GR: Correlation of standard diagnostic studies with surgically proven lumbar disc rupture. *South Med J* 80(1):44–46, 1987.

56. Kortelainen P, Puranen J, Koivista E, Lahde S: Symptoms and signs of sciatica and their relation to the localization of the lumbar disc herniation. *Spine* 10(1):88–92, 1985.

57. Bernard TN, Kirkaldy-Willis WH: Recognizing specific characteristics of nonspecific low back pain. *Clin Orthop* 217:266, 1987.

58. Dietemann JL, Sick H, Woilfram-Gabel R, Cruz da Silva R, Koritke JG, Wackenheim A: Anatomy and computed tomography of the normal lumbosacral plexus. *Neuroradiology* 29:58–68, 1987.

59. White SH, Leslie IJ: Pain in scrotum due to intervertebral disc protrusion. *Lancet* (March 1):504, 1986.

60. Nachemson AL: The lumbar spine, an orthopaedic challenge. *Spine* 1(1):59–69, 1976.

61. Bernini PM, Simeone FA: Reflex dystrophy. *Spine* 6(2):180–184, 1981.

62. Farfan HF: *Mechanical Disorders of the Low Back.* Philadelphia, Lea & Febiger, 1973, pp 15, 24, 44, 49, 135, 145.

63. Helfet AJ, Gruebel-Lee DM: *Disorders of the Lumbar Spine.* Philadelphia, JB Lippincott, 1978, pp 46–47, 72.

64. Bogduk N: The anatomy of the lumbar intervertebral disc syndrome. *Med J Aust* 1:878, 1976.

65. Tsukada K: Histologische Studien über die Zwischenwirbelscheibe des Menschen. *Altersvanderugen Mitt Akad Kioto* 25:1–29, 207–209, 1932.

66. Shinohara H: A study on lumbar disc lesions. *J Jpn Orthop Assoc* 44:553, 1970.

67. Malinsky J: The ontogenetic development of nerve terminations in the intervertebral discs of man. *Acta Anat* 38:96, 1959.

68. Hirsch C, Inglemark BG, Miller M: The anatomical basis for low back pain. Studies on the presence of sensory nerve endings in ligamentous, capsular and intervertebral disc structures in the human lumbar spine. *Acta Orthop Scand* 1:33, 1963–1964.

68a. Yoshizawa H, O'Brien J, Smith WT, Trumper M: The neuropathology of intervertebral discs removed for low-back pain. *J Pathol* 132:95–104, 1980.

69. Sunderland S: Anatomical paravertebral influence on the intervertebral foramen. In: *The Research Status of Spinal Manipulative Therapy.* Bethesda, MD, National Institute of Neurological

and Communicative Disorders and Stroke, NINCDS Monograph No. 15, DHEW No. 76-998, 1975, p 135.

70. Edgar MA, Ghadially JA: Innervation of the lumbar spine. *Clin Orthop* 115:35–41, 1976.

71. Lazorthes G, Poulhes J, Espagno J: Etude sur les nerfs sinu-vertébraux lumbaires le nerf de roofe existe-t-il? *CR Assoc Anat* 34:317, 1948.

72. Vernon-Roberts B, Pirie CJ: Degenerative changes in the intervertebral discs of the lumbar spine and their sequelae. *J Rheumatol Rehabil* 16: 13, 1977.

73. Cailliet R: *Low Back Pain Syndrome*. Philadelphia, FA Davis, 1962, pp 4–5.

74. Puschel J: Der Wassergehalt normaler and degenerieter Zuracken Werbelscheben. *Beitr Pathol* 84:123, 1930.

75. DePukey P: The Physiological oscillation of the length of the body. *Acta Orthop Scand.* 6:338d, 1935.

76. Hendry NGC: The hydration of the nucleus pulposus and its relation to intervertebral disc derangement. *J Bone Joint Surg* 40B:132, 1958.

77. Finneson BE: *Low Back Pain*. Philadelphia, JB Lippincott, 1973, pp 25, 27, 31, 33–37, 96, 264, 265.

78. Morris JM, Lucas DB, Bresler B: Role of the trunk in stability of the spine. *J Bone Joint Surg* 43A:327, 1961.

79. Gresham JL, Miller R: Evaluation of the lumbar spine by diskography. *Orthop Clin* 67:29, 1969.

80. Hoelein BF: *Canine Neurology: Diagnosis and Treatment*. Philadelphia, WB Saunders, 1965.

81. Epstein BS: *The Spine, A Radiological Text and Atlas*, ed 3. Philadelphia, Lea & Febiger, 1969, pp 35, 38, 554.

82. Keele CA, Neil E: *Samson Wright's Applied Physiology*, ed 10. London, Oxford University Press, 1961, p 51.

83. Lecuire J. et al.: 641 operations for sciatic neuralgia due to discal hernia, a computerized statistical study of the results. *Neurochirugie* 19:501–512, 1973.

84. Turek S: *Orthopaedics—Principles and Their Applications*. Philadelphia, JB Lippincott, 1956, chap 27, p 748.

85. Ritchie JH, Fahrni WJ: Age changes in the lumbar intervertebral disc. *Can J Surg* 13:65, 1970.

86. Yong-Hing K, Kirkaldy-Willis WH: The pathophysiology of degenerative disease of the lumbar spine. *Orthop Clin North Am* 14(13):501–503, 1983.

87. Lora J, Long D: So-called facet denervation in the management of intractable back pain. *Spine* 1(2): 121–126, 1976.

88. Arns W, et al.: Conservative therapy of lumbar intervertebral disc lesions. *Dtsch Med Wochenschr* 101:587–589, 1976.

89. Macnab I, et al.: Chemonucleolysis. *Can J Surg* 14: 280–289, 1971.

90. Macnab I: Negative disc exploration. *J Bone Joint Surg* 53A:891–903, 1971.

90a. Seligman JV, Gertzbein SD, Tile M, Kapasouri A: 1984 Volvo Award in Basic Science: computer analysis of spinal segment motion in degenerative disc disease with and without axial loading. *Spine* 9(6):566–573, 1984.

90b. Scull ER: Joint biomechanics and therapy: contribution or confusion? In Glasgow EF, Twomey LT, Scull ER, Kleynhans AM, Idczak RM (eds): *Aspects of Manipulative Therapy*, ed 2. New York, Churchill-Livingstone, 1985, pp 1–15.

91. Andersson GBJ: The biomechanics of the posterior elements of the lumbar spine. *Spine* 8(3):326, 1983.

92. Miller JAA, Haderspeck KA, Schultz AB: Posterior elements in lumbar motion segments. *Spine* 8(3):331–337, 1983.

93. Jayson MIV: Compression stresses in the posterior elements and pathologic consequences. *Spine* 8(3):338, 1983.

94. Adams MA, Hutton WC: The mechanical function of the lumbar apophyseal joints. *Spine* 8(3): 327–329, 1983.

95. Pearcy MJ: Stereo radiography of lumbar spine motion. *Acta Orthop Scand* 56(Suppl 212):9–44, 1985.

96. Panjabi MM, White A: Basic biomechanics of the spine. *Neurosurgery* 7(1):76–77, 1980.

97. Gregerson GG, Lucas DB: An in vivo study of the axial rotation of the human thoraco-lumbar spine. *J Bone Joint Surg* 49A:247, 262, 1967.

98. Lumsden RM II, Morris JM: An in vivo study of axial rotation and immobilization at the lumbosacral joint. *J Bone Joint Surg* 50A:1591–1602, 1968.

98a. Adams MA, Hutton WC: The mechanical function of the lumbar apophyseal joints. *Spine* 8(3): 327–329, 1983.

99. Adams MA, Hutton WC: The effect of posture on the lumbar spine. *J Bone Joint Surg* 67B:625–629, 1985.

100. Fahrni WH: Conservative treatment of lumbar disc degeneration: our primary responsibility. *Orthop Clin North Am* 6(1):93–103, 1975.

101. Fromelt K, Cox JM, Schreiner S: Activities causing injury to the lumbar spine: a computer study. *JACA* 17:3–16, 1983.

102. Kraemer J, Kolditz D, Gowin R: Water and electrolyte content of human intervertebral discs under variable load. *Spine* 10(1):69–71, 1985.

103. Thery Y, Bonjean P, Calen S, Roques JC: Anatomical and roentgenological basis for the study of the lumbar spine with the body in the suspended position. *Anat Clin* 7:161–169, 1985.

104. Pope MH, Bevins T, Wilder DG, Frymoyer JW; The relationship between anthropometric, postural, muscular, and mobility characteristics of males ages 18–55. *Spine* 10(7):644–648, 1985.

105. Heliovaara M: Body weight, obesity, and risk of herniated lumbar intervertebral disc. *Spine* 12(5): 469, 1987.

106. Vanharanta H, Heliovaara M, Korpi J, Troup JDG: Occupation, work load and the size and shape of lumbar vertebral canals. *Scand J Work Environ Health* 13, 1987.

107. Mellin G: Correlations of spinal mobility with degree of chronic low back pain after correction for age and anthropometric factors. *Spine* 12(3):464, 1987.

108. Biering-Sorensen F: Physical measurements as risk indicators for low back trouble over a one-year period. *Spine* 9(2):106, 1984.

109. Eisenstein S: Lumbar vertebral canal morphometry for computerized tomography in spinal stenosis. *Spine* 8(2):187–189, 1983.

110. Brinckmann P: Injury of the annulus fibrosus and disc protrusions: an in vitro investigation on human lumbar discs. *Spine* 11(2):149–153, 1986.

111. Devanny JR: An orthopaedist talks about low back syndromes. *Semin Neurol* 6(4):411–413, 1986.

112. Giles LGF, Taylor JR; Innervation of lumbar zygapophyseal joint synovial folds. *Acta Orthop Scand* 58:43–46, 1987.

113. Mooney V, Robertson J: The facet syndrome. *Clin Orthop* 115:149–156, 1976.

114. Hadley LA: *Anatomico-Roentgenographic Studies of the Spine.* Springfield, IL, Charles C. Thomas, 1976.

115. Wyke BD: The neurology of joints: a review of general principles. *Clin Rheumatic Dis* 7:223–239.

115a. Kos J, Wolf J: Les menisques intervertébraux et leur Rˆole possible dans les blocages vertébraux. *Annales de Medicine Physique* 15:203–217, 1978.

115b. Giles LGF, Taylor JR: Intra-articular synovial protrusions in the lower lumbar apophyseal joints. *Bull Hosp Joint Dis Orthop Inst* 42:248–255, 1986.

116. Larsen JL: The posterior surface of the lumbar vertebral bodies. Part 2. An anatomic investigation concerning the curvatures in the horizontal plane. *Spine* 10(10):901–906, 1985.

117. Adams MA, Dolan P, Hutton WC: The stages of disc degeneration as revealed by discograms. *J Bone Joint Surg* 68B:37, 1986.

118. Resnick D: Common disorders of the aging lumbar spine: radiographic-pathologic correlation. In *Spine Update 1984.* San Francisco, Radiology Research and Education Foundation, 1984, pp 35–42.

119. Golimbu C, Firooznia H, Rafil M: The intravertebral vacuum sign. *Spine* 11(10): 1040–1042, 1986.

120. MacGibbon B, Farfan H: A radiologic survey of various configurations of the lumbar spine. *Spine* 4(3):258–266, 1976.

121. Luyendijk W: The localization of protruded lumbar discs in advancing age. *Acta Neurochir* 85: 168–171, 1987.

122. Fernand R, Fox DE: Evaluation of lumbar lordosis: a prospective and retrospective study. *Spine* 10(9):799–803, 1985.

123. Saraste H, Brostrom L-A, Aparisi T, Axdorph G: Radiographic measurement of the lumbar spine—a clinical and experimental study in man. *Spine* 10(3):236, 1985.

124. Hansson T, Bigos S, Beecher P, Wortley M: The lumbar lordosis in acute and chronic low back pain. *Spine* 10(2):154–155, 1985.

125. Macnab I: The mechanism of spondylogenic pain. In Hirsch C, Zotterman Y (eds): *Cervical Pain.* New York, Pergamon Press, 1972, pp 89–95.

126. Gracovetsky S, Farfan H, Helleur C: The abdominal mechanism. *Spine* 10(4):317–324, 1985.

127. Hemborg B, Moritz U: Intra-abdominal pressure and trunk muscle activity during lifting. II. Chronic low back patients. *Scand J Rehabil Med* 17: 5–13, 1985,.

128. Deleted in text.

129. Macintosh JE, Valencia F, Bogduk N, Munro RR: The morphology of the human lumbar multifidus. *Clin Biomech* 1(4):196–204, 1986.

130. Jowett RL, Fidler MW, Troup JD: Histochemical changes in the multifidus in mechanical derangements of the spine. *Orthop Clinics North Am* 6(1): 157, 1975.

131. Valencia FP, Munro RR: An electromyographic study of the lumbar multifidus in man. *Electromyogr Clin Neurophysiol* 25:205–221, 1985.

132. Macintosh JE, Bogduk N: The qualitative biomechanics of the lumbar back muscles. *Proc Anat Soc Aust N Zealand* 1(4):205–213.

133. Brickley-Parsons D, Glimsher M: Is the chemistry of collagen in intervertebral discs an expression of Wolff's law: a study of the human lumbar spine. *Spine* 9(2):148–158, 1984.

134. Lowther DA: The effect of compression and tension on the behavior of connective tissues. In Glasgow CF, Twomey LT, Scull CR, Kleyhans AM, Idczak RM (eds): *Aspects of Manipulative Therapy.* New York, Churchill-Livingstone, 1985, pp 16–20.

135. Pearce RH, Grimmer BJ, Adams ME: Degeneration and the chemical composition of the human lumbar intervertebral disc. *J Orthop Res* 5: 198–205, 1987.

136. Twomey L, Taylor J: Age changes in lumbar intervertebral discs. *Acta Orthop Scand* 56:496–499, 1985.

137. Weiss S, Quennel R, Jayson M: Abnormal connective tissue degrading enzyme patterns in prolapsed intervertebral discs. *Spine* 11(7):695–700, 1986.

138. Crock H: Internal disc disruption: a challenge to disc prolapse fifty years on. *Spine* 11(6):650–653, 1986.

139. Nachemson A, Lewin T, Maroudas A, Freeman M: In vitro diffusion of dye through the end-plates

and the annulus fibrosus of human lumbar intervertebral discs. *Acta Orthop Scand* 41(6):589–607, 1970.

140. Eismont FJ, Wiesel SW, Brighton CT, Rothman RH: Antibiotic penetration into rabbit nucleus pulposus. *Spine* 12(3): 254, 1987.

141. Naylor A, Happey F, Turner RL, Shentall RD, West RD, Richardson C: Enzymatic and immunological activity in the intervertebral disc. *Orthop Clin North Am* 6(1):51–58, 1975.

142. Elves MW, Bucknill T, Sullivan MF: In vitro inhibition of leucocyte migration in patients with intervertebral disc lesions. *Orthop Clin North Am* 6:1, 1975.

143. Gertzbein SD: Degenerative disc disease of the lumbar spine. *Clin Orthop* 126:68–71, 1977.

144. Eyre DR: Biochemistry of the intervertebral disc. *Int Rev Connect Tissue Res* 8:227–289, 1979.

145. Marshall LL, Trethewie ER: Chemical radiculitis. *Clin Orthop* 129(November–December):61–67, 1977.

146. Saal JA: Electrophysiologic evaluation of lumbar pain: establishing the rationale for therapeutic management. *Spine: State of the Art Reviews* 1(1): 21–28, 1986.

147. Wald NJ, Nanchahal K, Thompson SG, Cuckle HS: Does breathing other people's tobacco smoke cause lung cancer? *Br Med J* 293(November): 1217–1223, 1986.

148. Luck TC, Prochazka AV: All veterans are smokers—a false perception. *Clin Res* 35(1):131A, 1987.

149. Holm S, Nachemson A: Nutrition of the intervertebral disc: acute effects of cigarette smoking: an experimental animal study. *Orthop Trans* 8:415, 1984.

150. Cox JM, Trier KK: Exercise and smoking habits in patients with and without low back and leg pain. *J Manipulative Physical Ther* 10:239–244, 1987.

151. Kelsey J, Githens P, O'Conner T, Ulrich W, Calogero J, Holford T, et al.: Acute prolapsed lumbar intervertebral disc: an epidemiologic study with special reference to driving automobiles and cigarette smoking. *Spine* 9:608–613, 1984.

152. Frymoyer JW, Pope MH, Clements JH, Wilder DG, MacPherson B, Ashikaga T: Risk factors in low back pain. *J Bone Joint Surg* 65A:213–218, 1983.

153. Svensson H: Low back pain in relation to other diseases and cardiovascular risk factors. *Spine* 8: 277–285, 1983.

154. Svensson HO, Andersson GBJ: Low back pain in forty to forty-seven year old men: work history and work environment factors. *Spine* 8:272–276, 1983.

155. Gytelberg F: One-year incidence of low back pain among male residents of Copenhagen aged 40–59. *Dan Med Bull* 21:30–36, 1974.

156. Frymoyer JW, Pope MH, Costanza MC, Rosen JC,

Goggin JE, Wilder DG: Epidemiologic studies of low back pain. *Spine* 5:419–423, 1980.

157. Urban JPG, Holms S, Maroudas A, Nachemson A: Nutrition of the intervertebral disc: an in vivo study of solute transport. *Clin Orthop* 129: 101–114, 1977.

158. Kamijok, Tsujimaya H, Obara H, Katsumata M: Evaluation of seating comfort. *Society of Automotive Engineers Technical Paper Series* 820761:1–6, 1986.

159. Daniell HW: Osteoporosis of the slender smoker. *Arch Intern Med* 136:298–304, 1976.

160. Hollo I, Gergely I, Boross M: Influence of heavy smoking upon the bone mineral content of the radius of the aged and effect of tobacco smoke on the sensitivity to calcitonin of rats. *Aktuel Gerontol* 9:365–368, 1979.

161. Hansson T, Roos B: Microcalluses of the trabeculae in lumbar vertebrae and their relation to the bone mineral content. *Spine* 6:375–380, 1981.

162. Biering-Sorenson F: Low back trouble in a general population of 30-, 40-, 50-, and 60-year-old men and women: study design, representativeness and basic results. *Dan Med Bull* 29:289–299, 1982.

163. Giles LGF, Taylor JR: Low back pain associated with leg length inequality. *Spine* 6(5):510–521, 1981.

164. Giles LGF, Taylor JR: Lumbar spine structural changes associated with leg length inequality. *Spine* 7(2):159–162, 1982.

165. Friberg O: Biomechanics and clinical significance of unrecognized leg length inequality. *Manuel Medizin* 21(4):83, 1983.

166. Gofton JP: Studies in osteoarthritis of the hip: Part IV. Biomechanics and clinical considerations. *Can Med Assoc J* 104:1007–1011, June 5, 1971.

167. Cox JM: *Low Back Pain: Mechanism, Diagnosis, and Treatment*, ed 4. Baltimore, Williams & Wilkins, 1985, pp 122–123.

168. Cailliet R: *Low Back Pain Syndrome*, ed 3. Philadelphia, FA Davis, 1983, pp 72–74.

169. Chamberlain WE: Measurements of differences in leg length. In Merrill V (ed): *Atlas of Roentgenographic Positioning*, Vol 1. St. Louis, CV Mosby, 1967.

170. Giles LGF, Taylor JR: Low back pain associated with leg length inequality. *Spine* 6(5):510–520, 1981.

171. Kirby RL, Hamilton RD, MacLeod DA: Assessing disturbances of standing balance by relating postural sway to the base of support. In: *Proceedings of the Ninth International Congress of Physical Medicine and Rehabilitation, Jerusalem, 1984*, p 283.

172. Shirazi-Adl A, Ahmen AM, Shrivastava SC: Mechanical response of a lumbar motion segment in axial torque alone and combined with compression. *Spine* 11(9):914, 1986.

173. Shirazi-Adl A, Ahmed AM, Shrivastava SC: A fi-

nite element study of a lumbar motion segment subjected to pure sagittal plane moments. *J Biomech* 9:4, 1986.

174. Hutton WC, Adam MA: Mechanical factors in the etiology of low back pain. *Orthopedics* 5(11): 1461–1465, 1982.

175. Posner I, White AA, Edwards WT, Hayes WC: A biomechanical analysis of the clinical stability of the lumbosacral spine. *Spine* 7(4):374–389, 1982.

176. Ehni G, Weinstein P: *Lumbar Spondylosis.* Chicago, Year Book, 1977, pp 19, 137.

177. Dyck P, Pheasant HC, Doyle JB, Rieder JJ; Cauda equina compression. *Spine* 2(1): 77, 1977.

178. Raney F: The effects of flexion, extension, Valsalva maneuver, and abdominal compression on the myelographic column. International Society for the Study of the Lumbar Spine. San Francisco Meeting, June 5–8, 1978.

179. Pilling JR: Water soluble radiculography in the erect position, a clinical radiological study. *Clin Radiol* 30:665-670, 1979.

180. Matthews JA, Yates DAH: Treatment of sciatica (Letter to the Editor). *Lancet* (March):352, 1974.

181. Wilmink JT, Penning L: Influence of spinal posture on abnormalities demonstrated by lumbar myelography. *Am J Neuroradiol* 4:656–658, 1983.

182. McNeil T, Warwick D, Andersson G, Schultz A: Trunk strengths in attempted flexion, extension, and lateral bending in healthy subjects and patients with low-back disorders. *Spine* 5(6): 529–538, 1980.

183. Adams MA, Hutton WC: Has the lumbar spine a margin of safety in forward bending? *Clin Biomech* 1:3–6, 1986.

184. Soni A, Sullivan J, Herndon W, Gudavalli M: Migratory pattern of vertebral motion in the lumbar spine. *Acta Orthop Scand* 56(Suppl 212):1985.

185. Penning L, Wilmink JT: Biomechanics of lumbosacral dural sac: a study of flexion-extension myelography. *Spine* 6(4):398–408, 1981.

186. Breig A: Adverse mechanical tension in the central nervous system. Stockholm, Almqvist & Wilesell International, 1978.

187. Adams MA, Dolan P, Marx C, Hutton WC: An electronic inclinometer technique for measuring lumbar curvature. *Clin Biomech* 1:130–134, 1986.

188. Adams MA, Hutton WC: The effect of fatigue on the lumbar intervertebral disc. *J Bone Joint Surg* 65B:199–203, 1983.

189. Deleted in text.

190. Adams MA, Hutton WC: The effect of posture on the lumbar spine. *J Bone Joint Surg* 67B:625, 1985.

191. Mayer TG, Tencer AF, Kristoferson S, Mooney V: Use of noninvasive techniques for quantification of spinal range-of-motion in normal subjects and chronic low-back dysfunction patients. *Spine* 9(6): 588–595, 1984.

192. Penning L, Wilmink JT: Biomechanics of

193. Wilmink JR, Penning L, Van den Burg W: Role of stenosis of spinal canal in L4-L5 nerve root compression assessed by flexion-extension myelography. *Neuroradiology* 26:173–181, 1984.

194. Epstein JA: Diagnosis and treatment of painful disorders caused by spondylosis of the lumbar spine. *J Neurosurg* 17:991–1011, 1960.

195. Schlesinger EB, Taveras JM: Factors in the production of "cauda equina" syndromes in lumbar discs. *Trans Am Neurol Assoc* 78:263–265, 1953.

196. Penning L, Wilmink JT: Posture dependent bilateral compression of L4 or L5 nerve roots in facet hypertrophy: a dynamic CT-myelographic study. *Spine* 12(5):488–500, 1987.

197. Knuttson F: Volum und Formvariationen des Wirbelkanals bei Lordosierung und Kyphosierung und ihre Bedeutung für die myelographische Diagnostik. *Acta Radiol* 23:431–443, 1942.

198. Taylor AR: Mechanism and treatment of spinal cord disorders associated with cervical spondylosis. *Lancet* 1:717–722, 1953.

199. Marras WS, Wongsam PE: Flexibility and velocity of the normal and impaired lumbar spine. *Arch Phys Med Rehabil* 67:213–217, 1986.

200. Lee CK, Langrana NA: Lumbosacral spinal fusion: a biomechanical study. *Spine* 9(6):574–581, 1984.

201. Twomey LT, Taylor JR: Sagittal movements of the human lumbar vertebral column: a quantitative study of the role of the posterior vertebral elements. *Arch Phys Med Rehabil* 64(3):322, 1983.

202. Farfan HF, Cossett B, Robertson GH, Wells RV, Kraus H: The effects of torsion on the lumbar intervertebral joints, the role of torsion in the production of disc degeneration. *J Bone Joint Surg* 52A:468 and 494–496, 1970.

203. Hirsch C, Schajowicz F: Studies on the structural changes in the lumbar annulus fibrosus. *Acta Orthop Scand* 22:184, 1953.

204. Maigne R: Low back pain of thoraco-lumbar origin. *Arch Phys Med Rehabil* 61:389–395, 1980.

205. Pearcy MJ, Tibrewal SB: Axial rotation and lateral bending in the normal lumbar spine measured by three-dimensional radiography. *Spine* 9(6): 582–587, 1984.

206. Liu YK, Goel VK, Dejong A, Njus G, Nishiyama K, Buckwalter J: Torsional fatigue of the lumbar intervertebral joints. *Spine* 10(10):894–900, 1985.

207. Stokes I: Surface strain on human intervertebral discs, University of Vermont, Department of Orthopaedics and Rehabilitation, Burlington, VT. *J Orthop Res* 5:348–355, 1987.

208. Kapandji I: The physiology of the joints (Letter to the editor). *J Orthop Sports Phys Therapy* 3(6):40, 1986.

209. Paris SV: Physiological signs of instability. *Spine* 10(3):277, 1985.
210. Lindblom K: Intervertebral disc degeneration considered as a pressure atrophy. *J Bone Joint Surg* 39A:933–944, 1957.
211. Brown T, Hansen R, Yorra A: Some mechanical tests on the lumbosacral spine with particular reference to the intervertebral discs: a preliminary report. *J Bone Joint Surg* 39A:1135, 1161–1162, 1957.
212. Eagle R: A pain in the back. *New Scientist* (October 18):170–173, 1979.
213. Hickey DS, Hukins DWL: Relation between the structure of the annulus fibrosus and the function and failure of the intervertebral disc. *Spine* 5(2):106–116, 1980.
214. Miller J: Empirical approaches to the validation of manipulation. Paper delivered at University of Michigan College of Osteopathic Medicine, April 30–May 1, 1983.
215. Lorenz M, Patwardhan A, Vanderby R: Load bearing characteristics of the lumbar spine in normal and surgically altered spinal segments. *Spine* 8(2):122–128, 1983.
216. Carrera CG: Lumbar facet injection in low back pain and sciatica. *Radiology* 737:665–667, 1980.
217. Dory M: Arthrography of the lumbar facet joints. *Radiology* 140:23–27, 1981.
218. Eklund J, Corlett EN: Shrinkage as a measure of the effect of load on the spine. *Spine* 9(2):189–194, 1984.
219. Tencer AF, Mayer TG: Soft tissue strain and facet face interaction in the lumbar intervertebral joint, Part II. Calculated results and comparison with experimental data. *J Bioengineering* 105(August):210, 1983.
220. Skipor AF, Miller JA, Spencer DA, Schultz AB: Stiffness properties and geometry of lumbar spine posterior elements. *J Biomechanics* 18(11):829, 1985.
221. Deleted in text.
222. Deleted in text.
223. Yang KH, King AI: Mechanism of facet load transmission as a hypothesis for low back pain. *Spine* 9(6):557–565, 1984.
224. Nachemson A: Lumbar intradiscal pressure: experimental studies on post-mortem material. *Acta Orthop Scand* 43(Suppl):2, 1960.
225. Magnuson PB: Differential diagnosis of causes of pain in the lower back accompanied by sciatic pain. *Ann Surg* 119:878, 1944.
226. Weinstein PR, Ehni G, Wilson CB: *Lumbar Spondylosis, Diagnosis, Management, and Surgical Treatment.* Chicago, Year Book, 1977, p 68.
227. Panjabi MM, Krag MH, Chung TQ: Effects of disc injury on mechanical behavior of the human spine. *Spine* 9(7):707–713, 1984.
228. Adams MA, Hutton WC: Gradual disc prolapse. *Spine* 10(6):524–531, 1985.
229. Dunlop RB, Adams MA, Hutton WC: Disc space narrowing and the lumbar facet joints. *J Bone Joint Surg* 66B:706–710, 1984.
230. Spencer DL, Miller JAA, Bertolini JE: The effect of intervertebral disc space narrowing on the contact force between the nerve root and a simulated disc protrusion. *Spine* 9(4):422–426, 1984.
231. Lewin T: Osteoarthritis in lumbar synovial joints. *Acta Orthop Scand* 73(Suppl)1–111, 1964.
232. Harrison MHM, Schagowicz F, Trueta J: Osteoarthritis of the hip: a study of the nature and evaluation of the disease. *J Bone Joint Surg* 35A:398, 1953.
233. Arnoldi CC: Intervertebral pressures in patients with lumbar pain. *Acta Orthop Scand* 43:109, 1972.
234. Giles LGF, Taylor JR: Osteoarthrosis in human cadaveric lumbo-sacral zygapophyseal joints. *J Manipulative Physiol Ther* 8:239–243, 1984.
235. Aoki J, Yamamoto I, Kitamura N, Sone T, Itoh H, Torizuka K, Takasu K: End plate of the discovertebral joint: degenerative change in the elderly adult. *Radiology* 164(2):411–414, 1987.
236. Anderson KH, Mosdal C: Epidural application of cortico-steroids in low back pain and sciatica. From Haase J: *Proceedings of the 38th Annual Meeting. Acta Neurochir* 84 (3–4):145–146, 1987.
237. Adams MA, Hutton WC: The effect of posture on the lumbar spine. *J Bone Joint Surg* 67B:625–629, 1985.
237a. Fahrni WH, Trueman GE: Comparative radiological study of the spine of a primitive population with North Americans and Northern Europeans. *J Bone Joint Surg* 47B:552–555, 1965.
238. Nachemson AF, Andersson GBJ, Schultz AB: Valsalva maneuver biomechanics: effects on lumbar trunk loads of elevated intraabdominal pressures. *Spine* 11(5):276–479, 1986.
239. Adams MA, Hutton WC: The effect of posture on the role of the apophyseal joints in resisting intervertebral compressive forces. *J Bone Joint Surg* 62B:358–362, 1980.
240. Miller JA, Schultz AB, Warwick DN, Spencer DL: Mechanical properties of lumbar spine motion segments under large loads. *J Biomech* 19(1):79–80, 1986.
241. Fairbank J, Pynsent P, Poortvliet J, Phillips H: Influence of anthropometric factors and joint laxity in the incidence of adolescent back pain. *Spine* 9(5):461–464, 1984.
242. Adams MA, Dolan P, Hutton WC: Diurnal variations in the stresses on the lumbar spine. *Spine* 12(2):130, 1987.
243. Cox JM: Statistical data on facet facings of the lumbar spine and tropism. *ACA J Chiropractic* 14(4):S-39, 1977.
244. Cyron BM, Hutton WC: Articular tropism and stability of the lumbar spine. *Spine* 5(2):168–172, 1980.

245. Badgley CE: The articular facets in relation to low-back pain and sciatic radiation. *J Bone Joint Surg* 23A:481–496, 1941.

246. Willis TA: Lumbosacral anomalies. *J Bone Joint Surg* 41A:935–938, 1959.

247. Putti V, Logroscino D: Anatomia dell'artritismo vertebrale apofisario. *Chir Organi Mov* 23: 317–321, 1937–1938.

248. Malmivaara A, Videman T, Kuosma E, Troup JDG: Facet joint orientation, facet and costovertebral joint osteoarthrosis, disc degeneration, vertebral body osteophytosis, and Schmorl's nodes in the thoracolumbar junctional region of cadaveric spines. *Spine* 12(5):458–463, 1987.

249. Van Schaik JPJ, Verbeist H, Van Schaik FDJ: The orientation of laminae and facet joints in the lower lumbar spine. *Spine* 10(1):59, 1985.

250. Kenesi C, Lesur E: Orientation of the articular process at L4, L5, and S1 possible role in pathology of the intervertebral disc. *Anat Clin* 7(43):17, 1985.

251. McGlean B, Hibbert C, Evans C, Porter RW: *The Lumbar Apophyseal Joints in an Archaeological Collection.* British Association of Clinical Anatomists, 1982.

252. Cercueil JP, Lemaire JP, Grammont P, Mabille JP: Anomalie rotatoire de la colonne lombaire par asymetric des articulaires postérieures. *J Radiol* 63(2):107–113, 1982.

253. Cox JM, Aspegren DD, Trier KK: Facet tropism: plain film determination compared with CT. To be published.

254. Bardsley JL, Hanelin LG: The unilateral hypoplastic lumbar pedicle. *Radiology* 101:315–317, 1971.

255. Feldman F: Miscellaneous localized conditions: a whirlwind review of "oh my aching back" syndrome. *Semin Roentgenol* 14:58–74, 1979.

256. Hadley HA: Congenital absence of pedicle from cervical vertebra: report of three cases. *Am J Roentgenol Radium Ther* 55:193–197, 1946.

257. Farfan HF, Sullivan JD: The relation of facet orientation to intervertebral disc failure. *Can J Surg* 10:179–185, 1967.

Suggested Readings

Andersen KH, Mosdal C: Epidural application of cortico-steroids in low back pain and sciatica. *Acta Neurochir* 84(3–4):145, 1987.

Aspegren DD, Cox JM, Trier KK; Short leg correction: a clinical trial of radiographic vs. non-radiographic procedures. *J Manipulative Physiol Ther* 10:233–237, 1987.

Farfan HF, Huberdeau RM, Dubow HI: Lumbar intervertebral disc degeneration: the influence of geometrical features on the pattern of disc degeneration—a post mortem study. *J Bone Joint Surg* 54A:492–510, 1972.

Keyes DC, Compere EL: The normal and pathological physiology of the nucleus pulposus of the intervertebral disc: an anatomical, clinical and experimental study. *J Bone Joint Surg* 14A:897, 1961.

Macintosh JE, Bogduk N: The morphology of the human lumbar multifidus. *Clinical Biomechanics* 1: 196–213, 1986.

Mayer TG, Smith SS, Kondraske G, Gatchel RJ, Carmichael TW, Mooney V: Quantification of lumbar function. Part 3. Preliminary data on isokinetic torso rotation testing with myoelectric spectral analysis in normal and low back pain subjects. *Spine* 10(10): 912–920, 1985.

Panjabi MM, Krag MH, Chung TQ: Effects of disc injury on mechanical behavior of the human spine. *Spine* 9(7):707–713, 1984.

Tibrewal SB, Pearcy MJ: Lumbar intervertebral disc heights in normal subjects and patients with disc herniation. *Spine* 10(5):452–454, 1985.

3

Neurophysiology of Nerve Root Compression

James M. Cox, D.C., D.A.C.B.R.

Tis man's worse deed

To let the things that have been

Run to waste

And in the unmeaning present

Sink the past.

> **—Lowell**

Throughout chiropractic history, interest has centered on the compression of nerve roots exiting the cauda equina and passing through the intervertebral foramen as a potential cause of human disease. It is appropriate that this text contain a chapter that discusses some of the modern concepts of nerve root compression, taking into account theories of mechanical and chemical irritation. The question of why some patients have nerve root compression without symptoms, while others with seemingly minimal compression have marked pain symptoms, must be addressed. It may be the very basis of chiropractic's past and future contribution to the healing arts.

We will discuss some authors who feel that the size of the vertebral canal and its lateral recesses determine the vulnerability of the nerve root to compression from any acquired abnormality, and others who feel that the size of the thecal sac is the prime determinant of potential nerve root compression. The question as to how much pressure creates what type of symptomatology is an important issue today and will continue to be un-

til the answers are collected. The question of pain-producing entities, that is, protrusions of the intervertebral discs, the vascular supply of the nerve root and the nociceptive and proprioceptive properties of the intervertebral disc, must be discussed. Neural trophic influence—by the delivery of specific proteins to target organs via a nerve from the brain—is being studied. The dorsal root ganglion, whether it be a passive transmitter or an active processor of impulse, is the subject of important clinical questions today.

DISC PROTRUSION NOT ALWAYS PAIN PRODUCING

Wiesel et al. (1) stated that 36% of patients who have never had low back or leg pain were found to have CT scans read as abnormal by neuroradiologists. Furthermore, they stated that 24% of people with no history of back pain or sciatica had abnormal myelograms as well. This creates two questions: how much pressure on the nerve root is required to create clinical symptoms, and why some patients have differing degrees of symptoms from similar nerve root compressive forces. At our clinic, we have seen cases where a repeat CT scan, taken with the patient asymptomatic, has shown no reduction in the size of the disc protrusion compared to that seen on the symptomatic CT scan, and we have also seen cases with varying degrees of reduction of the disc bulge while the patient still attained total relief of low back and leg pain. We will present three such cases from our clinical records to begin this chapter.

CASE 1

This is a case showing the reduction of disc protrusion on pre- and post-treatment CT scan. This patient was totally relieved of low back and leg pain, but you can see that there was far less than 100% reduction of the disc protrusion. Figure 3.1 reveals that the L5-S1 intervertebral disc protrusion occupied 38% of the sagittal diameter of the vertebral canal in June 1986. Following complete relief of low back and leg pain, in January 1987, the percentage occupied by the intervertebral disc protrusion was still 38% (Fig. 3.2).

Figure 3.3 reveals that in June 1986, the L4-L5 disc protrusion occupied 50% of the sagittal diameter of the vertebral canal. In January of 1987, however, the intervertebral disc protrusion occupied 37.5% of the total canal; this is a 12.5% reduction in the size of the disc protrusion (Fig. 3.4).

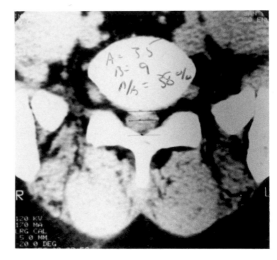

Figure 3.2. Six months later, following complete relief of the low back and leg pain symptoms, the patient shows the same 38% disc protrusion at the L5-S1 level.

CASE 2

A 32-year-old white male was involved in an automobile accident. Prior to this he had never had low back or leg pain. Following the accident, he developed low back pain and eventual left lower extremity pain in the distribution of the L5 and S1 dermatomes, especially the S1 dermatome. We saw the patient 11 months following the automobile accident. In that time, he had been treated by his family doctor, who referred him to a neurosurgeon when he failed to respond to drug therapy. This was 10 months following the injury. The neurosurgeon recommended that surgery be performed due to the positive CT scans at the L4-L5 and L5-S1 disc spaces, both of which revealed intervertebral disc protrusions.

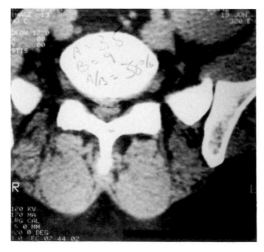

Figure 3.1. At L5-S1, 38% of the sagittal diameter of the vertebral canal is occupied by the disc protrusion when the patient's low back and leg pain symptoms are severe.

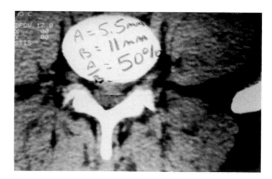

Figure 3.3. L4-L5 shows 50% of the sagittal diameter of the vertebral canal to be occupied by the disc protrusion when the low back and leg pain symptoms are severe.

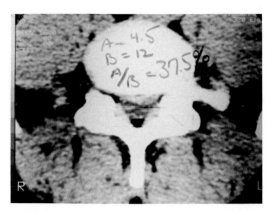

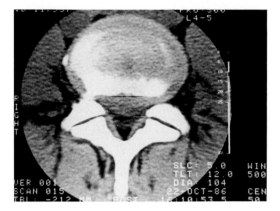

Figure 3.4. Following complete relief of low back and leg pain, the L4-L5 disc seen in Figure 3.3 is reduced to 37.5% of the canal diameter.

Figure 3.5. The L4-L5 disc protrusion occupies 50% of the vertebral canal diameter when this patient is in low back and left sciatic pain.

Ten months following the injury, and prior to surgery, the patient chose to have a chiropractic consultation for possible conservative treatment of his disc protrusions. Our examination revealed that the leg pain and back pain were aggravated by Déjérine's triad. The patient complained of night pain. The ranges of motion were limited only by 10° of extension and 10° of left lateral flexion. Straight leg raising produced no low back pain; however, Bechterew's sign or sitting straight leg raising sign did produce low back pain. There was no sign of motor weakness. The deep reflexes at the ankle and knee were +2 bilaterally, and there was no sensory deficit on pinwheel examination. Circulation of the lower extremities appeared adequate. The original CT scans, revealing the bulging L4-L5 and L5-S1 discs, are shown in Figures 3.5 and 3.6.

Treatment was started 11 months following the initial onset of pain. It consisted of flexion distraction manipulation of the L4-L5 and L5-S1 disc spaces. Physical therapy was given in the form of positive galvanism and alternating hot and cold to these disc areas and the sciatic nerve distribution on the left lower extremity. Tetanizing current to the paravertebral muscles was utilized. The patient was placed in a lumbar support and given home exercises consisting of knee-chest exercises and intraabdominal increasing of pressure. He was told to avoid sitting as well as bending and twisting at the waist. He attended low back wellness school to learn how to perform the proper bending and lifting in daily life without aggravating his back.

After 3 weeks of this care, the patient was over 50% relieved of his low back and left leg pain. At that time, he was started on Nautilus exercise regimens, and he rapidly regained muscle strength to the lumbar and abdominal areas. At the beginning of his Nautilus work, he could perform lumbar extension at approximately 10 pounds of pressure, and he eventually was able to lift

well in excess of 150 pounds at 15 repetitions, with three sets of repetitions at each session. These sessions were held three times weekly during the course of care. The patient continued the stretching of very tight hamstring muscles, which responded well even though they showed extreme shortness at the beginning of this care. This patient returned to work 5 weeks following the onset of treatment and has worked ever since. He was gradually weaned from his lumbar support and was told to only wear it in stressful situations that necessitated heavy lifting or repetitive bending or twisting. During the course of his healing, he had slight discomfort at the end of a work day, but this was relieved by rest and performing his exercises.

Figures 3.7 and 3.8 are repeat CT scans performed 4 months following the original CT scan and 3 months following the institution of our conservative flexion dis-

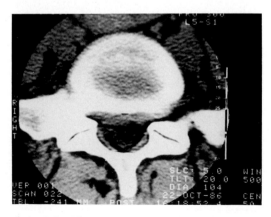

Figure 3.6. The L5-S1 disc protrudes into the vertebral canal to occupy 30% of the canal when the patient has low back and sciatic pain.

traction manipulation. By measuring the disc protrusion percentage occupying the vertebral canal, we determine that there had been no change in the size of the disc bulge, although there had been total relief of the patient's symptoms. Therefore, we note that the patient does maintain disc herniations at the L4-L5 and L5-S1 levels; however, he is totally asymptomatic. As has been discussed elsewhere in this chapter, we know that fully one-third of people who have never had low back or leg pain will reveal such disc protrusions.

Discussion of Cases 1 and 2

Here we have seen two patients with large disc protrusions, true sciatic radiculopathy, who under treatment obtained complete relief of symptoms although a large disc protrusion was still present. Certainly, some degree of tightness was created within the vertebral canal by the presence of this foreign element of disc material, but only when a certain degree of compression was reached were symptoms produced.

To further discuss the reduction of disc protrusion by conservative treatment, the cause of nerve root irritation, and its effective relief by conservative care, this author and Donald D. Aspegren, D.C., published a paper in the *Journal of Manipulative and Physiological Therapeutics*. At this time, excerpts from that paper will be presented to enlighten the reader on the conservative reduction of disc protrusions and how disc protrusion may be determined from diagnostic imaging.

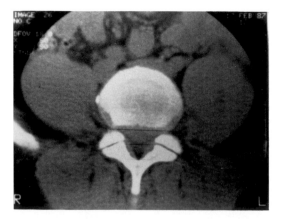

Figure 3.7. Following total relief of both low back and leg pain, CT scan of this patient still shows 50% of the L4-L5 vertebral canal to be occupied by the disc protrusion.

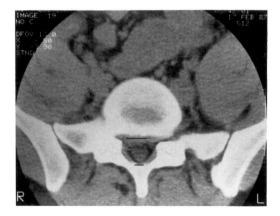

Figure 3.8. Likewise, the L5-S1 disc still bulges into the canal to occupy the same 30% of its diameter when the patient is asymptomatic.

A HYPOTHESIS INTRODUCING A NEW CALCULATION FOR DISCAL REDUCTION: EMPHASIS ON STENOTIC FACTORS AND MANIPULATIVE TREATMENT[a]

Measurement of a Disc Protrusion by CT Scan

We offer a technique to measure the disc protrusion size and to evaluate change in size of the bulge. These measurements were then correlated to the patient's subjective and clinical objective findings.

The technique involves obtaining three consecutive, parallel 2-mm cuts through the disc with the gantry angulation set to obtain axial scans in the plane of the disc. Of course, perpendicular sections to the rostrocaudal axis may be best in some cases. In this particular case, the same three cuts were made on each of three dates: January 1985, when the pain led to hospitalization and CT; June 1985, when the pain worsened; and August, when the pain was absent. The first measurement *(A)* is from the posterior vertebral body to the most posterior aspect of the disc bulge (Figs. 3.9 and 3.10). The second measurement *(B)* is from the posterior edge of the vertebral body to the posterior spinal canal where the laminae join with the spinous process (Figs. 3.9 and 3.10). These two measurements are used to form a percentage, $(A/B) \times 100$ (Table 3.1). The three disc-bulge-to-spinal-canal percentages obtained on each of the three CTs (Figs. 3.11–3.22) were then averaged for each date (Table 3.1).

[a] Modified from JM Cox, DD Aspegren: A hypothesis introducing a new calculation for discal reduction: emphasis on stenotic factors and manipulative treatment. *Journal of Manipulative and Physiological Therapeutics*, vol 10, issue 6, pp 287–294, © by the National College of Chiropractic, 1987.

Table 3.1.
Disc Protrusion Measurements[a]

Gantry Angulation	January 9	June 5	August 23
3rd angled gantry	$\frac{2.1}{5} = 42\%$	$\frac{5}{10} = 50\%$	$\frac{3.1}{9} = 34\%$
2nd angled gantry	$\frac{1.5}{5} = 30\%$	$\frac{4}{8} = 50\%$	$\frac{2.5}{7} = 36\%$
1st angled gantry	$\frac{2}{4} = 50\%$	$\frac{4}{9} = 44\%$	$\frac{2}{6} = 33\%$
Average	40.6%	48%	34%

[a]From Cox JM, Aspegren DD: A hypothesis introducing a new calculation for discal reduction: emphasis on stenotic factors and manipulative treatment, *Journal of Manipulative and Physiological Therapeutics,* vol 10, issue 6, pp 287–294, © by the National College of Chiropractic, 1987.

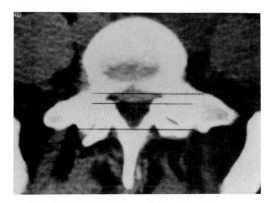

Figure 3.9. CT scan showing the line drawn along the posterior vertebral body, along the posterior disc bulge and at the junction of the spinous process and laminae (posterior vertebral canal border.) (From Cox JM, Aspegren DD: A hypothesis introducing a new calculation for discal reduction: emphasis on stenotic factors and manipulative treatment, *Journal of Manipulative and Physiological Therapeutics,* vol 10, issue 6, pp 287–294, © by the National College of Chiropractic, 1987.)

In January 1985, the three percentages averaged to 40.6%. The June 1985 slices, done prior to initiation of therapy, had increased to 48.0%, while in August 1985, after therapy and relief of symptoms, a marked reduction in the average disc-canal percentage was demonstrated at 34%.

The sagittal diameter of the spinal canal may be measured on CT with cursors placed on the posterior surface of the vertebral body and the anterior surface of the lamina.

In our case presentation, the patient had a sagittal L5 vertebral canal of 18 mm with the L5 body of 38 mm. This was a 2:1 ratio (2, 3) of body to canal, while the canal was well above accepted stenotic levels of 12 mm (2, 4–7). Our patient did not have vertebral canal stenosis by Eisenstein's measurement (2, 8–13). There was some facet arthrosis but not hypertrophic lateral recess changes. We did have disc protrusion dimensions as reported in Figures 3.11–3.22. We saw that a 14% reduction in disc protrusion size gave complete relief.

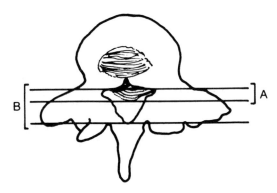

Figure 3.10. Schematic showing *A* as the disc bulge measured in millimeters and *B* as the sagittal vertebral canal diameter in millimeters. A/B = percentage of vertebral canal occupied by the disc protrusion. (From Cox JM, Aspegren DD: A hypothesis introducing a new calculation for discal reduction: emphasis on stenotic factors and manipulative treatment, *Journal of Manipulative and Physiological Therapeutics,* vol 10, issue 6, pp 287–294, © by the National College of Chiropractic, 1987.)

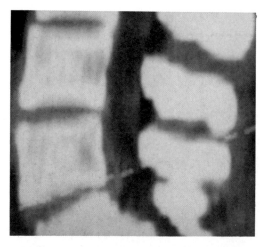

Figure 3.11. Third angled gantry parallel to the L5-S1 disc space. (From Cox JM, Aspegren DD: A hypothesis introducing a new calculation for discal reduction: emphasis on stenotic factors and manipulative treatment, *Journal of Manipulative and Physiological Therapeutics,* vol 10, issue 6, pp 287–294, © by the National College of Chiropractic, 1987.)

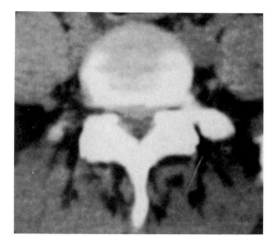

Figure 3.12. January 9 disc bulge at L5-S1 from Figure 3.11 gantry. (From Cox JM, Aspegren DD: A hypothesis introducing a new calculation for discal reduction: emphasis on stenotic factors and manipulative treatment, *Journal of Manipulative and Physiological Therapeutics,* vol 10, issue 6, pp 287–294, © by the National College of Chiropractic, 1987.)

We know that there was far from complete reduction of the disc protrusion, and certainly, we know that the size of the canal and dural sac did not change, nor the facet hypertrophy reduce. A conclusion is that the disc reduction lowered the nerve root pressure below threshold pressure for pain production.

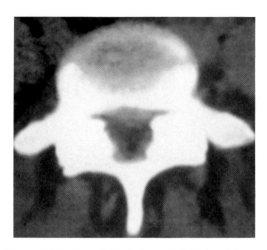

Figure 3.13. June 5 disc bulge at L5-S1 from Figure 3.11 gantry. (From Cox JM, Aspegren DD: A hypothesis introducing a new calculation for discal reduction: emphasis on stenotic factors and manipulative treatment, *Journal of Manipulative and Physiological Therapeutics,* vol 10, issue 6, pp 287–294, © by the National College of Chiropractic, 1987.)

The authors believe that disc tissue bulge is importantly measured by this disc-canal percentage, which can give an idea of disc increase, decrease, or maintenance of size. Other plain film measurements for stenosis of the bony canal are well documented for accuracy (4, 2–7, 10, 14–17). No one has offered measurements

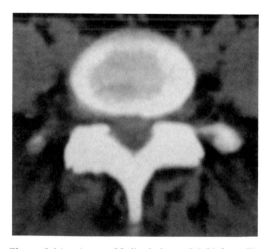

Figure 3.14. August 23 disc bulge at L5-S1 from Figure 3.11 gantry. (From Cox JM, Aspegren DD: A hypothesis introducing a new calculation for discal reduction: emphasis on stenotic factors and manipulative treatment, *Journal of Manipulative and Physiological Therapeutics,* vol 10, issue 6, pp 287–294, © by the National College of Chiropractic, 1987.)

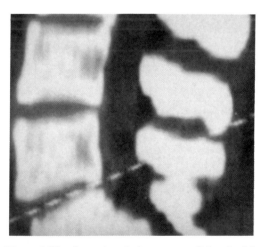

Figure 3.15. Second angled gantry parallel to the L5-S1 disc space. (From Cox JM, Aspegren DD: A hypothesis introducing a new calculation for discal reduction: emphasis on stenotic factors and manipulative treatment, *Journal of Manipulative and Physiological Therapeutics,* vol 10, issue 6, pp 287–294, © by the National College of Chiropractic, 1987.)

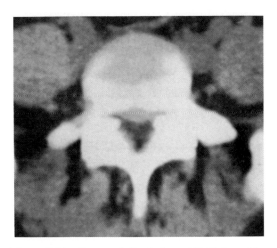

Figure 3.16. January 9 disc bulge at L5-S1 from Figure 3.15 gantry. (From Cox JM, Aspegren DD: A hypothesis introducing a new calculation for discal reduction: emphasis on stenotic factors and manipulative treatment, *Journal of Manipulative and Physiological Therapeutics,* vol 10, issue 6, pp 287–294, © by the National College of Chiropractic, 1987.)

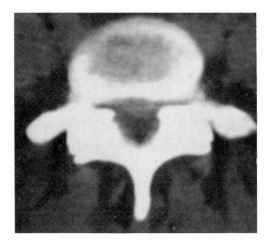

Figure 3.17. June 5 disc bulge at L5-S1 from Figure 3.15 gantry. (From Cox JM, Aspegren DD: A hypothesis introducing a new calculation for discal reduction: emphasis on stenotic factors and manipulative treatment, *Journal of Manipulative and Physiological Therapeutics,* vol 10, issue 6, pp 287–294, © by the National College of Chiropractic, 1987.)

of disc bulge size to monitor patient treatment progress. With the acceptance of mensuration procedures as outlined for stenosis of the canal, our CT measuring system is an extension of such methods.

Need for measurement systems for stenosis has recently been shown by the work of Schonstrom et al. (18,

19) with the introduction of a new measurement for the transverse area of the dural sac on CT scan. They believed that bony measurements alone did not reliably identify patients with spinal stenosis, the dural sac transverse area being the most accurate method of identifying stenosis, with the critical size for the dural sac below

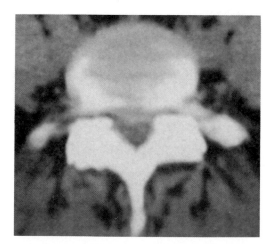

Figure 3.18. August 23 disc bulge at L5-S1 from Figure 3.15 gantry. (From Cox JM, Aspegren DD: A hypothesis introducing a new calculation for discal reduction: emphasis on stenotic factors and manipulative treatment, *Journal of Manipulative and Physiological Therapeutics,* vol 10, issue 6, pp 287–294, © by the National College of Chiropractic, 1987.)

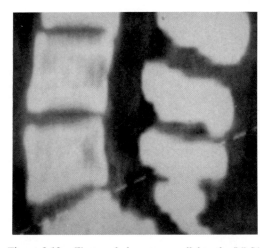

Figure 3.19. First angled gantry parallel to the L5-S1 disc space. (From Cox JM, Aspegren DD: A hypothesis introducing a new calculation for discal reduction: emphasis on stenotic factors and manipulative treatment, *Journal of Manipulative and Physiological Therapeutics,* vol 10, issue 6, pp 287–294, © by the National College of Chiropractic, 1987.)

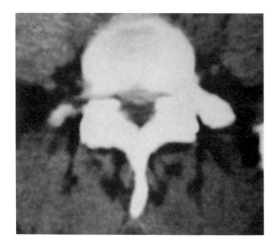

Figure 3.20. January 9 disc bulge at L5-S1 from Figure 3.19 gantry. (From Cox JM, Aspegren DD: A hypothesis introducing a new calculation for discal reduction: emphasis on stenotic factors and manipulative treatment, *Journal of Manipulative and Physiological Therapeutics,* vol 10, issue 6, pp 287–294, © by the National College of Chiropractic, 1987.)

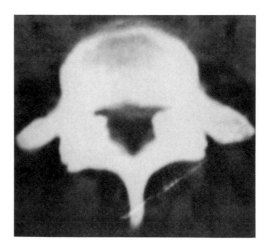

Figure 3.21. June 5 disc bulge at L5-S1 from Figure 3.19 gantry. (From Cox JM, Aspegren DD: A hypothesis introducing a new calculation for discal reduction: emphasis on stenotic factors and manipulative treatment, *Journal of Manipulative and Physiological Therapeutics,* vol 10, issue 6, pp 287–294, © by the National College of Chiropractic, 1987.)

100 mm. Further, they found the most common causes of spinal stenosis to be intervertebral disc and ligamentum flavum soft tissue encroachment as well as facet degeneration and hypertrophic changes (18). By careful manometric monitoring of highly pressure-sensitive catheters in the dural sac of seven spines removed at autopsy, Schonstrom et al. (19) found that circumferential restricting of the transverse area of the intact cauda equina at 60 to 80 mm caused a build-up of pressure in the dural sac. Once that critical size was reached, even a *minimal* further reduction of the area caused a distinct pressure increase among the nerve roots.

The dural sac can tolerate a degree of compression above which additional pressure increases create symptoms. The compression of the cauda equina was most commonly due to intervertebral disc protrusion or ligamentum flavum hypertrophy (18). We can correlate our disc canal percentage reduction with relief of pain as possibly lowering the dural sac and nerve root pressure.

Documenting disc bulge reduction by the disc canal percentage is one means of monitoring the stenotic effect of disc lesions. In the past, we have heard and read that the disc bulge was still present following a given treatment. Yet not only total reduction but also partial reduction can bring relief of pain.

Conclusion

Recognition of the need for investigation of disc herniation reduction following conservative care is called for. Teplick and Haskin (20) discuss 11 cases of spontaneous regression of herniated lumbar disc on CT scan and call

for further investigation of conservative treatment effects on disc herniation. Many others (21–39) have shown reduction of disc herniation on myelography, epidurography, or CT scan, or clinical relief when flexion distraction manipulation, bracing in flexion and hanging or upright gravity reduction systems are ap-

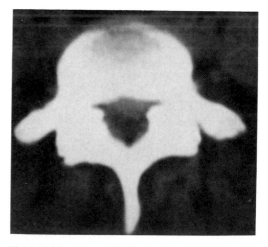

Figure 3.22. August 23 disc bulge at L5-S1 from Figure 3.19 gantry. (From Cox JM, Aspegren DD: A hypothesis introducing a new calculation for discal reduction: emphasis on stenotic factors and manipulative treatment, *Journal of Manipulative and Physiological Therapeutics,* vol 10, issue 6, pp 287–294, © by the National College of Chiropractic, 1987.)

plied as therapy. Also, Naylor et al. (40), Gertzbein (41), Rydevik et al. (42), Elves et al. (43), and Eyre (44) inculpate the chemical irritations (radiculitis) of the nerve by discal biodegradation products as much as the mechanical irritation. This has been called the autoimmune mechanism involved with the inflammatory tissue reaction seen around degenerative discs. This results in intraneural edema and impaired intraneural microcirculation leading to functional changes of motor and sensory deficits.

This paper offers a CT measuring system to determine the percentage of the vertebral canal occupied by a disc bulge; changes in size of the disc herniation can be evaluated later by repeating the identical CT views.

Stenosis is the problem within the vertebral canal leading to nerve root compression. Controversy exists over what is the most important factor in stenosis—the bony vertebral canal size or the dural sac area. Regardless, soft tissue stenosis by intervertebral disc protrusion, ligamentum flavum thickening, or facet degenerative change is involved, with further narrowing of the vertebral canal or intervertebral foramen and the resultant pressure increase in the dural sac or nerve roots. Depending on the degree of developmental stenosis present, the amount of acquired stenosis becomes important. The person with preexisting bony stenosis or a large dural sac may develop marked nerve root compression with minimal disc or soft tissue lesion, whereas someone with a large bony canal and small dural sac may have minimal or no sign of symptoms of nerve root compression when such acquired factors appear.

A case was presented with a 14% reduction of a disc protrusion following chiropractic manipulation as measured on CT scans before and after care. Less than total disc herniation reduction resulted in total relief of sciatica in this patient.

Perhaps patients can tolerate a degree of nerve root compression by soft tissue encroachment, depending on the amount of developmental stenosis of the vertebral canal or the size of the dural sac; but if the pressure reaches sufficient levels, symptoms appear. Study in this area is important and progressing.

ASSOCIATION BETWEEN NERVE ROOT COMPRESSION AND DISEASE STATES

Before we look at modern research on this question of nerve root compression, let's first look at some other instances of association between nerve root compression in the human spine and elements of organic disease. To begin with, a study from the Duke University Medical Center described a previously healthy 21-year-old black woman with a C1-C2 subluxation, spontaneously developed, in association with inflammatory bowel disease, namely Crohn's disease. The study

stated that this heretofore unreported association should be considered: namely, the association of clinically silent or undiagnosed inflammatory bowel disease with atlantoaxial subluxation (45).

An association between significant coronary stenosis and thoracic osteophytosis was found in a study in which 31 (43%) of 72 patients with thoracic osteophytosis had significant coronary stenosis, as compared with only three of 20 patients (15%) with normal coronary arteries who had accompanying thoracic osteophytosis. It was concluded from this study that the presence of thoracic osteophytosis is a specific predictor of coronary atherosclerosis (85%) in this small population, but this was not felt to be a sensitive enough conclusion to be confirmatory of this relationship (46).

Beal (47) performed a study on 108 patients in the cardiac service of a hospital to identify any relationship between heart disease and dysfunction of the spine. A palpatory examination was conducted of the segmental vertebral motion and muscle tension over the transverse processes of the upper thoracic spine. A typical pattern of somatic dysfunction was observed to involve at least adjacent spinal segments in the area of T1 to T5 on the left side. The results were compared with those for a group of patients with gastrointestinal disease, who were observed to have similar evidence of somatic dysfunction but at vertebral levels associated with the autonomic nerve supply of the particular viscera involved. A group of 25 patients with diagnosed cardiac or gastrointestinal disease were examined in a blind study to determine the predictive value of the selected findings for the cardiac disease. These palpatory findings were found to have a predictive value of 75% for indicating the presence of cardiac disease.

Suarez et al. (48) studied 97 consecutive male patients admitted to a hospital for comprehensive lumbar pain evaluation, arriving at a diagnosis including herniated nucleus pulposus, spinal stenosis, segmental instability, and idiopathic lumbar syndrome. By including a comprehensive neurological examination as a part of the routine investigation of these patients with lumbar pain complaints, the researchers assembled data that indicated that abnormalities of visceral function have diagnostic significance equal to that of other neurological deficits. Their data indicated that lumbar disease can itself produce significant urinary bladder and sexual dysfunction, and hence it is incumbent upon clinicians investigating lumbar problems to also obtain a comprehensive genito-urinary appraisal.

History of Chiropractic Concepts of Disease Causation

The 1895 origin of chiropractic included the concept of a spinal subluxation being not only a cause of pain but equally a cause of organic disease. The dispute over this latter concept has led to a major division between chiropractic and other branches of medicine; an attempt to bridge this academic gap has led the chiropractic profession to accept primarily a role, in more recent years, as a provider of treatment of musculoskeletal disease, centered upon the spinal column and its altered kinematics. However, the chiropractic profession must maintain a scientific approach to the organic disease potential created by nerve root compression. The above citations of relationships between organic disease and spinal dysfunction are proof of this need.

Chiropractic Principles Revisited

Let's look at some early chiropractic concepts and rejudge them with a structured investigative methodology in order to determine if there can be any future study that will benefit treatment of human disease. Palmer (49) wrote that chiropractic is founded on anatomy—osteology, neurology, and body function. It is a science—a knowledge of health and disease reduced to law and embodied into a system. The origin of chiropractic rests largely with the treatment of a janitor, Harvey Lillard, who had been deaf for 17 years, unable to hear even the ticking of a watch. Palmer found out that the man's deafness had followed an episode of exerting himself in a cramped, stooping position that caused his back to "give way," which was followed immediately by deafness. Finding a vertebra out of its normal position, Palmer replaced the vertebra, and the man's hearing was immediately restored (49). This sounds like a preposterous clinical event, but it is noteworthy that Bourdillion (50), in his book *Spinal Manipulation*, quotes this case history of Palmer and states that he has reproduced the same finding with spinal manipulation. Bourdillion is a past president of the North American Academy of Manipulative Medicine.

Forster (51) states that chiropractic is based upon five fundamental premises:

1. That a vertebra may become subluxated;
2. That this subluxation induces impingement on the contents of the intervertebral foramen;
3. That, as a result of this impingement, the irritability of the corresponding segment of the spinal cord and its connecting spinal and autonomic nerves is reduced, and the conduction of the nerves is impaired;
4. That, as a result thereof, certain parts of the organism are deprived of their innervation in whole or in part, and become functionally or organically diseased or predisposed to disease;
5. That adjustment of a subluxated vertebra removes the impingement on the structures passing through the intervertebral foramen, thereby restoring to diseased parts their full quota of innervation and rehabilitating them functionally and organically.

The principle of manipulating vertebrae certainly did not start with Palmer. In his own text (49), Palmer states that the basic principle, and the principles of chiropractic that have been developed from it, are not new. They are as old as the vertebrae. He stated that he was not the first person to replace subluxated vertebrae, for this art had been practiced for thousands of years. This author (J.M.C.) recalls having read of adjustments described by Hippocrates, and an adjustment of the sacroiliac joints from the days of the Roman empire. What Palmer claimed was that he was the first to replace displaced vertebrae by using the spinous and transverse processes as levers with which to reduce the subluxated vertebrae to their normal position. Further, he created a science that was new to the healing arts.

Palmer (49) admits that his first knowledge of spinal manipulation was received from Dr. Jim Atkinson, who lived and practiced in Davenport, Iowa. Thus we can see that what Palmer actually did was to organize into a specific branch of the healing arts the concepts and principles of spinal manipulation. It is from that point that organized chiropractic must advance its science.

Medicine Now Reveals Great Interest in Chiropractic Principles

Before proceeding, this author would like to ask you to remember the quotation at the beginning of this chapter: "'Tis man's worse deed / To let the things that have been / Run to waste / And in the unmeaning present / Sink the past."

Wiltse (52), when giving the 1985 presidential address to the North American Spine Society, stated that his members must remember that many of the great advances in medicine have been made by people outside of it. Medicine's history is replete with instances of this. Midwives were scorching the cloth they laid over the umbilicus of newborns centuries before Lister or Semmelweis were heard of. Perhaps, Wiltse stated, medicine should take a lesson from this in dealing with spinal manipulation. The explanations given as to how manipulation works may be wrong by medicine's lights, but its practitioners must be doing something right, or 10 million people a year would not be filling their offices. He stated that medicine must at least learn about spinal manipulation and that interest in chiropractic principles of healing will make those principles increasingly more important and deserving of study.

BASIC NERVE ROOT ANATOMY AND PHYSIOLOGY

Consequences of Neurotrophic Nerve Deformation

Korr (53) states that the most distressing consequences of the biomechanical impairments of the musculoskeletal system which are amenable to manipulative therapy are those mediated by the nervous system. These include pain and other sensory manifestations and motor and autonomic disturbances. The neural phenomena concerning the transport and exchange of macromolecular materials, namely, axonal transport and neurotrophic relations between neurons and target cells, are also of vital interest.

TROPHIC FUNCTION OF NERVES

In recent years, scientists have ceased to be self-conscious and apologetic about the use of the word *trophic* in connection with nerves. Neural phenomena have always been explained in terms of impulses, electrical potentials, and frequencies; and it was unsettling to the scientific world to discuss factors other than impulses and reflexes as influences on target tissues supplied by nerve fibers.

Korr (53) inquires about the simple muscle atrophy following a severed nerve supply. He states that as long as protoplasmic continuity is maintained in the axon from perikaryon to motor end plate, even if it is nonconducting, the neuronal trophic influence continues to be exerted. The longer the nerves are attached to the muscle, the longer the time before post-denervation changes appear. This would indicate that what matters is the amount of nerve substance still available to the muscle, and that when it has been exhausted, trophic support ends. Thus, the crucial factor is not the fact that the nerve has been severed, stopping its impulses, but rather, for what length of time the trophic support is available to the muscle.

Among the components axonally transported to muscle by nerves are proteins, phospholipids, enzymes, glycoproteins, neurotransmitters and their precursors, mitochondria, and other organelles. While rates of approximately 1 mm/day have been found to be common to many mammalian nerves, it is now known that there are several rates of transport, up to several hundred millimeters per day, different cargoes being carried at different rates.

AXOPLASMIC TRANSPORT

The demonstration of multiple delivery waves raised a new set of questions. Are different proteins axonally transported and delivered in each of the periods? Can specific proteins be traced from the medulla, through the nerve, to the tongue muscle? Do all of the protein fractions carried in the axon reach the muscle, or is there some selection? Are the proteins that are delivered to the muscle different from those synthesized by the muscle itself (53)? Research shows:

1. Rabbits that had been prepared as in previous investigations were sacrificed for tissue specimens at peak times in each "wave" (delivery of proteins via the axon), namely days 1, 12, 22, and 34, to maximize the yields of radioactive protein.
2. The proteins extracted from the tissues were first divided by centrifugation into soluble and insoluble portions (the insoluble being those associated with particular cellular elements), each of which was assayed for radioactivity.

Observations were as follows:

1. Of the 12 conspicuous "spikes" of soluble radioactive proteins evident in the medulla

(hypoglossal nerve cells) on day 1, only two to three were evident in the nerve, the rest not appearing until day 12.

2. The proteins reaching the muscle in the first wave, on day 1, were almost exclusively insoluble. Those studying axonal transport had also generally agreed that insoluble or structural proteins are carried in the rapid transport system.

3. With certain exceptions, electrophoretic fractions were traceable from hypoglossal neurons through nerve to muscle.

4. Each wave carried a different mixture of proteins, as observed in nerve and muscle, although there were fractions common to consecutive waves because of the overlap previously mentioned.

5. Proteins synthesized by the muscle were different from those delivered by the nerve.

From these observations and from earlier studies, the following conclusions are made:

1. Some proteins synthesized in the hypoglossal nerve cells are held for up to 12 days before being dispatched into axons.

2. Each of the four waves carries a different complement of protein synthesized in the perikaryon, with some admixture due to overlap of the waves.

3. While there is continuity of transport from one part of the nerve to the next, there is discontinuity of transfer from nerve to muscle.

4. Transfer of proteins from nerve to muscle is a different, apparently slower, process than transport along the nerve.

5. The neuron supplies proteins that are not manufactured by the muscle.

With increased support and elaboration, the hypothesis, first stated as a question, is offered: that trophic influences of nerves on target organs depend, at least in substantial part, on the delivery of specific neuronal proteins by axonal transport and junctional transfer.

Hence, in considering the neurological impact on human health of postural and biomechanical defects in the body framework that are amenable to manipulative therapy, we can no longer limit ourselves to disturbances in impulse traffic. Conspicuous and distressing as are the resultant pain and the motor, sensory, and autonomic dysfunctions, the more subtle and insidious trophic consequences of disturbances in axoplasmic composition and transport are no less important (53).

Rydevik et al. (42) discusses the biomechanical aspects of nerve root deformation induced by compression. The functional changes induced by compression can be caused by mechanical nerve fiber deformation but also may be a consequence of nerve root microcirculation, leading to ischemia and intraneural edema. Intraneural edema and demyelinization seem to be critical factors for the production of pain in association with nerve root compression.

The dorsal and ventral nerve roots approach, inside the dural root sheath, the intervertebral foramen. The dorsal root continues into the dorsal root ganglion, which usually is located within the central portion of the intervertebral foramen. More distally, the roots join to form the spinal nerve, which continues into the peripheral nerve (Fig. 3.23).

Nerve Root Compared to Peripheral Nerve

The nerve roots lack a perineurium, whereas peripheral nerves have a well-developed epineurium wherever they are subjected to mechanical forces such as compression and tension. Nerve roots, having no such well-developed epineural connective tissue, are more susceptible to mechanical deformation than are peripheral nerves. Nerve roots are protected, to some extent, by the cerebrospinal fluid, which acts with the dura and arachnoid membrane to mechanically protect them (54).

Nerve Root Blood Supply

An adequate supply of oxygen to nerve fibers via intraneural microcirculation is necessary for nerve function.

The dorsal root ganglion receives its blood supply from spinal branches from each segmental artery (55). Figure 3.24 shows the nerve roots within the cauda equina, the motor and sensory components of the spinal nerve, and the dorsal root ganglion lying within the intervertebral foramen.

We will discuss the vulnerability of the dorsal root ganglion to compressive reaction later in this chapter. Interference with the blood supply of the nerve root or the dorsal root ganglion can lead to disturbed nerve root function. Nerve root

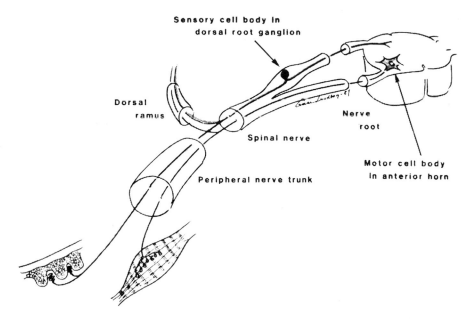

Figure 3.23. Schematic drawing of the arrangement of nerve roots, spinal nerve, and peripheral nerve, including the target organs of the neurons. The axons are long cellular extensions from the nerve cell bodies, located in the anterior horn of the spinal cord or in the dorsal root ganglia. (Reproduced with permission from Rydevik B, Brown MD, Lundborg G: Pathoanatomy and pathophysiology of nerve root compression. *Spine* 9(1):8, 1984.)

compression may interfere with the blood supply to the nerve root (56, 57).

Rydevik et al. (58) studied the intraneural microcirculation under graded compression of a rabbit tibial nerve. It was found that the first sign of impairment of intraneural blood flow was stasis in epineural vessels, appearing at pressures as low as 20 to 30 mm Hg. Such compression at higher pressures or for prolonged periods of time may damage the endoneural blood vessels, resulting in an increased permeability or a breakdown of the blood-nerve barrier and, consequently, formation of an endoneurial edema (59, 60). This has been compared to a "closed compartment syndrome" in which the microcirculation of the nerve fascicles is jeopardized and a posttraumatic ischemia of the injured nerve established. A corresponding mechanism may operate in the case of nerve root compression at the level of the intervertebral foramen, or a tight sheath surrounding the nerve roots and spinal nerve where these nervous components are enclosed in a rigid bony canal (Fig. 3.24). The dorsal root ganglion contains more permeable microcirculation than peripheral nerves, and may be easily subjected to endoneurial edema by compression. The ganglion has a tight capsule, and

therefore any such edema could increase the pressure on the ganglion quite easily (61).

Dorsal Root Ganglion

The dorsal root ganglion as a mediator for low back pain in an animal model was investigated. Low-frequency vibration, a known mechanical cause of low back pain, was investigated. Quantitative results suggest a significant effect on substance P, one of several neurotransmitters located in the dorsal root ganglion. The functional results of these changes are currently under investigation.

Research implicating the dorsal root ganglion as a modulator of low back pain was first alluded to by Lindblom and Rexed in 1948 (62). Their cadaveric studies focused on dorsal root ganglion compression as a result of dorsal-lateral lumbar disc protrusion. In some of the compressions, enlarged facet joints were found to be an accessory factor in causing nerve injury, and such bony enlargements can no doubt cause similar dorsal root ganglion damage quite independent from disc herniation.

The dorsal root ganglion is a vital link between the internal and external environment and the

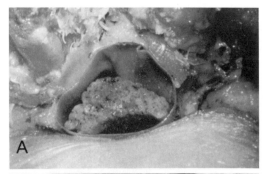
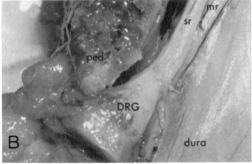
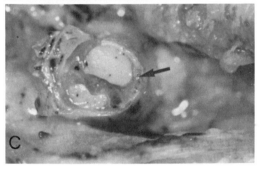

Figure 3.24. **A**, Cross-section, demonstrating the cauda equina in the spinal canal. The intervertebral disc is seen at bottom. **B**, Dorsal view of the nerve roots inside the dural sheath, following removal of the lamina and opening of the dura. The nerve root complex, comprising motor root (*mr*), sensory root (*sr*), and dorsal root ganglion (*DRG*), is located beneath the pedicle (*ped*), which has been divided. **C**, Cross-section through the root sheath (*arrow*) just central to the ganglion. The two roots are located within the tight sheath, which in turn is running in a rigid bony canal. (Reproduced with permission from Rydevik B, Brown MD, Lundborg G: Pathoanatomy and pathophysiology of nerve root compression. *Spine* 9(1):8, 1984.)

spinal cord. The primary sensory role of the spinal cord is to receive afferent stimuli in the form of action potentials and to relay the information transmitted to and from the brain. The particular mechanism of pain transmission has attracted much active research. The classic hypothesis that the effect of nerves on target organs is mediated by chemicals released from those nerves was first studied in the peripheral nervous system and was proven to be valid in the central nervous system as well. One of the most important advances in the field of neurochemistry has been the discovery of chemically defined pathways within the central nervous system. While, early on, only seven chemically identified neurotransmitters had been documented, many other transmitters have now been identified, some of which are designated "putative" because their involvement in synaptic transmission in the central nervous system is still unresolved. Furthermore, the discovery of a new family of chemicals, the neuroactive peptides, in the brain, spinal cord, and dorsal root ganglion has enormously expanded the list of candidate neurotransmitters of neuromodulators (63).

The cells in the dorsal root ganglia were originally divided into two classes according to their diameters. The large cells give rise to large myelinated fibers and the small cells to the unmyelinated (C) and finely myelinated (A) fibers. The central terminations of these primary afferent fibers, derived from the small cells, end mainly in the substantia gelatinosa, lamina II of the spinal cord. Several peptides, including calcitonin gene-related peptide and substance P, have been localized to a subpopulation of small dorsal root ganglion cells. To date, calcitonin gene-related peptide is thought to be the most abundant peptide in the dorsal root ganglion.

SUBSTANCE P

Substance P and other peptides are therefore likely to play a significant role in the processing of cutaneous sensory information in the dorsal horn of the spinal cord.

In proposing a role for substance P in the dorsal root ganglion, it has been assumed that its depletion, as in injured sensory nerves, results from decreased synthesis and/or axonal transport. Substance P is only one of several dorsal root ganglion neuropeptides that may play a role in nociceptor transmission. It was first discovered in 1931, but today its physiological role remains incompletely elucidated. Understanding the physiology of substance P depends much on the interpretation of the radioimmunoassay results and, clearly, there is a need for careful characterization, although surprisingly few assay methodology papers have been published (63).

The bulk of substance P (approximately 80%) is synthesized in small dorsal root ganglion cells and is transported along dorsal root afferent fibers to terminals located in laminae 1 and 2 in the most dorsal part of the dorsal horn. The evidence for this is based on the accumulation of substance P-reactive material proximal to a ligation of a dorsal root and on the profound decrease of substance P in the segment of the dorsal horn to which the dorsal root projects (63).

Dorsal Root Ganglion as an Origin of Pain-Producing Impulses

Nerve impulses were recorded in dorsal roots or in the sciatic nerve of anesthetized rats. It was shown by making sections, by stimulation, and by collision that some ongoing nerve impulses were originating from the dorsal root ganglia and not from the central peripheral ends of the axons. In a sample of 2731 intact or acutely sectioned myelinated sensory fibers, 4.75% + 3.7% contained impulses generated within the dorsal root ganglia. Slight mechanical pressure on the dorsal root ganglion increased the frequency of impulses (64).

Unmyelinated fibers were also found to contain impulses originating in the dorsal root ganglion.

Fine filament dissection of dorsal roots and of peripheral nerves, as well as collision experiments, showed that impulses originating in dorsal root ganglia were propagated both orthodromically into the root and antidromically into the peripheral nerve. It was also shown that the same axon could contain two different alternating sites of origin of nerve impulses: one in the sensory ending, and one in the ganglion. These observations suggest that the dorsal root ganglion, with its ongoing activity and mechanical sensitivity, could be a source of pain-producing impulses and could particularly contribute to pain in those conditions of peripheral nerve damage where pain persists after peripheral anesthesia or where vertebral manipulation is painful.

DORSAL ROOT GANGLION AN ACTIVE PAIN GENERATOR

Nystrom and Hagbarth (64) recorded from sensory nerve fascicles central to amputation neuromas in two patients, and found considerable ongoing activity that was not silenced by local anesthesia of the neuroma. There are reasons to suspect that the dorsal root ganglia might have contributed to this ectopic barrage, and Wall and Devor (64) state that De Santis and Duckworth identified dorsal root ganglia as a source of discharge in rat muscle nerves damaged by freeze lesions. Further, they state that Kirk had previously shown in cat and rabbit that transection of the spinal nerve immediately peripheral to the dorsal root ganglion produces firing in dorsal root filaments. In contrast to axons (excluding sensory endings), which are highly resistant to impulse generation following mechanical impact and, even after having been cut across, normally produce only a brief injury discharge, dorsal root ganglion cells produce a very prolonged discharge with relatively gentle mechanical compression (64).

It is generally presumed that afferent signals received by the spinal cord in normal animals arise exclusively in sensory nerve endings. The results described here show that, at least under experimental conditions, the dorsal root ganglion constitutes a second source of afferent impulses. Specifically, dorsal root ganglia contribute a tonic, low-level (about four impulses per second in 5% of sciatic nerve afferent fibers), spontaneous background discharge.

There seems no doubt from these results that afferent impulses may originate from dorsal root ganglion cells. In fact, the possibility that dorsal root ganglion cells might be a significant source of afferent barrage under certain circumstances has already been shown by Howe et al. with their demonstration of the relatively low mechanical threshold of normal dorsal root ganglia. They did not, however, discuss the possibility that there may be spontaneous discharge. The finding that chronic peripheral nerve section exaggerates the tendency of axotomized dorsal root ganglion cells to fire spontaneously also confirms the conclusions of Kirk and of De Santis and Duckworth, as cited by Wall and Devor (64), based on results from quite different preparations.

The high degree of excitability of normal dorsal root ganglion cells and its enhancement by chronic nerve injury may have important clinical significance. The Lasègue sign, pain in the leg on straight leg raising, could be the consequence of shifting tension on the dorsal root ganglia, which are mechanically stressed by the maneuver. It appears conceivable that the afferent barrage is being affected by manipulation of the dorsal root ganglia. The increase in ganglion discharge in cases of chronic nerve injury could partly account for prolonged intractable pains and paresthesias that may follow nerve damage, including phantom limb sensation and pain.

The mechanism and exact site of ectopic spontaneous impulse generation in dorsal root ganglia is not known for certain. Circumstantial evidence, however, places it in the axon hillock region.

The radicular pain of sciatica, as stated by Howe et al. (65), was ascribed by Mixter and Barr to compression of the spinal root by a herniated intervertebral disc. It was assumed that root compression produced prolonged firing in the injured sensory fibers and led to pain perceived in the peripheral distribution of those fibers.

This concept has been challenged on the basis that acute peripheral nerve compression neuropathies are usually painless. Furthermore, animal experiments have rarely shown more than several seconds of repetitive firing in acutely compressed nerves or nerve roots. It has been suggested that "radicular pain" is actually pain referred to the extremity through activation of deep spinal and paraspinal nociceptors (65).

CHRONICALLY IRRITATED NERVE ROOTS ARE MOST SENSITIVE

Experiments on cat lumbar dorsal roots and rabbit sural nerves have confirmed that acute compression of the root or nerve does not produce more than several seconds of repetitive firing. However, long periods of repetitive firing (5 to 25 minutes) follow minimal acute compression of the normal dorsal root ganglion. Chronic injury of dorsal roots or sural nerve produces a marked increase in mechanical sensitivity; several minutes of repetitive firing may follow acute compression of such chronically injured sites. Such prolonged responses could be evoked repeatedly in a population of both rapidly and slowly conducting fibers. Since mechanical compression of either the dorsal root ganglion or of chronically injured roots can induce prolonged repetitive firing in sensory axons, it is concluded that radicular pain is due to activity in the fibers appropriate to the area of perceived pain.

Although repeated or maintained compression of the roots did not produce prolonged activity, a minor chronic injury altered the response to a subsequent acute compression (65).

REPETITIVE DISCHARGE

Data show that minor compression of the dorsal root ganglion invariably produces repetitive firing lasting several minutes. Occasionally a discharge lasting as long as 25 minutes can be detected in small multifiber filaments dissected from dorsal rootlets. Similar forces can produce several seconds or, rarely, a few minutes of repetitive firing when chronically damaged dorsal roots are compressed at the site of prior trauma, but not at sites along the root or nerve other than the chronically injured region. The forces sufficient to excite these responses are similar in both situations. They are of small magnitude and can be slowly applied. This abnormal response can be triggered repetitively without changing stimulus parameters. Such forces are insufficient to excite normal dorsal roots unless applied rapidly. In the normal dorsal root, it is more difficult to repeatedly elicit the same response from the same region. Furthermore, an adequate initial force, when repeated, usually results in irreversible damage to the axons.

Injured nerves (end-bulb neuromas and incontinuity regenerating nerves) have a markedly increased sensitivity to mechanical stimulation. Minor movements can result in 15 to 30 seconds of repetitive firing. Evidence for slightly longer periods (2 to 3 minutes) of activation in response to acute compression of chronically injured roots has been seen. The usual response to compression of the chronically injured region is 15 to 30 seconds of repetitive firing in both large and small fibers. This mechanical sensitivity may represent the physiological equivalent of Tinel's sign (65).

It seems likely that compression of the dorsal root ganglion is important in the generation of the radicular pain of an acute herniated intervertebral disc. Typically, the patient with this syndrome describes the sudden onset of pain in the back and leg which radiates into the foot. The dermatome in which the pain is perceived usually predicts the compressed spinal root. Neurological deficit, if present, usually occurs in the same dermatome. The pain persists much longer than the momentary response seen in the acute compression of a normal nerve root and is more consistent with the slowly adapting response seen following dorsal root ganglion compression. This radicular pain can often be relieved by immobilization or complete bed rest; minor movements or coughing reactivate the pain.

Anatomical studies have shown that the lumbar dorsal root ganglion can be trapped easily between a herniated disc and the facet. Small and repeated movements of the joint could intermittently traumatize the dorsal root ganglion. The dorsal root ganglion in the lumbar region lies directly over the lateral portion of the disc. In an autopsy study, in all cases of herniated lumbar discs, the dorsal root ganglion was compressed, distorted, and manifested various degrees of degeneration (65).

Smyth and Wright described the reproduction of radicular pain in patients who had undergone laminectomies for the removal of herniated disc. In these patients, they looped a nylon suture around the root at the time of surgery and brought the ends out through the skin. Postoperatively they were able to precisely reproduce the preoperative radicular pain by very gentle traction on the suture. They noted that the injured or involved root was much more sensitive to this manipulation than an adjacent normal or uninvolved root. Murphey reported similar findings (65).

The ease of activation and prolonged response of Aa and C fibers in response to dorsal root ganglion compression implies that the radicular pain associated with a herniated intervertebral disc, and perhaps other intraspinal masses, is due initially to compression of the dorsal root ganglion. The subsequent development of mechanical sensitivity in the chronically injured nerve roots may also contribute to the production of continuing radicular pain. Studies demonstrate that radicular pain can be due to activity in the fibers appropriate to the region of pain, and need not be a referred phenomenon (65).

DORSAL ROOT GANGLION PRODUCES REPETITIVE FIRING OF IMPULSES

The middle of an axon is not usually a site of impulse generation; it is a region of impulse replication, where impulses originating elsewhere are faithfully reproduced in one-for-one fashion. Nonetheless, it is not so specialized that it cannot generate impulses upon compression. For example, because of rudimentary mechanosensitivity of axons, compression of the ulnar nerve at the elbow produces paresthesia. This ectopic generation of nerve impulses appears to operate in the manner of most mechanoreceptors: a generator

potential is developed, and the repetitive firing patterns that result are those expected from the pacemaker-like rhythmic firing mode in which depolarization is converted into firing rate. Although repetitive firing in normal peripheral nerves and dorsal roots is usually quite transient even with sustained compression, dorsal root ganglion cells and chronically injured axons are capable of producing sustained repetitive firing on sustained compression, as we have described elsewhere (66).

The dorsal root is extremely sensitive to pressure. In peripheral nerves, the Aa fibers that mediate impulses from the muscle spindle and the Golgi apparatus, as well as efferent motor impulses, are the most pressure-sensitive structures. According to this hypothesis, slight pressure on these fibers in the dorsal roots and ganglia results initially in reduced inflow of afferent impulses from muscle and tendon receptors. This is in agreement with the anatomical arrangement in the intervertebral foramina. As a result, the central nervous system responds with an increase in outflow of efferent impulses. This in turn gives rise to sustained increase in muscle tone, leading to myalgia and tendonitis (67).

SCIATICA, CLAUDICATION, AND GROIN PAIN DUE TO DORSAL ROOT GANGLION IRRITATION

A series of patients with leg pain, whose dorsal root ganglia were located more proximal than usual and lay within the nerve root canal, was reported (68). These proximal ganglia became entrapped in a space that, although slightly narrowed, would have accommodated a normal nerve root without causing symptoms.

There were 11 patients, two men and nine women. Their ages ranged from 28 to 60, and over half were in the 4th and 5th decade. Most of these patients presented with an exceptionally long history of symptoms prior to diagnosis (average 7 years).

Pain was aggravated by the standing position in seven patients. Seven complained of intermittent claudication. The pain radiated down the leg in a sciatic distribution in all patients and extended to the ankle or foot in eight. Radiation to the groin was reported in three patients, two with compression of the L5 ganglion and one with compression of both the L5 and S1 ganglia.

Physical examination was entirely normal in

three patients. Straight leg raising was limited to 70° in the affected lower limb in four patients, significantly reduced to 60° in one, and reduced to 30° in another. There was muscle weakness or wasting in four patients, and sensory abnormalities were present in three. The ankle reflex was depressed in three patients and absent in one.

All 11 patients underwent surgical decompression. Subarticular entrapment of the L5 dorsal root ganglion was found in six patients, both L5 and S1 dorsal root ganglion entrapment in three, and S1 dorsal root ganglion entrapment alone in two (68).

SUBSTANCE "P" PRODUCED IN DORSAL ROOT GANGLION

The neuropeptide known as substance P is known to be synthesized in cell bodies of the dorsal root ganglia. This neuropeptide is also known to modulate sensory, nociceptive transmission postsynaptically in the dorsal root ganglia, nerve roots, and substantia gelatinosa of the spinal dorsal horn that the cell bodies innervate. These results were determined by using both immunohistochemistry and radioimmunoassay. This study suggests that substance P may modulate nociception when lumbar nerve roots are stimulated mechanically (69).

The dorsal root ganglion normally lies within the lateral portion of the intervertebral foramen and is not directly compressed by a bulging disc prolapse or a bony spur that may compromise the nerve root (70). This ganglion contains cell bodies of first-order sensory neurons. The chemical response to mechanical deformation of the dorsal root ganglion may hold significance for some of the unknowns in the etiology of low back pain.

Stimulation and release of the neuropeptide substance P, or similar agents, by pathophysiological mechanisms has been postulated to explain the pain of spinal nerve root pathology. Proximal flow of substance P from the dorsal root ganglion to the spinal cord certainly occurs (70). Substance P is one of the neurotransmitters produced in the cell bodies of the dorsal root ganglion. This neuropeptide probably acts as a neuromodulator of pain signals at synapses in the region of the substantia gelatinosa where pain perception is first integrated in the spinal cord. The appearance of substance P in this area may be the first chemical signal of exteroceptive pain in the spinal cord.

The abundance of substance P immunoreactive nerve terminals in the substantia gelatinosa of the dorsal horn of the spinal cord suggests that substance P is contained in primary afferent fibers that penetrate this region—as well as the dorsolateral funiculus radially—and terminate in the dorsal horn.

The increased amounts of substance P produced after mechanical stimulation provide a possible neurophysiological explanation for the nociceptive effects produced by mechanical compromise of the spinal nerve roots. Dorsal root ganglion irritation associated with various syndromes of mechanical compromise seem able to produce increased amounts of substance P, which is known to have central effects modulating nociceptive afferent transmission. A delay between mechanical stimulation and the appearance of substance P centrally, where it may modulate neurotransmission, may also be important. It is interesting to speculate whether this may be an explanation for the well-known clinical observation that after a disc prolapse there may be a period of several days before sciatic pain is experienced, even though back pain may be immediately apparent following the disc protrusion (69).

Sympathetic Trunk Compressed by Osteophytosis of Thoracic Spine

The presence of osteophytes compressing the sympathetic structures in the thorax was found in 655 (65.5%) of 1000 cadavers. In 60.4% of the affected cases, the compression was on the right side, and in 36.9% it was bilateral although the right side was more severely affected. In 2%, the compression was on the left only. The highest frequency of compression was at the T8-T10 level. The sympathetic trunk itself (ganglia and cord) was affected only by osteophytes of vertebrae at the lowest thoracic levels; however, bony excrescences due to costovertebral joint arthritis were frequently found impinging on the sympathetic trunk and its rami communicantes, with similar frequencies on both sides (71).

We assume that symptoms will result either from irritation (stimulation) of the sympathetic structures or from inhibition (paralysis), according to the degree of compression. In our opinion, many pathological conditions might be explained by compression of osteophytes on sympathetic structures (71).

Effects of Nerve Fiber Compression

Thirty to fifty mm Hg probably creates some degree of nerve fiber deformation (72, 73). According to Hahnenberger (72) and Ochoa (73), these changes are probably reversible if the compression is released after a single trauma. Sustained compression at these pressure levels or repeated compression is likely to create disturbances in nerve structure and function (73). Higher pressures may lead to different kinds of nerve lesions, either segmental demyelination or, in cases of severe trauma, loss of axonal continuity, leading to wallerian degeneration. A nerve root lesion associated with a herniated nucleus pulposus probably creates demyelination and wallerian degeneration.

Rydevik (58) placed a small inflatable cuff around peripheral nerves in animals and demonstrated that compression at 30 mm Hg and higher could block axonal transport. Chronic nerve entrapments with long-standing blockage of axonal transport can lead to wallerian degeneration of the axons distal to the lesions. These axons may regenerate, however, a process that in humans may take place at a speed of about 1 mm/day in optimal conditions.

Critical Pressure Levels

A pressure of 30 to 50 mm Hg applied to a peripheral nerve results in changes in intraneural blood flow, vascular permeability, and axonal transport. There have been no measurements performed in vivo on the pressure levels acting on a nerve root due to, for example, a herniated disc. One may extrapolate some data, however, from existing knowledge on the pressures generated by swelling of the nucleus pulposus. It has been demonstrated in vitro that specimens of nucleus pulposus may generate pressures of several hundred millimeters of mercury if exposed to free fluid within the confined space (74–76). If a sequestered fragment of nucleus pulposus is displaced into the foramen, one may speculate that the nearby nerve root could be compressed at high pressure levels by the swelling disc fragment. The validity of this hypothesis remains to be proven experimentally, however (42). The "edge effect" (Fig. 3.25) in neural damage by compression refers to the injuries seen in nerve fibers and intraneural blood vessels at the edges of the compressed segment, with sparing in the center (60,

77). Compression of a nerve at high pressure may induce intraneural damage, leading to functional deterioration at the compressed segment, but with preserved axonal continuity and nerve function proximal and distal to the compressed segment.

Compression of normal peripheral nerve or nerve root may induce numbness but usually does not cause pain. *Experimental investigations on human peripheral nerves in vivo have indicated that the numbness induced is a result of ischemia, not mechanical nerve fiber deformation, of the compressed segment. If a nerve root—or a peripheral nerve—is the site of chronic irritation, however, even minor mechanical deformation may induce radiating pain. This has been demonstrated by placing sutures or inflatable catheters around nerve roots at the time of surgery for herniated discs and postoperatively inducing stretching or compression of the nerve root.* Lindblom and Rexed (62) investigated a large number of postmortem specimens of the lumbar spine with special reference to the relations between disc herniations and nerve root compression. They found that the dorsal root ganglion often was deformed by the pressure from the intervertebral disc. The dorsal root ganglion thus is frequently compressed by herniated intervertebral discs, and experimental data indicate that compression of this nerve structure may induce radiating pain.

Obviously, mechanical factors are involved in nerve root injury in connection with intervertebral disc herniations. It also has been speculated that breakdown products from the degenerating nucleus pulposus may leak out to the root and induce a "chemical radiculitis." Nachemson (78) has measured pH in intervertebral discs intraoperatively and found very high hydrogen ion concentration in some patients who had extensive adhesion formation around the nerve root. Such changes in the tissue electrolyte balance may in various ways lead to pain. Autoimmune mechanisms also have been proposed to be involved in the inflammatory tissue reactions seen around degenerating discs.

The nerve fibers react to trauma with demyelination or axonal degeneration, leading to changes in nerve function. Another important causative factor for the functional deterioration is the impairment of intraneural microcirculation and the formation of intraneural edema. In cases of chronic compression, intra- and extraneural fibrosis may develop, which leads to further tissue irritation and the establishment of a chronic inflammatory process (Fig. 3.26).

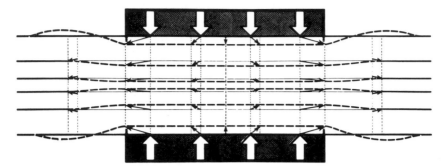

Figure 3.25. Schematic drawing, demonstrating the displacement of nerve tissue, which can be induced by circumferentially applied pressure. The pressure application leads to a bidirectional displacement of nerve tissue from the compressed nerve segment towards the noncompressed parts of the nerve. The interrupted lines show the positions of different tissue layers during compression. The *arrows* are vectors that indicate the displacement of nerve tissue components as a result of the applied pressure. Note that the displacement is maximal at the edges of the compressed segment. The diagram is based upon computations performed by Professor Richard Skalak, Columbia University, New York, N.Y. (Reproduced with permission from Lundborg G, Rydevik B: Läkartidn [Sweden] 79: 4035, 1982.)

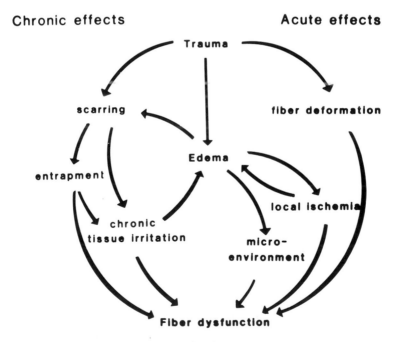

Figure 3.26. Proposed sequence of events leading to changes in nerve root function as a cause of acute and chronic compression. The dysfunction of the nerve fibers can be either loss of function or increased sensitivity to further mechanical stimulus. (Reproduced with permission from Rydevik B, Brown MD, Lundborg G: Pathoanatomy and pathophysiology of nerve root compression. *Spine* 9(1):8, 1984.)

The functional changes seen may be either loss of nerve function, seen as muscle weakness or sensory deficit, or a state of hyperexcitability of the nerve tissue. These two conditions may be present at the same time, meaning that nerve fibers may have a decreased conduction velocity at the site of injury, still being hypersensitive to further mechanical stimulus at the injured segment. The hyperexcitability can give rise to positive symptoms from the respective nerves, that is, pain, paresthesia, and possibly muscle fasciculations.

Conclusion

The anatomical complex of nerve root, ganglion, and spinal nerve may be involved in pathological processes in association with disc herniation and spinal stenosis. Compression of the nerve tissue may induce structural damage to the nerve fibers, impairment of intraneural blood flow, and formation of intraneural edema as well as axonal transport block (42).

The following discussion of the effects of compression on spinal nerve roots is based on the work of Seth Sharpless (54):

1. Dorsal roots are far more susceptible to compression block than is the peripheral (sciatic) nerve. When pressure is applied for 3 minutes followed by 3-minute recovery periods, 100 mm Hg must be applied to the sciatic nerve to achieve the same conduction block that can be produced in spinal roots by 20 mm Hg.

2. Pressure as slight as 10 mm Hg, maintained for 15 to 30 minutes, reduces the compound action potentials of dorsal roots to about half of their initial values. With such small pressures, nearly complete recovery occurs in about 30 minutes.

3. It is probable that the compression block produced even by such small pressures is due to mechanical deformation rather than ischemia, since the larger fibers are blocked first, whereas anoxia is believed to affect small fibers first.

4. It has been shown elsewhere (MacGregor et al., 1975) (54) that a pressure vessel model of a nerve predicts that large fibers would be most compressed, which may account for their susceptibility to blockage. The pressure vessel model might also account for the progressive character of compression block, assuming a viscous flow of the fiber contents.

5. The slow onset of compression block would have adaptive value, since transient increments of pressure which occur in confined spaces during extremes of motion would have little effect.

6. Spinal nerves acquire a structural feature that protects them from compression block before they enter the intervertebral foramina. The sheath does not appear to play an important role. The nature of this protective feature is still unknown.

Comparison of Normal and Chronic Nerve Root Irritability

Compression of a normal nerve root may be associated with numbness and motor weakness but does not usually cause pain. However, if the nerve tissue is chronically irritated, mechanical deformation may induce radiating pain. Thus, intraneural inflammation seems to be a factor of importance in the pathogenesis of pain production in nerve root compression syndromes. It is debated whether such intraneural inflammation is the result of an inflammatogenic effect of nucleus pulposus on nerve tissue ("chemical radiculitis") or is an effect of mechanical nerve root deformation by the herniated disc (79).

Injection under pressure of normal saline into a degenerated lumbar disc elicits pain that the patient experiences as identical to lumbago. The moment the pressure on the syringe is released, the pain disappears. It returns each time the pressure is increased. Identical experiments on a normal disc produce no pain. The amount of liquid that can be introduced into a normal nucleus pulposus is very small (80).

Nerve Root Compression Necessary to Cause Pathology

It is interesting to note the amount of pressure needed to create pathological compression in the human body. An example of this is carpal tunnel syndrome.

A number of experimental studies have been designed to evaluate the functional response of the median nerve at the wrist to various degrees of acute local compression in healthy volunteers and hypertensive patients. The relative significance of ischemia and mechanical deformation in early nerve compression, the critical threshold pressure for nerve conduction impairment, and the clinical sensibility testing system most accurate for evaluating and following patients with acute and chronic compressive neuropathies have been determined using a human model for median nerve compression in the carpal tunnel.

Between 40 and 50 mm Hg, there exists a critical threshold pressure in normotensive people at which peripheral nerve is acutely jeopardized. The critical pressure threshold is higher in hypertensive patients. The threshold exists at 30 mm Hg below diastolic blood pressure and 45 mm hg below mean arterial blood pressure in both normotensive and hypertensive individuals. The correlation between systemic blood pressure and the function of the nerve in response to local compression favors the concept that reduced microvascular perfusion plays the major role in the early stages of low-pressure nerve compression. In acute and chronic compression neuropathy, threshold tests (Semmes-Weinstein pressure, vibratory sensibility) detect the earliest abnormalities of nerve function (81).

Here we note that, at values of compression between 40 and 50 mm Hg, the peripheral median nerve will react pathologically. This is similar to the pressures found necessary to be applied to the spinal nerve root in order to create ischemic disease.

Nerve Fiber Compression by Disc Herniation

According to a study by Lindblom and Rexed (62), when a protrusion of the intervertebral disc bulges dorsolaterally into the intervertebral canal, it will first press upon the ventral root fibers and then on the whole of the spinal ganglion and the spinal nerve, while at the same time it pushes up the entire nervous structure against the dorsolateral margin of the intervertebral canal in the region of the intervertebral joint.

The region where the disc protrusion compresses the nerve always proved to be somewhere on the distal half of the spinal ganglion and the first centimeter of the spinal nerve. The deformation ranged from a slight flattening at a circumscribed area on the nerve to a severe hollowing out of a long stretch of it. In cases with slight pressure, the ventral root bundles seemed to be more resistant than the ganglion, but with increasing pressure both ventral root bundles and ganglion become flattened.

The basic effect of the compression is degeneration of a greater or lesser number of the nerve fibers. The damage does not occur as a massive, single trauma to the nerves but as many repeated small traumata. Furthermore, each trauma is not restricted to a sharply localized point but exerts its effect over a relatively large area. As a result, the degenerating nerve fibers are usually diffusely strewn all over the cross section in smaller or greater numbers in proportion to the severity and duration of the compression. Also, the standing of the degeneration varies from fiber to fiber, some showing signs of a fresh, others of an earlier lesion. This gives rise to another characteristic feature of these nerve injuries: as soon as a nerve fiber begins to degenerate, there occur reactive regenerative processes.

The damage to the sensory fibers is, of course, very similar in appearance to that of the motor fibers. However, degeneration is apparently much more infrequent and not as severe. There may be several reasons for this. One is that small myelinated and nonmyelinated fibers are very numerous among the sensory fibers. The pressure acts on these nerve fibers in the distal part of the ganglion or in the first stretch of the spinal nerve. Distally, they almost immediately mix with the motor fibers, which, of course also are damaged in these cases, and it may happen that some degenerations are wrongly ascribed to motor instead of sensory fibers. There is also the possibility that motor nerve fibers on the whole are more damaged than the sensory ones, since the ventral root fibers lie closer to the protrusion. As a last factor, there is the possibility that the motor nerve fibers generally are more vulnerable than the sensory ones. In any case, the amount of degeneration has always been estimated with great caution, and it may in reality be greater than has been assumed here.

The spinal ganglion itself and its nerve cells show more obvious reaction to the pressure. The spinal ganglion as a whole is often deformed to a greater or lesser extent.

A remarkable alteration of the nerve roots at their entry into the intervertebral foramina is noted. This alteration is evidently quite unrelated to the injury caused by the protruding discs. In the small funnel-shaped space, formed when the dura mater closes in on the roots, there could be seen in some cases a pathological thickening and proliferation of the arachnoidea. In the most extreme cases, the circumscribed proliferations resulted in severe deformation of the nerve roots and were connected with cystic formations in the root fascicles themselves (62).

PAIN GENERATION DYSFUNCTION BY ANATOMICAL STRUCTURES OF THE LUMBAR SPINE

Due to the nociceptive nerve ending presence within the annulus fibrosus of the disc, annular tears can cause pain in the low back, buttock, sacroiliac region, and lower extremity. This pain can occur in the absence of nerve root compression by a disc protrusion, while disc protrusion that does not compress the nerve root can cause an inflammatory response and secondary radiculitis by chemically induced inflammatory neural pain (82).

Facet arthropathy can cause low back, buttock, and lower extremity pain because of the abundant nerve supply to the zygapophyseal joints and their potential pain generation (82).

Basic Anatomy and Pathophysiology of Lumbar Nerve Injury

The motor (i.e., ventral) nerve root and sensory (i.e., dorsal) nerve root pass dorsal and lateral to the intervertebral disc.

The dorsal nerve roots have a larger diameter than the ventral nerve root and therefore a greater susceptibility of the sensory axons to compressive forces. The S1 nerve roots are approximately 170 mm long, while the L1 nerve roots are 60 mm long. The nerve roots as well as the spinal nerves are composed of axons that have arisen within the substance of the spinal cord and course to their final destination in the periphery. These axons may exceed 100 cm in length (82).

Spinal nerve roots lack the connective tissue protection that sheaths peripheral nerves. This sheathing has considerable mechanical strength and possesses properties to form a barrier to diffusion of certain molecules. The spinal nerve roots, therefore, are at a disadvantage mechanically and possibly biochemically. The nerve roots are surrounded, however, by cerebrospinal fluid, and this, together with the dura, does give the spinal nerve roots an element of mechanical protection. The dura of a spinal nerve root appears to be continuous with the epineurium of the periph-

eral nerve. It must be kept in mind that the nerve root complex must be extraordinarily mobile.

Nerve roots must change length dependent upon the degrees of flexion, extension, lateral bending, and rotation of the lumbar spine. Lumbar nerve roots limited in motion by fibrosis of either intraspinal or extraspinal origin will create traction upon the nerve root complex, causing ischemia and secondary neural dysfunction. This fact must also be kept in mind during the rehabilitation process. Flexibility exercises must be designed to maintain nerve root mobility.

Intraneural blood flow is markedly affected when the nerve is stretched about 8% over the original length. Complete cessation of all intraneural blood flow is seen at 15% elongation.

The dorsal root ganglion, because of its fibrous capsule as well as its rich vascular supply, may be more susceptible to changes in intraneural blood flow as well as to the development of secondary intraneural edema with consequent fibrotic change. This may explain sensory loss on gross neurological examination (82).

Sunderland (57) has also stated that spinal nerves will tolerate remarkable degrees of deformation provided that the deformation occurs slowly and does not alter the blood supply. Normal spinal nerves appear to have a high tolerance to mechanical deformation. Damaged nerve fibers are more susceptible to deformation and ischemia. Therefore, a patient with a long-standing radiculopathy will tolerate less instability and mechanical stress than the patient with a healthier nerve root.

Compression of a normal nerve root usually induces a sensation of numbness but not pain. However, mechanical deformation of a previously compressed nerve does cause pain. The dorsal root ganglion appears to be the most sensitive to mechanical deformation (57).

Spinal Fixation

The long-lasting nature of certain abnormal autonomic and musculoskeletal activity patterns has been recognized for many years. In clinical practice, the aftereffect of periods of abnormal afferent input has often been termed the "neural scar" due to the seemingly permanent changes that many physicians have observed even after long periods of treatment. Possible causes of such changes could be peripheral alterations or changes within the nervous system itself. Recent work on long-lasting changes in the excitability of the spinal reflex pathways has shown that relatively short periods (15 to 30 minutes) of fairly intense afferent input to the spinal reflex pathways can cause increases in the neural excitability which last for several hours. This phenomenon is known as *spinal fixation*. The work (83) reported here extends these findings to show that, in rats, stimulation periods of from 45 to 90 minutes which cause no observable locomotion problems can have effects on reflex excitability which are seen up to 72 hours later, following normal living patterns and locomotion. Thus, the excitability alterations are apparently masked by descending brain influences but remain despite such activity. The implications of this work for manipulative therapy and clinical observations of the effects of abnormal function included the necessity to take possible long-lasting reflex alterations into account in determining ongoing therapy.

The body of evidence on spinal fixation began with the work of DiGiogio in 1929 (83). The effect she noted, now known as spinal fixation, was one of altered posture following central nervous system (CNS) damage. By creating a small lesion in the cerebellum of an anesthetized dog, she could create a postural imbalance: the limbs on one side would actively flex and remain in that position. If the spinal cord was then severed, thus disconnecting the damaged cerebellum from the spinal reflex centers, the limbs would retain the flexed posture, provided a sufficient time (3 to 4 hours) had elapsed from the time of the lesion. It appeared that the disrupted outflow from the cerebellum to the spinal centers had created a site of altered activity in the spinal reflex arcs, which maintained the postural imbalance in the absence of the instigating stimulus (83).

DiGiogio (83) found that a number of CNS lesions would produce the postural changes that would become fixated. Most importantly, it was found that the time required to fix the postural changes seemed to be about 45 minutes. That is, once the lesion was produced and the limbs flexed, about 45 minutes had to elapse before cutting the spinal cord would result in retention of the limb flexion.

The next series of studies by DiGiogio was performed to find out if the cause of the flexion had to come from cerebellar lesions or whether other inputs could fixate the flexion. Stimulation was applied directly to the hind limb of anesthetized rats for varying periods in different groups. The outcome of these studies showed that the fixation effect could be achieved even more readily by direct cutaneous stimulation than by central lesions. In fact, the effect was seen in all subjects in at least 5 minutes less than with the lesion. The fixation could also be obtained in animals in which the spinal cord had first been severed, then the hind limb stimulated. This study showed that the cerebral cortex and brainstem were not necessary for the observed alteration in the spinal reflex excitability. In fact, the animals in which the spinal cord was severed prior to hind limb stimulation showed fixation of the flexion in only 30 minutes, thus indicating that the absence of the brain shortened the alteration process.

It was evident from these studies that some alteration of the reflex arcs was possible with both central and peripheral stimulation, but it was not evident that the alteration was within the spinal cord.

Groves and Thompson (83) delineated the basic neural mechanisms for the phenomena now known as *reflex habituation* (a decrease in reflex output after repeated activation) and *sensitization* (an increase in output), showing both effects to be mediated within the spinal cord and of neural origin.

Conclusively, the phenomena being studied were the product of alterations of the spinal reflex circuits and not of peripheral alterations.

At present, it is unclear whether the effects of severe alterations produced by intense patterns of input to reflexes can be increased or decreased. Periods of normal or even subnormal input should tend to restore the reflex to its normal excitability range. Thus, manipulative therapy that tends to restore free motion, reduce muscle tension and so forth, and thus decrease abnormal and overactive afferent input should at least allow the affected reflex paths to regain more appropriate excitability levels. The spinal reflexes should be considered as active participants in the symptoms treated with manipulative therapy and their role in these symptoms recognized in the treatment (83).

Sacral Nerve Root Compression Produces Genitourinary Problems

Organic pathology of the lumbar spine, compromising the sacral nerve roots, can produce symptoms of erectile and bladder dysfunction. This study reports experience with 97 consecutive male patients admitted to the hospital for comprehensive lumbar pain evaluation. Lumbar diagnosis included herniated nucleus pulposus, spinal stenosis, segmental instability, and idiopathic lumbar spine syndrome.

By including a comprehensive neurological evaluation as a part of the routine investigation of the males with lumbar pain complaints, data have been gathered that indicate that abnormalities of visceral function have diagnostic significance equal to that of other neurological deficits. These data indicate that lumbar disease can itself produce significant bladder and sexual dysfunction, and hence, it is incumbent upon all clinicians investigating lumbar problems to also obtain a comprehensive genitourinary appraisal (48).

Theoretical Concepts Explaining Relief of Spinal Pain by Manipulative Therapy

Repetitive mechanical stimulation (once every 3 seconds) for 30 seconds has been found to cause a rapid block of sensitized nociceptors in the inflamed ankle joint of a rat (83a). This lasted for several minutes until the afferents again conducted pain impulses. Manipulative therapy may reduce nociceptive input in much the same way, and reduction of intraarticular pressure by manipulative maneuvers may be the mechanism whereby afferent input is reduced. Intraarticular pressure has been seen to be reduced for a few minutes under passive manipulative procedures of the apophyseal joints, thus reducing afferent discharge (84).

Although controversial, the gate control theory stated that selective stimulation of somatic large-diameter afferent fibers in peripheral nerves would suppress the rostral transmission of painful stimuli. Muscle guarding alleviation in joint pain may be the result of joint nociceptive blockage by passive range of motion allowing reduced afferent firing (85). Pain on motion manipulation may be the result, not the cause, of resistance of the joint to motion; elimination of painful muscle guarding is due to relief of painful afferent transmission allowing return of motion (86). One to two minutes of repetitive or maintained passive motion of a joint or pressure over the joint has been found to result in a decrease to total failure in the ability of normal joint afferents to conduct painful impulses (87).

CONUS MEDULLARIS INTERSEGMENTAL MOTOR SYSTEM

An epispinal system of motor axons virtually covers the ventral and lateral funiculi of the human conus medullaris between the L2 and S2 levels. These nerve fibers apparently arise from motor cells of the ventral horn nuclei and join spinal nerve roots caudal to their level of origin. In all observed spinal cords, many of these axons converged at the cord surface and formed an irregular group of ectopic rootlets that could be visually traced to join conventional spinal nerve roots at a level one to several segments below their original segmental level; occasional rootlets join a dorsal nerve root. As almost all previous reports of nerve root interconnections involved only the dorsal roots and have been cited to explain a lack of an absolute segmental sensory nerve distribution, it is believed that these intersegmental motor fibers may similarly explain a more diffuse efferent distribution than has previously been suspected (88).

Microvessel Irritation of Nerves
PERIPHERAL NERVES

If a peripheral nerve is to function properly, two basic requirements must be met: (*a*) its connection with the mother cells in the central nervous system must remain undisturbed; and (*b*) it must receive a continuous and adequate supply of oxygen through the intraneural vascular system. While transection of a nerve results in loss of excitability in its distal parts within 3 to 8 days, complete ischemia is followed by a rapid deterioration of nerve function within 30 to 90 minutes. However, if blood flow is then reestablished, recovery of nerve function occurs coincident with the restoration of the intraneural blood flow.

BLOOD VESSELS OF NERVES ARE PAIN SENSITIVE

The vasa nervorum are innervated by sympathetic nerves, and stimulation of the lumbar part of the sympathetic chain of a rabbit results in a marked vascular response in the tibial nerve. Immediately after stimulation, there is vasoconstriction in the intraneural microvascular bed and a general slowing down of the blood flow. The arteriolar constriction is so extensive that some of the vessels are hardly visible and only a few erythrocytes are occasionally seen passing through them. In some capillaries, the flow comes to a complete standstill, and occasionally during the period of stimulation there is retrograde flow in some capillaries (59).

EFFECT OF ISCHEMIA

The effect of ischemia on nerve function has been studied extensively both clinically and experimentally, and detailed reviews of the literature were presented by Adams, Richards, Blunt, Lundborg and Branemark, and Lundborg (59). Within 30 to 90 minutes of the onset of ischemia, there is a complete deterioration of nerve function, but it was shown in animal studies that ischemia for 5 or 6 hours or less may be followed by rapid recovery of nerve function. When ischemia of an extremity is induced by means of a tourniquet, the nerve segment distal to the cuff becomes ischemic, while the segment under the cuff is subjected to mechanical compression as well as ischemia.

The perineurium also appears to be resistant to longstanding ischemia. In studies of human femoral nerves and of peripheral nerves of experimental animals, the perineurial barrier was found to tolerate as much as 24 hours of ischemia (59).

Experimental compression lesions of peripheral nerves were induced by applying pressure directly to exposed rabbit nerve trunks. The results indicate that a slight trauma to a nerve (e.g., 50 mm Hg for 2 hours) induced an epineural edema by increasing the permeability of the epineural vessels, which were more susceptible to compression trauma than the endoneurial vessels (60).

NERVE ROOTS

Spinal nerve roots in general and the human lumbosacral spinal nerve roots in particular are structurally, vascularly, and metabolically unique regions of the nervous system. Peculiarities of their intrinsic vasculature and supporting connective tissue may account for suspected "neuroischemic" responses to pathological mechanical stresses and inflammatory conditions associated with degenerative disease of the lower spine.

The painful and disabling consequences of degenerative disease in the lower spine are most frequently the manifestation of a mechanical stress on the lumbosacral spinal nerve roots. Considering the prevalence of neurovascular involvement in low back disorders, the current knowledge of the finer structure of the lumbosacral nerve roots and their vascular relations is surprisingly scant (89).

In past studies in which vascular injection showed the more conspicuous elements of the true radicular blood supply, it was assumed that the direction of arterial flow throughout the extent of the root was always toward the cord. This was an understandable misconception, as a nearly complete injection of the human spinal root arteries, particularly those of the lumbosacral region, reveals that each root is supplied by longitudinal arteries that show a fairly consistent caliber throughout their course, and the usual terminal tapering, which would suggest the direction of blood flow, is lacking.

In the lumbosacral region, the largest nerve roots of the spinal cord must emerge from the few centimeters of the abruptly tapering conus medullaris. They leave the root zone as individually distinct fiber bundles that, because of their propinquity, shortly become combined into the common bundle that is characteristic of the lumbosacral root. An extension of the pial covering of the cord ensheathes the rootlets individually as they emerge and continues to follow them throughout their course as root fascicles.

Considering the dual source of nutrition and the protective adaptations found in the lumbosacral nerve root vasculature, it may seem paradoxical that many symptoms of low back problems appear to have a neuroischemic basis. Since the root is usually fixed at the intervertebral foramen, entrapments or additional displacements may tend to increase the linear stresses on the root substance, thus having a more extensive effect along a greater length of its microvasculature than a simple epidural compression at a given point.

The mechanisms whereby the tension interrupts the blood flow are open to speculation, but a plausible effect may result from the straightening of the interwoven collagen bundles. As a child's "finger puzzle" increases its interwoven constrictive grip the more one tries to pull the fingers free, the ultimate results of a pathological tension on a nerve or nerve root may be a constrictive pressure at the microvascular level that can affect a considerable length of the vascular bed. Thus, the thin-walled radicular veins may be readily collapsed and may effectively block the afferent side of the nutritional circuit (89).

PAIN DUE TO MECHANICAL NERVE ROOT COMPRESSION

While the so-called disc syndrome is a well-established clinical entity, there does not appear to be any experimental evidence showing that a herniated nucleus pulposus pressing on a lower lumbar nerve root does in fact cause sciatica.

Inman and Saunders (90), commenting on the concept that sciatica is caused solely by pressure on the nerve root, stated that this is not borne out by the existing experimental evidence on the effects of pressure on nerves, and that there is no experimental evidence to indicate that pressure alone upon the nerve root initiates pain of this characteristic type.

From a series of 22 patients with sciatica due to intervertebral disc pressure, eight were chosen. Each of these patients had classic sciatica, and in each an unequivocal disc herniation pressing on the fifth lumbar and first sacral roots was demonstrated at operation (90). The disc material was removed through a small aperture cut in the ligamentum flavum. An effort was made to center this aperture directly over the protruding disc. When the disc material was removed, a loop of nylon thread was passed around the involved root and its two ends brought to the surface. It was so placed that, when the slack was taken up, the loop pressed on the root at the same place as the disc had. It tended to maintain this relation to the root because of its passage through the small aperture in the ligamentum flavum directly above. It was hoped that, by pulling on this nylon thread in order to bring it in contact with the root, the effects of disc pressure would be closely simulated.

The experiment was performed on the first postoperative day in three patients, on the 14th day in one, and on the 10th day in the remaining four. In all these eight patients, symptoms were completely relieved by removal of the disc.

In 11 patients, 10 of whom had herniated discs, the ligamentum flavum, interspinous ligament, and annulus fibrosus were tested instead of a nerve root or the dura mater. In eight patients, one nylon suture was passed through the ligamentum flavum and one through the interspinous ligament. In two patients, the ligamentum flavum was tested; in the last, the annulus fibrosus alone was tested.

It has been established that the nerve root need only be touched to cause sciatica. It would also appear that, if touched repeatedly or continuously, the root becomes hypersensitive (90).

EFFECTS OF NERVE ROOT COMPRESSION

The following material is presented with permission of Michael Feuerstein, Ph.D., associate professor of Psychiatry and Anesthesiology at the University of Rochester School of Medicine and Dentistry, and his coauthors. It is an excellent treatise on chronic low back pain, and it is a pleasure to present it here.

Biobehavioral Mechanisms of Chronic Low Back Pain[b]

Pain has been defined as "an unpleasant sensory and emotional experience associated with actual or potential tissue damage, or described in terms of such 'damage' "(1). . . .

Chronic back pain is often defined as a disorder of the skeletal muscles, vertebrae, or intervertebral discs of the lower back, and has been characterized by "varying degrees of discomfort and aching or back stiffness with difficulty bending, decreased back mobility, skeletal muscle spasm and tenderness, concern or preoccupation with the back and with general concomitant disabilities" (2).

Chronicity has been conceptualized in different ways (3). This review will consider the acute back pain patient as one who experiences a debilitating episode but who recovers within 2 to 6 weeks with appropriate therapy. On the other hand, the chronic patient, the major subject of this review, is defined as having experienced pain over a period of at least 6 months, whether the pain is continual or recurrent during this period and whether demonstrable organic pathology is present (3). . . .

EPIDEMIOLOGY

. . . Magora (4) estimates that 12.9% of bank clerks, post office clerks, bus drivers, policemen, nurses, farmers, and both light and heavy industrial workers experience back pain for at least 3 days per year. Bonica (3) estimates that 7.1% of the United States' population

---

[b] Modified with permission from *Clinical Psychology Review*, vol 7, Feuerstein MJ, Papciak AS, Hoon PE: Biobehavioral mechanisms of chronic low back pain, Copyright 1987, Pergamon Journals, Ltd.

currently suffers from chronic low back pain (CLBP). Other estimates of the proportion of the population suffering from CLBP are variable, ranging from 4% to 18% in the general population (5) and to 30% in industrial communities (6–8).

Chronic low back pain patients constitute a substantial portion of the physically limited or impaired population. In the United States, among all chronic conditions, impairment of the back and spine is the most frequent cause of activity limitation in persons under 45 years and ranks fourth (9) after heart disease, arthritis, and rheumatism in persons aged 45–64. Of currently employed persons in the labor force with limitation of activity due to chronic conditions, impairment of back or spine was the leading cause of impairment (8, 10).

Absence-from-work statistics also suggest a high prevalence of back pain. In United States industry, Rowe (11) found 4 hours/person/year were lost because of CLBP, a figure second only to hours lost due to upper respiratory infections. Also in the United States, Anderson (12) reports a loss of 10 million days per year due to back pain, whereas in Sweden and Britain (13), 2 million and 13 million days of work are lost, respectively. Frymoyer et al. (14) estimate that low back pain accounts for $11 billion in lost wages per year in the United States. Among manual workers, back pain may account for 63% of sickness absence (10) or between 10%–30% of all medical claims (13). The significance of the chronicity of low back pain is shown in a typical industry in Washington (15), where employees who were absent from work for more than 6 months had only a 50% chance of ever achieving productive employment again. Absenteeism for longer than 1 year reduced the probability to 25%, and the chances of a worker ever returning to productive employment were negligible after 2 years of absence.

Low back pain patients account for 2%–4% of doctors' patients (16), and back symptoms are the second leading symptom for patients visiting physicians (17). Statistics from Britain show the typical course of back pain difficulty in a general population: 1.1 million consult a physician for back pain during the course of a year, each patient averaging three consultations (16). Twenty-two to 43% (17) of these are referred to a hospital at one time in their lives, and 6 to 14% of these are admitted. Five-tenths of 1% undergo surgery (16).

CHARACTERISTICS

Nagi, Riley, and Newby (5) found that the frequency of back pain reports increases with age, and prevalence data reported by Biering-Sorenson (18) suggest that the prevalence rate may increase by 50% or more for both men and women between the ages of 30 and 60. Nagi et al. (5) reported that higher frequencies of back pain were associated with less formal education and separated, divorced,

or widowed persons. Roland (8) and Cypress (17) found the incidence higher among men. Frymoyer et al. (14) report a relationship between severe back pain and cessation of sports participation after adolescence and cigarette smoking, and Cypress (17) reports that the back patient is frequently obese. Blue collar workers, nurses (4), and heavy industrial workers tend to have a higher incidence of back pain (6).

One out of five back pain patients will be severely disabled, two will be able to work but will have to change jobs, and two will remain in their original jobs but will be limited in their type and amount of work (19). Thus, 85% of back pain patients have little-to-moderate limitation of activity (5), which is consistent with the finding that 40% of back pain reports are only "slightly serious."

The range of a back pain episode is from 9–32 days (16, 20). Eleven percent of the industrial population have pain with a duration of less than 6 months, while 5% experience pain for greater than 6 months (21), meeting the reviewer's definition of chronicity. Roland (8) examined the natural history of back pain and found that only 5% of those with back pain consult a physician. Of this group, 60% will have been in pain less than 1 week, with only one-quarter of the patients consulting a physician for more than 2 weeks after their initial visit. In addition, only 10% will consult for longer than 4 weeks. These data indicate that acute back pain is much more common than chronic back pain.

PATHOPHYSIOLOGY

The pathophysiology of CLBP is complex (22). Roland (8) points out that the underlying condition in the majority of patients is best described as "non-specific mechanical back pain." It is clear that, given the number of potential causal factors, the diagnosis of back pain from medical factors alone is difficult and uncertain in accuracy. Additional complicating factors in diagnosis include: (a) the relative inaccessibility of the spine for examination, and (b) the low correlation of pathological changes in the spine with symptoms of LBP. It has been estimated that only 20% to 30% of patients with low back pain are found to have "objective" signs of disease (23). Unfortunately, there is virtually no data concerning the relative frequency of the various medical diagnoses. There is, however, general agreement regarding the most common diagnoses. Common causes of back pain include: (a) lumbosacral sprains and strains (24) associated with fatigue, obesity, inadequate muscle tone, or pregnancy (21); (b) herniated disc, axial skeletal joint dysfunction (25), and injuries of the bone, joint, or ligament (21); (c) myofacial [sic] syndromes (muscle spasm) (25); and (d) degenerative disease of the spine (osteoarthritis, including ankylosing hyperostosis) (25). The reliability with which diagnosticians agree on these classifications has not been empirically demonstrated. . . .

Table 3.2.
Pathway Following Onset of Pain/Injury [a]

Evaluation/Treatment Process	Outcome

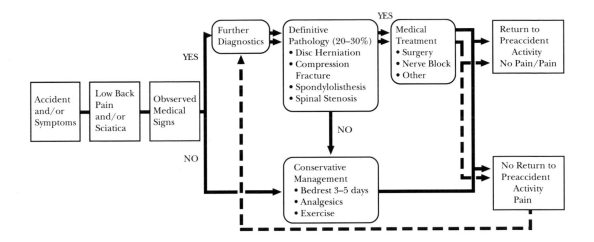

[a]Reprinted with permission from *Clinical Psychology Review*, vol 7, Feuerstein MJ, Papciak AS, Hoon PE: Biobehavioral mechanisms of chronic low back pain, Copyright 1987, Pergamon Journals, Ltd.

BIOBEHAVIORAL ``MECHANISMS''

Table 3.2 provides a schematic representation of the sequence of events that a typical low back pain patient experiences following onset of reported pain or injury. As indicated, only a minority of patients (20%–30%) have definitive pathology necessitating a more invasive procedure. The majority of individuals (80%) experience a low back pain episode, follow a conservative treatment regimen, and within 6 weeks return to work either with or without pain (23). Twenty percent, however, do not return to work within the 6-week period. It is this group that continually recycles through the health care system (*broken line* on table) for repeated diagnostic and treatment procedures. Generally, the longer the reported pain, the more likely a complex set of environmental, cognitive, and emotional factors are operative. These 20% account for 80% of the total costs to society for back pain (23). Recurrence of symptoms are [*sic*] observed in 50% of those who return to work during the first 2–3 years after the acute episode.

References for "Biobehavioral Mechanisms of Chronic Low Back Pain"

1. International Association for the Study of Pain: Pain terms: a list and notes on usage. *Pain* 6: 249–252, 1979.
2. Vazuka FA: Etiology and mechanisms in the development of low back syndrome. In Nodine JH, Moyer JH (eds): *Psychosomatic Medicine* Philadelphia, Lea & Febiger, 1962.
3. Bonica JJ: Pain research and therapy: past and current status and future needs. In Ng LKY, Bonica JJ (eds): *Pain, Discomfort, and Humanitarian Care*. North Holland, Amsterdam, Elseviera, 1980, pp 1–46.
4. Magora A: Investigation of the relation between low back pain and occupation. *Occupational Medicine* 39:465–471, 1970.
5. Nagi SZ, Riley LE, Newby LG: A social epidemiology of back pain in a general population. *J Chronic Dis* 27:769–779, 1973.
6. Anderson JAD, Duthie JJR, Moody BP: Social and economic effects of rheumatic diseases in a mining population. *Ann Rheum Dis* 21:342–352, 1962.
7. Anderson JAD, Duthie JJR: Rheumatic complaints in dockyard workers. *Ann Rheum Dis* 22: 401–409, 1963.
8. Roland MO: The natural history of back pain. *Practitioner* 227:1119–1122, 1983.

9. Kelsey JL, White AA: Epidemiology and impact of low back pain. *Spine* 5:133–142, 1980.
10. Anderson JA: Low back pain: cause and prevention of long-term handicap (a critical review). *International Rehabilitation Medicine* 3:89–96, 1981.
11. Rowe ML: Low back pain in industry: a position paper. *J Occu Med* 11:161–169, 1969.
12. Anderson JA: Back pain in industry. In Jayson M (ed): *The Lumbar Spine and Back Pain.* London, Pitman, 1976, pp 29–46.
13. Chaffin DB, Park KS: A longitudinal study of low back pain as associated with occupational weight lifting factors. *Am Ind Hyg Assoc J* 34:513–524, 1973.
14. Frymoyer JR, Pope MH, Clements JH, Wilder DG, MacPherson B, Ashikaga T: Risk factors in low back pain: an epidemiological survey. *J Bone Joint Surg* (65–68):213–218, 1983.
15. McGill C: Industrial back problems: a control program. *Journal of Occupational Medicine* 10:174–178, 1968.
16. Benn RT, Wood PHN: Pain in the back: an attempt to estimate the size of the problem. *Rheumatology and Rehabilitation* 14:121–128, 1975.
17. Cypress BK: Characteristics of physician visits for back symptoms: a national perspective. *Am J Public Health* 73:389–395, 1983.
18. Biering-Sorenson F: Low back trouble in a general population of 30-, 40-, 50-, and 60-year-old men and women. *Dan Med Bull* 29:289–299, 1982.
19. Wood PHN: Epidemiology of back pain. In Jayson J (ed): *The Lumbar Spine and Back Pain.* New York, Grune and Stratton, 1976.
20. Wood PHN, McLeish CL: Statistical appendix: digest of data on the rheumatic diseases. *Ann Rheum Dis* 33:93, 1974.
21. Brown JR: *Low Back Pain Syndrome: Its Etiology and Prevention.* Toronto, Labour Safety Council of Ontario, 1977.
22. Hickson, N: Back problems in general practice. *Aust Fam Physician* 12:345–346, 348, 1983.
23. Nachemson A: Work for all. *Clin Orthop* 179:77–85, 1983.
24. Finneson B: *Low Back Pain.* Philadelphia, JB Lippincott, 1980.
25. Loeser JD: Low back pain. *Res Pub Assoc Res Nerv Ment Dis* 58:363–377, 1980.

Pain Receptors in Low Back Pain

Livermore (91) states that there are two basic types of sensory nerve fibers. They are: (*a*) type A—large, myelinated fibers that conduct impulses quickly and tend to conduct modalities of touch and pressure; and (*b*) type C—fine, unmyelinated fibers that conduct impulses slowly and transmit pain and temperature perception. Peripheral sensory fibers carry both A and C fibers and run with the motor portion of the nerve.

The course of a pain impulse is as follows: peripheral sensory ending → common root at intervertebral level via ventral ramus → dorsal root → dorsal root ganglion cell bodies → spinothalamic tracts (lateral carries type C fibers for pain and temperature, anterior carries A fibers for touch and pressure) → thalamus (for organization and modification) (91).

There are two types of pain sensation: (*a*) deep pain (splanchnic pain—associated with C fiber irritation—dull, deep, aching, diffuse pain that follows myotomes and sclerotomes. Referred pain is close to site of pathological condition. Pain is of later onset—more disabling, difficult to localize. (*b*) Superficial pain—called *somatic* pain—sharp, localized. Type A fibers carry it. Pain follows dermatome (91).

Ligamentous Nerve Root Fixation in the Vertebral Canal

The anatomy of 54 pairs of lumbosacral nerve roots was described in nine fresh adult cadaver specimens, with particular attention given to the fixation of the nerve roots to surrounding skeletal and ligamentous structures in the lumbar spine. Dural ligaments were identified fixing the dura and nerve roots at their exit from the main dural sac to the posterior longitudinal ligament and vertebral body periosteum proximal to the intervertebral disc. Distal fixation occurs at the intervertebral foramen where the epineural sheath of the spinal nerve is attached. The overall arrangement is one that tends to hold the existing nerve root anteriorly in the spinal nerve (92).

Mechanical analysis of this anatomical arrangement explains how pressure can be applied to the extrathecal nerve root by a disc protrusion without compression of the nerve root against the posterior elements. The possible role of the dural ligaments in the pathogenesis of the sciatica syndrome is discussed.

The extrathecal intraspinal lumbar nerve root is relatively fixed in the spinal canal. Because of this fixation, the extrathecal nerve root cannot easily slip away from a disc protrusion, whereas the nerve root lying freely in the thecal sac can.

Trolard (92), in 1893, described and illustrated a "ligamentum sacral anterius durae matrin'' as an anterior midline series of bands that fastened the dura to the posterior longitudinal ligament in the lower lumbar and sacral regions. Hofmann (92), in 1898, more extensively described several dural ligaments, including a "ligamenta anteriora dura matris" similar to Trolard's earlier description.

This anatomical arrangement means that traction forces applied to the lumbosacral nerves are resisted by the intervertebral foraminal attachments and the dura, in effect insulating the intrathecal nerve roots from the traction forces.

A new finding is an additional attachment by a ligamentous band running from the sheath of the extrathecal foramen. This ligamentous attachment may provide additional fixation of the nerve root to the spine distal to the intervertebral disc.

We are therefore suggesting that when a contact force is present on the nerve root, tension forces are developed, with the forces shared by the dural ligaments just proximal to the disc and the well-known foraminal attachments distal to the disc. Thus, traction forces are exerted on the attachments of the dural ligaments (the posterior longitudinal ligament and vertebral periosteum) and the pedicular periosteum and connective tissue at the foraminal exit of the spinal nerve.

Thus, a disc protrusion is a necessary but not sufficient condition for a contact force to be exerted on the nerve root. The pressure distribution in the nerve root as a result of this contact force, which would determine the pattern of vascular compromise of the nerve root, would depend upon the contact area of force application, the tissue properties, and the particular geometric configurations involved.

Simple mechanical considerations also suggest that the dural ligaments are situated such that pressure exerted by the disc on the nerve root can be transmitted via these ligaments to the posterior longitudinal ligament and vertebral periosteum. These very structures have been shown previously to produce a characteristic component of sciatic pain when subjected to traction forces (92).

Furcal Nerve

Attention must be paid to the furcal nerve when analyzing lumbosacral radicular symptoms, especially when neurological findings are atypical and the responsible level cannot be assessed (93). An anatomical and clinical study (93) of the furcal nerve showed the following: the furcal nerve was found in all dissections, and it arises at the L4 root level in most dissections (93%); the furcal nerve has its own anterior and posterior root fibers and its own dorsal nerve root ganglion. This proves that the furcal nerve is an independent nerve root. Neurological symptoms suggestive of two roots being involved are frequently due to furcal nerve compression.

Neurological symptoms implying involvement of two roots may be due to four causes. First, two roots may be compressed by a single lesion. Second, two lesions may be present. Third, there may be an anomaly of root emergence with two nerve roots emerging through the same foramen. Finally, the furcal nerve may be involved.

When a single nerve root block produces motor weakness and sensory deficits in two nerve root areas, and when the other three possibilities are not demonstrated by the myelographic findings, the furcal nerve should be examined (93).

Counterirritation Principles

The inhibitory effects of acute pain produced by Lasègue's maneuver on the lower limb nociceptive flexion reflexes induced by electrical sural nerve stimulation were explored in patients complaining of sciatica as a result of an identified unilateral disc protrusion. Lasègue's maneuver on the affected side produced a typical radicular pain and resulted in a powerful depression of nociceptive reflexes elicited either in the normal or in the affected lower limb. Simultaneously, patients reported relief of the electrically induced pain. In contrast, painless Lasègue's maneuver on the normal side had no effect on these parameters. These results confirm other reports that have shown that experimental pain thresholds can be increased by a conditioning painful stimulus applied to other areas of the body (94–97).

Furthermore, it has been shown that various modalities of experimentally induced pains, "heat, cold, pressure," applied to heterotrophic body areas can depress simultaneously the nociceptive flexion reflex activity and pain sensation due to sural nerve stimulation. All of these observations are probably relevant to counterirritation phenomena, defined as a paradoxical pain-relieving effect of pain elicited from other regions of the body (94). Thus they provide experimental support for the use of intense cold for the treatment of clinical pain, such as ice massage of the hand for the relief of dental pain (94).

Articular Neurology

All the synovial joints of the body (including the apophyseal joints of the vertebral column) are provided with four varieties of receptor nerve endings (Table 3.3). Three of the varieties of receptor (types I, II, and III) are corpuscular mechanoreceptors (i.e., biological transducers) that are stimulated by increases in tension in the tissue in which they are embedded. The type IV variety is represented by nonencapsulated unmyelinated nerve fibers that provide the articular nociceptive system, which is normally inactive but becomes active when abnormally high tensions develop in the articular tissues, or when the nerve terminals are exposed to high concentrations of irritant chemical substances in the tissue fluid that bathes them (98).

Experimental electroneurographic studies of the impulse traffic in single afferent fibers in articular nerves have revealed that when joints are immobile, there is a tonic discharge at low frequency from some of the low-threshold type I mechanoreceptors in response to the small static tension that then prevails throughout the joint capsule (98). Such studies also reveal that when a joint is moved by manipulation, in any direction, there is a diphasic response from the mechanoreceptors located in the region of the joint capsule that is thereby stretched. This consists of an initial brief burst of impulses from the type II receptors that melts into a prolonged increase in type I receptor activity whose parameters are determined by the amplitude and velocity of the joint movement. At the same time, there is a reduction in, or abolition of, the tonic discharge from the type I receptors in the opposing region of the joint capsule, which is simultaneously relaxed. As a result of this coordinated adjustment of their discharge frequency, the type I receptors signal the direction, amplitude, and velocity of joint movements, while the type II receptors in the stretched region of joint capsule merely signal that a movement has been initiated. On the other hand, when traction is applied axially through a joint, the mechanoreceptors on all aspects of the joint capsule are thereby stimulated simultaneously, and should traction be sustained, the frequency of the type I receptor discharge remains proportional to the applied traction force. The type II receptors fire only briefly at the moment of imposition of the traction force, while the type III receptors in the joint ligaments do not fire at all unless the traction force is considerable (98).

Central Effects of Articular Mechanoreceptor Activity

The afferent discharges derived from articular mechanoreceptors (and especially from the type I and type II receptors embedded in the joint capsules) are of particular importance to manipulative therapists by virtue of the threefold effects they produce when they enter the neuraxis in response to joint manipulation or traction (or in response to active joint movement). These effects are as follows:

Reflexogenic Effects. It is through this mechanism that changes in muscle tone (involving both facilitation and inhibition of motor unit activity), which have long been empirically familiar to practitioners of manipulative therapy, are developed.

Perceptual Effects. These are the reason that patients whose articular mechanoreceptors are destroyed by joint trauma, inflammation, or degenerative disease processes manifest impairment of postural and kinesthetic sensibility in the regions of their body thus affected.

Pain Suppression. Of even more practical importance to manipulative therapists is the pain-suppressive effect exerted by stimulation of articular mechanoreceptors. Since massage, compression, vibration, and stretching stimulate embedded mechanoreceptors, and there is a close morphological relationship between the mechanoreceptor and nociceptive receptor systems in the somatic tissues, it therefore seems likely that it is primarily through controlled stimulation of peripheral tissue mechanoreceptors by the application of static or phasic forces that manipulative therapists are able to produce relief of pain, especially pain arising from mechanical or chemical abnormalities in joint tissues.

It should now be clear that passive manipulation of, or the application of traction through, limb and spinal joints has many reflexogenic and perceptual consequences. Not least of these in a clinical context is the relief of pain as a result of production of presynaptic inhibition of nocicep-

Table 3.3.
Characteristics of Articular Receptor Systems[a]

Type	Morphology	Location	Parent Nerve Fibers	Behavioral Characteristics
I	Thinly encapsulated globular corpuscles (100 μM × 40 μm), in tridimensional clusters of 3 to 8 corpuscles	Fibrous capsules of joints (in superficial layers)	Small myelinated (6–9 μm)	Static and dynamic mechanoreceptors: low-threshold, slowly adapting
II	Thickly encapsulated conical corpuscles (280 μm × 120 μm), individual or in clusters of 2 to 4 corpuscles	Fibrous capsules of joints (in deeper subsynovial layers). Articular fat pads	Medium myelinated (9–12 μm)	Dynamic mechanoreceptors: low-threshold, rapidly adapting
III	Thinly encapsulated fusiform corpuscles (600 μm × 100 μm), individual or in clusters of 2 to 3 corpuscles	Applied to surfaces of joint ligaments (collateral and intrinsic)	Large myelinated (13–17 μm)	Dynamic mechanoreceptors: high-threshold, slowly adapting
IV	(a) Tridimensional plexuses of unmyelinated nerve fibers	Fibrous capsules of joints; articular fat pads; adventitial sheaths of articular blood vessels		
	(b) Free unmyelinated nerve endings	Joint ligaments (collateral and intrinsic)	Very small myelinated (2–5 μm) and unmyelinated (<2 μm)	Nociceptive mechanoreceptors: very high-threshold, nonadapting; chemosensitive (to abnormal tissue metabolites) nociceptive receptors

[a]Reproduced with permission from Wyke BD: Articular neurology and manipulative therapy. In Glasgow EF, Twomey LT, Scull ER, Kleynhans AM, Idczak RM (eds): *Aspects of Manipulative Therapy.* Edinburgh, Churchill Livingstone, 1985, p 73.

tive afferent transmission through the synapses in the basal spinal nucleus because of the mechanoreceptor stimulation that is inevitably associated with all manipulative procedures (98).

Conclusion. Thus degenerative, inflammatory, or traumatic affections of the joints result in loss of the mechanoreceptor (but not the nociceptor) system in the joints in question, giving rise to reflex disorders of posture and movement, and to impairment of postural and kinesthetic sensation. Furthermore, since progressive degenerative loss of mechanoreceptor afferent nerve fibers in all peripheral nerves (including those innervating the joints of the limbs and spine) is an inevitable consequence of advancing age, it seems highly likely that this plays a significant part in producing the disorders of posture and gait that are experienced by elderly people, as well as contributing to their diminished pain tolerance. It may also explain why some manipulative thera-

peutic procedures are less effective in relieving joint pain in elderly patients than they are in younger people.

CHEMICAL RADICULITIS

Marshall et al. (99) describe a new pathological concept termed *chemical radiculitis.* This lesion occurs when the annulus fibrosus has been weakened by intervertebral disc degeneration and finally ruptures under the stress of some traumatic episode. Nuclear fluid is, at that time, of waterlike consistency. It is ejected into the peridiscal tissues and tracks down to the nerve root. Because of its glycoprotein component, nuclear fluid is highly irritant to nerve tissue, and sudden severe sciatic pain results.

Liberation of nuclear fluid from the sealing annulus fibrosus capsule converts the glycoprotein of nuclear fluid into an antigen role, which results in antibodies detectable in high titer in the bloodstream after a 3-week interval. This is an autoimmune reaction. Chemical radiculitis can explain some or possibly all cases of acute or chronic inflammatory change around the nerve root.

Walk (99) suggested that there were two neurological syndromes caused by the lumbar intervertebral disc: (*a*) compression of the nerve by the disc; and (*b*) irritation of the nerve by the perineural spread of the contents of the nucleus pulposus occurring through a disc rupture.

If chemical radiculitis is to be accepted as a viable theory, several important factors need to be verified, such as: (*a*) Can nuclear fluid reach the nerve root? Lindblom and Rexed (89) dissected 160 cadavers and demonstrated a connecting pathway from the nucleus via the annular rupture to the root. (*b*) Is nuclear fluid in a liquid form at some stage of the degenerative process? This has been noted by many individual observers at operation and verified by Armstrong and Walk. Armstrong (89) states that he has incised the annulus on occasions and that the fluid has squirted out of the wound.

If the immunological research proves to be correct, a rupture of the annulus with consequent liberation of nuclear fluid into the tissues will be followed by a high serum titer to glycoprotein. Thus, for the very first time, a serum test will be available for the detection of a valid disc lesion 3 weeks after the initial pain. Armed with this knowledge, the correct immediate treatment, as above, can be administered.

Chemical radiculitis is an inflammatory condition of the nerve root due to the rupture of the annulus fibrosus and dissemination of disc fluid along the nerve root sheath. The inflammatory component of disc fluid is glycoprotein. The inflammation is a reaction to repeated injuries of the spinal column, as, for example, in occupational lifting of heavy loads. Rupture of the annulus fibrosus and liberation of disc fluid into the tissues also evokes circulating antibody response and autoimmune reaction. A high titer to glycoprotein at 3 weeks after an acute attack of back pain is evidence of the presence of a significant disc lesion. In selected cases, immediate relief from pain has occurred after administration of cortisone or a suitable cortisone derivative. Prolonged rest may be contraindicated because of the risk of formation of radicular adhesions (99, 100).

Although an inflammatory component in degenerative disc disease is known to occur, the chronicity of this process requires further evaluation. An autoimmune mechanism as a possible cause of prolonged signs and symptoms once the nucleus pulposus is herniated has been considered. Clinical evidence for this is found in patients who develop recurrent signs and symptoms at the same level following surgery. Factors important in the autoimmunity theory are:

1. Degenerative disc disease of the lumbar spine is mediated in some patients by an inflammatory component.
2. The chronicity of the inflammation may have an autoimmune basis.
3. The leukocyte migration-inhibition test demonstrated the presence of a cellular immune response in patients whose discs were found to be sequestrated at the time of surgery.
4. No human humoral antibody could be demonstrated (101).

Piriformis Muscle Syndrome Caused by Chemical Irritant

Sciatic neuritis is now believed to result from irritation of the sciatic nerve sheath, which is caused by biochemical agents released from an inflamed piriformis muscle where the two structures meet at the greater sciatic foramen. The symptoms of piriformis syndrome present almost identically to lumbar disc syndrome, except for the consistent absence of true neurological findings. Diagnosis is accomplished by palpation of myofascial trigger points within the piriformis muscle. Treatment, which consists of a conservative approach employing local anesthetics and osteopathic manipulation, is without significant risk. Reducing muscle spasm, restoring joint motion, and keeping the patient ambulatory and in motion are keys to successful treatment (102).

SUMMARY

Degenerative changes in cartilage set off a series of well-defined pathoanatomical reactions in surrounding structures. This applies to the synovial joints as well as to the intervertebral discs. The structures adjoining the cartilaginous area become the focus of vascularization, which at times results in the formation of granulation-like tissue. In discs, this vascular reaction does not occur until the degenerative process has reached the outer layers of the annulus, where a capillary network is present. The disc itself is avascular. An extensive capillary network can also be seen as an ingrowth into a degenerated disc.

The chemical components of the material in discs are not constant. It seems likely that morphological changes in the disc may release polysaccharide-bound proteins into surrounding structures outside the annulus, where these substances act as foreign elements, since the lack of vascular communication with the disc normally keeps them enclosed inside the intervertebral space. It is possible that the response could be interpreted as autoimmunization, that is, the production of a reactive inflammation. Animal experiments with transplantation of disc material to other areas have produced results that are not incompatible with this theory. Therefore it is felt that we should pay attention to the chemical and immunological aspects of disc reactions on surrounding structures if this novel concept of low back pain is to achieve increased biological relevance.

If we continue to accept the disc as the origin of symptoms, this must be ascribed to certain properties of the disc which are active during a certain period of life but at a later stage are lost. It is not inconceivable that the physical properties of the disc produce more severe mechanical disorders at the beginning of the degenerative process than during its late stages, when the disc has collapsed and lost most of its function. This theory is supported by numerous morphological and mechanical data. If we could, in some way, affect the degenerative process by speeding up the conversion of the intervertebral disc into a fibrous structure of different behavior, we might have succeeded in finding a solution to the problem (80).

The chemical irritation of the nerve root in association with disc prolapse is the likely cause of the very acute pain following injury. This view has arisen from the frequent operative finding of a swollen, inflamed nerve root without bone pressure. The chemical content of the nerve root includes glycoprotein. Previously, it was shown that the carbohydrate capsule of the pneumococcus liberates histamine and other H substances from perfused organs in much the same way as venom. Direct tests of nucleus pulposus pharmacologically show the presence of 1 to 4 µg of histamine per gram, but no tryptamine and no slow-reacting substance or kinin. Extract of the glycoprotein from human nucleus pulposus releases considerable quantities of histamine, edema

fluid, protein, and another amine with four times the mobility of histamine from the isolated perfused lung of the guinea pig. Acute pain in disc injury is due to local irritation of the nerve root producing edema and release of protein and H substances at the site of injury. Relief of pain by cortisone accords with these findings, since cortisone inhibits the peripheral response to H substances (94).

We have seen not only that the mechanical compression of the nerve root is a source of low back and sciatic radiculopathy, but also that chemical radiculitis is a new and scientifically equally exciting cause of nerve root irritation. What effects such mechanical and chemical irritants will have on trophic function of nerves is yet to be learned. Certainly chiropractors can be excited about the interest in an area of the human anatomy, the spinal nerve root, that has been the primary focus of their contribution to the healing arts for almost 100 years.

Chiropractic Adjustment and Manipulation Defined

Lastly in this chapter, allow me to present definitions of manipulation I have compiled:

1. "A sudden, small, high velocity maneuver" (Edwards, 1969);
2. "Methods for reduction of positional abnormalities (subluxations), increasing movement at a locked joint and/or the reduction of disc lesions with each therapeutic maneuver requiring the attainment of motion between vertebral segments to achieve its goal" (Goldstein, 1975);
3. "A maneuver employing long levers for the active, passive, and resistive movement of the body without the use of dynamic thrust, aimed at remobilizing parts of the vertebral column" (Janse, 1975);
4. "A rotational stress on the lumbar spine, and the short amplitude, high velocity thrust is designed to gap or cavitate the facet joints—producing a dramatic 'click' " (Fisk, 1977);
5. "Small amplitude, high velocity movements going beyond normal active ranges of motion" (Jayson, 1981);
6. "An assisted passive motion applied to the spinal apophyseal and sacroiliac joints" (Kirkaldy-Willis, 1985);
7. "A carefully graded and directed thrust applied across the joint space" between "the

passive range of motion" and "the limit of anatomical integrity" (Kirkaldy-Willis, 1985).

The last definition to be presented here is my own: Flexion distraction manipulation is a form of spinal manipulative therapy allowing the following benefits: (*a*) it increases the intervertebral disc height to remove annular distortion in the pain-sensitive peripheral annular fibers; (*b*) it allows the nucleus pulposus to assume its central position within the annulus and relieves irritation of the pain-sensitive annular fibers; (*c*) it restores vertebral joints to their physiological relationships of motion; and (*d*) it improves posture and locomotion while relieving pain, improving body functions, and creating a state of well-being.

The future will find this chapter to be but a beginning of the search for the explanation of how the nervous system affects health and disease and how manual therapy interrelates with this cycle of disease. It has been an excitement and privilege of this author to present this chapter. It is probably the most important of this text.

References

1. Wiesel S, Tsourmas N, Feffer H, Citrin C, Patronas N: A study of computer-assisted tomography: the incidence of positive CAT scans in an asymptomatic group of patients. *Spine* 9(6):549, 1984.

2. Epstein BS, Epstein J, Lavine L: The effect of anatomic variations in the lumbar vertebrae and spinal canal on cauda equina nerve root syndromes. *Am J Roentgenol Radium Ther Nucl Med* 91:105, 1964.

3. Jones RAC, Thomson JLG: The narrow lumbar canal, a clinical and radiological review. *J Bone Joint Surg* 50B:595, 1968.

4. Verbiest H: Fallacies of the present definition, nomenclature, and classification of the stenoses of the lumbar vertebral canal. *Spine* 2:1, 1976.

5. Kirkaldy-Willis WH, Paine KWE, Candioix J, et al.: Lumbar spinal stenosis. *Clin Orthop* 99:30–50, 1974.

6. Cox J: *Low Back Pain: Mechanism, Diagnosis, Treatment.* Baltimore, Williams & Wilkins, 1985, pp 186–200.

7. Gargano FP, Jackson RE: Transverse axial tomography of the spine. *CRC Crit Rev Clin Radiol Nucl Med* 8:279–328, 1986.

8. Rydevik B, Lundborg G, Nordborg C: Intraneural tissue reactions induced by internal neurolysis. *Scand J Plast Reconstr Surg* 10:3–8, 1976.

9. Rydevik B, McLean WG, Sjostrand J, Lundborg G: Blockage of axonal transport induced by acute, graded compression of the rabbit vagus nerve. *J Neurol Neurosurg Psychiatry* 43:690–698, 1980.

10. Eisenstein S: Measurement of the lumbar spinal canal in 2 racial groups. *Clin Orthop* 115:42–45, 1976.

11. Leiviska T, Videman T, Nurimen T, Troup JDG: Radiographic versus direct measurements of the spinal canal at lumbar vertebrae L3-L5 and their relations to age and body stature. *Acta Radiol Diag* 26:403–411, 1985.

12. Winston K, Rumbaught C, Colucci V: The vertebral canals in lumbar disc disease. *Spine* 9: 414–417, 1984.

13. Hellovaara M, Vanharanta H, Korpi J, Troup JDG: Herniated lumbar disc syndrome and vertebral canals. *Spine* 11:433–435, 1986.

14. Van Akkerveeken PF, O'Brien JP, Park WM: Experimentally induced hypermobility in the lumbar spine. *Spine* 4:236–241, 1979.

15. Ullrich OG, Binet E, Sanecki MG, et al.: Quantitative assessment of the lumbar spinal canal by computed tomography. *Radiology* 134, 137–143, 1980.

16. Huizinga J, Heiden JA, Vinden PJJG: The human vertebral canal: a biometric study. Konniinkijke Nederladse Akademic van Weteushappen. Proceedings of the Section of Sciences 1952:C55:22.

17. Postacchini F, Ripani M, Carpano S: Morphometry of the lumbar vertebrae. *Clin Orthop* 172: 296–303, 1983.

18. Schonstrom NSR, Bolender NF, Spengler DM: The pathomorphology of spinal stenosis as seen on CT scan of the lumbar spine. *Spine* 10:806–811, 1985.

19. Schonstrom N, Bolender NF, Spengier DM, Hansson TH: Pressure changes within the cauda equina following constriction of the dural sac: an in vitro experimental study. *Spine* 9:604–607, 1984.

20. Teplick JG, Haskin ME: Spontaneous regression of herniated nucleus pulposus. *AJNR* 6:331–335, 1985.

21. Hirschberg GG: Treating lumbar disc lesion by prolonged continuous reduction of intradiscal pressure. *Tex Med* 70:58–68, 1975.

22. Neugebauer J: Re-establishing of the intervertebral disc by decompression. *Med Welt* 27:19, 1976.

23. Tien-You F: Lumbar intervertebral disc protrusion, new method of management and its theoretical basis. *Chin Med J* (Eng) 2:183–194, 1976.

24. Gupta RC, Ramarao SV: Epidurography in reduction of lumbar disc prolapse by traction. *Arch Phys Med Rehabil* 59:322–327, 1978.

25. Tsung-Min L, Tsung-min Li, Chiang-hua W, Chen-chung Y, Kuo-hsiu C, Kuei-fu T, et al.: Verticle suspension traction with manipulation in lumbar intervertebral disc protrusion. *Chin Med J* 3:407–412, 1977.

26. Burton C: The gravity lumbar reduction therapy program. *J Musculoskeletal Med* (December): 12–21, 1986.

27. Tkachenko SS: Closed one-stage reduction of acute prolapse of the intervertebral disc. *Ortop Travmatol Protez* 34:46–47, 1973.

28. Mathews JA, Yates DAH: Treatment of sciatica. *Lancet* 1:352, 1974.

29. Pomosov DV: Treatment of slipped discs by a closed reduction method. *Voen Med Zh* 7:76–77, 1976.

30. Edwards JP et al.: A comparison of chiropractic technics as they relate to the intervertebral disc syndrome. *Dig Chiro Econ* (November/December):92–101, 1977.

31. Potter GE: A study of 744 cases of neck and back pain treated with spinal manipulation. *J Can Chiro Assoc* (December):154–156, 1977.

32. Sharubina I: Effectiveness of using medical gymnastics together with traction in a swimming pool in the overall treatment of discogenic radiculitis. *Vopr Kurortol Fizioter Lech Fiz Kult* 38:536–557, 1973.

33. Raney FL: The effects of flexion, extension valsalva maneuver, and abdominal compression on the large volume myelographic column. International Society for the Study of the Lumbar Spine, San Francisco Meeting, June 5–8, 1978.

34. Pilling JR: Water soluble radiculography in the erect posture: a clinico-radiological study. *Clin Radiol* 30:665–670, 1979.

35. DeSeze S, Levernieux J: Les tractions vertébrales: premiers étude experimentales et resultats thérapeutiques d'après un expérience de quatre années. Semaine ole hospitales, Paris. 27:2085, 1951.

36. Larsson V, Choler V, Lindstrom A, et al.: Autotraction for treatment of lumbago-sciatica: a multicenter controlled investigation. *Acta Orthop Scand* 51:791–798, 1980.

37. Cyriax J: *Textbook of Orthopaedic Medicine*, ed 7. London, Bailliere Tindall, 1978.

38. Cyriax J: *Textbook of Orthopaedic Medicine*, 8, ed, vol 1. London, Bailliere Tindall, pp 315–316.

39. Lossing W: Low back pain and the Cottrell 90/90 Backtrac system. *Orthotics and Prosthetics* 37:31–38, 1983.

40. Naylor A, Happey F, Turner RL, Shentall RD, West RD, Richardson C: Enzymatic and immunological activity in the intervertebral disc. *Orthop Clin North Am* 6:51–58, 1975.

41. Gertzbein SD: Degenerative disc disease of the lumbar spine. *Clin Orthop* 129:68–71, 1977.

42. Rydevik B, Brown MD, Lundborg G: Pathoanatomy and pathophysiology of nerve root compression. *Spine* 9:7–15, 1984.

43. Elves MW, Bucknill T, Sullivan MF: In vitro inhibition of leucocyte migration in patients with intervertebral disc lesion. *Orthop Clin North Am* 6:1, 1975.

44. Eyre DR: Biochemistry of the intervertebral disc. *Int Rev Connect Tissue Res* 8:227–289, 1979.

45. Jordan JM, Obeid LM, Allen NB: Isolated atlantoaxial subluxation as the presenting manifestation of inflammatory bowel disease. *Am J Med* 80(March):517, 1986.

46. Cox J, Gideon D, Rogers F: Incidence of osteophytic lipping of the thoracic spine in coronary heart disease: results of a pilot study. *J Am Osteopath Assoc* 82:837–838, 1983.

47. Beal MC: A study of viscerosomatic reflexes. *Manuelle Medizin* 21(4):93, 1983.

48. Suarez GM, Larocca H, Baum NH: Sexual and bladder dysfunction in patients with lumbar pain syndromes (Abstract). *J Urol* 135(4):264, part 2, 1986. American Urological Association 81st Annual Meeting, May 18–22.

49. Palmer DD: *The Science, Art, and Philosophy of Chiropractic.* Portland, OR, Portland Printing House, 1910, pp 11, 12, 18, 28.

50. Bourdillion J: *Spinal Manipulation,* ed 2. East Norwalk, CT, Appleton-Century-Crofts, p 5.

51. Forster AL: *Principles and Practice of Chiropractic,* ed 3. Chicago, IL, National Publishing Association, 1923, p 1.

52. Wiltse L: The 1985 Presidential Address: North American Spine Society, an amalgamation for progress. *Spine* 11(6):654, 1984.

53. Korr IM: Neurochemical and neurotrophic consequences of nerve deformations. In Glasgow EF, Twomey LT, Scull ER, Kleynhans AM, Idczak RM (eds): *Aspects of Manipulative Therapy.* Edinburgh, Churchill Livingstone, 1985, pp 64–70.

54. Sharpless SK: Susceptibility of spinal roots to compression block. In Goldstein M (ed): *The Research Status of Spinal Manipulative Therapy.* NINCDS monograph no. 15, DHEW Publication NIH 76–998, 1975, pp 155–161.

55. Bergmann L, Alexander L: Vascular supply of the spinal ganglia. *Arch Neurol Psychiatry* 46:761–782, 1941.

56. Bentley FH, Schlapp W: The effects of pressure on conduction in peripheral nerves. *J Physiol* 72–82, 1943.

57. Sunderland S: *Nerves and Nerve Injuries,* ed 2. Edinburgh, Churchill Livingstone, 1978.

58. Rydevik B, Lundborg G, Bagge U: Effects of graded compression on intraneural blood flow—an in vivo study on rabbit tibial nerve. *J Hand Surg* 6:3–12, 1981.

59. Lundborg G: Structure and function of the intraneural microvessels as related to trauma, edema formation, and nerve function. *J Bone Joint Surg* 57A:938–945, 1975.

60. Rydevik B, Lundborg G: Permeability of intraneural microvessels and perineurium following

acute, graded experimental nerve compression. *Scand J Plast Reconstr Surg* 11:179–189, 1977.

61. Arvidson B: A study of the perineurial diffusion barrier of a peripheral ganglion. *Acta Neuropathol* (Berl) 46:139–144, 1979.

62. Lindblom K, Rexed B: Spinal nerve injury in dorsolateral protrusions of lumbar discs. *J Neurosurg* 5:415–425, 1948.

63. Weinstein J: Mechanisms of spinal pain: the dorsal root ganglion and its role as a mediator of low-back pain. *Spine* 11(10):999–1001, 1986.

64. Wall PD, Devor M: Sensory afferent impulses originate from dorsal root ganglia as well as from the periphery in normal and nerve injured rats. *Pain* 17:321–337, 1983.

65. Howe JF, Loeser JD, Calvin WH: Mechanosensitivity of dorsal root ganglia and chronically injured axons: a physiological basis for the radicular pain of nerve root compression. *Pain* 3:25–41, 1977.

66. Howe JF, Calvin WH, Loeser JD: Impulses reflected from dorsal root ganglia and from focal nerve injuries. *Brain Res* 116:139, 1976.

67. Johannson B: Practical experience of intervertebral joint dysfunction as a possible cause of disturbed afferent nerve activity influencing muscle tone and pain. *Manuelle Medizin* 21(4):90–91, 1983.

68. Vanderlinden RG: Subarticular entrapment of the dorsal root ganglion as a cause of sciatic pain. *Spine* 9(1):19, 1984.

69. Badalamente MA, Dee R, Ghillani R, Chien P, Daniels K: Mechanical stimulation of dorsal root ganglia induces increased production of substance P: a mechanism for pain following nerve root compromise? *Spine* 12(6):552–555, 1987.

70. Marks JL: Brain peptides: is substance P a transmitter of pain signals? *Science* 205:886–889, 1979.

71. Nathan H: Osteophytes of the spine compressing the sympathetic trunk and splanchnic nerves in the thorax. *Spine* 12(6):527–532, 1987.

72. Hahnenberger RW: Effects of pressure on fast axoplasmic flow: an in vitro study in the vagus nerve of rabbits. *Acta Physiol Scand* 104:229–308, 1978.

73. Ochoa J: Histopathology of common mononeuropathies. In Jewett DL, McCarroll HR Jr (eds): *Nerve Repair and Regeneration.* St. Louis, CV Mosby, 1980, pp 36–52.

74. Charnley J: The imbibition of fluid as a cause of herniation of the nucleus pulposus. *Lancet* I: 124–127, 1952.

75. Hendry NGC: Hydration of the nucleus pulposus and its relation to intervertebral disc derangement. *J Bone Joint Surg* 40B:132–144, 1958.

76. Urban JPG: *Fluid and Solute Transport in the Intervertebral Disc.* Thesis, London University, London, England, 1977.

77. Ochoa J, Fowler TH, Gilliatt RW: Anatomical changes in peripheral nerves compressed by a pneumatic tourniquet. *J Anat* 113:433–455, 1972.

78. Nachemson A: Lumbar spine: orthopaedic challenge. *Spine* 1(1):59, 1976.

79. Rydevik B, Brown MD, Ehira T, Nordborg C, Lundborg G: Effects of graded compression and nucleus pulposus on nerve tissue: an experimental study in rabbits. In: *Proceedings of the Swedish Orthopaedic Association, Goteberg, Sweden, August 17, 1982. Acta Orthop Scand* 54:670–671, 1983.

80. Hirsch C: Etiology and Pathogenesis of low back pain. *Israel J Med Science* 2:362–369, 1966.

81. Szabo RM, Gelberman RH: Peripheral nerve compression: etiology, critical pressure, threshold and clinical assessment. *Orthopedics* 9:1461–1466, 1984.

82. Saal JA: Electrophysiologic evaluation of lumbar pain: establishing the rationale for therapeutic management. *Spine: State of the Art Reviews* 1(1): 21–28, 1986.

83. Patterson MM, Steinmetz JE: Long-lasting alterations of spinal reflexes: a potential basis for somatic dysfunction, active processor not passive transmitter. *Manual Medicine* 2:38–42, 1986.

83a. Giulbaud G, Iggo A, Tegner R: Sensory receptors in ankle joint capsules of normal and arthritic rats. *Exp Brain Res* 58:29–40, 1985.

84. Giovanelli-Blacker B, Elvey R, Thompson E: The clinical significance of measured lumbar zygapophyseal intracapsular pressure variation. In: *Proceedings of the Fourth Biennial Conference, Manipulative Therapists Association of Australia, Brisbane, 1985.*

85. Lewit K: The muscular and articular factor in movement restriction. *Manual Medicine* 1:83–85, 1985.

86. Jull, GA, Bogduk NM: Manual examination: an objective test of cervical joint dysfunction. In: *Proceedings of the Fourth Biennial Conference, Manipulative Therapists Association of Australia, Brisbane, 1985.*

87. Clark FJ: Information signalled by sensory fibres in medial articular nerve. *J Neurophysiol* 38: 1464–1472, 1975.

88. Parke WW, Watanabe R: Lumbosacral intersegmental epispinal axons and ectopic ventral nerve rootlets. *J Neurosurg* 67:269–277, 1987.

89. Parke WW, Watanabe R: The intrinsic vasculature of the lumbosacral spinal nerve roots. *Spine* 10(6): 508–515, 1985.

90. Smyth MJ, Wright V: Sciatica and the intervertebral disc. *J Bone Joint Surg* 40A:1401, 1402, 1417, 1958.

91. Livermore NB: Low back pain syndrome: a clinical overview. In *Spine Update 1984.* San Francisco, Radiology Research and Education Foundation, pp 23–34.

92. Spencer DL, Irwin GS, Miller JAA: Anatomy and significance of fixation of the lumbosacral nerve roots in sciatica. *Spine* 8(6):672–673, 676–678, 1983.

93. Kikuchi S, Hasue M, Nishiyama K, Ito T: Anatomic features of the furcal nerve and its clinical significance. *Spine* 11(10):1002–1007, 1986.

94. Willer JC, Barranquero A, Kahn MF, Salliere D: Pain in sciatica depresses lower limit nociceptive reflexes to sural nerve stimulation. *J Neurol Neurosurg Psychiatry* 50:1–5, 1987.

95. Duncker K: Some preliminary experiments on the mutual influence of pain. *Psychol Forsch* 21: 311–326, 1937.

96. Hardy JD, Goodell H, Wolff HG: The influence of skin temperature upon the pain threshold as evoked by thermal radiation. *Science* 114: 149–150, 1951.

97. Parsons CM, Goetze FR: Effect of induced pain as pain threshold. *Proc Soc Exp Biol Med* 60:327–329, 1945.

98. Wyke BD: Articular neurology and manipulative therapy. In Glasgow EF, Twomey LT, Scull ER, Kleynhans AM, Idczak RM (eds): *Aspects of Manip-ulative Therapy*. Edinburgh, Churchill Livingstone, 1985, pp 72–77.

99. Marshall LL, Trethewie ER, Curtain CC: Chemical radiculitis. *Clin Orthop* 129(November–December) 61–66, 1977.

100. Marshall LL, Trethewie ER: Chemical irritation of nerve root in disc prolapse. *Lancet* (August 11): 320, 1973.

101. Gertzbein SD, Tile M, Gross A, Falk R: Autoimmunity in degenerative disc disease of the lumbar spine. *Orthop Clin North Am* 6(1):67–73, 1975.

102. Steiner C, Staubs C, Ganon M, Buhlinger C: Piriformis syndrome: pathogenesis, diagnosis, and treatment. *J Am Osteopath Assoc* 87(4):318–323, 1987.

Suggested Reading

Brown MC, Hardman VJ: A reassessment of the accuracy of reinnervation by motoneurons following crushing or freezing of the sciatic or lumbar spinal nerves of rats. *Brain* 110:695–705, 1987.

4

Leg Length Inequality[a]

Dana J. Lawrence, D.C.

The secret of being miserable is to have the leisure to bother about whether

you are happy or not.

—George Bernard Shaw

Since its inception, the chiropractic profession has devoted a great amount of its time and energy to the study of human biomechanics. Much of this study has centered upon the pelvis and sacroiliac joints, in recognition of this region's importance for gait, locomotion, and weight bearing. One critical component of this study has been in the area of leg length insufficiency (LLI).

It is certain that few such areas of study have been as rife with controversy. Since the measurement of leg length is important to a number of different chiropractic adjustment systems, the need for in-depth research is of paramount concern for the future validation of chiropractic tenets. Thus, the chiropractic profession has had an important role to play in this particular discipline of research.

Tremendous, intuitive leaps of knowledge are rare in human biomechanics; rather, the knowledge base slowly and organically develops from work done by others. This chapter will detail the developments that have occurred in the study of LLI.

Traditionally, study of LLI has occurred in five different areas (1). Initially, all study was done relative to the presence of an anatomical, or structural, LLI, that is, a congenital or possibly acquired actual difference in the length of the limb. Only later did research begin to focus on functional, or apparent,

LLI. Functional LLI is believed to be due to changes in pelvic musculature and biomechanics. It is this area of study that has produced such controversy, because it is the measurement of functional LLI that is at the core of some chiropractic diagnostic and adjustive systems. To date, few studies have shown that such measurement is reliable; none have ever been shown to be valid. There is some debate as to whether the use of the term "functional leg length insufficiency" is appropriate, because in general the measurement of that entity is used to describe changes in pelvic biomechanics and not an actual change in limb length (1). It may be that, in light of such a lack of good supportive ev·dence, the chiropractic profession can take the lead in using new descriptive terminology to describe this phenomena; the term *pelvic insufficiency* is but one possible new term that might be used.

MAJOR AREAS OF LLI STUDY

There are five major areas of study in leg length insufficiency research. They include:

1. The development and use of certain radiographic procedures to document the presence of LLI;
2. The construction of various orthopedic devices that might be used to determine the presence of LLI;
3. Inter- and intraexaminer reliability studies testing the reliability of various measurement systems, including radiographic systems, tape

[a] Adapted from DJ Lawrence: Chiropractic concepts of the short leg: a critical review, *Journal of Manipulative and Physiological Therapeutics*, vol 8, pp 157–161, © by the National College of Chiropractic, 1985.

measure systems, and visual observation systems;

4. The use of the above systems to attempt to differentiate between structural and functional LLI; and

5. The ultimate goal of seeing how the presence of LLI will manifest itself clinically, and how it will affect or alter normal biomechanics.

Radiographic Measurement Systems

Radiographic assessment procedures are considered to be the most accurate method of determining and documenting the presence of LLI. It must be kept in mind that these procedures will only determine whether a structural LLI is present. The first researchers to study the use of radiography for LLI measurement were Rush and Steiner (2). They placed the patient in an upright standing posture and directed the central beam of the x-ray through the level of the femoral heads. One problem with this was that it failed to take into account a phenomenon of projectional x-ray distortion known as the parallelogram effect. Therefore, Gofton and Trueman (3) modified the procedures developed by Rush and Steiner. Very simply, they made sure that patient positioning was such that the feet were directly under the femur heads; this entailed positioning the feet so that they were about 7 inches apart. This same study also showed that rotation of the pelvis of up to 18° produced no error when the femur heights were equal, while a difference of 18 mm in femur head height produced only a 1.5-mm error with the same 18° pelvic rotation. Others who have used and modified this system have included Clarke (4), Willman (5), Henrard (6), Giles (7), and Friberg (8).

Green and his colleagues, in an early and influential study, utilized an orthoroentgenographical system that took three radiographic exposures of the entire lower extremity. The sectional views were made at 90° to the ankle, knee, and hip of a patient lying in a supine position (9). The system was later modified by Goldstein and Dreisinger (10).

Drs. Farinet, Piasco, and Boffa developed a system known as panoramic teleradiography to measure LLI (11). Pugh utilized a procedure known as slit scanography to x-ray the entire lower extremity (12). However, these various systems, as developed by the people listed above, did have certain methodological problems. La-

dermann has shown that these radiographic procedures failed to take into account the effects of gravity on the body and its compressible tissues. The chiropractic profession has long been interested in the effects of posture on human biomechanics, and it was felt that the procedures listed above did not adequately address this issue (13). Thus, most radiographic procedures used by the chiropractic profession are performed in the postural, or upright standing, position (14–19).

Gaux (17), working with Henrard and others, used a procedure that modified Gofton and Trueman but determined only the presence and amount of inequality without actually measuring the length of the limb. This was done in an attempt to correlate the presence of LLI with the later onset of degenerative joint disease in the hip. The radiograph was taken with the patient in the upright position; it used a plumbline to find the center of the patient for x-ray marking. Cagnoli (18) did much the same but also added a restraint around the knees to help prevent motion and projectional distortion.

As stated above, the chiropractic profession has worked to develop postural systems of limb length mensuration. Gonstead (20) and Reinert (21) did early pioneering work in this area. One well-documented system, developed by Winterstein, was found to compare highly with the standard procedure of using femoral head views. Winterstein's method used an 84-inch focal film distance with full-spine radiography (22, 23). This procedure had actually grown out of the initial work of Gofton and Trueman (3) and others (2, 7), so that patient positioning was standardized and the parallelogram effect was minimized. Here, the central ray was directed through the xiphoid process of the patient. Obviously, this would produce divergence of the central ray at the level of the femoral heads, so Winterstein devised a millimetric measurement procedure to correct for this. The correlation between this method using the correction factor and the standard femoral head views was found to be 0.955, which was significant at $P = 0.0001$ (23).

Finally, a very interesting paper by Huurman et al. reports on the use of computerized axial tomography to measure leg length (24). Their procedure used a scout scanogram that had originally been developed by Helms and McCarthy (25). A series of cursors were then used to mark landmarks, and distances were measured by a computer program that was provided with the equipment. The program made several measurements and then provided an average for its read-outs. This system compared favorably with standard orthoroentgenographic systems but used less exposure to ionizing radiation. This, then, becomes important for future studies on leg length inequality.

Orthopedic Devices

Obviously, the above procedures all required exposure to ionizing radiation. In an attempt to discover other ways to assess the presence of leg length insufficiency, other researchers began to construct devices that could determine the presence of LLI. Sandra Jones, while working to document the presence of scoliosis, found that the elaborate lucite screen she used to assess scoliosis could also be used to determine LLI (26). The screen measured 130 cm by 50 cm, was marked in 10-cm increments, and had a plumb line dividing the screen. Spaces were cut at the bottom to accommodate the patient's feet. Leg length measurement could be decided by measuring the distance on the screen between the floor and the anterior superior iliac spines, and then watching for changes in leg length as shoe lifts were inserted. Anatomical landmarks were marked on the patient's body.

Hirschberg and Robertson constructed an aluminum device that was to be placed on the patient's iliac crests. The bars of the device could slide and telescope, so that it could be placed on people of differing sizes. A bubble level was housed on the top crossarm of the device, and by moving off center, the level would indicate the presence of LLI. Shoe lifts were then used to raise the short leg until the bubble level was even (27).

Using the basic idea of Hirschberg and Robertson, the podiatrists Okun, Morgan, and Burns developed a device they named the Orthotractor (28). This device is described by the authors as a "biological protractor" that could measure the angle formed between any two symmetrical bony landmarks. The Orthotractor is able to accurately assess the angle of pelvic tilt; then, by trigonometric principles, it is able to measure the amount of LLI. Also, according to the authors, this device is able to differentiate between structural and functional leg length deficiencies. In their initial study with the Orthotractor, nearly 88% percent of the people tested were found to have LLI.

A simple measurement system that utilizes a series of graduated wooden step blocks was developed by Schilgen (29). By varying the heights of the various steps, and by examining the heights of the iliac crests after so doing, Schilgen found he could assess the presence of LLI accurately. He later modified the original device, upgraded it, and called it an "ossometer" (30).

One of the pioneers in this work, Gofton, used a very simple assessment system (31). All he did was place his fingers on the patient's iliac crests, note their levelling and the presence of scoliosis in the patient, and then place wooden blocks under the patient's foot until the pelvis became level to the ground. He stated that he could detect differences as small as 1/2 inch by using this method.

When studies are done using the systems and devices listed above, nearly all report about the same percentage of short leg in the experimental populations. This turns out to be somewhere around 80% or greater, a number that seems to be supported by other studies that have asked the same question (1, 32–36).

Further information came from a more unlikely source: orthopedic surgeons. As part of the procedures and protocols used to make decisions relative to performing leg-lengthening surgery, growth charts and nomograms were developed that could give some prediction to how quickly a child might be expected to grow. The initial straight-line growth charts were created by Todd (37) and Anderson et al. (38, 39). Hechard and Carlioz (40) and Mosely (41) later modified and improved upon these original designs. These nomograms were found to favorably compare to more established nomographic methods of determining future long bone limb growth (42–45).

In a more recent study, Hosek has developed a computer-aided gravity weight line analyzer that, while not strictly used for leg length assessment but rather for studies of postural sway with LLI, may find future application in measuring LLI (46).

Necessarily, the development of all these orthopedic devices, while interesting in itself, means little if the devices and other measurement systems are not tested in reliability and validity studies.

Comparison Reliability Studies

Standard measurement systems include such procedures as: radiographic procedures; iliac crest palpation; visual observation; use of orthopedic devices; and tape measurement systems, such as anterior superior iliac spine (ASIS) to medial malleolus. In one study, Clarke (47) compared three of these procedures. He tested ASIS to medial malleolus, femoral radiograph, and iliac crest palpation. The radiographic assessment was found to be the most reliable procedure, while the two other procedures were much less reliable overall.

This study agreed with a study performed by Venn, Wakefield, and Thompson (48). They tested the reliability of tests commonly used by chiropractors, including pelvic x-ray, ASIS to medial malleolus tape measure, and a visual procedure known as a "quick check," which observed leg length while the patient's legs were fully extended when prone, flexed when prone, and extended when supine. The inter-rater reliability for the "quick check" was found to be low between three examiners; also, there was low agreement between the x-ray and the tape measurements. The visual system also did not correlate well with the other two procedures. With a total agreement of only 64%, which was found not significant, the authors questioned the use of the procedures as a diagnostic technique.

DeBoer and his colleagues found the opposite in their study of intra- and inter-rater reliability using tape measurement of a patient in the prone position (49). In the first part of the study, they found that, overall, between 72% and 82% of their experimental population had a short leg. This agreed with other studies (2, 38, 39). They also found a high rate of agreement between examiners. Though DeBoer concluded that it appeared that the procedures tested were at least reliable, he could make no conclusion concerning the validity of the test. The values were consistent, but the clinical utility of the test remained open to debate.

This was essentially the same conclusion reached by Woehrle (50) in his study comparing two tape measurement systems: ASIS to medial malleolus, and inferior aspect of the greater trochanter to anterior aspect of the lateral femoral condyle and then to the inferior aspect of the lateral malleolus. For each procedure, the intra- and inter-rater reliability was found to be significant, and when the two tests were themselves compared, they also showed a high degree of agreement.

Woerman and Binder-MacLeod tested five different measurements (51). They started with two different x-ray measurements, using split scanography and anteroposterior (AP) standing radiographs to obtain valid measurements. Indirect methods tested included use of lift blocks, ASIS to lateral malleolus measurement, and iliac

crest height palpation. The method using lift blocks was found to be the most accurate and precise of all the measurement systems used, excluding x-ray. The ASIS to lateral malleolus method was also found to have a high degree of accuracy. This study also noted the fact that obesity might be a factor that could ultimately affect the accuracy of the measurements being performed. It raised the issue of how various factors might alter biomechanics, which will be discussed later in this chapter.

Gogia and Braatz (52) performed a study examining the reliability and validity of one tape measurement system, ASIS to medial malleolus. They first compared it to x-ray, using slit scanography, and then performed intra- and inter-rater studies on the test. They concluded that the tape system was both reliable and valid, having very high degrees of correlation statistically. This study then goes beyond that of DeBoer to finally comment on the validity of a measurement system.

In a study by Andrew and Gemmell, a particular chiropractic system, that used by Activator Methods, was tested (53). This used a predominantly visual system in which the leg length was observed while the patient lay prone with legs extended. The mean pairwise agreement was 69%, with chance agreement pairwise at 52%. The study concluded that, while agreement was above chance, more than just this test needed to be used. Expansion of the method used to observe and measure leg length was later reported by Mc-Alpine (54, 55).

It is certain that continuing studies will be performed. The jury seems to be mixed when discussing the reliability and validity of the systems chiropractors use to assess LLI. It must be noted that most of these systems make little comment upon the difference between structural and functional LLI; however, any study using tape measurement may be looking at both types of LLI. The data at present remain perplexing.

Clinical Biomechanics of LLI

Quite a few researchers have noted a relationship between the presence of LLI, low back pain, and scoliosis (7, 8). Giles and Taylor had noted that LLI in excess of 1 cm could be associated with asymmetrical changes in both subchondral bone and joint cartilage in the lumbar facet joints in the presence of scoliosis due to postural defects (56). He found that the cartilage was thicker on the concave side of the curvature, but the subchondral bone was thicker on the convex side of the scoliotic curvature. He was unable to determine how age-dependent this might be.

In the above study, Giles and Taylor utilized histological examination of the joint cartilage and subchondral bone using tissue-specific dyes. In a separate but related work, they examined radiographic evidence of structural changes within the lumbar spine when LLI was present (57). Starting by using a measurement system developed by Dietz and Christensen (58), and making comparisons to a control group without LLI, Giles and Taylor made several noteworthy observations. For one, in the presence of LLI, concavities developed in the vertebral end plates of lumbar vertebrae, causing those vertebrae to become wedged in appearance, and thus later leading to the production of traction spurs in the lumbar spine. Giles and Taylor concluded that the intervertebral discs might be undergoing asymmetrical degeneration due to the traction and stretching forces on the convex side of a scoliosis. In another study, Giles found that there were changes in the angles of facet joints when LLI was present. This also could contribute to the asymmetrical stresses that were occurring in the lumbar spine (59).

Delacerda and McCrory performed an experiment in which they measured oxygen uptake and consumption in people with LLI (60). They found that LLI had a negative effect on oxygen usage with a constant submaximal work load, and also found little effect on the same usage during the acceleration to maximum work load. In a later study with his colleague Wikoff, Delacerda found that shoe lift therapy did help to reduce the total kinetic energy at the submaximal work load (61). This study also suggested that the biomechanical efficiency of gait and ambulation could be improved by the correction of LLI.

Bolz and Davies found, in a study that used fairly complex and technically sophisticated equipment, that overall muscle strength on the side of the short leg was significantly less than that on the side of the longer limb (62). The conclusions they drew from this study suggested to them that they might benefit by examining leg length insufficiency against such parameters as reaction time, balance ability, and upper extremity and trunk muscle strength. Klein was also able to show differences in muscle strength in the presence of limb length deficiency, here using as his experimental population high-school athletes

(63–65). In one of these studies, which examined how gait was altered in the presence of LLI, Klein was able to postulate a mechanism to suggest why the potential for knee injury was increased in this population of athletes (65). What he found was that, on the side of LLI, the ankle was very commonly pronated as the foot was planted on the walking surface. This then forced the foot outward, causing the knee to go into valgus and producing an excessive amount of tibial torsion. Thus, the tension on medial knee ligaments such as the medial collateral ligament was unduly increased. Also produced was a good deal of sacroiliac stress. Necessarily, this would result in a much greater chance of producing injury to the knee.

Bailey studied the neurological changes in LLI that occurred as the result of the alteration of gait and ambulation (66). More recently, D'Amico and colleagues looked at the alteration of several more gait parameters occurring in the presence of LLI. In this study, an electrodynographic analysis was performed on 17 patients with confirmed LLI. Force sensors were placed on each foot which could register forces generated between the foot and the ground. The study showed that the ground reaction forces were higher on the side of long leg, that the long leg had a cadence of 10% less than the short leg, and that more time was spent bearing weight on the long leg side (67).

Botte identified several neurological abnormalities that could occur as a result of the unleveling of the pelvis that accompanies a short leg (68). Included among these abnormalities were myofascial pain syndrome, sciatica, and low back pain. Both Friberg (8) and Giles and Taylor (7) concurred; Friberg showed a very high relationship between these conditions and the presence of LLI. Significantly, in this study both the sciatica and the hip symptomatology were more common on the side of long leg, which would seem to support the work performed by D'Amico (67). Friberg was able to decrease symptomatology with the use of shoe lifts. Since the hip could be affected by LLI, it was not surprising to find that there could be lumbar and low back symptoms developed as well.

In a study that examined electromyographic evidence in LLI, Taillard concluded that LLI less than 1 cm would not produce a change in body statics or gait parameters (69). Lawrence et al. found interesting conclusions in a study that examined shifts of weight bearing in the presence of

LLI (70). In the study, when a patient had a short leg of 6 mm or less, there was a tendency for weight to shift toward the side of the short leg. With limb length differences of greater than 6 mm, the tendency was to shift weight toward the long leg side. The authors theorized that this was due to compensatory involvement of the gluteus medius muscle attempting to right the body and compensate for the increasing list of the patient.

Kujala and colleagues studied the relationship between the presence of LLI and patellofemoral joint incongruence in the production of knee exertion injuries (71). The incongruences examined included patella alta, patellar apicitis, presence of genu valgus, and lateral patellar displacement. Most assessments were made radiologically. They found no relationship of genu valgus with LLI, even though they feel that the presence of LLI will affect the lower limb in several ways. They did find a relationship between the presence of patella alta and LLI, along with other indices.

Bandy and Sinning used electrogoniometry (an electronic joint motion measurement procedure) to study how heel lifts could be used to help correct lower limb length differences (72). The elgons (electrogoniometric devices) were placed on the patient at standardized locations, and the patient was asked to walk or jog on a treadmill with and without heel lifts. The elgons measured maximal flexion and extension during the support and swing phases of gait, the range of motion, the duration of movement, and the angular velocity of each joint. They were able to conclude that the addition of a heel lift did not appear to significantly alter the biomechanical measures of gait; and also, the use of a heel lift did tend to cause more symmetrical motion for the maximal angle of hip extension and the range of motion of the swing phase of the ankle in plantar flexion, with asymmetrical motion of the flexion phase of the knee.

LLI Effects on Posture

Several papers have examined how the presence of LLI can have an effect on posture. Mahar et al. looked at how a simulated LLI altered the mean center-of-pressure position in postural sway. They felt that LLI of as little as 1 cm could induce significant postural shift and increase the amount of postural sway (73). They therefore measured people on a force platform transducer barefoot, and with varying amounts of lifts placed under

the foot to create an LLI. They found that, with a 1-cm leg length discrepancy, the center of pressure shifted toward the long leg side to a significant extent. This was in a mediolateral direction; there was no anteroposterior effect. This seems to accord well with the work of Lawrence et al. (70). Mahar et al. concluded that LLI of 1 cm could be biomechanically important.

Winter and Pinto reported on the causes and treatments of pelvic obliquity, noting that one cause was the presence of LLI (74). In their detailed paper, they discussed predominantly the surgical approaches to correcting these obliquities, noting procedures for surgical correction of LLI where necessary. Ames noted the involvement of LLI in the static determination of posture (75). This was particularly in relationship to the production of low back pain. Taking an opposite tack to that developed by Winter and Pinto, Ames discussed the conservative approaches to therapy that could be used. Reid and Smith combine both approaches in their own paper (76). Here, they develop a simple grading system for LLI, discuss the clinical implications of its presence, and then explain several treatment protocols. Reid and Smith list LLIs of up to 3 cm as a mild discrepancy and state that these have not yet been convincingly linked to pain syndromes. They conclude their paper by discussing the use of orthotics in the management of LLI.

Pick looked at the relationship between abnormal heel cord tension and LLI (77). He manually dorsiflexed the patient's ankle to note the resistance in the Achilles tendon tension. This was then correlated to the presence of LLI. Though there were several flaws in this study, particularly in a lack of standardized procedures used by the various examiners, a correlation was found between the side of short leg and abnormally high heel cord tension. This study might bear repeating under stricter protocols.

Subotnick, who has written eloquently on LLI, published a paper that differentiates the various types of limb length discrepancies (78). He also spends time explaining the symptomatology that may accompany LLI. Many other researchers have raised the question of how much LLI is needed to produce symptoms and pain (79–83). There seems to be little agreement on the exact amount, but all seem to agree that LLI will definitely at some point lead to symptom production. There does seem to be mild consensus that LLI of less than 20 mm will not produce the noted symptoms (84–86). As an example of this variability, Gross studied how much LLI could cause a problem and found that some people with LLI in excess of 2.5 cm still were able to perform quite athletically; most under 2.0 cm never noted a problem at all (87). He concluded that clinical judgment was still to be used as the best indicator, since prediction in these cases proved not fruitful.

Finally, there have been some studies that looked at LLI from a surgical and clinical viewpoint. Friberg first found that amputees who were given lower limb prostheses were found to have a high degree of LLI (functionally, of course) as a result; in other words, they had not been fitted properly and were suffering various biomechanical problems as a result (88).

Friberg also examined the relationship between LLI and stress fractures in the leg and foot (89). She believed that the presence of LLI in a nonathlete would not cause difficulty, but in the athlete it might contribute to the production of significant problems, since it was known that LLI as slight as 10 mm caused a remarkable increase in the activity of several muscle groups, leading to the fact that complete rest for those muscles became a near impossibility (90). The study found that there was a high relationship between limb length discrepancy and the presence of a stress fracture on the long leg side. The greater the discrepancy, the higher the correlation.

Gibson then looked at how an LLI produced by a femoral fracture could later influence the growth of the spine. The major problem created was a scoliotic curvature, which could be corrected by the proper application of a shoe lift (91). O'Brien and colleagues looked at how early closure of the femoral epiphyses could produce growth disturbances that would later lead to production of LLI. These were at the proximal end of the femur, and were found to follow certain patterns (92). Fergusson examined the use of Syme's amputation for children with significant LLI and ultimately recommended the procedure for younger children with an abnormal foot and LLI (93).

CONCLUSION

For an area of such seemingly limited interest among different disciplines, the area of leg length insufficiency has had a great amount of quality research and examination performed. It will continue to remain a controversial area, particularly because the chiropractic profession continues to rely upon the visual examination for the presence of a functional short leg. There are schools of thought that claim that, medical and chiropractic writings notwithstanding, it is impossible to create a functional short leg; the presence of limited sacroiliac motion coupled with a strong pubic symphysis and the presence of the sacroiliac and sacrotuberous ligaments cannot allow the type of motion that would essentially "swing" the acetabulum forward and up in the nutational movement of the sacrum and pelvis. The term "functional short leg" leads to too many problems in understanding, and there is now a movement to use the term "pelvic insufficiency" instead; this may be more realistic, in that the chiropractic use of the term "functional short leg" is nearly universally used to describe pelvic changes.

Heufelder said, as recently as 1976, that the problem of leg length difference is not sufficiently known by either general physicians or radiologists (94). This is fortunately no longer the case, and future work cannot but help to make our understanding of the perplexing problem even better.

References

1. Lawrence DJ: Chiropractic concepts of the short leg: a critical review. *J Manipulative Physiol Ther* 8: 157–161, 1985.
2. Rush A, Steiner WA: A study of lower extremity leg length inequality. *Am J Roentgenol* 55:616–623, 1946.
3. Gofton JP, Trueman GE: Studies in osteoarthritis of the hip and leg length disparity. *CMAJ* 104: 791–799, 1970.
4. Clarke GR: Unequal leg length: an accurate method of detection and some clinical results. *Rheum Phys Med* 11(8):385–390, 1972.
5. Willman WK: Radiographic technical aspects of the postural study. *J Am Osteopath Assoc* 76:739–744, 1977.
6. Henrard JC, Bismuth V, deMaulmont C, Gaux JC: Inégalité de longeur des membranes inférieurs. Mesure par une méthode radiologique simple. Application aux enquêtes épidémiologiques. *Revue de Rheumatisme* 41:773–779, 1974.
7. Giles LGF, Taylor JR: Low-back pain associated with leg length inequality. *Spine* 6(6):510–521, 1981.
8. Friberg O: Clinical symptoms and biomechanics of lumbar spine and hip joint in leg length inequality. *Spine* 8(6):643–650, 1983.
9. Green WT, Wyatt GM, Anderson M: Orthoroentgenography as a method of measuring the bones of

the lower extremity. *J Bone Joint Surg* 28A:60–65, 1946.

10. Goldstein LA, Dreisinger F: Spot orthoroentgenography. *J Bone Joint Surg* 32A:449–452, 1950.

11. Farinet G, Piasco D, Boffa W: Studies radiologico con teleradiographie panoramica della dismetria degli arti nefia scoliosi. *Radiol Med* 60.903–906, 1982.

12. Pugh DC: Scanography for leg length measurement: an easy satisfactory method. *Radiology* 87:130–133, 1966.

13. Ladermann JP: About inequalities of the lower extremity. *Ann Swiss Chiropractic Assoc* 6:37–59, 1976.

14. Gibson PH, Papaioanou T, Kenwright J: The influence on the spine of leg length discrepancy after femoral fracture. *J Bone Joint Surg* 65B:584–587, 1983.

15. Friberg O: Leg length asymmetry in stress fracture: a clinical and radiologic study. *J Sports Med* 22:485–488, 1982.

16. Marstrander F: Benlengdeforskjell og skjevhet i ryggens fundament. *Tidsskr Nor Laegfaren* 100:435–436, 1980.

17. Gaux JC, Henrard JC, deMaulmont C, Blery M, Bismuth V: Mesure de l'inégalité de longeur des mcmbrancs inférieurs par une methode radiologique simple. *J Radiol Electrol* 55:615–616, 1974.

18. Cagnoli H: Un procédé radiographique simple de mesure de la différence de longeur des membranes inférieurs. *Rev Chir Orthop* 58(8):817–819, 1972.

19. Roesler H, Rompe G: Beinlangendifferenz und Verkurzungsausgleich. *Z Orthop* 110:623–628, 1972.

20. Herbst RW: *Gonstead Chiropractic Science and Art.* Sci-Chi Publications, 1964.

21. Reinert O: *Chiropractic Procedures and Practice.* St. Louis, MO, Marian Press, 1962.

22. Winterstein JF: *Chiropractic Spinography.* Lombard, IL, National College of Chiropractic, February 1970.

23. Lawrence DJ, Pugh J, Tasharski CC, Heinze W: Evaluation of a radiographic method determining short leg mensuration. *J Am Chiro Assoc* 18:57–59, 1984.

24. Huurman WW, Jacobsen FS, Anderson JC, Chu WK: Limb-length discrepancy measured with computerized axial tomographic equipment. *J Bone Joint Surg* 69A:699–705, 1987.

25. Helms CA, McCarthy S: CT scanograms for measuring leg length discrepancy. *Radiology* 151:802, 1984.

26. Jones SL: Measurement screen for leg length and scoliosis. *Phys Ther* 56:188–190, 1976.

27. Hirschberg GG, Robertson KB: Device for determining difference in leg length. *Arch Phys Med Rehabil* 53:45–46, 1972.

28. Okun SJ, Morgan JW, Burns MJ: Limb length discrepancy: a new method of measurement and its

clinical significance. *J Am Podiatry Assoc* 72(12):595–599, 1982.

29. Schilgen L: Eine neue, vereinfachte Mebmoglichkeit zar Bestimung der Beinlangendifferenz: die Mebtreppe. *Z Orthop* 111:805–808, 1973.

30. Schilgen L: Beinlangendifferenzmessung mit dem "Ossometer." *Z Orthop* 113:818–820, 1975.

31. Gofton JP: Studies in osteoarthritis of the hip. Part IV. Biomechanics and clinical considerations. *CMAJ* 104:1007–1011, 1971.

32. Redler I: Clinical significance of minor inequalities in leg length. *New Orleans Med Surg J* 104:308, 1952.

33. Nichols PJ: Short leg syndrome. *Br Med J* 18:1863–1865, 1960.

34. Kerr HE, Grant JH, McBain RN: Some observations on the anatomical short leg in a series of patients presenting themselves for treatment of low back pain. *J Am Osteopath Assoc* 42:437, 1942–1943.

35. Beal MD: A review of the short leg problem. *J Am Osteopath Assoc* 50:109, 1950.

36. Pearson WM: Survey of 200 weight bearing x-ray studies. *J Osteopathy* 45:18, 1938.

37. Todd TW: *Atlas of Skeletal Maturation.* St. Louis, CV Mosby, 1937.

38. Anderson M, Green WT, Messner NB: Growth and prediction of growth in the lower extremities. *J Bone Joint Surg* 45A:1–14, 1963.

39. Anderson M, Green WT: Length of the femur and tibia. *Am J Dis Child* 75:279–290, 1948.

40. Hechard P, Carlioz H: Méthode pratique de provision des inégalités de longeur des membres inférieurs. *Rev Chir Orthop* 64:81–87, 1978.

41. Mosely CF: A straight line graph for leg length discrepancies. *Clin Orthop* 136:33–40, 1978.

42. Tanner JM, Whitehouse RM, Marshall WA, Healy MJR, Goldstein H: *Assessment of Skeletal Maturity and Prediction of Adult Height (TW2 Method).* London, Academic Press, 1975.

43. Bayley N, Pinneau SR: Tables for predicting adult height from skeletal age: revised for use with the Greulich-Pyle hand standards. *J Pediatr* 40:423, 1952.

44. Greulich WW, Pyle SI: *Radiographic Atlas of Skeletal Development of the Hand and Wrist.* Stanford, Stanford University Press, 1950.

45. Stinchfield AJ, Reidy JA, Barr JS: Prediction of unequal growth of the lower extremities in anterior poliomyelitis. *J Bone Joint Surg* 31A:478, 1949.

46. Hosek RS: Computerized leg check: a computer-aided gravity weight line analyzer. *Today's Chiropractic* (January–February):9–13, 1985.

47. Clarke GR: Unequal leg length: an accurate method of detection and some clinical results. *Rheum Phys Med* 11:385–390, 1972.

48. Venn EK, Wakefield KA, Thompson PR: A comparative study of leg length checks. *Eur J Chiro* 31:68–80, 1983.

49. DeBoer KF, Harmon RO, Savoie S, Tuttle CD: In-

ter- and intra-examiner reliability of leg length differential measurement: a preliminary study. *J Manipulative Physiol Ther* 6(2):61–66, 1983.

50. Woehrle J: Reliability testing of leg length measurements (Abstract). *Phys Ther* 64(5), 1984.

51. Woerman AL, Binder-MacLeod SA: Leg length discrepancy assessment: accuracy and precision in five clinical methods of evaluation. *J Orthop Sports Phys Ther* 5(5):230–239, 1984.

52. Gogia PP, Braatz JH: Validity and reliability of leg length measurements. *J Orthop Sports Phys Ther* 8(4):185–188, 1986.

53. Andrew S, Gemmell H: Inter-examiner agreement in determining side of functional short leg using the activator methods test for short leg. *J Chiro Assoc Oklahoma* 5(1):8–9, 1987.

54. McAlpine JE: Measurement of the functional short leg phenomena. Part 1. *Today's Chiropractic* (September–October):23–26, 1984.

55. McAlpine JE: Measurement of the functional short leg phenomena. Part 2. *Today's Chiropractic* (January–February):19–21, 1985.

56. Giles LGF, Taylor JR: The effect of postural scoliosis on lumbar apophyseal joints. *Scand J Rheumatol* 13:209–220, 1984.

57. Giles LGF, Taylor JR: Lumbar spine structural changes associated with leg length inequality. *Spine* 7:159–162, 1982.

58. Dietz GW, Christensen EE: Normal "cupids bow" contour of the lower lumbar vertebra. *Radiology* 121:577–579, 1976.

59. Giles LGF: Lumbosacral facetal 'joint angles' associated with leg length inequality. *Rheumatol Rehabil* 20:233–238, 1981.

60. Delacerda FG, McCrory ML: A case report: effect of leg length differential on oxygen consumption. *J Orthop Sports Phys Ther* 3:17–20, 1981.

61. Delacerda FG, Wikoff OD: Effect of lower extremity asymmetry on the kinematics of gait. *J Orthop Sports Phys Ther* 3(3):105–107, 1982.

62. Bolz S, Davies GJ: Leg length differences and correlation with total leg strength. *J Orthop Sports Phys Ther* 3(3):105–107, 1982.

63. Klein KK, Buckley JC: Asymmetries of growth in the pelvis and legs of growing children: summation of a three year study 1967–1969. *Am Corrective Ther J* 22(2):53–55, 1968.

64. Klein KK: Developmental asymmetries of the weightbearing skeleton and its implication in knee stress and knee injury. *Athletic Training* 13(2):78–80, 1978.

65. Klein KK: Developmental asymmetries in the weightbearing skeleton and its implications in knee stress and knee injury: a continuing report. *Athletic Training* 18:207–208, 1982.

66. Bailey HW: Theoretical significance of postural imbalance, especially the "short leg." *J Am Osteopath Assoc* 77:452–455, 1978.

67. D'Amico JC, Dinowitz HD, Polchaninoff M: Limb length discrepancy: an electrodynographic analysis. *J Am Podiatric Med Assoc* 75:639–643, 1985.

68. Botte RR: An interpretation of the pronation syndrome and foot types of patients with low back pain. *J Am Podiatric Assoc* 71(5):243–253, 1981.

69. Taillard W: Colonne lombaire et inegalité des membres inférieurs. *Acta Orthopedia Belgica* 35:601–613, 1969.

70. Lawrence DJ, Baker J, Driscoll DR, Tasharski CO, Heinze W: Lateralization of weight in the presence of structural short leg: a preliminary study. *J Manipulative Physiol Ther* 7:105–108, 1984.

71. Kujala UM, Friberg O, Aalto T, Kvist M, Osterman K: Lower limb asymmetry and patellofemoral joint incongruence in the etiology of knee exertion injuries in athletes. *Int J Sports Med* 8:214–220, 1987.

72. Bandy WD, Sinning WE: Kinematic effects of heel lift use to correct lower limb length differences. *J Orthop Sports Phys Ther* 7(4):173–179, 1986.

73. Mahar RK, MacLeod DA, Kirby RL: Simulated leg-length discrepancy: its effect on mean center-of-pressure position and postural sway. *Arch Phys Med Rehabil* 66:822–824, 1985.

74. Winter RB, Pinto WC: Pelvic obliquity: its causes and its treatment. *Spine* 11(3):225–234, 1986.

75. Ames RA: Posture in the assessment, diagnosis and treatment of chronic low back pain. *J Australian Chiro Assoc* 15:21–31, 1985.

76. Reid DC, Smith B: Leg length inequality: a review of etiology and management. *Physiotherapy Canada* 36(4):177–182, 1984.

77. Pick MG: Evidence of nontraumatic heel tension and associated short leg. *Source* 4(1):7–8, 1987.

78. Subotnick SI: The short leg syndrome. *J Am Podiatric Assoc* 66(9):720–723, 1976.

79. D'Aubigne RM, Duboussett J: Surgical correction of large length discrepancies in the lower extremity of children and adults: an analysis of twenty consecutive cases. *J Bone Joint Surg* 53A:411–430, 1971.

80. Duthie RB, Ferguson AB: *Mercer's Orthopedic Surgery*. Baltimore, Williams & Wilkins, 1973.

81. Goff CW: *Surgical Treatment of Unequal Extremities*. Springfield, IL, Charles C Thomas, 1960, p 38.

82. Anderson WV: Lengthening of the lower limb, its place in the problem of limb length discrepancy. In Graham WD (ed): *Modern Trends in Orthopaedics*. London, Butterworths, 1967, vol 5, pp 1–22.

83. Poirier H: Epiphyseal stapling and leg equalization. *J Bone Joint Surg* 50B:61–69, 1968.

84. Ingelmark BE, Lindstrom J: Asymmetries of the lower extremities and pelvis and their relation to lumbar scoliosis. *Acta Morphol Scand* 5:221–234, 1963.

85. Marsk A: Studies in weight distribution upon the lower extremities in individuals in the standing position. *Acta Orthop Scand* 27 (Suppl):31, 1958.

86. Heripret G, Perves A, Taussig G: Inégalités de longeur des membres inférieurs: prévision et indi-

cations générales pendant la croissance. *Rev Chir Orthop* 58(8):733–739, 1972.

87. Gross RH: Leg length discrepancy: how much is too much? *Orthopedics* 1(4):307–310, 1978.

88. Friberg O: Biomechanical significance of the correct length of lower limb prosthetics: a clinical and radiological study. *Prosthet Orthot Int* 8:124–129, 1984.

89. Friberg O: Leg length asymmetry in stress fractures: a clinical and radiological study. *J Sports Med* 22:485–488, 1982.

90. Morscher E: Etiology and pathophysiology of leg length discrepancies. *Prog Orthop Surg* 1:9–19, 1977.

91. Gibson PH, Papaioannou T, Kenwright J: The influence of leg-length discrepancy after femoral fracture. *J Bone Joint Surg* 65B:584–587, 1983.

92. O'Brien TO, Millis MB, Griffin PP: The early identification and classification of growth disturbances of the proximal end of the femur. *J Bone Joint Surg* 68A:970–980, 1986.

93. Fergusson CM, Morrison JD, Kenwright J: Leg-length inequality in children treated by Syme's amputation. *J Bone Joint Surg* 69B:433–436, 1987.

94. Heufelder P: Die Beinlangendifferenz: Statistik einer allgemeinpraxis untersuchungen seit 1976. *Z Orthop* 119:469–474, 1981.

5

Sacroiliac Joint

There are two things to aim at in life: first, to get what you want; and after that,

to enjoy. Only the wisest of mankind achieve the second.

—Logan P. Smith

Part One
ANATOMY

Chae-Song Ro, M.D., Ph.D.

INTRODUCTION

The sacroiliac joints (SIJ) are different from other joints in the body in many ways. The effects of gravity on body weight cause the load of the body to be transmitted through the lumbosacral joint and then divided equally onto both SIJs (Fig. 5.1) (1). Humans are bipedal; the SIJs of the human carry at least twice the load from weight bearing and locomotion carried by the SIJs of quadrupedal animals. In the quadruped, the pelvis is oriented rectangular to the vertebral column; however, in the bipedal human, the pelvis is parallel with the spinal column, serves as its base, and thus carries all the weight of the superincumbent body. In the quadruped, the SIJs are syndesmotic (2). In the human, the SIJ reveals half the area to be a synovial joint and half the area to be syndesmotic (Figs. 5.1 and 5.2) (3). The human pelvis needed to enlarge in order to balance the bipedal body posture. In order to adapt to bipedal requirements for mobility and stability, the human SIJs have far greater variation and asymmetry. The joint structures and surface contours change frequently with age, sex, and the mechanical loads placed on them (4, 5). The female SIJ needs more mobility than the male, due to the special requirements of pregnancy and parturition. The hormone relaxin causes vastly increased mobility of the female SIJ during the later stages of pregnancy and childbirth; the hormone causes ligamentous relaxation in the pelvic basin. The male pelvis requires more stability and usually contains strong ligamentous support, some bony interlocking, and earlier ankylosis (Figure 5.3).

There is a great deal of controversy surrounding SIJ classification, function, mobility, and cartilage type. There is still question as to whether the joint is diarthrodial (a synovial joint) or amphiarthrodial, though the weight of evidence is on the joint being diarthrodial (6–9). However, greater than half of the area of the posterosuperior part of the joint is covered by a strong interosseous ligament. This is unique to the SIJ and throws doubt onto the idea of the joint being purely diarthrodial.

In the days of Hippocrates, early thought on the function of the SIJ centered around its role in childbirth. Today, many authors believe that its main role is in the transmission of weight from the upper body into the lower extremities. Janse, among others, stated that it was for avoiding the exaggerated swinging and tilting of the pelvis that occurred as the center of gravity shifted during gait (9–11). It does provide some compensatory movement for the lumbosacral joint (12) as well as for all the joints of the trunk and lower extremity (13).

MOBILITY AND STABILITY

When studying mobility, it had long been found that the change of the length of the true conjugate in the pregnant woman by changing posture was due to both SIJ and symphysis pubis movement. SIJ motion was later confirmed by the finding that the sacral promontory "nodded" in nutational movement when examined by lateral radiography (14). Others demonstrated SIJ mobility during surgical exposure of the joint. In clinical examination using motion palpation, it was noted that the posterior superior iliac spines moved in predictable ways. This led several researchers to study SIJ motion by embedding tiny

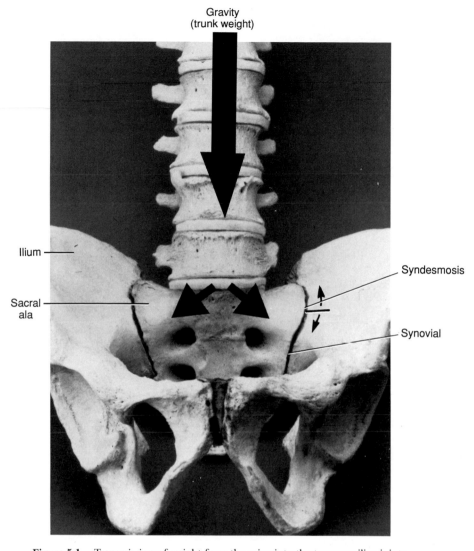

Figure 5.1. Transmission of weight from the spine into the two sacroiliac joints.

metal balls in various locations near the joint, and then digitizing the motion as studied by radiographic methods. Mathematical formulae to calculate three-dimensional position changes were then developed. It is now generally accepted that motion occurs in both the sacrum and the ilium; however, this motion is only in the range of 1 to 2 mm, and is thus very hard to measure.

Where the axis of rotation for motion is located has long been debated as well (10). Since the SIJ joint anatomy varies according to age, sex, mechanical load, and other factors, most authorities believe there is no one such axis.

The SIJ needs both mobility and stability. Often, one has to sacrifice one for the other. Men generally require more stability; women more mobility. One who carries a greater mechanical load needs more stability. Younger individuals require more mobility, while older people need more stability. For stability, the SIJ needs bony interlocking and ankylosis (Fig. 5.4). The SIJ undergoes degeneration earlier than most other joints, though the reasons for this are not completely understood. Some believe it is a result of a greater need for stability, some believe it is due to disuse degeneration,

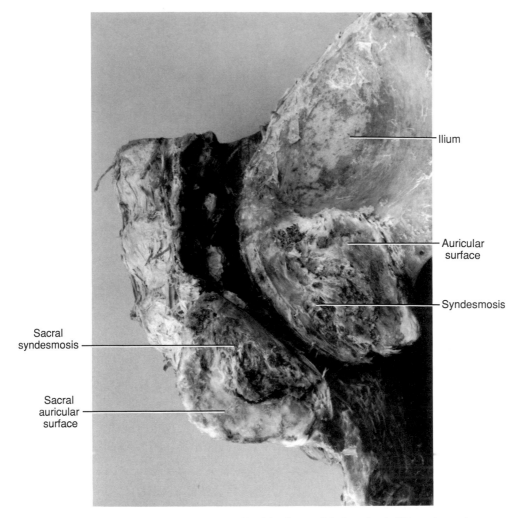

Ilium

Auricular
surface

Syndesmosis

Sacral
syndesmosis

Sacral
auricular
surface

Figure 5.2.   Half the area of the sacroiliac joint is synovial; the other half is syndesmotic.

and some believe it is simply the inevitable result of aging.

Most researchers believe that the sacral auricular surface is covered by hyaline cartilage and the iliac auricular surface is covered by fibrocartilage (6, 15, 16, 17). The answer is decided only by the amount of fibrous tissue and the orderliness of the chondrocyte arrangement. Some authors have found that infants have hyaline cartilage on both surfaces. It is also known that iliac cartilage degenerates earlier (8). In old age, sacral cartilage also becomes fibrous (3). Biochemically, it has been found that the cartilage of both sides of the joint contains type II collagen; this is evidence that hyaline cartilage exists on both sides of the joint (3).

DEVELOPMENT OF THE
SACROILIAC JOINT

The fins of a fish have no connection with its vertebral column, since they are embedded in muscle. But they are connected to each other by a primitive pelvic symphysis. The amphibian pelvic girdle is connected to a "sacral rib." The SIJ of a quadriped is syndesmotic (2, 18). For the biped, the hind legs carry out a dual role of weight bearing and locomotion (18). As the human evolved, to compensate and balance the load, the SIJ had to turn around to align straight with the vertebral column. This caused the curvature of the spinal column to change. The fascia lata had to be strengthened, and the tensor fascia lata had to be

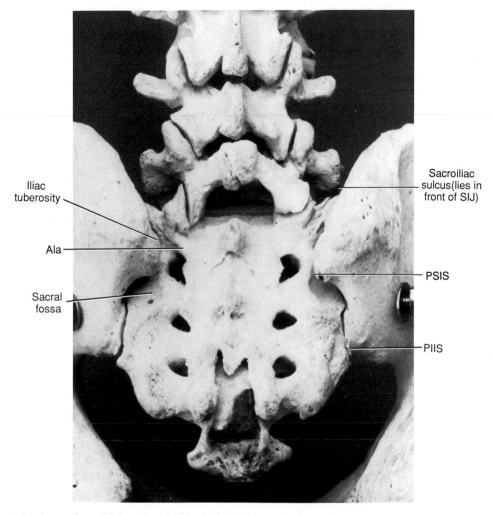

Figure 5.3. Areas of possible bony interlocking include (*a*) between the sacral ala and depression of the iliac tuberosity; (*b*) between the tubercle of the tuberosity and the sacral fossa; and (*c*) between the posterior rim of the sacral auricular surface and the sulcus between the iliac tuberosity and iliac auricular surface.

developed. The interosseous ligaments were strengthened. Bony interlockings had to be developed. Half of the SIJ needed to be synovial, while the rest remained syndesmotic.

The SIJ starts developing during the 7th week of fetal life, with the ilia moving up behind the sacrum. At the 8th week, mesenchyme forms a three-layered structure. At the 10th week, multiple cavities are formed, separated by fibrous septa; this is different from other joints. These septa disappear by the time the fetus reaches term (19). The sacral cartilage is three times thicker than the iliac cartilage. The septum may be added like a disc. The cavitation process is

completed by the 34th week; other joints are completed by the 12th week.

Until puberty, the auricular surface is flat and oriented vertically and straight (13). It moves in any direction, being restricted only by ligaments. After puberty, the horizontal limb, which is longer than the vertical limb, is formed for stability (7). A longitudinal ridge is formed in the center of the iliac auricular surface to meet a corresponding groove in the sacral auricular surface (Fig. 5.5). This arrangement limits motion and increases stability. During the 3rd decade, the interosseous ligaments are strengthened; bony tubercles and corresponding fossae develop to

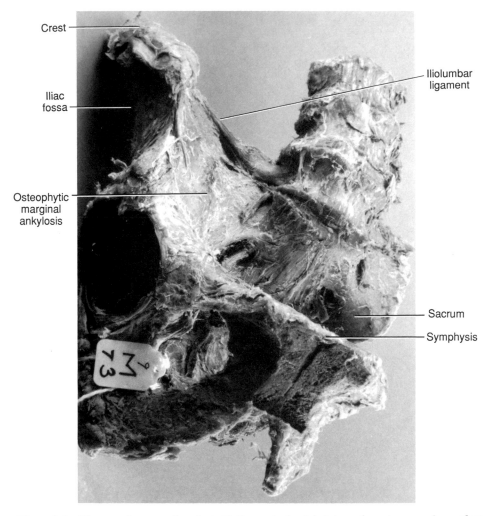

Figure 5.4. The most frequent site of *osteophytic marginal ankylosis* is on the anterosuperior surface.

increase stability by interlocking. From the 4th decade in men, and 5th decade in women, marginal osteophytes begin to develop, particularly on the superior margin of the anterior capsule. These also add stability to the joint. Cartilage will also undergo degeneration, further adding to marginal ankylosis. This may ultimately cause total fibrous ankylosis. After the 8th decade, mobility of the joint is usually lost.

STRUCTURES OF THE SACROILIAC JOINT

The joint surfaces on the medial end of the ilium and the lateral end of the sacrum articulate to make the joint itself. The sacrum is wedge shaped,

with its base wider than its apex. Its anterior surface is wider than its posterior surface. Without ligamentous support, the sacrum could "fall" anteriorly but never posteriorly. Half of the area of the joint surface is synovial, and the remaining half is syndesmotic. The synovial part is shaped auricularly (Fig. 5.6). The average area is 25 mm × 50 mm. The superior limb is oriented anterosuperiorly, and the inferior limb is oriented posteroinferiorly. The iliac surface is covered by fibrocartilage. The apex of the convex portion of the ilium faces the arcuate line of the ilium. The end of the inferior limb is the posterior inferior iliac spine (PIIS). On the center of the surface of the ilium is a longitudinal ridge.

On the sacral auricular surface, the superior

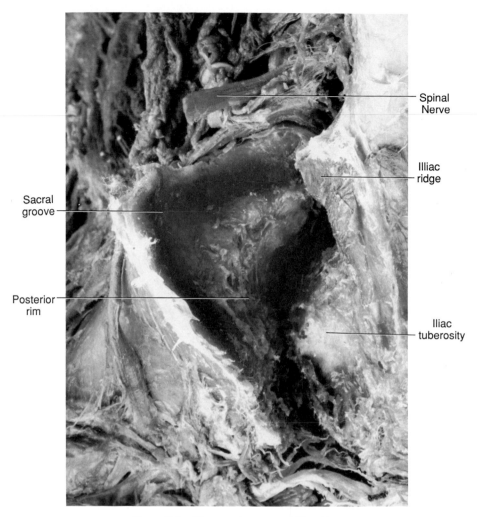

Spinal
Nerve

Illiac
ridge

Sacral
groove

Posterior
rim

Iliac
tuberosity

Figure 5.5. The *sacral groove* and *iliac ridge.*

limb occupies two-thirds of the anterior alar margin (Fig. 5.7). The apex of the convex portion is at the level of the first sacral foramen. The inferior limb ends near the second sacral lateral tubercle. On the center of the sacrum is a longitudinal groove that corresponds to the ridge on the auricular surface of the ilium. The posterior rim of the lower portion is very thick. The ridge continuing posteriorly to the second lateral tubercle is called the sacral tuberosity. An accessory synovial surface is occasionally found there which articulates with the accessory synovial surface on the iliac tuberosity (20–22). Some authors believe accessory joints resist the main joint, though one of the authors of this chapter (Ro) believes it helps with gliding motion.

The space between the iliac and sacral surfaces is about 2 mm. The ventral margin of the synovial part is covered by a synovial membrane and a fibrous capsule. The ventral sacroiliac ligament is a thickened fibrous capsule. It is particularly thick at the apex of the convex portion and around the PIIS. On the dorsal margin of the auricular surface, the capsule merges with the interosseous ligaments.

The part of the SIJ that is syndesmotic occupies the posterosuperior portion of the joint. The size of this area is similar to that of the auricular surface. There are many bony interlockings for stability. The interosseous ligaments are extremely strong (Fig. 5.8). They do, however, allow some gapping to occur by extending their length.

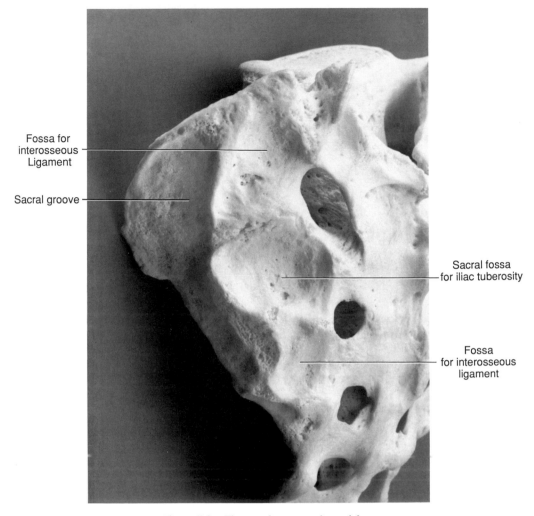

Fossa for interosseous Ligament

Sacral groove

Sacral fossa for iliac tuberosity

Fossa for interosseous ligament

Figure 5.6. The *sacral groove* and *sacral fossa*.

The thickened quarter of the iliac crest located in its posterior aspect is called the iliac tuberosity. It is covered by interosseous ligaments and is oval in shape. At its posterior end is the posterior superior iliac spine (PSIS). Located between the iliac tuberosity and the dorsal margin of the auricular surface of the ilium is a deep sulcus that corresponds to the sacral tuberosity for interlocking the joint (4). On the superolateral aspect of the iliac tuberosity is a depression; this interlocks with the sacral alar tuberosity. On the sacrum, behind the auricular surface and about at the center of the semicircular shape of the synovial part, is another deep fossa that meets with the highest portion of the iliac tuberosity. This forms an axial articulation (23).

The iliac tuberosity pivots in the fossa to cause the iliac ridge to move in the sacral groove. There are depressed areas above and below the fossa. These areas are for attachment of the interosseous ligaments from the iliac tuberosity. The interosseous ligaments have both superficial and deep layers. The deep layer contains a cranial band and a caudal band. The cranial band is shorter and is oriented transversely. It prevents the sacrum from tipping or "falling" anteriorly. The caudal band is longer, at about 12 mm, and is directed vertically (Fig. 5.9). It pulls the sacrum up. Janse found another cranial group directed upward (9). The posterior sacroiliac ligament (50 mm long) covers the interosseous ligaments. Between these two groups of ligaments lie nerves and blood ves-

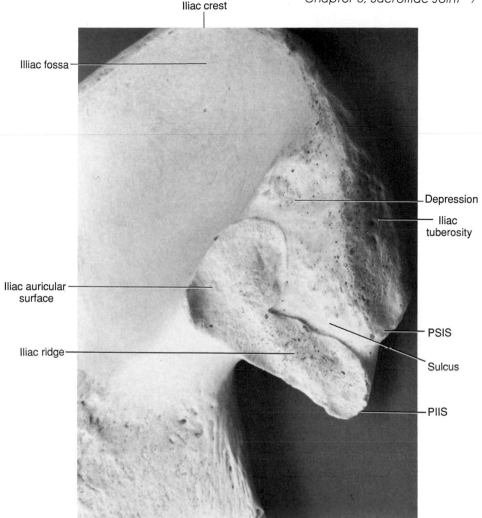

Iliac crest

Illiac fossa

Depression

Iliac tuberosity

Iliac auricular surface

PSIS

Iliac ridge

Sulcus

PIIS

Figure 5.7. The *iliac ridge* and *auricular surface*.

sels. The sacroiliac ligament also contains cranial and caudal bands; the fetus, however, has no caudal group. This ligament also resists the sacral nodding motion.

The SIJ also has accessory ligaments (6, 24). Iliolumbar ligaments connect the iliac crest and the transverse processes of the L5 vertebrae. Part of the iliolumbar ligament makes the lumbosacral ligament, which attaches to the anterosuperior part of the sacrum; it resists lateral movement and sacral nodding. The sacrospinous ligament runs from the lateral margin of the sacrum and coccyx to the ischial spine. The sacrotuberous ligament arises from the PSIS, the PIIS, the lateral sacral crest, and the lateral margin of the coccyx to attach to the ischial tuberosity. These last two

ligaments serve to prevent the coccyx from moving, backward and up, when the sacrum moves anteriorly and inferiorly.

There are no typical intrinsic muscles for the SIJ. There are, however, about 40 muscles that can influence SIJ motion (10). Several of these muscles attach to three points, including the sacrum and ilium (15, 16); these include the erector spinae group, the multifidi, the iliopsoas, the gluteus maximus, and the piriformis (18). SIJ motion can also be created by muscles that (*a*) flex or extend the vertebral column; (*b*) tilt the pelvic ring anteriorly or posteriorly; (*c*) cause flexion-extension, abduction-adduction, and supination-pronation in the hip and thigh, such as the sartorius (which pronates the innominate) and the pirifor-

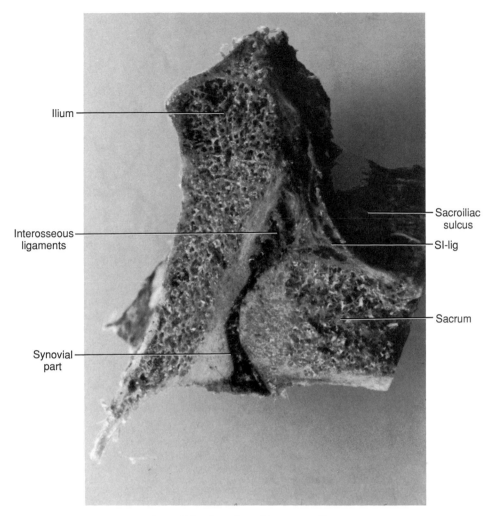

Figure 5.8. Location of *interosseous ligaments.*

mis (which supinates it). The rectus abdominis muscle tilts the pelvic ring posteriorly, while the erector spinae group tilts it anteriorly. The rectus femoris muscle and the hamstring group cause the innominate to rotate medially or laterally by causing flexion and extension of the thigh, respectively. The quadratus lumborum causes gapping of the SIJ at its inferior end; tensor fascia latae and adductor muscles create gapping at the superior end.

Some authors believe the SIJ to be innervated by all of the posterior primary division (PPD) of L1 to S4, while others include only some of those levels. The interosseous ligaments and the posterior sacroiliac ligaments are innervated by PPD of S1 and S2 only (25). Very few authors will

include the PPD of L5 (dorsal ramus) (7, 22), although this author (Ro) has found the PPD of L5 running all the way down between the interosseous ligament and the posterior sacroiliac ligament (Fig. 5.10).

The anterior sacroiliac ligaments are innervated by the anterior primary division (APD) of L2 to L4. The iliolumbar ligament is innervated by the APD of L1. The sacrospinous and sacrotuberous ligaments are innervated by PPD of S1 to S3. Solonen states that innervation will vary in each individual, with even a single person capable of having asymmetric innervation (25). It is true that the SIJ receives nerve branches from many segments, which is why the SIJ can both receive and send more referred pain (26–28). The SIJ,

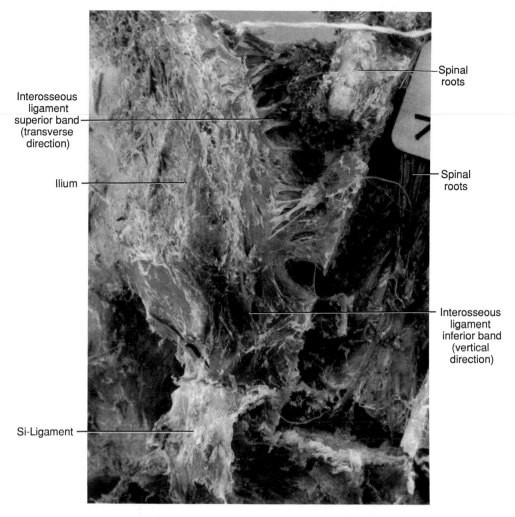

Interosseous
ligament
superior band
(transverse
direction)

Ilium

Si-Ligament

Spinal
roots

Spinal
roots

Interosseous
ligament
inferior band
(vertical
direction)

Figure 5.9. *Superior* and *inferior bands* of the interosseous ligaments.

along with the temporomandibular joint, is the most richly endowed with proprioceptors in the body (7, 13). This is, of course, due to the fact that the joint needs to monitor movement and position in order to keep the body balanced and upright for gait.

The histological makeup of SIJ cartilage is quite complex. Sacral cartilage is three times thicker than iliac cartilage. Larger, round, paired chondrocytes are distributed throughout the hyaline matrix; this is mainly homogeneous with very little fibrous tissue (17). The cells are arranged in columns parallel with the surface. Iliac cartilage is thin (1 mm), and contains smaller spindle-shaped chondrocytes clumped in the fibrous matrix. The cell column is oriented at right angles to the

surface (29). Hyaline cartilage is best used for motion, while fibrous cartilage is best for compression (22). During fetal development, both sides of the joint contain hyaline cartilage. After birth, the amount of fibrous tissue in iliac cartilage increases. It also degenerates earlier (30). Sacral cartilage degenerates later; it becomes fibrous much later as well. Walker examined the biochemical makeup of cartilage (3). He found that both sacral and iliac cartilage are hyaline cartilage with type II collagen peptides and glycosaminoglycans (16). Under 30 years of age, all is normal. At this age, radiographic changes of narrowed joint space, subchondral sclerosis, erosion, ankylosis (31), osteophyte formation, subchondral cysts, and asymmetry (32) are probably

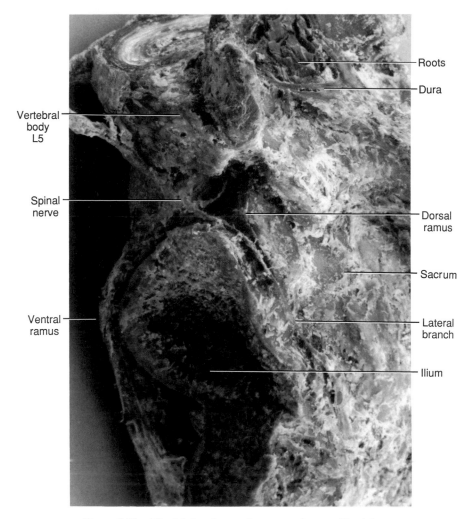

Figure 5.10. The L5 *dorsal ramus* innervates the sacroiliac joint.

pathological. After 40 years of age, these findings (except for erosion and ankylosis) are not considered pathological (33, 34). Scintigraphy using technetium phosphate appears to be a more effective procedure than CT to detect early inflammatory changes (35–41). As the ankylosis progresses, however, the radioactivity falls progressively (42–44). Also, nonsteroidal antiinflammatory drugs diminish SIJ uptake in scintigraphic procedures. Also, the procedure is not useful in assessing the immature SIJ (19, 45, 46).

SACROILIAC JOINT MOVEMENT

It is extremely difficult to study SIJ motion. Direct palpation is impossible. The joint moves only a few millimeters and in a three-dimensional manner (5). It is variable in shape and symmetry. Many forces, including gravity, ground reaction, and muscular action, combine to affect and influence motion. Because the joint has both synovial and syndesmotic components, there are many possible movements and combination types. Since the pelvic ring mechanism is so very complex, even knowledge of force interaction isn't sufficient to explain motion in the joint. As an example, it has been found that removal of a small bone piece from the iliac crest, to be used for a fusion procedure, has led to fracture of the pubic arch (22). The SIJ and symphysis pubis are interdependent functional units in the pelvic ring (47–50).

Hippocrates believed that the SIJ was immobile except during pregnancy. Even today, there are authors who still believe the joint to be immobile except during that part of pregnancy when the hormone relaxin, which relaxes the pelvic ligaments selectively, is circulating in the body (19). In 1889, Walcher found that the true conjugate of the pregnant woman increased by 8 to 13 mm. Since that time, researchers have also noted that the true conjugate length can increase or decrease with posture, even without pregnancy occurring (14). This is due as much to the pubic symphysis as to the SIJ. Other authors found that the "Walcher position" (extension) increased the pelvic inlet, while the lithotomy position (flexion) increased pelvic outlet (51–52).

Sacral promontory movement was then studied radiographically. This led to the finding of sacral nodding (nutational motion) occurring about 5 to 6 mm around a transverse axis 5 to 10 cm below the promontory; the rotating angle was 4° to 12°, with 8° being the average (6, 13, 14, 53). There was a combined translation upward and downward with the rotation. This seems to be generally agreed upon. However, these researchers also wanted to define iliac movement relative to the sacrum. PSIS motion was studied using motion palpation, and it was not a simple linear movement. ASIS-PSIS inclination as measured with an inclinometer was found to be approximately 11° (52).

Colachis, in 1963, implanted Kuschner pins to use as radiographic markers (53). The deduced path from the initial point to the end point could be different from the actual path of the motion. The motion was then studied cineradiographically (9). Since the length of the pin created problems, 0.8-mm-diameter tantalum balls were implanted instead (19, 54). Since rotation is three-dimensional and should be measured by the degree of angle, biplanar orthogonal radiography was attempted, with the two films perpendicular to each other (51, 55, 56). This was done with double images on the same film and stereoradiographically. Frigerio, in 1974, used a combination of stereoradiography and mathematical modeling to determine that the movement of the ilium relative to the sacrum was an average of 2.7 mm (12.0 mm maximum) (57). The movement between the innominates themselves was up to 26 mm. In 1978, Egund, using stereophotogrammetric and mathematical modeling, found 2° of rotation and 2 mm of translation (58). Miller found much the same results. Drerup, in 1987,

used rasterographic surface measurement, surface curvature analysis of the PSIS dimple, and computer mathematical analysis to reconstruct the true spatial position of the joint; he found PSIS dimple displacement of ±1.5 mm and a torsional angle of ±1.5° (59).

ANATOMICAL STRUCTURES FOR MOVEMENT

The synovial part of the SIJ is semicircular in shape. The center is in the syndesmotic part behind the synovial region, where the iliac tuberosity and sacral fossa interlock and where the transverse axis passes through (23, 60). The iliac tuberosity pivots in the sacral fossa to make the iliac ridge move in the sacral groove. The direction of motion will be either anterosuperior (AS) or posteroinferior (PI) (61–63). This corresponds to Gonstead's listings of AS or PI (64, 65).

There is another, shorter, course of movement. The SIJ has a saddle shape, with two ways of motion (4). The iliac ridge rotates on the sacral groove obliquely in an inferolateral (IL) or superomedial (SM) direction (66). The axis of rotation passes obliquely from the lower end of the auricular surface to its upper end (67). Gonstead's EX and IN listings apparently mean straight-line motion, not rotary or oblique (61). The use of diagnostic terminology such as anterior or posterior innominate does not exactly express the SM or IL movement; these actually mean pronation or supination in the oblique direction (10, 68, 69). The sacral auricular surface is 2 mm narrower than the iliac. The sacral groove has space for rolling 2 mm up or down. When the iliac ridge moves only 2 mm, the ASIS will move about 10 mm by pronation or supination. The syndesmotic part of the joint will be gapping when the ilium moves inferolaterally and closing when it moves superomedially (55). There is about 5.6 mm of sacral promontory nutational motion and about 2 mm of the sacral auricular surface gliding up or down. This seems to be generally accepted (6, 14, 67). As noted above, the SIJ is a saddle joint, and although 2 mm gliding is a very small motion, it is rotation.

POSSIBILITY OF SACROILIAC JOINT DISORDERS

Most authors believe that the SIJ is very strong and has very little motion (70). Thus, subluxation or fixation should be rare (19). Logan, among others, believed that all vertebral disorders originated from the fact that one side of the lumbosacral joint became lower than the other (61, 71, 72). This could lead to abnormalities of sacral nutational motion. An anatomical leg length difference could lead to SIJ disorder (22, 73–76), as could trauma and repeated locus minoris (11, 25, 70, 77, 78). The most frequent disorders of the SIJ occur as a result of pregnancy and childbirth. They are PI sacral fixation, and osteitis condensans ilii around the PIIS, which is also common (79, 80). Anterosuperior sacral fixation is rare, because gravity tends to pull the sacrum down. Inferolateral (pronated) ilium or an anterior innominate are also possible; superomedial fixations are rare (a supinated ilium).

RELATIONSHIPS WITH NEIGHBORING JOINTS

The lumbosacral joint, SIJ, symphysis pubis, and hip joints act as one interdependent functional unit (10, 50, 81, 82). In particular, the SIJ and symphysis pubis have a close relationship (83, 84). SIJ dysfunction must always be noted in combination with pelvic torsion. There are many methods to detect pelvic torsion. Winterstein used a method of drawing landmarks on a precisely taken radiograph (85). It allowed for accurate measurement of torsion.

SYMPTOM AND STRUCTURE

It is generally believed that spinal x-ray findings do not correlate well to spinal symptomatology (54). The range of compensation is very wide in the spinal system (75). If pelvic torsion is well-compensated, there will be no symptoms. In 1970, Lewit found that more than 40% of young schoolchildren (aged 6 and 7) have pelvic torsion but suffer no symptoms (22). Problems in structure could alter function; problems in function might affect structure (86). Gillet noted that soft tissue adaptation is the real problem relevant to symptomatology (87, 88). Examination and treatment of the soft tissues is believed to be the best way to manage spinal and SIJ problems (61, 89, 90). The most pain-sensitive regions of the SIJ are in the area of the PIIS and sacroiliac sulcus (22). The anterior and posterior sacroiliac ligaments are located there. A piriformis syndrome can re-

sult when the spastic piriformis muscle pulls the pronated innominate back (91).

INITIATION OF MOVEMENT

The forces for SIJ motion are gravity, ground reaction force, and muscle power. SIJ motion is initiated by the muscles of the vertebral column, thighs, and respiration (10, 13, 51). The vertebral column muscles initiate SIJ motion of the sacrum relative to the ilium by changing posture (lying, sitting, standing) and by changing the shape of the spinal column (flexion, extension, side bending, and rotating) (52, 53, 92). The movement is due to change in the center of gravity, with the apex of the lordotic curve moving up or down and causing the sacrum to nutate and the ilium to flare. As a result, the auricular surfaces move anterosuperiorly to posteroinferiorly, and superomedially or inferolaterally; the two PSIS will approximate and separate. On side bending or rotation, both iliac and sacral auricular surfaces move together, gapping at different times the anterior or posterior part of the joint as well as the upper or lower margins.

The thigh muscles initiate SIJ motion of the ilium relative to the sacrum, again by altering posture and causing motion of the thigh (rather than the spine, as above). Here, motions will include thigh flexion, extension, supination, pronation, abduction, and adduction (93). The two thighs can act together or independently. Abduction and adduction create SIJ gapping but no shearing of cartilage.

Respiration aids SIJ motion during inspiration and expiration (13). During inspiration, the erector spinae muscles contract and the rectus abdominis relaxes in order to decrease abdominal pressure (94). The pelvic diaphragm also relaxes to decrease abdominal pressure. When the erector group pulls the posterior part of the pelvic ring up and the rectus abdominis is relaxed, the pelvic ring will be tilted anteriorly. This causes the sacral promontory to move backward and superior (AS sacrum and PI ilium). During expiration, the erector group relaxes, the rectus abdominis contracts, and the pelvic diaphragm contracts. Action of the rectus abdominis pulls the symphysis pubis up and tilts the pelvic ring posteriorly. Abdominal pressure is increased. This causes the sacral promontory to move anteriorly and inferiorly (PI sacrum and AS ilium) (95, 96). This is one reason why those who practice sacrooccipital technique (SOT) attempt to correct SIJ motion abnormalities by using deep respiratory procedures (61, 97, 98).

ADDITIONAL COMMENTS

Most authors state that the posterior region of the SIJ is innervated by dorsal rami of S1 and S2 only (25). One author (Ro) found that the PPD of L5, lateral branch, ran all the way down between the interosseous ligaments and the dorsal sacral ligaments (7, 22).

After 30 years of age, ligaments become weakened, the work load on the joint increases, and the SIJ needs bony interlocking. The iliac tuberosity and sacral fossa create a deep interlocking. This is also the axial articulation for rotation of the auricular surfaces. One can find traces of the eminence of the iliac tuberosity pivoting in the sacral fossa (23, 60). There are two more interlockings that occur. One is of the alar tuberosity and the depression behind the iliac tuberosity; the other is of the sulcus between the iliac tuberosity and iliac auricular surface with the sacral tuberosity. Ro found that this last interlocking disfigured the left-side iliac tuberosity by widening the sulcus (Fig. 5.11). This only occurred on the left side, was present in about 75% of the iliac tuberosities examined, and never occurred on the right. Reasons for this are not clear, though it may be due to short leg length on the left. Janse found that body weight was carried by the short leg (9), though this has been disputed. One thing that is clear is that the sacral tuberosity pushes the iliac tuberosity upward.

Few authors discuss the gapping that can occur in the SIJ (55, 67). Those that do so mention the fact that gapping helps motion of a synovial joint. It is possible that the gapping of the posterosuperior part of the joint is more important than the rotation of the synovial part (89). It helps balance body posture by tilting the pelvis. Also, this gapping motion, when combined with the synovial part of rotation, makes it extremely difficult to accurately measure SIJ motion.

The SIJ makes rotary movement in an AS or PI direction combined with gliding movement up or down (29). This gliding can also be considered as rotation; the SIJ, in a sense, may be considered a saddle joint with two axes (Fig. 5.12). The SIJ alters its structure depending upon whether it needs more mobility or stability. Early degeneration of the joint may be age related or due to the need for greater stability (3). Very likely, the largest reason for degeneration is disuse; this may be preventable by exercise. Gillet noted that the sitting posture greatly approximated the two PSIS, more so than in standing or recumbency. This may be because sitting pushes up the posterior part of the pelvic ring, while the sacrum is fixed and can't move (99).

It is well known that disorders of the SIJ can be seen in association with enteric disorders (100–108). Crohn's disease, psoriasis, Reiter's syndrome, and other inflammatory bowel diseases can cause low back and SIJ pain (19, 109–112). This is probably referred pain, since it has been found that injection of anesthetic into the SIJ has helped to relieve lower abdominal pain and involvement.

Some authors have noted that dominance of eye or "handedness" has a close relationship to iliac movement (19, 52). *Gray's Anatomy* stated that, when a person is standing on one leg, the

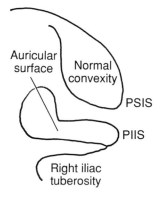
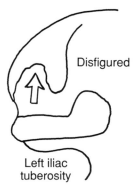

Figure 5.11. Disfigurement of iliac tuberosity.

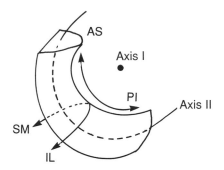

Figure 5.12. Saddle shape of SIJ, showing two paths of motion: a long course and a short course.

anced and adjusted by SIJ motion. When the SIJ is dysfunctional, walking can become stiff and awkward.

The rate of SIJ dysfunctions is high in fetuses from diabetic mothers (114). Some animal experiments with insulin injection produced SIJ malformations.

Both pain and functional limitation are usually thought of as symptoms (22). Usually the patient with no pain and with a certain degree of function is regarded as symptom-free (61). It seems as though chiropractors emphasize function, in terms of range, direction, and strength. When Colachis pinned the PSIS of volunteer students, half of them complained of toothache-like pain, while the other half complained of posterior thigh pain (22). The reason for the toothache pain is not known.

When Kapandji did force analysis of the SIJ, he noted that the ground reaction force on the SIJ acted in two directions (115). Similarly, the gravitational force also must be acting in two directions. One force vector pushes the ilium laterally, and by lever action with the acetabulum as the fulcrum; the other vector moves the ischial tuberosity medially (Fig. 5.13).

Marginal osteophytic ankylosis of the SIJ is fairly common, along with fibrous ankylosis. Full bony ankylosis is not as common, though some authors disagree (50). Rheumatoid arthritis of the SIJ is rare (116).

gluteus medius and minimus exert such powerful traction on the hip bone that the pelvis is actually raised slightly on the unsupported side (6). There may still be some "sagging" of the ilium from the weight of the hanging leg, though it may only be as little as a couple of millimeters. To balance this, the pelvis is actually raised a little.

The biomechanics of walking is very complicated (10, 113). It involves flexion/extension and abduction/adduction of the thigh and flexion/extension, lateral bending and rotation of the vertebral column. All of these motions are bal-

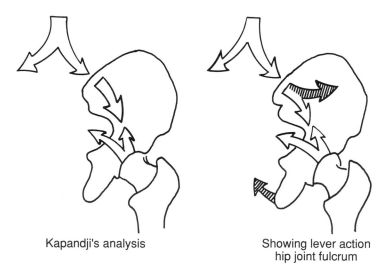

Kapandji's analysis

Showing lever action
hip joint fulcrum

Figure 5.13. Force analysis.

Part Two
CLINICAL CONSIDERATIONS

Dana J. Lawrence, D.C.

ORTHOPEDIC ASSESSMENT OF THE SACROILIAC JOINT

Yeoman Test

In the Yeoman test, the patient lies prone while the doctor stands at the side of the table. The doctor applies pressure over the sacroiliac (SI) joint using the cephalad hand while stabilizing the pelvis on the side being tested. The knees are then flexed to 90° on the side tested, and the doctor passively extends the thigh of the patient by taking the patient's knee off the table using a medial knee contact. A positive finding is either pain in the SI joint or reduplication of symptoms, which is probable evidence of a sacroiliac lesion. This test acts as it does by placing a stretching stress on the anterior sacroiliac ligament and thus placing a stress into the SI joint (117).

Gaenslen Test

The patient lies supine and the doctor stands on the homolateral side of the table. The patient is instructed to flex the thigh and knee of the side *not* being tested, and to hold that thigh and knee against the abdomen using his or her hands. The remaining leg and thigh are then extended off the table. The doctor places his cephalad hand on the flexed knee and his caudad hand on the knee of the hyperextended leg. A force is placed on these two structures, gently moving them further into the pattern created. Again, pain or reduplication of symptoms is considered evidence of a sacroiliac lesion. With the knee and thigh flexed, the lumbar spine and pelvis are "fixed" against the table, so that the hyperextension of the tested leg causes the pelvis on that side to rotate in the sagittal plane. The ligamentous attachments act on the ilium, as do various muscular attachments, to create the stress that then produces the pain (118).

Piriformis Stretch Test

With the patient lying supine, the doctor flexes the patient's knee and thigh to 90° and then internally and externally rotates the thigh. As is typical of sacroiliac orthopedic procedures, the positive finding is pain or reduplication of symptoms. Here, this is evidence of a lesion of the piriformis muscle. The procedure creates an extreme stretch of the piriformis and also brings the muscle into close contact with the sciatic nerve. The knee flexion removes the possibility that the hamstring muscles are creating the pain (119–120).

Anterior Iliac Compression Test

The patient lies on his or her side and the doctor stands behind the patient. The doctor places his or her cephalad forearm on the iliac crest of the patient, using the caudal hand to stabilize the patient's body. The doctor then exerts pressure over the anterior aspect of the iliac crests. This test approximates the anterior superior iliac spines and puts a distraction force into the SI joint. Pain or symptom production is indicative of an SI lesion (121).

Patrick Test

This is also known as the FABERE test, the Patrick-FABERE test, or the "sign of 4" test. It consists of having the doctor flex (*F*), abduct (*AB*) and externally rotate (*ER*) the thigh and knee of the patient so that the leg is placed in a position that is similar to the figure "4." In that position, the thigh is externally rotated further, while the opposite ASIS is stabilized on the table. This procedure places a stress on the hip joint; positive findings are pain and symptom production.

Anvil Test

This is a second test for the possibility of a hip joint lesion. Here, the doctor strikes the extended sole of the foot of a patient who lies supine with the leg extended. This places a compressive force into the hip joint, which is then responsible for the pain or symptoms that are generated.

Trendelenburg Test

In this test, the patient is standing, with the doctor standing behind the patient and observing as the patient completes the maneuver. The patient will lift a leg and flex the thigh onto the abdomen. During this procedure, the doctor observes the movement of the posterior superior iliac spine on the side being lifted. Normally, when a person lifts a leg in the manner described by the test, the hip on that side will drop slightly due to the contraction of the gluteus medius muscle, and the hip on the unsupported side will elevate. A positive finding in this test would be the reverse: if the pelvis on the unsupported side drops, the gluteus medius on the side tested is weak. If this should be the case, it is likely that the patient will also demonstrate the Trendelenburg gait, in which the patient will lurch out over the affected side in an attempt to compensate for the weakness in the muscle. There are many possible reasons for weakness in the gluteus medius muscle, including such entities as slipped capital femoral epiphysis, coxa valga, fracture of the greater trochanter, and congenital dislocation of the hip, as well as certain neurological conditions such as poliomyelitis (121, 122).

NEUROLOGICAL ASSESSMENT OF THE SACROILIAC JOINT

Basic assessment of the neurological levels of the sacroiliac joint includes muscle testing, reflex testing, and sensory assessment of dermatomal levels. In the neurological level of the S1 nerve root, the appropriate muscles to test include the gastrocnemius-soleus group, the peroneus longus and brevis, and the gluteus maximus. These groups can be tested both manually and functionally (123). Functionally, the gastrocnemius-soleus group can be simply tested by having the patient walk on his or her toes.

The peronei may be functionally tested by having the patient walk on the medial borders of his or her feet; the peronei are evertors of the ankle and foot. To functionally test the gluteus medius, one need only ask the patient to stand up from a sitting position, but without using his or her hands. Procedures for the manual testing of these muscle groups have long been standardized and can be found in several good texts (120, 123).

The Achilles reflex must be tested when lesions involving the SI nerve root are suspected. This is accomplished by having the patient seated with the leg hanging free. A small amount of dorsiflexion of the ankle is created by the doctor, and the Achilles tendon will then be struck with a re-

flex hammer. This should produce a sudden plantar flexion of the foot.

The S1 dermatome supplies the posterolateral thigh, lateral leg, lateral foot into the small toe, and a part of the plantar surface of the foot.

The S1 nerve root is a major one because it will be affected by prolapse of the L5 disc. Neurological levels of S2 to S4 are somewhat harder to assess because they are not so affected by disc prolapse (although a large prolapse of the L5 disc may involve the S2 nerve root along with S1) and also because there are no major muscles that can be tested. The S2 and S3 nerve roots do supply innervation for the intrinsic muscles of the foot, and one might examine the toes for evidence of clawing if these nerve roots are damaged. The S2 to S4 nerve roots are important in the maintenance of bladder function, however.

As well, the S2 to S4 nerve root levels have no deep tendon reflexes associated with them. They do have the superficial anal reflex associated, though. In this test, the skin surrounding the anus is touched. The normal response is contraction of the anal spincter. The dermatomal levels supplied by these four nerve roots circumferentially ring the anus, with S2 being the outermost ring, S3 in the middle, and S4 and S5 directly surrounding the opening of the anus.

MOTION PALPATION OF THE SACROILIAC JOINT

The process and mechanics of motion palpation have been described by many individuals (88, 124, 125). In general, the procedure screens and examines spinal pelvic and extraspinal articulations for the presence or absence of the nonvoluntary motion known as joint play, or paraphysiological space. Motion palpation procedures have been particularly effective in helping to evaluate sacroiliac motion and in helping to determine proper adjustive procedures and protocols.

When examining the sacroiliac joint, the articulations between the sacrum, both ilia, the fifth lumbar vertebra and the symphysis pubis must all be considered, since pelvic motion requires all to work in combination. In the process of motion palpation, only iliac motion within the sacrum is usually considered. The sacroiliac joint moves about three separate axes of motion: one in flexion, a second in extension, and the third as the sacrum flexes and extends about a central axis. The sacrum appears to rotate around a central vertical axis. The sacral alae also move superiorly and inferiorly, suggesting a gyroscopic or nutational motion similar to a figure eight described in three dimensions. The sacroiliac ligaments, which are among the strongest in the human body, along with the irregular shape of the sacral articulations, limit motion to only a few millimeters (55).

Motion of the sacroiliac joint is examined in flexion and extension using an anterior-to-posterior orientation. There has traditionally been some confusion as to what exactly constitutes flexion and extension of the sacroiliac joint; for our purposes here, we will use the side being tested (the side on which the hand contacts by the doctor are made) as the point of reference. If we are contacting the right sacroiliac joint, regardless of whether we are contacting the upper or lower joint, if the right leg is lifted, that will be called "flexion"; if the left leg is then lifted, that will be deemed "extension."

During all of the following procedures, the patient will be standing and will place his or her arms in front of him or her on a wall or chair to provide stabilization during the leg lifting process. The doctor will be standing or kneeling behind the patient, making the necessary hand contacts on the upper or lower sacroiliac joint.

Flexion of the Upper Sacroiliac Joint

For all descriptions of the procedures in this section, we will be using the right sacroiliac joint as our reference; we are testing the right sacroiliac joint for all four ranges of motion, separating the joint into two components, upper and lower.

For flexion of the right upper sacroiliac joint, the doctor's right thumb will contact the right posterior superior iliac spine (PSIS) of the patient. The left thumb is placed upon the second sacral tubercle. The patient will then lift the right leg up, a procedure called the Trendelenburg gait. The normal response here would be to see the right thumb move slightly inferior, medial and posterior, indicative of the innominate motion. The left thumb should not move, since the sacrum is essentially "tied" to the opposite innominate, which itself cannot move or the patient would fall backward. As in all of these procedures, lack of the proper motion indicates fixation.

Extension of the Upper Sacroiliac Joint

The doctor's thumb contacts are the same as noted above. However, in this setup, the patient will lift the left leg in the Trendelenburg gait. In this situation, the left thumb should fall inferiorly slightly; the right thumb will not move. Here, as the left leg is lifted, the right leg bears all weight of the body, and thus the right innominate must be "fixed" and stable to prevent the patient from falling.

Flexion of the Lower Sacroiliac Joint

The thumb contacts are now moved. The right thumb is placed on the right ischial tuberosity of the patient, while the left is placed upon the apex of the sacrum. The patient performs the Trendelenburg gait with the right leg. The right thumb should move forward and laterally to a small degree; when the leg is lifted, the normal response of the sacrum is to swing its lower part forward.

Extension of the Lower Sacroiliac Joint

The hand contacts are as noted directly above. The Trendelenburg gait is performed with the left leg. When this is done, the thumb on the sacral apex (the left thumb, in this case) should move away from the right thumb by about ½ inch. Lack of separation of the two thumbs would indicate fixation.

With the above information in hand, it becomes easy for a chiropractor to select an appropriate manipulative or adjustive procedure for the sacroiliac joint, one that is designed to induce the motion that has been lost. Such procedures will be delineated later in the text.

BIOMECHANICS

Understanding the biomechanics of the sacroiliac joint has proved to be a very frustrating task. Analysis of motion planes has been complicated by the irregular shapes of the joint surfaces; however, much good work has been accomplished, and today we have a good general idea of the way the sacroiliac joint moves.

Work done by Frigerio, published in 1974,

demonstrated for the first time that the sacroiliac joint was capable of a small amount of motion and thus was to be classified as amphiarthrodial. In his study, Frigerio adapted a system of stereoradiography whereby two orthogonal x-ray beams were taken and were then mathematically analyzed using appropriate procedures designed to pinpoint objects in three-dimensional space from two-dimensional films. This allowed him to accurately reconstruct the position of the sacroiliac joint in space and then to correlate relative motion of the joint itself. He concluded that he seemed to have resolved a major controversy in manipulative medicine, in that he was able to show movement up to over 1 cm in translation of the innominates as well as in rotation and flexion. He did point out that future studies should be done with even greater precision; it would thereby be possible to produce an in vivo model of sacroiliac mechanics (57).

Several studies focused on the measurement of pelvic landmark motion on the ilium and sacrum. If the relative distances between the structures changed with a change of body position, it was taken as evidence of motion in the sacroiliac joint itself. One of the very first to perform such studies was Ashmore (126), who used as her measurement points the distance between the posterior superior iliac spines when related to body position. She found that these distances changed and were greater in the upright position than in a position in which the patient was bent forward. John Mennell found similar findings in patients when he compared the upright seated posture against a prone measurement (127).

Halladay, who made a series of measurements in cadaveric samples, noted that the symphysis pubis, when it moves, also produced movement of the sacroiliac joint; also, that only unilateral motion of the sacroiliac joint could produce motion of the symphysis pubis, while motion of both joints did not (128). He also noted that rotation of the sacrum under the L5 vertebrae would cause the ilia to rotate backward on the side of sacral rotation, while the symphysis pubis would move upward and forward; he believed all of this would occur during the normal gait cycle of walking.

Colachis, in a series of measurements, concluded that the greatest motion of the sacroiliac joint occurred in forward bending from the upright position (53).

Drerup used a rasterstereographic procedure to help investigate motion and anatomical displacement of structures in the sacroiliac joint (59). The first necessary step was to use the procedure to help identify the location of anatomical landmarks with a great deal of precision and accuracy (129). In the study noted above, the landmarks chosen were the lumbar dimples, which are in close relation to the posterior superior iliac spines; thus, motion of the dimples can be used as an indicator of pelvic motion. In the study, an artificial pelvic tilt was created, and they noted than a near perfect correction between landmark and pelvic motion ($r=0.99$).

Pitkin (130) used an inclinometer to measure the angle of inclination between the posterior superior iliac spine and the anterior superior iliac spines. He chose to make such measurements with the patient placed in three different positions: regular stance, and with either the right or left leg on a block $1\frac{1}{2}$ inches in height. From this study, Pitkin decided that two motions could occur at the sacrum: flexion/extension (where the ilium is essentially fixed), and lateral bending with rotation (in which it is the ilium that moves, with the sacrum following the motion). These motions occurred in the way they did in part due to the presence of the various sacroiliac ligaments. This agrees with the findings of James Mennell (127) and his son John (131), who also noted the presence of two motions of the sacrum.

There has been a great deal of debate about where the axis of rotation in the sacrum lies. Very early on, Farabeuf suggested that the axis of rotation was located through a transverse axis passing through the interosseous ligament (132). Bonnaire later suggested that this transverse axis passed through the sacral tubercle (133). Pitkin noted that the axis for flexion and extension also fell through the interosseous ligament (130). Others have suggested different locations, including through the iliac tubercle (14), around the femoral head (134), etc. Finally, the pubic symphysis became important for its role in the nutational motion of the sacroiliac joint. As Jolliot has said, this confirmed the functional relationship of all the joints in the pelvis; she has suggested that it is important to differentiate the motion of the sacroiliac joint from the flexion and extension of the sacrum that occurs with motion of the spine (135).

Strachan (92, 136, 137) performed a study in which a cadaveric ilium was placed in a concrete block to fix it. With pins placed in the ilium to help determine motion, the sacroiliac joint was observed as motion was induced in the trunk of the cadaver. Strachan made several observations. One observation was that when the lumbar spine was extended during motion, the sacrum also extended upon the fixed ilium. The unfixed ilium (on the contralateral side of measurement) did indeed follow the sacrum, but there was only a limited amount of motion. A second observation was that when the lumbar spine was rotated, the sacrum also rotated to the same side, while there was a concomitant lateral flexion to the opposite side. A third finding related that the lumbar spine, when flexed, produced flexion of the sacrum on the ilium that was prevented from moving. The mobile (contralateral) ilium also followed the sacrum, but there was much less overall flexion than on the fixed side. When the lumbar spine was laterally bent, the sacrum laterally flexed to the same side. The coupled rotation here was little noted and not consistent. Finally, Strachan found that when the spine was tractioned, the sacrum would move into extension; conversely, compression of the spine caused sacral flexion.

DonTigny has noted that the basic function of the sacroiliac joints is to lessen the concussion that can occur with rapid changes of body weight redistribution; this occurs in each of two directions (113). When this occurs, the sacroiliac joint will rotate around a transverse axis. Wilder felt that the sacroiliac joint also had a role to play in the absorption of energy, since the possible motion required both joint separation and ligamentous stretching (55). DonTigny, again, noted that the sacroiliac joints help to absorb shear forces.

SACROILIAC SYNDROMES

The sacroiliac joint is subject to several different processes that may damage it. Sprain is common, and sacroiliac joint subluxation can occur. Sprain may occur with heavy loads placed upon the joints, with a fall, or with blows to the sacroiliac joint. The pain that occurs will be felt unilaterally over the sacroiliac joint and can radiate into the ipsilateral hip or buttocks. The pain will be made worse by movement of the joint or by axial loading of the joint. Upon palpation, the joint is extremely tender, particularly near an area just inferomedial to the posterior superior iliac spine. When examining the patient for global motions, the ability to extend the area may produce some pain, while forward bending into flexion is typically not painful, nor is recovery to the upright

position from the flexed position. Lateral bending may be painful but is not universally so, particularly if the motion is very smoothly performed. Straight leg raise testing produces pain at approximately 70° of flexion. There are no muscular changes noted, and reflex testing will be normal.

Pain from sacroiliac joint lesions other than sprain will typically be dull in nature and perceived in the region of the buttocks. It may radiate into the area of the anterior groin, the posterior thigh, the knee, or even the lower abdomen, causing possible misdiagnosis as an intraabdominal lesion (138, 139). Neurological symptoms are rare, so paresthesias are not often seen. Maitland has noted that when patients suffer from mechanical lesions of the sacroiliac joint, the pain is usually unilateral and will be exacerbated by motions that produce stress on the joint (139). He classifies disorders of the sacroiliac joint into several different groups: (*a*) inflamatory lesions; (*b*) infectious lesions; (*c*) mechanical lesions; (*d*) degenerative lesions; and (*e*) osteitis condensans ilii.

INFLAMMATORY SIJ PROBLEMS

There are a great many inflammatory disorders that affect the sacroiliac joint. Most of these fall under the general heading of the seronegative arthropathies, such as ankylosing spondylitis, Reiter's syndrome, psoriatic arthritis, and so on. In such cases, a combination of radiographic and laboratory tests can be used to confirm the presence of the particular disease. Each disease has its own characteristics under these procedures, such as the predisposition of ankylosing spondylitis to start in the sacroiliac joint and migrate superiorly up the spine.

Infections within the sacroiliac joint are caused most frequently by staphylococcus bacteria, as well as tuberculous or brucellar infection. X-ray can once again be used to show typical changes, and bone scans will be quite useful in demonstrating the "hot spot" appearance of such infections. Aspiration biopsy is needed to culture the organism, and medical referral is then necessary for appropriate treatment.

Maitland claims that mechanical lesions of the sacroiliac joint are not common, and consist of both hypo- and hypermobility lesions (139). Causes of hypomobility lesions include rotational stress on the joint, pregnancy, and trauma, as well as unequal leg length. Hypermobility lesions are due only to an unstable symphysis pubis, or to pregnancy (which also affects the symphysis pubis via the release of the hormone relaxin, which is designed to soften the symphysis in preparation for the passage of the baby through the vaginal canal).

Degenerative changes may occur within the sacroiliac joint as well as in any other joint in the body. The changes that occur in the joint are similar to those in other joints as well; there will be pitting of the bone accompanied by subchondral sclerosis and osteophytic changes. This condition has a tendency to occur as we age, in concert with greater amounts of stress placed upon the joint, such as increasing weight or damage from such conditions as fracture or biomechanical abnormality.

Osteitis condensans ilii is a condition in which bone condenses along the ilium near the sacroiliac joint. The cause of this condition is not known, though it does seem to be more frequent in women, particularly during pregnancy. It may be associated with increased stress, with ankylosing spondylitis (140), with urinary tract infection, and with circulatory problems. It can lead to low back pain. On radiograph, there is a characteristic triangular area of sclerosis located near the medial ilium.

Schafer has noted that sacroiliac subluxation may produce irritative microtrauma to the articular structures, induction of spinal curvatures, induction of spinal and/or pelvic subluxation and fixation, and biomechanical abnormalities in stance and locomotion (141). Evaluation of the sacroiliac joint for the presence of such subluxation or fixation will need to combine both static and dynamic palpation as well as plumb line analysis. There may be tenderness upon palpation of the posterior superior iliac spine when there is innominate rotation; conversely, it is necessary to perform a full motion palpation procedure to properly evaluate the joint for motion abnormalities or fixation. Both procedures need to be done to best evaluate the joint with regard to the presence of subluxation of fixation.

MANIPULATION AND ADJUSTMENT OF THE SACROILIAC JOINT

The chiropractic profession has long prided itself for its studies into the biomechanics and management of the sacroiliac joint. Many different forms of manipulative procedures have been developed and advocated for managing sacroiliac disrelationships, and an entire book could be devoted to the subject. In this chapter, we will look at the use of both flexion distraction procedures and some high-velocity adjustive techniques that can be used to manage the sacroiliac joint.

Flexion Distraction Protocols

The basic protocol for the use of flexion distraction therapy in the management of sacroiliac joint dysfunction is to use the positioning of the innominates as the guide to proper use of the technique.

ANTERIOR INNOMINATE

When the innominate ilium portion is anterior and the ischium is posterior, the following findings will be noted:

1. Long leg on mensuration;
2. A low ilium and an anterior ilium on visual examination;
3. Probably, spasm of the gluteus medius and minimus muscles and the quadriceps muscles and weakness on testing of the gluteus maximus muscle, the hamstring muscle, and the gracilis muscle;
4. Possibly, internal rotation of the foot due to spasm of the gluteus medius and minimus muscles and/or weakness of the gluteus maximus muscle and piriformis muscle;
5. Possibly, external rotation of the foot due to spasm of the gluteus maximus muscle and piriformis muscle and/or weakness of the gluteus medius and minimus muscles;
6. Bilateral anterior ilia or the anterior pelvis on x-rays. The pelvic outlet is vertically increased in height, and the obturator foramina are smaller.

Treatment of the anterior innominate is accomplished in the following way:

1. Balance the gluteal muscles by strengthening the gluteus maximus muscle and relaxing the gluteus medius and minimus muscles.
2. Strengthen the hamstring muscles and relax the quadriceps muscles as shown in Chapter 15.
3. Balance the piriformis muscle by applying pressure on its insertion at the greater trochanter.

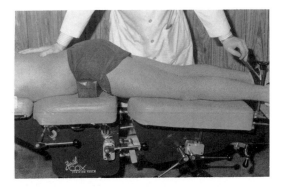

Figure 5.14. Unilateral correction being applied to the anterior ilium.

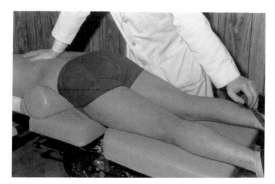

Figure 5.15. Dutchman roll is placed under the ilia for correction of a bilateral anterior pelvis.

4. Place a block under the anterior superior iliac spine (ASIS) and apply traction to the innominate (Fig. 5.14). This can be done while a disc lesion, facet syndrome, or other low back condition is being reduced. If both innominates are anterior (anterior pelvis), a Dutchman roll can be placed under the ilia, and both ilia can be distracted simultaneously (Fig. 5.15).
5. Maintain hand contact on the L5 spinous process with cephalad pressure for 20 seconds while pumping the caudal section of the table up and down 2 inches. This 20-second distraction is repeated three times.

POSTERIOR INNOMINATE

When the innominate ilium portion is posterior and the ischium is anterior, the following findings will be noted:

1. Short leg on mensuration;
2. A high and posterior ilium on visual examination;
3. Probably, spasm of the gluteus maximus muscle, weakness of the gluteus medius and minimus muscles, the gracilis muscle, and possibly the quadriceps muscles, tenderness of the gracilis muscle over the medial tibial insertion, and good strength in the hamstring muscles on testing;
4. Possibly, inward or outward rotation of the feet according to the muscle changes described in item 4 in the section on the anterior innominate;
5. Enlargement of the obturator foramen and lessening of the pelvic outlet vertical height on x-rays (Figs. 5.16–5.18).

Treatment of the posterior innominate is accomplished the following way:

1. Balance the gluteal muscle by relaxing the gluteus maximus muscle and strengthening the gluteus medius and minimus muscles as described in Chapter 15.
2. Relax the hamstring and strengthen the quadriceps muscles.

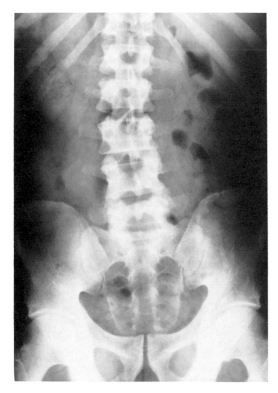

Figure 5.16. X-ray showing bilateral posterior ilia.

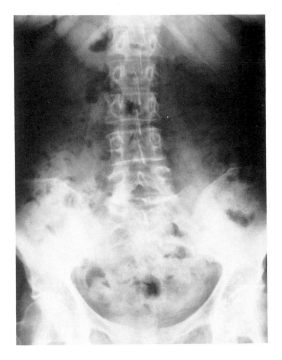

Figure 5.17. X-ray showing bilateral posterior ilia.

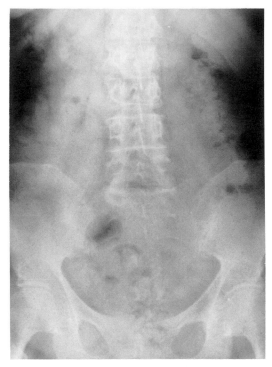

Figure 5.18. X-ray showing bilateral posterior ilia.

3. Balance the piriformis muscle, after foot rotation and testing.
4. Place a block under the acetabulum, and apply traction to the innominate (Fig. 5.19). This can be done while a disc lesion, facet syndrome, or other low back condition is being treated.
5. Maintain hand contact on the L5 spinous process with cephalad pressure for 20 seconds while pumping the caudal section of the table up and down 2 inches. This 20-second distraction is repeated three times.

High-Velocity Adjustive Protocols

A great many adjustive procedures exist for the management of sacroiliac joint dysfunction. They revolve around contacts upon either the innominate or the sacrum; the decision as to which should best be used is an art unto itself and has not been adequately addressed in the literature, though the proponents of the diagnostic procedure known as motion palpation, developed by such individuals as Mennell, Gillet, and Faye, offer perhaps the best current rationale for the choice of contacts. The procedures offered here are applicable to both static and dynamic considerations and are simply representative of the genre; others exist as well and may be equally effective.

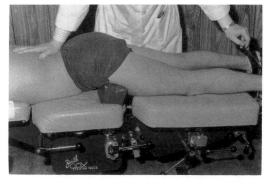

Figure 5.19. Unilateral or bilateral correction of the posterior ilium being applied.

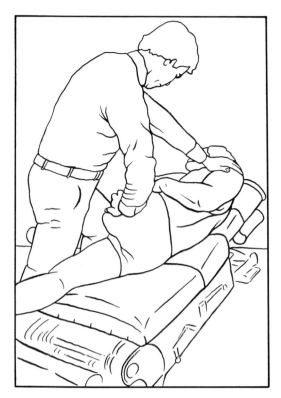

Figure 5.20. Ischial-popliteal-deltoid technique for anterior innominate subluxation.

ANTERIOR INNOMINATE

In this technique, the patient is placed in a side-lying position, with the side of the involved anterior innominate placed up. The patient's upper leg is brought off the table, and the doctor stands between the patient's legs. The doctor's stance is described as a "fencer's stance," and the doctor's outside leg is placed so that the doctor's knee is in the popliteal fossa of the leg hanging off the table. The doctor's cephalad hand is placed on the patient's upper shoulder for stabilization; the caudal hand makes a pisiform contact upon the ischial tuberosity of the patient on the side placed up. The thrust in this procedure is delivered by the doctor thrusting anteriorly on the ischial tuberosity, while simultaneously driving the upper leg forward. This procedure thus drives the upper innominate posteriorly by using both the leg and the ischial tuberosity as levers (Figs 5.21 and 5.22).

POSTERIOR INNOMINATE

Adjustment of a posterior-based innominate is a basic chiropractic procedure. Here, the patient is again placed in a side-lying position, with the involved side placed up. The patient's upper leg is flexed, and the foot is placed in the popliteal space of the patient's lower leg. The doctor makes a lateral thigh-to-thigh contact on the patient's upper leg. The cephalad hand is placed on the upper shoulder, while a pisiform contact is made on the upper posterior superior iliac spine (PSIS). The line of drive is anterior on the PSIS, while the doctor also performs a "body drop" on the patient's upper leg (Figs 5.22 and 5.23).

ANTERIOR SACRUM

For this procedure, the patient lies prone in an antigravity position, or with a Dutchman's roll placed under the abdomen. The doctor stands on the side of the anterior sacrum, in a "fencer's stance" facing the foot of the table. A pisiform contact is made with the cephalad hand on the contralateral sacral apex; this contact is supported by the caudal hand, which will place a web contact on the contact hand: the little finger is placed into the web of the thumb and index finger, the second through fourth fingers lie obliquely across the dorsum of the contact hand, and the thumb wraps around the wrist. This wrist is kept neutral, with no flexion or extension in it. The thrust is delivered in line with the arms.

POSTERIOR SACRUM

Here again, the patient is placed with the affected side placed up while in a side-lying position. The patient's lower arm is placed under the head; the upper arm rests on the lateral body wall. The doctor makes a lateral thigh-to-thigh contact, with a contact made by the caudal hand on the upper base of the sacrum between the iliac crest and the second sacral tubercle. The cephalad hand is placed on the patient's upper shoulder. The thrust will drive the sacral base anteriorly, while the wrist torque is slightly in an upward (or radial) direction. There is a simultaneous "body drop" with this technique as well.

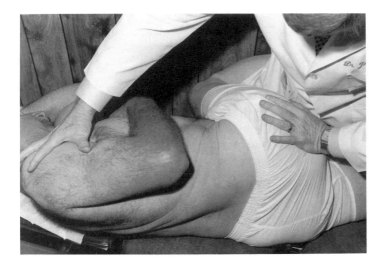

Figure 5.21. In adjustment of the anterior ilium subluxation, the patient lies on the side with the involved sacroiliac joint up, and the patient's knee is flexed. The doctor places his patella into the popliteal fossa of the patient's knee and applies flexion traction to the ilium through the femoral traction. The patient's shoulder is stabilized, and rotation to the lumbar spine is avoided by making no downward pressure to the patient's knee as the doctor applies flexion to the femur. At the end of distraction, a thrust by the doctor's contact hand on the patient's ischium is made in a cephalad direction. At the same time the cephalad thrust is applied to the ischium, the patient's femoral traction is increased by the forward lifting of the knee by the doctor's popliteal pressure. This combination of cephalad femoral and ischial thrust creates the adjustment of the anteriorly subluxed ilium in relation to the sacrum.

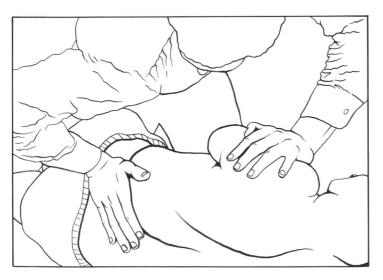

Figure 5.22. Thigh-ilio-deltoid technique for posterior innominate subluxation.

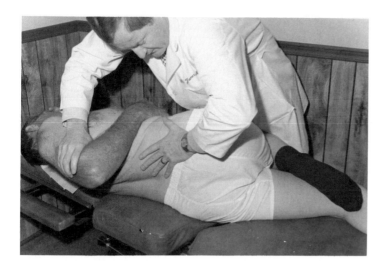

Figure 5.23. In adjustment of the posterior ilium subluxation, the patient lies on the side with the involved sacroiliac joint up, and the patient's knee is flexed. The doctor flexes the patient's hip and knee joints by applying force with his thigh against the patient's leg. At the same time, the posterior superior iliac spine is contacted with the doctor's pisiform hand contact. An anterior thrust is applied to the ilium as the doctor's thigh applies a cephalad traction to the ilium by having the doctor apply increasing flexion to the hip and knee joint. The patient's shoulder is stabilized with the doctor's free hand, and rotation is avoided at the lumbar spine by not applying any downward force to the patient's thigh. This allows the posterior ilium to be brought anterior without inflicting any rotation forces to the lower lumbar spine.

References for Parts 1 and 2

1. Miller JAA, et al.: Load displacement behavior of sacroiliac joint. *J Orthop Res* 5:92–101, 1987.
2. Romer AS: *The Vertebral Body,* ed 4. Philadelphia, WB Saunders, 1970, pp 182–187.
3. Walker JM: Age-related differences in human sacroiliac joint, a histological study. *J Orthop Sports Phys Ther* 7(6):325–334, 1986.
4. Weisl H: The articular surface of sacroiliac joint and their relation to the movement. *Acta Anat* 22: 1–14, 1954.
5. Hinwood JA: Sacroiliac joint biomechanics. *Dig Chiro Econ* 25(5):41–44, 1983.
6. Williams PL, Warwick R: *Gray's Anatomy,* 36th British ed. Philadelphia, Lea & Febiger, 1980, pp 473–475, 601.
7. Otter R: A review study of differing opinions expressed in the anatomic literature. *Eur J Chiro* 33: 221–242, 1985.
8. Duffy PM: Adult sacroiliac joint cartilage, a histological study. *Proceedings of the Anatomical Society of Great Britain and Ireland* 9(2):250–251.
9. Janse J: The clinical biomechanics of sacroiliac mechanism. *ACA J Chiropractic* 12(January, Suppl 1), 1978.
10. Mitchell FL: *Structural Pelvic Function.* Year Book, 1965, vol 2, pp 178–199.
11. Buddingh CC: The stubborn low back. *Dig Chiro Econ* (July/August):72–73, 1980.
12. Diakow PRP: Post-surgical sacroiliac syndrome. *J Can Chiro Assoc* 27(1):19–21, 1983.
13. Beal MC: The sacroiliac problem, review of anatomy, mechanics and diagnosis. *J Am Osteopath Assoc* 82(June):667–673, 679–685, 1982.
14. Weisl H: The movement of the sacroiliac joint. *Acta Anat* 23:80–91, 1955.
15. McGill SM: A biomechanical perspective of sacroiliac pain. *Clinical Biomechanics* 2:145–151, 1987.
16. Paquin JD: Biomechanical and morphological study of cartilage from adult human sacroiliac joint. *Arthritis Rheum* 26(7):887–895, 1983.
17. Bowen V, Cassidy JD: Macroscopic and microscopic anatomy of sacroiliac joint from embryonic life. *Spine* 6(6):620–628, 1981.
18. Simkins CS: Anatomy and significance of sacroiliac joint. In: *AAO Year Book, 1952,* pp 64–69.
19. Bellamy N: What do we know about sacroiliac joint. *Arthritis Rheum* 12(3):282–309, 1983.
20. Hadley LA: Accessory sacroiliac joint. *J Bone Joint Surg* 34A(1):149–155, 1952.
21. Ehara S: The accessory sacroiliac joint, a common anatomic variant. *AJR* 150:857–859, 1988.
22. Grieve GP: The sacroiliac joint. Norfork & Norwich Hospital, 1975, pp 384–401,.
23. Bakland O, Hansen J: The axial sacroiliac joint. *Anatomica Clinica* (University of Oslo, Norway) 6: 29–36, 1984.
24. Weisl H: The ligaments of sacroiliac joint exam-

ined with their particular reference to function. *Acta Anat* 20(3):201–213, 1954.

25. Solonen KA: Sacroiliac joint in the light of anatomical, radiological and clinical study. *Acta Orthop Scand* (Suppl 27):160–162, 1957.

26. Pitkin HC: Sacrarthrogenic telalgia. *J Bone Joint Surg* 18A(1), 1936.

27. Norman GF: Sacroiliac condition simulating intervertebral disc syndrome. *WJSO & G* (August): 401–402, 1956.

28. Koffman DM: Technical excellence, the next key to our survival. *Dig Chiro Econ* (July/August):53, 1984.

29. Sashin D: A critical analysis of anatomy and pathology of sacroiliac joint. *Bull Hosp Joint Dis* 891–910, 1929.

30. Resnick D: Sacroiliac joint in renal osteodystrophy. *J Rheum* 2(3):287–295, 1975.

31. Resnik CS: Radiology of disorder of sacroiliac joint. *JAMA* 253(19):2863–2866, 1985.

32. Cone RO: Roentgenographic evaluation of sacroiliac joint. *Orthop Rev* 12(1):95–105, 1983.

33. Volger JB: Normal sacroiliac joint. *Radiology* 151(2), 1984.

34. Jajic I: The prevalence of osteoarthrosis. *Clin Rheumatol* 6:39–41, 1987.

35. Lontle BC: The scintigraphic investigation of sacroiliac disease. *J Diag Nucl Med* 18(6):529–533, 1977.

36. Namey TC: Nucleographic studies of axial spondarthritides. 1. Quantitative sacroiliac scintigraphy in early HLA-B27 associated sacroiliitis. *Arthritis Rheum* 20(5):1058–1064, 1977.

37. Scott DL: An evaluation of the techniques of sacroiliac scintiscanning. *Rheum Rehab* 19:76–82, 1980.

38. Webb J: Fluorine 18 isotope scans in early diagnosis of sacroiliac joint. *Med J Aust* 2:1270–1274, 1971.

39. Dick WC: The use of radioisotopes in normal and diseased joints. *Arthritis Rheum* 1(4):301–325, 1972.

40. Davis M: Comparison of 99m-TC-labeled phosphate agents for skeletal imaging. *Nucl Med* 6(1): 19–31, 1976.

41. Hoffer PB: Radionucleic joint imaging. *Nucl Med* 1(6):121–137, 1976.

42. Whelan MA: Computed tomogram of normal sacrum. *AJR* 139:1183–1195, 1982.

43. Borlaza GS: Computed tomogram of the evaluation of sacroiliac arthritis. *Radiology* 139(May): 437–440, 1981.

44. Elhabal M: Tomographic examination of sacroiliac joint in adult patients with rheumatoid arthritis. *J Rheum* 6(4):417–425, 1979.

45. Dunn EJ: Pyogenic infection of sacroiliac joint. *Clin Orthop* 118(July/August):113–117, 1976.

46. Bose RN: Ankylosing spondylitis: treatment. *American Chiro* (May/June):50, 1982.

47. Walheim GG: Motion of symphysis in pelvic instability. *Scand J Rehab Med* 16:163–169, 1984.

48. LaBan MM: Symphyseal and sacroiliac joint pain associated with symphysis instability. *Arch Phys Med Rehabil* 59:470–472, 1978.

49. Grieve E: Lumbopelvic rhythm and mechanical dysfunction of sacroiliac joint. *Physiotherapy* 67(6): 171–173, 1981.

50. Sandoz RW: Structural and functional pathology of pelvic ring. *Ann Swiss Chiro Assoc* 101–155, 1978.

51. Wood J: Motion of sacroiliac joint. *Palmer College Research Forum* (Spring):1–16, 1985.

52. Pitkin HC: A study of sacral mobility. *J Bone Joint Surg* 18A:365–374, 1936.

53. Colachis SC: Movement of sacroiliac joint in adult male. *Arch Phys Med Rehabil* 44(September): 490–497, 1963.

54. Dulhunty JA: Sacroiliac subluxation, facts, fallacies and illusions. *J Austr Chiro Assoc* 15(3):91–99, 1985.

55. Wilder DG: The functional topography of sacroiliac joint. *Spine* 5(6):575–579, 1980.

56. Lawson TL: The sacroiliac joint anatomic plain x-ray and CT analysis. *J Comput Assist Tomogr* 6(2): 307–314, 1982.

57. Frigerio NA: Movement of sacroiliac joint. *ACA J Chiropractic* 8(November, Suppl)161–166, 1974.

58. Egund N: Movement of sacroiliac joint, demonstrated with roentgen stereophotogrammetry. *Acta Radiol Diag* 19(Fasc 5):833–846, 1978.

59. Drerup B: Movement of human pelvis and displacement of related anatomical landmarks on body surface. *J Biomech* (Britain) 20(19):971–977, 1987.

60. Valojerdy MR: The irregularities on the articular surface and their relationship to movement. *Proceedings of Anatomical Society of Great Britain* 247–248, 1988.

61. Maltezopoulos V: A comparison of four chiropractic systems in diagnosis of sacroiliac malfunction. *Eur J Chiro* 32:4–42, 1984.

62. Grove AB: *Chiropractic Techniques, A Procedure of Adjusting*. Madison, WI, Straus Printing, 1979, pp 92–106.

63. Pierce WV: Pelvic technique. *Dig Chiro Econ* (January-February):46–50, 1983.

64. Herbst RW: *Gonstead Chiropractic Science and Art*. CI-Chi Publication, 1968.

65. Cox WA: Gonstead system. *American Chiro* (July/August):68, 1988.

66. Duffield HJ: *Manipulation of Sacroiliac Joint*, pp 108–114.

67. Lavignolle B: An approach to functional anatomy of sacroiliac joint in vivo. *Anatomica Clinica* 5: 169–176, 1983.

68. Kirk CR, Lawrence DJ: *State Manual of Spinal and Pelvic Technique*. Lombard, IL, National College of Chiropractic, 1965, pp 113–143.

69. Gemmel HA: Low force sustained pressure for sacroiliac fixation. *American Chiro* (November): 28–32, 1987.

70. Schuchman JA: Sacroiliac strain syndrome, diagnosis and treatment. *Tex Med* 82(June):33–36, 1986.

71. Gemmel HA: The force necessary to correct fixation of sacroiliac joint. *Dig Chiro Econ* (September/October):12, 1986.

72. Logan HB: *Logan Basic Methods.* Florrisant, MO, Text Book, 1950, pp 91–95.

73. Kotheimer WMJ: Analysis of sacroiliac joint, a simple approach. *Dig Chiro Econ* (July/August): 10–12, 1985.

74. Bailey HW: Short leg and spinal anomalies. *J Am Osteopath Assoc* 36(7):319–327, 1937.

75. Fryette HH: Some reasons why sacroiliac lesions recur. *J Am Osteopath Assoc* 36(3):119–122, 1936.

76. Heymann WC: Consideration of diagnostic tests for sacroiliac lesions. *J Am Osteopath Assoc* 67: 1013–1069, 1968.

77. Abel MS: Sacroiliac joint change in traumatic paraplegics. *J Radiology* 55:235–239, August 1950.

78. Johnson JW: Sacroiliac strain. *J Am Osteopath Assoc* 63:1132–1148, August 1964.

79. Nykoliation JW: Osteitis condensans ilii, a stress phenomenon. *J Can Chiro Assoc* 28(1):21–24, March 1984.

80. Romanus R: *Pelvo-Spondylitis Ossificans.* Copenhagen, Munksgaard, and Chicago, Year Book, 1955.

81. Fidler MW: The effect of four types of support on segmental mobility of the lumbosacral spine. *J Bone Joint Surg* 65A:943–947, 1983.

82. Grieve EM: *Mechanical Dysfunction of Sacroiliac Joint.* Queens College, Glasgow, June 1982, pp 46–52.

83. Lichtblau S: Dislocation of sacroiliac joint. *J Bone Joint Surg* 44A:193–198, 1962.

84. Jenkins DHR: The operative treatment of sacroiliac joint subluxation and disruption of symphysis pubis. *British J Accid Surg* 10(2):139–141.

85. Winterstein JF: *Spinographic Evaluation of Pelvic and Lumbar Spine.* Lombard, IL, National College of Chiropractic, 1972.

86. Weiant CW: The past and future of chiropractic technique. *Dig Chiro Econ* (May/June):116–118, 1980.

87. Gillet H: *Osteopathic-chiropractic manipulation.* Bulletin No. 29 of European Chiropractors Union, 1981, pp 152–154.

88. Gillet H: *Motion Palpation.* Belgian Chiropractic Research Association Notes no. 1, 1975, pp 1–39.

89. Potter NA: Intertester reliability for selected clinical tests of sacroiliac joint. *Phys Ther* 65(11): 1671–1675, 1985.

90. Gatterman MI: Indication for spinal manipulation in treatment of back pain. *ACA J Chiropractic* 16(10):51–63, 1982.

91. Fligg DB: Piriformis technique. *J Can Chiro Assoc* 30(2):87–88, 1986.

92. Strachan WF: A study of mechanics of sacroiliac joint. *J Am Osteopath Assoc* 33(12):576–578, 1933.

93. Greenman PE: Innominate shear dysfunction in sacroiliac syndrome. *Manual Med* 2:114–121, 1986.

94. Epstein MC: Cause of low back problem. *Dig Chiro Econ* (January/February):52–54, 1983.

95. DeJarnette MB: *Sacro-Occipital Technique of Spinal Therapy.* pp 1–5, 1940.

96. DeJarnette MB: *Sacro-Occipital Technique of Chiropractic.* Private publication, 1952, pp 1–13.

97. DeJarnette MB: Cornerstone, interview with Dr. Jarnette about SOT. *American Chiro* (July/August):22–23, 28, 34, 1982.

98. DeJarnette MB: Sacro-occipital technique. *Today's Chiro* (May/June):97–98, 1986.

99. Bermis T: Validation of long sitting test on subject with sacroiliac dysfunction. *J Orthop Sports Phys Ther* 8(7):336–343, 1987.

100. Norman GF: Sacroiliac disease and its relationship to lower abdominal pain. *Am J Surg* 116(July):54–56, 1968.

101. Dekker BJ: Prevalence of peripheral arthritis, sacroiliitis and ankylosing spondylitis in patients suffering from inflammatory bowel disease. *Ann Rheum Dis* 37:33–35, 1978.

102. Lehman TJA: HLA-B-27 negative sacroiliitis, a manifestation of familial Mediterranean fever. *Pediatrics* 61(3):423–426, 1978.

103. Brodey PA: Radiographic change in sacroiliac joint in familial Mediterranean fever. *Radiology* 114:331–333, 1975.

104. Pettingale KW: Acute sacroiliitis due to salmonella okatie. *British Med* (June):1449, 1977.

105. Yazici H: A controlled survey of sacroiliitis in Behcet's disease. *Ann Rheum Dis* 40:558–559, 1981.

106. Steinberg CL: Brucellosis as a cause of sacroiliac arthritis. *JAMA* 138(1):15–19, 1947.

107. Carter ME: Sacroiliitis in Still's disease. *Ann Rheum Dis* 21:105–120, 1962.

108. Davis P: Quantitative scintigraphy of sacroiliac joint with Crohn's disease. *Arthritis Rheum* 21(2): 234–237, 1978.

109. Russell AS: The sacroiliitis of acute Reiter's syndrome. *J Rheum* 4(3):293–296, 1977.

110. McEwen C: Ankylosing spondylitis accompanying ulcerative colitis, regional enteritis, psoriasis and Reiter's disease. *Arthritis Rheum* 14(3):291–318, 1971.

111. Blower PW: Clinical sacroiliac joint test in ankylosing spondylitis and other causes of low back pain—2 studies. *Ann Rheum Dis* 43:192–195, 1984.

112. Gatterman MI: Contraindications and complications of spinal manipulative therapy. *ACA J Chiropractic* 15S(September):75–86, 1981.

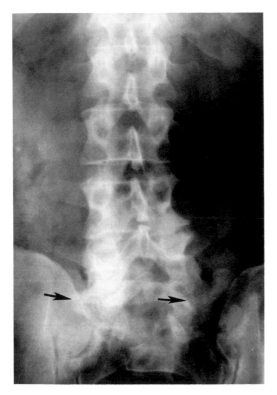

Figure 6.1. The *arrows* point to the overdeveloped, spatulated transverse processes of L5 that form the pseudoarticulations with the sacrum. Note the four lumbar segments above.

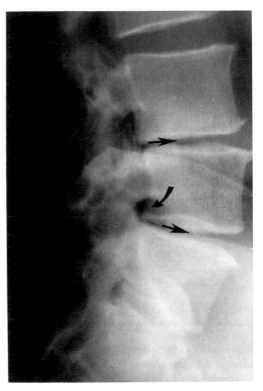

Figure 6.2. Lateral view of the patient in Figure 6.1 shows degenerative changes of the L3-L4 and L4-L5 discs (*straight arrows*) with traction spurs of the anterior and lateral body plates. Note the narrowing of the L4-L5 intervertebral foramen (*curved arrow*).

(6). The degeneration of the L5-S1 disc places the paramount responsibility for motion on the cephalad disc levels. These discs often are seen to degenerate in a domino effect, beginning at L4-L5 and moving upward.

Except for facet tropism, a change in the number of mobile vertebrae in the lumbar spine is the most significant congenital vertebral anomaly that can cause low back pain. Lumbarization of the first sacral vertebra (giving the individual, in effect, six lumbar vertebrae) increases the lever arm of the lumbar spine and causes greater stress on the lumbar spine and the lumbosacral joint. In contrast, sacralization of the fifth lumbar vertebra (reducing the number of mobile vertebrae in the lumbar region to four) is unlikely to cause symptoms when the entire vertebra is solidly incorporated into the sacrum. Occasionally, only one transverse process articulates with the sacrum, altering spinal mechanics and resulting in severe instability and stress (7).

Unilateral sacralization of a lumbar vertebra or lumbarization of a sacral vertebra produces a condition known as Bertolotti's syndrome (Fig. 6.4), which has been diagnosed with increasing frequency in the past 10 years. Unilateral contact places unusual stress on the spine, and the resulting torque movements often cause herniation of the disc one level above the sacralization or lumbarization. Herniation, in turn, produces symptoms of nerve root entrapment. In the patient with Bertolotti's syndrome, surgery to decompress the herniated disc should always include spinal fusion to weld the affected vertebrae together so that further torque stresses are eliminated.

Wigh (8) found that none of 42 patients who underwent disc surgery, and also had transitional segment, had any sign of disc protrusion at the level of the transitional segment. The disc at the transitional segment was hypoplastic, with the stress placed on the segment directly above.

Therefore, in an L5 transitional segment, the L4-L5 disc is under stress and will be found to be the level of protrusion, whether contained or non-contained.

CLASSIFICATION OF LUMBOSACRAL TRANSITIONAL VERTEBRAE

Based upon morphological and clinical characteristics with respect to herniated nucleus pulposus, a classification of lumbosacral transitional vertebrae was developed (9) (Fig. 6.5).

Type 1. Dysplastic Transverse Process. (*a*) Unilateral; (*b*) bilateral. A large transverse process, triangular in shape, measuring at least 19 mm in width is seen.

Type 2. Incomplete Lumbarization/Sacralization. (*a*) Unilateral; (*b*) bilateral. A large transverse process forms a pseudoarticulation between the transverse process and the sacrum. This appears to be a diarthrodial joint.

Type 3. Complete Lumbarization/Sacralization. (*a*) Unilateral; (*b*) bilateral. A true bony union exists between the spatulated transverse process and the sacrum.

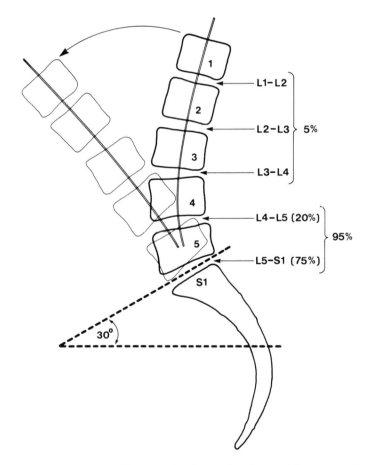

Figure 6.3. Segmental site and degree of lumbar spine flexion. The degree of flexion, noted at each segment of the lumbar spine as a percentage of total lumbar flexion, is indicated. The major portion of flexion (75%) occurs at the lumbosacral joint, 20% of flexion may occur at the L4-L5 interspace, and the remaining 5% is distributed between L1-L4. The forward-flexed diagram indicates the mere reversal past lordosis of total flexion of the lumbar curve. The lumbosacral angle is computed as the angle from a base parallel to horizontal and the hypotenuse drawn parallel to superior level of the sacral bone. The optimum physiological lumbosacral angle is in the vicinity of 30°. (From Weinstein PR, Ehni G, Wilson CB: *Lumbar Spondylolysis: Diagnosis, Management, and Surgical Treatment.* Chicago, Year Book, 1977, p 14. Originally based on Cailliet R: *Low Back Pain Syndrome* ed 2. Philadelphia, FA Davis, 1968.)

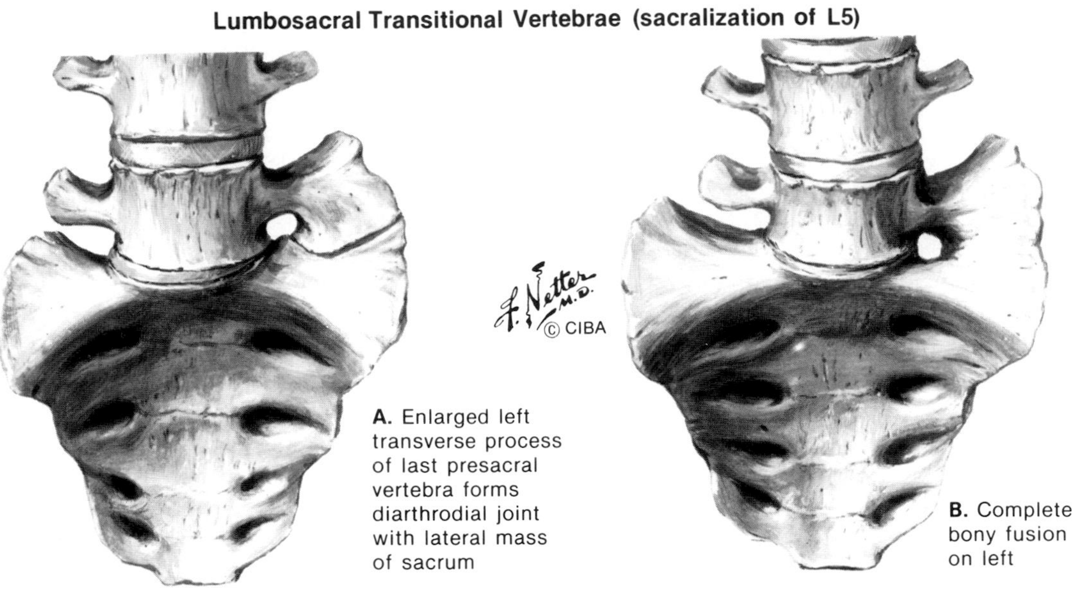

Lumbosacral Transitional Vertebrae (sacralization of L5)

A. Enlarged left transverse process of last presacral vertebra forms diarthrodial joint with lateral mass of sacrum

B. Complete bony fusion on left

Figure 6.4. Illustration of lumbosacral transitional vertebrae (sacralization of L5) by Frank H. Netter, M.D. (Reproduced with permission from Keim HA, Kirkaldy-Willis WH: Clinical Symposia. *Ciba Found Symp* 32(6):9, 1980. © 1980, CIBA Pharmaceutical Company, Division of CIBA-GEIGY Corporation. All rights reserved.)

Type 4. Mixed. The patients that fall into this category exhibit type 2 (pseudoarticulation) on one side and type 3 (bone fusion) on the other.

The terms *lumbarization* and *sacralization* were not used because the total number of vertebrae in the patients' spines could not be determined.

The sex distribution of lumbosacral anomaly showed a greater incidence in men (71.5%) than in women (28.5%).

Conclusion

The type 2 unilateral or bilateral pseudoarticulation between the transverse processes and sacrum has the highest incidence of disc herniation at the disc above the transitional segment. Types 1, 3, and 4 do not prove to produce any higher incidence of disc herniation above the transitional segment.

CASE PRESENTATIONS

CASES 1 AND 2

A 40-year-old white chiropractor (case 1) had had low back pain for several years, but in the last 4 years it had been getting progressively worse, to the point that at times his right leg gave out from under him when he was walking. He stated that both legs felt asleep.

Examination failed to reveal any motor or sensory change of the lower extremities. The straight leg raises were negative except for some shortness of the hamstring muscles. The deep reflexes were +2 bilaterally. The gluteus maximus and hamstring muscles were grade 5 of 5 strengths.

X-ray examination (Figs. 6.6 and 6.7) shows one of the most interesting studies I have ever seen. Figure 6.6 reveals a transitional fifth lumbar segment, namely a sacralized fifth lumbar vertebra. You will also note that there is hypertrophy of the right superior L4 articular facet. The pars interarticularis fracture is visualized on lateral projection.

Therefore, we see here a forward slippage of the fourth lumbar vertebral body on a transitional fifth lumbar segment. This is truly a Bertolotti's syndrome with actively degenerating disc tissue and annular fiber stress of the L4-L5 level.

Figures 6.8, 6.9, and 6.10 (case 2) reveal a transitional L5 segment and a true spondylolisthesis at L4. Cases 1 and 2 represent the only two cases I have seen in clinical practice of a transitional segment with spondylolisthesis at the segment above. Case 2 is courtesy of Alice Wright, D.C., of Hatfield, Pennsylvania.

In treatment of transitional L5 segment, a Dutchman flexion roll is placed under the L5 segment as shown in Figure 6.11. The contact is placed on the spinous process of L4 while flexion distraction is applied with the

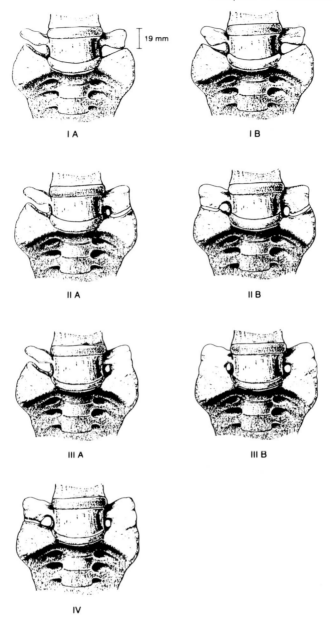

Figure 6.5. Classification of lumbosacral transitional vertebrae according to radiomorphological and clinical relevance with respect to lumbar disc herniation. (Reproduced with permission from Castellvi AE, Goldstein LA, Chan DPK: Lumbosacral transitional vertebrae and their relationship with lumbar extradural defects. *Spine* 9(5):493–495, 1984.)

caudal section of the table. A description of technique application to patients with and without spondylolisthesis above the level of transitional segment is shown in the legend of Figure 6.11.

Figure 6.12 shows the spinous process contact made while the lumbar segments are individually placed in lateral flexion. A flexion roll is left in place to maintain slight flexion of the lumbar spine so as to prevent further stenosis of the spondylolisthetic slip.

Figure 6.13 shows goading of the acupressure points

B22 through B49 prior to and following flexion distraction manipulation.

Figure 6.14 shows the application of tetanizing current to the paravertebral muscles following spinal manipulation. In addition, if the pain is severe, we will apply alternating hot and cold packs as well—heat applied for 10 minutes, and cold for 5 minutes.

Figure 6.15 shows that we place a belt on these patients for stabilization. This belt contains a memory foam insert that molds snugly against the lumbar spine regardless of the contour. We find that transitional segments do well when allowed to have this type of support while healing takes place. We start the patients on exercises to regain abdominal strength and stretch the hamstring muscles; in the case of spondylolisthesis in the transitional segment, we also prescribe knee-chest exercises.

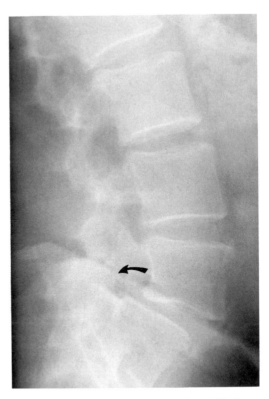

Figure 6.7. L4 is a true spondylolisthesis with the *arrow* denoting the pars interarticularis fracture.

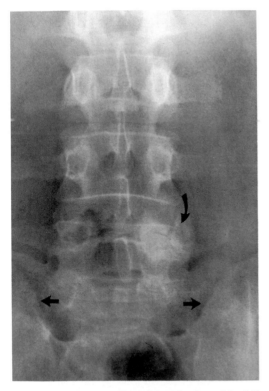

Figure 6.6. Note the bilateral sacralization of the fifth lumbar vertebral transverse processes (*straight arrows*). Also, the fourth lumbar right superior articular facet hypertrophy is shown by the *curved arrow*.

These exercises would be exercises 2, 5, and 9 of the Cox exercises, as shown in Chapter 12, "Care of the Intervertebral Disc."

CASE 3

A 32-year-old white male, 71 inches tall, weighing 182 pounds, was seen for low back pain and numbness in the right foot. This pain had started 2 years previously with low back and complete right lower extremity pain, but there had been relief of the leg pain except for numbness in the right foot. The patient had been treated by a chiropractor, who gave him this relief, for approximately 4 months. He then developed a severe antalgic posture approximately 1 month prior to seeing us. He also developed complete low back and right lower extremity pain but no testicle pain. He lost approximately 40 pounds of weight. It was suggested that he have a laminectomy.

Examination revealed flexion at 30° and extension at 10°, both of which were extremely painful. Straight leg raising was positive on the right at 40°, creating both low back and leg pain, while the left leg created a well-leg-raising sign at 80° with right low back pain. The right L5-S1 dermatomes were hypesthetic to pinwheel examination. This patient could heel and toe walk normally; however, the right gluteus maximus muscle was approximately grade 4 of 5 strength in comparison to the left. Circulation in the lower extremities was within normal limits.

Radiographic examination (Figs. 6.16 and 6.17) reveals a degenerative spondylolisthesis of L5 on S1, and the partes interarticularis are bilaterally intact. Anterolateral lipping and spurring are noted at the body plates of L4-L5. The transverse process of L5 is spatulated on the right side. The facets at L4-L5 appear to be tropic. Review of a myelogram taken by the surgeon revealed a large, central-type disc prolapse at the L4-L5 level and a

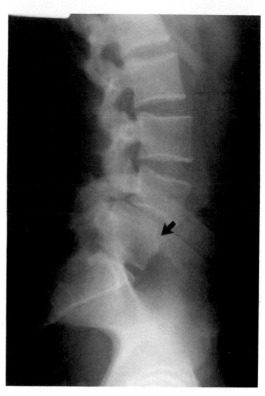

Figure 6.9. L4 is anterior on L5. Note the step defect (*arrow*) of the L5 anterior superior vertebral plate due to failure of epiphyseal development.

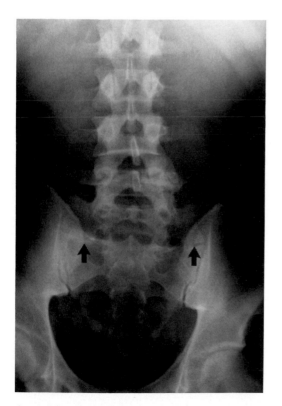

Figure 6.8. Both L5 transverse processes are overdeveloped and spatulated, forming pseudoarticulations with the sacrum (*arrows*). (This case is courtesy of Alice Wright, D.C., of Hatfield, Pennsylvania.)

smaller L5 right discal protrusion. Figure 6.18, an oblique view, reveals no pars interarticularis defect.

Treatment was instituted with the usual rule that, if at least 50% improvement was not obtained within 3 to 4 weeks of treatment, surgery would be recommended. Of course, if there should be any increased motor weakness or cauda equina symptoms, surgery would be recommended earlier. The results of flexion distraction manipulation were that, 6 days following the onset of treatment, the patient stated that he was "remarkably free of pain." He was started on Nautilus exercise consisting of extension. This patient had extremely short hamstring muscles, and stretching with proprioceptive neuromuscular facilitation was instituted. Treatment of the acupressure points B22 to B54 was utilized.

This is the only case of transitional segmentation with spondylolisthesis at the same level that this author has seen.

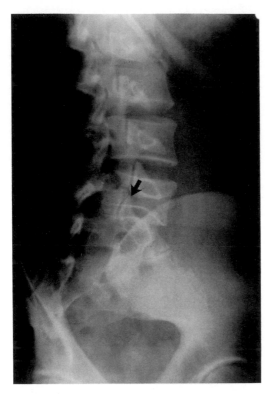

Figure 6.10. The *arrow* denotes the pars interarticularis fracture at L4.

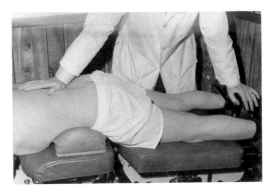

Figure 6.11. Distraction is applied to a patient with a transitional segment of L5. A flexion Dutchman roll is placed under the L5 level, and the thenar contact of the doctor's right hand contacts the spinous process of L4, the vertebra above the transitional segment. A downward tractive force is applied to the caudal section of the table, while the spinous process is vectored cephalad. This force is applied until the doctor feels the space between the spinous processes under the contact hand tauten or begin to separate. This application of tractive force is applied repeatedly at about five or six such applications per 20-second period of time until such time as the desired motion is sensed by the contact hand. We then place the segments through the other ranges of motion as shown in Figure 6.12. The above technique is applied to the transitional segment, without spondylolisthesis above the level of transitional segment, as shown in Figure 6.2, in which the patient has a degenerative disc and loss of the intervertebral foramen vertical diameter at L4-L5, forming a facet syndrome at the L4-L5 level. If a spondylolisthesis is present above the transitional segment, the same procedure of care is followed *except* that the contact hand will be on the spinous process of the vertebra above the spondylolisthetic segment. Figure 6.9 shows this type of case.

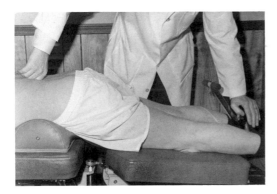

Figure 6.12. Lateral flexion is applied to the facet joints following the application of flexion distraction as shown in Figure 6.11. The spinous process is held firmly between the index finger and thumb as lateral flexion is applied with the caudal section of the Zenith-Cox instrument. The contact of the spinous process is done to ensure that the joints being adjusted are those directly caudal to the spinous contact. That is, if the fourth lumbar spinous process is contacted, only the facet joints between L4 and L5 are mobilized. *Remember,* in the absence of sciatica, the facets are moved through their full physiological ranges of motion. If sciatica is present, *only flexion is performed until 50% relief of the leg pain is attained.*

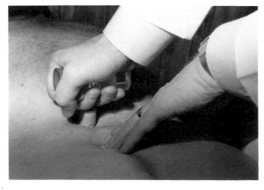

Figure 6.13. Acupressure points are treated with deep compression before and after the application of manipulative procedures to the vertebrae found at lesion. These acupressure points are outlined in the Chapter 12, "Care of the Intervertebral Disc."

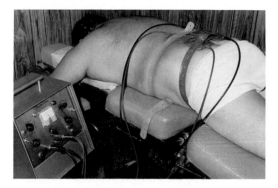

Figure 6.14. Tetanizing current is applied to the paravertebral muscles following manipulation, and sometimes prior to manipulation if muscle spasm is great.

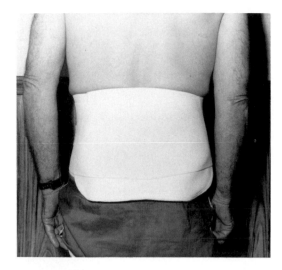

Figure 6.15. A lumbar support orthosis is worn for stabilization in patients with great pain, especially if instability of the segment above the transitional segment is found.

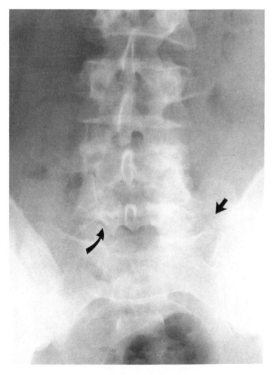

Figure 6.16. The posteroanterior x-ray study reveals the right transverse process of L5 to be spatulated (*straight arrow*), while the left superior sacral facet forms an articulation with the lamina of L5 (*curved arrow*).

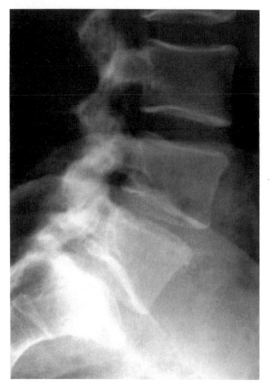

Figure 6.17. A lateral projection view of the patient in Figure 6.16 shows that L5 is anterior on the sacrum, a pseudospondylolisthesis at the level of a transitional segment. This is an unusual condition, since pseudospondylolisthesis occurs 90% of the time at the L4 segment.

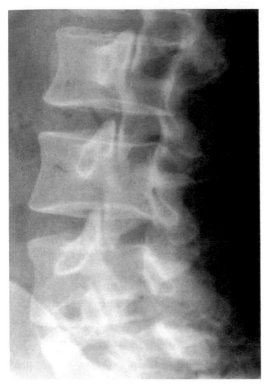

Figure 6.18. Oblique view shows that there is intact pars interarticularis at L5, the level of forward slippage shown in Figure 6.17.

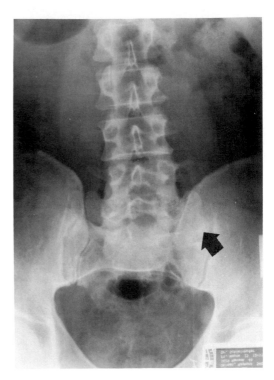

Figure 6.19. Left lateral flexion of the lumbar spine is seen, with left lateral flexion subluxation of L4 on L5 noted. The right transverse process of L5 is spatulated, forming a pseudoarticulation with the sacrum (*arrow*).

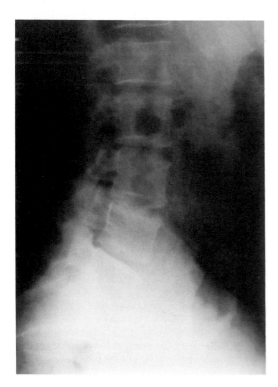

Figure 6.20. Note the rudimentary disc at L5-S1, the level of the transitional segment. The L4-L5 disc is degenerated as seen typically in Bertolotti's syndrome.

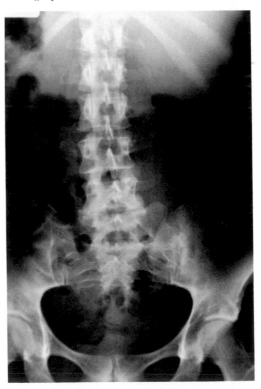

Figure 6.21. Both L6 transverse processes are spatulated, forming pseudoarticulation with the sacrum. Also note the L5-S1 disc thinning and left rotation subluxation of L5 on L6.

CASE 4

A 40-year-old male had had right L5 dermatome pain for approximately 1 month. He had seen a neurosurgeon and had a myelogram, and surgery was recommended.

Examination findings included straight leg raising positive on the right at approximately 20°. The deep reflexes were active and +2 equal bilaterally with no signs of motor weakness noted in the patient.

X-ray examination (Figs. 6.19 and 6.20) reveals a levorotatory list of the lumbar spine with L4 in left lateral flexion subluxation on L5 and a transitional segment of L5 on the sacrum. This transitional segment has a very large spatulated transverse process forming a pseudoarthrosis on the right side with the sacrum. Note the rudimentary disc at the L5-S1 level.

The diagnosis here is a Bertolotti's syndrome, meaning the combination of a transitional segment with an intervertebral disc protrusion above. To reiterate, this means that all the flexion and extension movement now must occur at the L4-L5 disc, although normally 75% of such

movement occurs at the L5-S1 disc, which is now rudimentary, partially fused at the sacrum, and incapable of motion. This will lead to early degenerative change at the L4-L5 disc, eventually causing protrusion and compression of the L5 nerve root. This case would represent a right L4 lateral disc protrusion.

Treatment consisted of 3 weeks of daily flexion distraction, which resulted in progressive relief of the leg pain. It is to be remembered that transitional segment, statistically shown by the 576 case studies documented in Chapter 1 of this book, requires more days and more visits than any other condition to achieve relief (1).

CASE 5

Figures 6.21 and 6.22 are anteroposterior and lateral views of the lumbar spine and pelvis which reveal spatulization of the L6 transverse process, forming pseudoarticulations with the sacrum and illia. Figure 6.22 shows the degenerated L5-L6 disc above the transitional sixth segment. You will note the loss of disc space and the traction spurring of both the L5 and L6

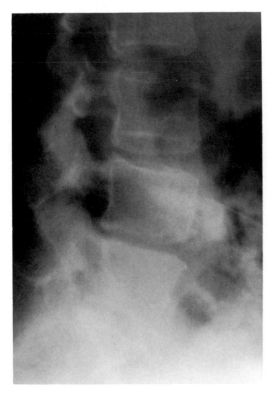

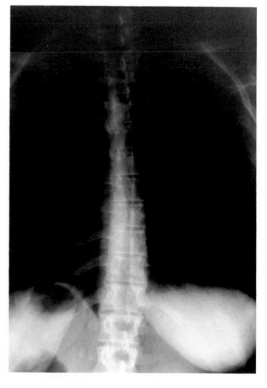

Figure 6.22. The L5-L6 disc is markedly degenerated in this 40-year-old female, with traction spurring present at the anterior lateral plates of L5-L6.

Figure 6.23. Note the dextrorotatory scoliosis of the thoracolumbar spine in the patient with the L6 transitional segment.

vertebral body plates. This is a good example of Bertolotti's syndrome.

Figure 6.23 reveals that this patient also has a dextrorotatory scoliosis of the thoracic spine.

This was a patient who had been involved in an automobile accident, sustained rotational-type injuries to the
lumbar spine, and developed back pain. It took approximately 6 weeks of manipulative and therapeutic care,
as outlined in this chapter, to give this patient maximum
relief.

CASE 6

A 33-year-old male was seen for low back pain subsequent to playing softball. He later bent forward,
coughed, and felt severe sharp pain in the lumbosacral
spine. He took muscle relaxants but continued to have
pain and stiffness.

Imaging studies are shown in Figures 6.24 through
6.30. These were taken 2 years previously to the current
injury, when this man had had left fifth lumbar nerve
root dysesthesia of the lower extremity and had under-

gone surgery to correct it. Figure 6.24 reveals the
spatulated transverse process of L5 as it forms a
pseudoarticulation with the sacrum. Figure 6.25 demonstrates the rudimentary L5-S1 disc that accompanies
the transitional segment. Figure 6.26, on oblique projection, further illustrates the underdeveloped facet
joints at the transitional segment. Figure 6.27 reveals
the discal protruding defect into the anterior dye-filled
subarachnoid space. Figure 6.28 is the postero-anterior
study that shows the filling defect due to the L4-L5 protrusion. Figure 6.29, oblique myelographic study, also
shows the defect. The CT scan in Figure 6.30 classically
shows asymmetrical left posterior protrusion of the left
L4-L5 disc into the lateral recess and intervertebral canal.

This is an excellent representation of Bertolotti's syndrome with which to end this chapter. At the time we
saw the patient, he had no leg pain. This patient did
heavy manual labor entailing repetitive bending and
lifting. He was placed on a strong regimen of abdominal, low back, and gluteus maximus muscle strengthening exercises. His hamstring muscles were especially
contracted, and proprioceptive neuromuscular facilitation technique was used in lengthening them.

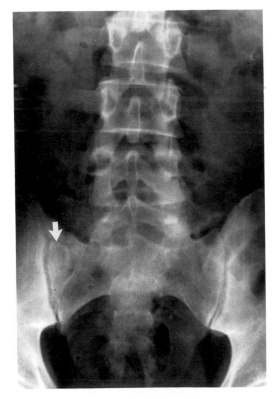

Figure 6.24. The spatulated transverse process (*arrow*) forms a pseudoarthrosis with the sacrum.

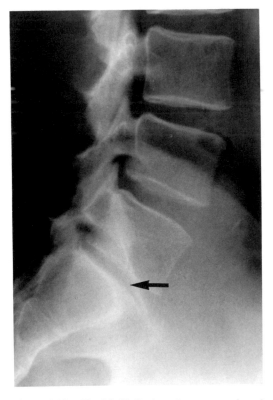

Figure 6.25. The L5-S1 disc is rudimentary, as is typical of the transitional segment (*arrow*).

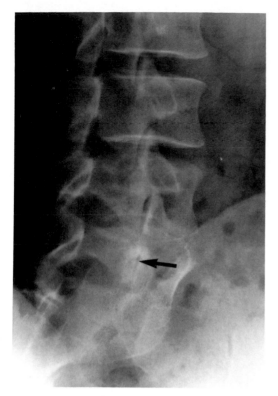

Figure 6.26. Oblique view shows the rudimentary facet joint formation (*arrow*) compared to the normal levels above.

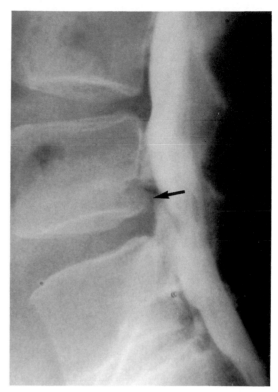

Figure 6.27. Lateral projection of the myelographic examination shows the filling defect (*arrow*) behind the L4-L5 disc space due to discal protrusion compressing the dye-filled subarachnoid space.

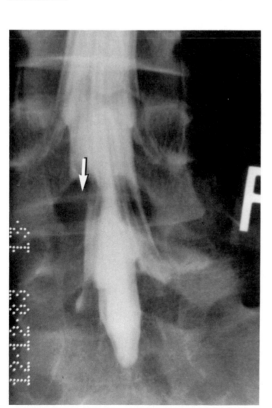

Figure 6.28. Posterior-anterior myelographic study shows the filling defect at L4-L5 (*arrow*).

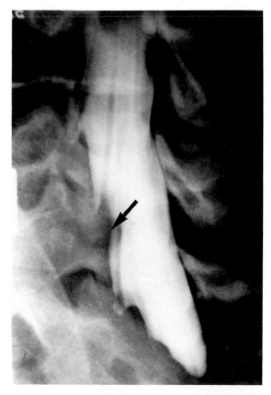

Figure 6.29. Oblique myelographic study shows the L4-L5 discal defect (*arrow*).

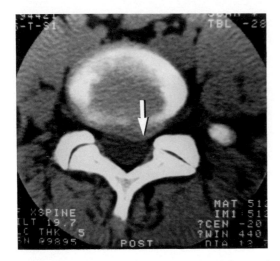

Figure 6.30. The CT scan shows the large, left central discal protrusion that stenoses the lateral recess and enters the intervertebral canal (*arrow*).

Flexion distraction manipulation at the L4-L5 level was administered, along with range-of-motion palpation and restoration of motion to the entire lumbar spine with lateral flexion, circumduction, and progressive rotation into the upper lumbar levels. This patient made good progress in 1 month of care, at the end of which he stated he felt better than at any time since his surgery 2 years previously.

References

1. Cox JM, Shreiner S: Chiropractic manipulation in low back pain and sciatica: statistical data on the diagnosis, treatment, and response of 576 consecutive cases. *J Manipulative Physiol Ther* 7:1–11, 1984.
2. Schwerdtner HP: Lumbosacral transitional anomalies as relapse causes in chirotherapeutic treatment techniques. *Manuelle Medizin* 24:11–15, 1986.
3. Bressler H, Deltoff M: Sacroiliac syndrome associated with lumbosacral anomalies: a case report. *J Manipulative Physiol Ther* 7:173, 1984.
4. Avrahami E, Cohn DF, Yaron M: Computerized tomography, clinical and x-ray correlations in the hemisacralized 5th lumbar vertebra. *Clin Rheumatol* 5(3):332, 1986.
5. Cailliet R: *Low Back Pain Syndrome*. Philadelphia, FA Davis, 1966.
6. Weinstein PR, Ehni G, Wilson CB: *Lumbar Spondylosis—Diagnosis, Management, and Surgical Treatment*. Chicago, Year Book, 1977, pp 14–15.
7. Keim HA, Kirkaldy-Willis WH: Clinical symposia. *Ciba Found Symp* 32(6):89, 1980.
8. Wigh RE: Transitional lumbosacral discs. *Spine* (March/April), 1981.
9. Castellvi A, Goldstein L, Chan D: Lumbosacral transitional vertebrae and their relationship with lumbar extradural defects. *Spine* 9(5):494, 1984.

7

Stenosis

James M. Cox, D.C., D.A.C.B.R.

True Education Makes for Inequality:

The Inequality of Individuality,

The Inequality of Success;

The Glorious Inequality of Talent, of Genius;

For Inequality, Not Mediocrity,

Individual Superiority, Not Standardization,

Is the Measure of the Progress of the World.

    —Felix E. Schelling

Lumbar spinal stenosis is narrowing of the lumbar spinal canal, the lateral recesses, and the intervertebral foramina by bone encroachment, soft tissue changes, or both (1). The narrowing may be congenital or acquired (2). A lateral recess stenosis is a narrowing of the lateral recess of the spinal canal; this is usually acquired. Lumbar spinal and lateral recess stenosis have solid anatomical and pathophysiological foundations leading to clinical findings of intermittent radicular symptoms such as pain, paresthesias, and weakness in the lower extremities induced by standing and walking. Lumbar spinal and lateral recess stenosis are indistinguishable pathophysiologically (3).

Figure 7.1 shows the various diameters of the vertebral canal. The lateral recess is bordered anteriorly by the vertebral body posterior surface, posteriorly by the superior articular facet, and laterally by the pedicle, while opening medially into the vertebral canal.

From Figure 7.1, it can be seen that the lateral recess can be encroached, or stenosed, by the following:

1. Facet joint hypertrophic degenerative changes, probably best seen in superior articular facet *arthrotic* hypertrophy entrapping a lumbar nerve root coursing through the lateral recess;
2. Posterolateral disc protrusion or prolapse;
3. Ligamentum flavum hypertrophy;
4. Spondylolisthesis (2);
5. Lumbar fusion secondary bone overgrowth;
6. Degenerative disc disease.

PATHOGENESIS OF SPINAL STENOSIS PAIN

Traction is produced on neural tissue as the spine rotates, flexes, or extends itself. Normal persons have sufficient room in the canal and lateral recesses for molding and gliding; hence, movement produces no clinical symptoms. However, if the size of the canal is further narrowed by bony or ligamentous proliferations, symptoms appear (1).

Pain may be the result of direct nerve impingement, but it has been postulated that very high-grade obstructions could at least partially block

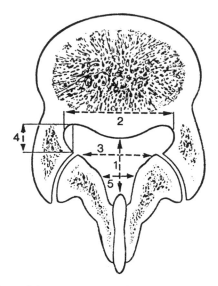

Figure 7.1. Cross-section of vertebral canal at L5 with various diameters. *1*, Sagittal diameter of spinal canal; *2*, interpeduncular distance; *3*, interfacet distance; *4*, lateral recess; *5*, interlaminar distance.

lymphatic and venous channels in the dura or its sleeves. This could cause a buildup of cerebrospinal fluid below the obstruction, collapsing the venous return and producing stagnant anoxia (4).

Axon reflexes via the autonomic nervous system are postulated to account for the pain (5).

It is the integration of causative factors causing nerve root irritation that helps to explain low back and leg pain symptoms. Stenosis may be the most important element in determining symptoms, their severity, response to treatment, and prognosis of recurrence. A patient may have a large disc protrusion but also a large-diameter vertebral canal and lateral recess and therefore have no symptoms, whereas the same disc protrusion may cause severe motor and sensory findings in a patient with a stenotic canal. Figure 7.2 demonstrates how the nerve roots lie snugly within the lateral bony recess prior to exiting the intervertebral foramina. The L5 and S1 nerve roots lying within the lateral recesses are more vulnerable to compression from a protruding intervertebral disc than the higher lumbar roots lying within a rounder vertebral foramen (Fig. 7.3).

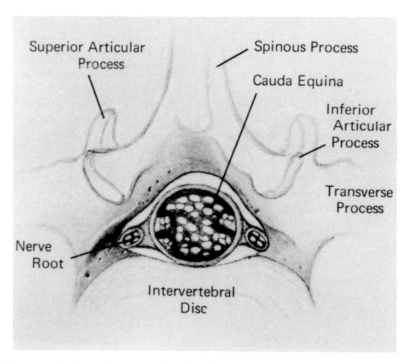

Figure 7.2. Prior to exiting from the intervertebral foramina, the nerve root lies at the lateralmost portion of the vertebral foramen. (Reproduced with permission from Finneson BE: *Low Back Pain,* ed 2. Philadelphia, JB Lippincott, 1980, p 9.)

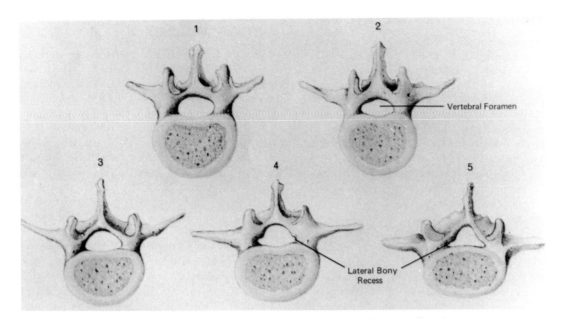

Figure 7.3. The five lumbar vertebrae. Note the *lateral bony recess* formed by the last two vertebrae. (Reproduced with permission from Finneson BE: *Low Back Pain,* ed 2. Philadelphia, JB Lippincott, 1980, p 8.)

Figure 7.4 exemplifies how a patent, non-stenotic canal can accommodate a relatively large disc protrusion without creating symptoms, whereas a stenotic lateral recess would compromise the nerve root with compression, creating marked pain and motor findings. Therefore, the same disc protrusion size would not be as important as the size of the canal it bulges into.

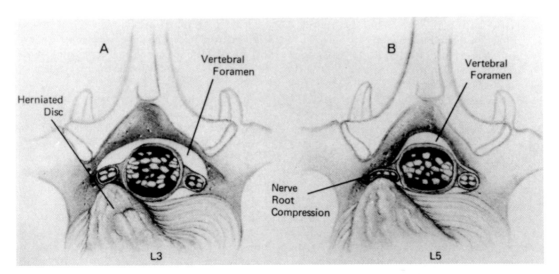

Figure 7.4. **A,** A relatively small intervertebral disc protrusion may not produce significant nerve root compression when the vertebral foramen is oval and may permit elevation of the root. **B,** When the nerve root lies within a lateral bony recess, even a small disc protrusion may produce severe root compression. (Reproduced with permission from Finneson BE: *Low Back Pain,* ed 2. Philadelphia, JB Lippincott, 1980, p 9.)

GROWTH FACTORS IN STENOSIS

Does infant malnutrition produce smaller adult spinal canals? Lumbar and thoracic vertebrae (n = 1073) from a prehistoric American Indian population (15 to 55 years of age) were measured for anteroposterior (AP) and transverse (TR) vertebral canal sizes, nerve root tunnel (intervertebral foramen) widths (NRT), vertebral heights (VH), vertebral osteophytosis (VO), and tibial lengths. They underwent a dietary change from hunting and gathering, with a protein-rich (PR) diet to maize agriculture, with a protein-deficient (PD) diet, between 950 and 1300 A.D. Multivariate analyses controlled for age, sex, culture, NRT, VH, VO, and wedging were done. Canal size was significantly smaller in the PD. AP diameters were generally and highly correlated with NRT, and thus both spinal stenosis and sciatica may have a developmental basis. Canal size was independent of statural components. Consequently, canal size is a most powerful tool in assessing the presence of infant malnutrition. Moreover, perhaps the association between canal size and low back pain (LBP) found in living populations has been underestimated, and this component of LBP is preventable (6).

Roaf (7) has provided rough estimates in inches for lumbar and thoracic spine growth from 2 to 16 years of age. The lumbar vertebrae and discs grow approximately twice as much as the thoracic. He suggests (without data) that, in the thoracic region, the posterior elements may grow faster than the anterior, and that this may be reversed in the lumbar region.

Using data from Porter et al. (8), Eisenstein (9), and Hinck et al. (10), it appears that at birth the canal is approximately 65% of its adult size, and by 5 years it is 90% of its adult size. In addition, within the canal, the anteroposterior (AP) diameters appear to be more advanced than the transverse (TR) vertebral canal.

First, the estimates of the association between low back pain (LBP) and canal size, derived from ultrasound readings, using a 15° oblique angle, suggest that only 2 mm (a decrease in canal size of about 15%) separates persons with and without LBP (8). The frequency of small TR diameters and LBP has been suggested to be 53% (11). Consequently, if AP diameters are most variable and most frequently associated with LBP, then even less than 2 mm may separate those persons with and without LBP. Indeed, more than 53% of patients with LBP may have AP spinal stenosis.

CAUSES OF NERVE ROOT SYMPTOMS

Today, the fact is being discussed that large portions of the population have disc protrusion yet have no symptoms. Weisel et al. (12) reported that three neuroradiologists, in a blind study, found 35% of 52 asymptomatic patients to have a herniated nucleus pulposus on computed tomographic (CT) scan. Further, it was pointed out that 24% of normal patients undergoing myelography, patients with no history of low back or sciatic pain, showed significant abnormalities. Perhaps the reason for the absence of pain in these "normal" individuals is absence of sufficient pressure on the nerve root by the herniated disc to elicit "pain." Also keep in mind that stenosis increases the probability of nerve root compression. A decrease in vertebral canal size by as little as 15% (2 mm) separates persons with and without back pain. Indeed, more than 53% of patients with low back pain may have spinal stenosis (11).

Rydevik et al. (13) showed that the functional changes induced by nerve root compression can be caused by mechanical nerve fiber deformation associated with intervertebral disc herniation and spinal stenosis; also, the changes may be a *consequence of changes in nerve root microcirculation*, leading to ischemia and formation of intraneural edema. Nerve root compression can, by different neurophysiological mechanisms, induce motor weakness and altered sensibility or pain. Intraneural edema and demyelination seem to be critical factors for the production of pain in association with nerve root compression. Rydevik compares the jeopardized microcirculation of the nerve to a "closed compartment syndrome" within the foramen.

While no in vivo measurements of the pressures that act on a human nerve root, as for example by a disc herniation, are known to this author or Rydevik, Rydevik (13) extrapolates from existing knowledge on the swelling pressure of a nucleus pulposus herniation. He states that the pressure demonstrated on in vitro nucleus pulposus specimens could reach several hundred millimeters of mercury if the specimen was exposed to free fluid within a confined space. A sequestered fragment in the foramen could be speculated to create high pressure levels in the nerve root, but the validity of the hypothesis needs to be proven. Yet when we consider that the peripheral nerve has a perineurium but nerve root does not, and that the peripheral nerve has a well-developed epineural connective tissue where it passes close to bone and joint, whereas the nerve root has a poorly developed epineural lining, we see that nerve roots are more susceptible to mechanical deformation than peripheral nerves (13).

A peripheral nerve, at 30 to 50 mm Hg compression, demonstrates change in intraneural blood flow, vascular permeability, and axonal transport (14, 15, 16, 17). The rabbit tibial nerve showed these changes at 20 to 30 mm Hg; with complete ischemia at 60 to 80 mm Hg and higher pressures resulting in delayed recovery of intraneural blood flow (13).

PAIN MECHANISMS IN NERVE ROOT COMPRESSION

Compression of normal peripheral nerve or nerve root may induce numbness but usually does not cause pain. *Experimental investigations of human peripheral nerves, in vivo, have indicated that the numbness induced is a result of ischemia, not mechanical nerve fiber deformation, of the compressed segment. If a nerve root—or a peripheral nerve—is the site of chronic irritation, however, even minor mechanical deformation may induce radiating pain. This has been demonstrated by placing sutures or inflatable catheters around nerve roots at the time of surgery for herniated discs and postoperatively inducing stretching or compression of the nerve root* (13).

We see that stenotic problems may create pressure levels on nerve roots but not be sufficient to cause motor or sensory findings. Thus, it seems that a nerve root can tolerate some degree of pressure from whatever the cause. Some persons who have never had pain reveal disc protrusion on CT or myelography, yet they could have a large vertebral canal, small dural sac, no ligamentum flavum or facet hypertrophy, and a small disc protrusion. This combination of factors could result in minimal pressure on the nerve root, not enough to cause symptoms. On the other hand, a person with a small vertebral canal, a large dural sac area, and facet lateral recess hypertrophic stenosis with ligamentum flavum thickening could have severe pain in the presence of a moderate or even small disc protrusion causing high compressive forces on the nerve root.

THECAL SAC SIZE IN STENOSIS

The need for measurement systems for stenosis has recently been shown by the work of Schon-strom et al. (18, 19) with the introduction of a new measurement for the transverse area of the dural sac on CT scan. They felt that bony measurements alone did not reliably identify patients with spinal stenosis; the dural sac transverse area is the most accurate method of identifying stenosis, with the critical size for the dural sac below 100 mm. Further, they found the most common causes of spinal stenosis to be intervertebral disc and ligamentum flavum soft tissue encroachment, as well as facet degeneration hypertrophic changes (18). By careful manometric monitoring of highly pressure-sensitive catheters in the dural sac of seven spines removed at autopsy, Schon-strom et al. (19) found that circumferential restriction of the transverse area of the intact cauda equina to 60 to 80 mm caused a buildup of pressure in the dural sac. Once that critical size was reached, even a *minimal* further reduction of the area caused a distinct pressure increase on the nerve roots.

These authors note that again we see that the dural sac can tolerate a degree of compression above which pressure increases create symptoms. The compression of the cauda equina was most commonly due to intervertebral disc protrusion or ligamentum flavum hypertrophy (18).

SIGNS OF DORSAL ROOT GANGLION COMPRESSION

Reports have been cited of a series of patients with leg pain whose dorsal root ganglia were located more proximal than usual and lay within the nerve root canal (20). These proximal ganglia became entrapped in a space that although slightly narrowed, would have accommodated a normal nerve root without causing symptoms (Fig. 7.5).

There were 11 patients, two men and nine women. Their ages ranged from 28 to 60 years, and over half were in the 4th and 5th decade. Most of these patients presented with an exceptionally long history of symptoms prior to diagnosis (average, 7 years).

Pain was aggravated by the standing position in seven patients. Seven complained of intermittent claudication. The pain radiated down the leg in a sciatic distribution in all patients and extended to the ankle or foot in eight. Radiation to the groin was reported in three patients, two with compression of the L5 ganglion and one with compression of both L5 and S1 ganglia.

Physical examination was entirely normal in

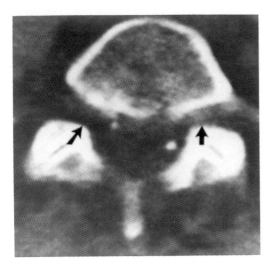

Figure 7.5. Subarticular entrapment of left L5 DRG (*straight arrow*) and asymptomatic right DRG (*oblique arrow*). (Reproduced with permission from Vanderlinden RG: Subarticular entrapment of the dorsal root ganglion as a cause of sciatic pain. *Spine* 9(1):21, 1984.)

three patients. Straight leg raising was limited to 70° in the affected lower limb in four patients, and significantly reduced to 60° in one and to 30° in another. There was muscle weakness or wasting in four patients, and sensory abnormalities were present in three. The ankle reflex was depressed in three patients and absent in one.

Operative Findings

The surgical treatment of subarticular entrapment of a dorsal root ganglion was identical to the treatment of nerve root compression in lateral spinal stenosis. The nerve root canal was unroofed by removing the medial third of the apophyseal joint and pars interarticularis. Hemilaminectomy of L5 and laminotomy of L4 and S1 were often necessary to obtain satisfactory decompression. Occasionally, the inferomedial portion of the pedicle was removed as well.

All 11 patients underwent surgical decompression. Subarticular entrapment of the L5 DRG was found in six patients, entrapment of both the L5 and S1 DRG in three, and entrapment of the S1 DRG alone in two (20).

CLASSIFICATION OF LUMBAR STENOSIS

I. Congenital
  A. Achondroplasia;
  B. Developmental—here the central canal is narrowed in both the sagittal and lateral dimensions (21). Short pedicles and overdeveloped lamina can cause the narrowing.
II. Acquired stenosis (degenerative)
  A. Thickened, irregular laminae (22);
  B. Ligamentum flaval hypertrophy (23);[a]
  C. Soft tissue hypertrophy—from mechanical instability and degenerative disease (24);[a]
  D. Posterior articular joint disease;
  E. Trefoil configuration;
  F. Intervertebral disc protrusion;
  G. Spondylolisthesis—with forward L5 displacement on the sacrum, the fifth lumbar nerve root may be kinked around the lower border of the pedicle or compressed by degenerative changes occurring between the pedicle and the upper sacral border (21);[a]
  H. Posterior intervertebral body plate hypertrophic osteophytes into foramina;
  I. Narrowing of lateral recess by hypertrophic articular processes.
III. Iatrogenic stenosis
  This occurs with excessive stress placed on a motion segment above a level of spinal fusion (25).[a] The interspinous ligament and ligamentum flavum become thickened, the spinous process base projects into the canal, and the laminae protrude ventrally.

  There may be proliferation of bone under the fused area, with thickening of the laminae and ligamentum flava associated with bulging of the posterior articular process. Disc herniation is common in both sets of circumstances.

  Laminectomy and discectomy may also cause progressive deterioration of the intervertebral disc, with consequent migration of the superior articular process and continued degenerative changes. Scar formation at the operative site may contribute to local stenosis (24).
IV. Foraminal (lateral recess) stenosis

---

[a] See case presentations at the end of this chapter, which depict these causes of stenosis.

Trauma or recurrent inflammation leads to hypertrophy and intrusion of the superior facet into the lateral recess (26).

Lumbar Degenerative Disc Disease Induced Stenosis

The triple joint complex, made up of the two posterior zygapophyseal joints and single anterior intervertebral disc, can be affected by trauma or degenerative disc disease. One of the joints of the complex begins the process of degeneration, and it may or may not be symptom producing. However, since the function of the three joints are so intertwined, changes in any one eventually affects the other.

With combined triple joint complex degeneration, there will be eventual loss of disc height and facet cartilage, with resultant ligamentous laxity of other ligamentous restraints. Stress will be transferred to levels above and below, where the process will repeat itself until multilevel spondylosis occurs (27). Nerve entrapment can occur at each level.

Algorithm of Stenosis Development

Panjabi (28) probably best develops the stages of stenosis in the following algorithm:

1. Asymmetric disc injury at one functional spinal unit (FSU);

2. Disturbed kinematics of FSUs above and below injury;

3. Asymmetric movements at facet joints;

4. Unequal sharing of facet loads;

5. High load on one facet joint;

6. Cartilage degenerative *or* facet atrophy and narrowing of IVF (intervertebral foramen).

CLINICAL CHIROPRACTIC PRINCIPLES OF STENOSIS

Many in the chiropractic profession remember the work of Earl Rich, D.C., radiologist for the Lincoln Chiropractic College, on pedicogenic spondylosis. This man, who died prior to the full impact of his efforts in this field being felt, contributed greatly to our understanding of a very important aspect of low back pain. The implications of Rich's work on pedicogenic stenosis in the study of the etiology of low back pain are being stressed today.

Lumbar spondylosis is the lipping or marginal vertebral osteophytic formation secondary to degenerative disc disease. It is not observed in the absence of disc degeneration and collapse (29, 30, 31); i.e., it is not noted in the presence of a normal disc. Vernon-Roberts and Pirie (32) believe that there is a direct relationship between the degree of disc degeneration, the marginal osteophyte formation on the vertebral bodies, and the apophyseal joint changes which suggest that disc degeneration is the primary event leading to degenerative spondylosis. Disc degeneration is the genesis of osteoarthrosis of the apophyseal joints, as well as of the spondylosis seen commonly in the lumbar spine. Figure 7.6 shows the spondylotic change seen so typically in the lum-

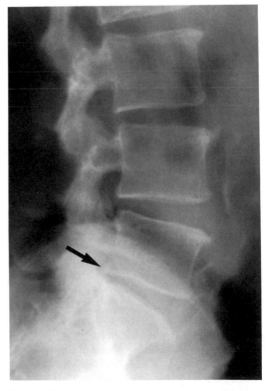

Figure 7.6. Radiograph of discogenic spondyloarthrosis at the L5-S1 level. The facet syndrome is present at both the L4 and the L5 level (*arrow*) with L5 posterior on sacrum.

bar spine, which follows collapse of the disc and protrusion of the annulus. According to Collins (33), spondylosis primarily refers to separation of the annulus fibers from their firmly embedded attachments to the margins of the vertebral bodies. Periosteal elevation stimulates osteoblastic activity, resulting in the anterolateral osteophytic change and the possible bridging that follow. Osteophytosis, therefore, is the spondylotic effect of intervertebral nuclear protrusion through the annulus, elevating the periosteum and resulting in subperiosteal osteogenesis.

The term arthrosis describes the sclerosis and loss of joint space that accompanies a synovial lined joint, namely, the articular facets. Thus, we refer to discogenic spondylosis as an early change in disc degeneration and to discogenic spondyloarthrosis as a later manifestation. Interestingly, according to Schmorl and Junghanns (34) the marginal osteophytes may appear within 4 to 8 weeks following injury. Remember, therefore, that the term osteoarthrosis of the spine is used to refer only to the degenerative changes occurring in the synovial lined joints, namely, the articular facets, not to changes occurring in the anterolateral vertebral plates following disc degeneration.

Symptoms of a Stenotic Canal

Until recently, the term *intermittent claudication* was believed to be associated with reduced blood flow to the lower extremities, resulting in hypoxia of the muscles with attendant cramping and pain in the lower extremities. The French applied this term to the atheroscleromatous plaqueing of the arteries in old carriage horses when these horses were unable to walk due to limp. This concept was applied to humans with similar plaqueing until vascular surgeons found that there was no interference with the blood supply of the lower extremities and further explanation for this phenomenon had to be made. Today, the term *neurogenic intermittent claudication* is used and applies to those conditions found in people who have such lower extremity pain and who have no ischemia to the leg muscles but have compression of the cauda equina in the lumbar spine.

In the conclusion to their article, Dyck et al. (35) state that the diagnosis of neurogenic intermittent claudication can be made on the clinical findings alone and that demonstration of a defor-

mity by myelography is not diagnostic proof of the syndrome.

The pain of intermittent claudication may be unilateral or bilateral and may be more severe in one leg than in the other. It is caused by or aggravated by walking or standing for a long period of time. The pain is relieved by flexion of the lumbar spine and is aggravated by extension of the spine. It is interesting to note that in 1911 Goldthwaite (36) was credited with paralysis of a patient when he placed that patient in a hyperextension plaster cast for the treatment of low back pain.

Figure 7.7 is a differential diagnostic chart of lower extremity pain as caused by arterial insufficiency and neurogenic claudication. According to Weinstein et al. (367), the most classic clinical symptom of a narrowed lumbar canal is aggravation of the pain in the lower extremities following exaggerated lordosis of the lumbar spine. This classic clinical symptom is one of numbness and tingling or a feeling that the legs are asleep. It may be brought on by standing, bending back-

Finding	Arterial Insufficient Claudication	Neurogenic Claudication
Arterial pulses of femoral, popliteal, post. tibial, and dorsalis pedis	One or more diminished	Normal
Pain in legs induced by	Exercise such as walking but not by posture change	Walking, standing kneeling, hyperextension
Relieved by	Rest	Bend forward, squat, flexion
Accompanied by low back, buttock, thigh pain	Rare	Common
Type pain	Cramping is severe if exercise is continued	Dysesthesia such as numbness, tingling, and burning
Comes at rest	No	Yes
Sensory loss	Rare	Mild
Leg raise	Normal	Normal
Arterial murmur	Yes	No
Plain x-ray findings	Arteriosclerosis of abdominal aorta or iliac and femoral vessels	Discogenic spondyloarthrosis

Figure 7.7. Differential diagnostic factors of intermittent claudication.

ward, or reaching overhead. Ehni (38) has shown that during myelography the extension of the lumbar spine produces total block of the column, whereas flexion permits the dye to pass through the lumbar spine.

An interesting diagnostic point was presented by Dyck et al. who said that the ankle reflex, when accompanying intermittent claudication, may be absent after exercise and present when at rest. Furthermore, Weinstin et al. (37) noted that there were two patients in the claudication groups who when ambulatory had urinary retention but following rest were able to void normally.

Although an exact neurological explanation for the changes in lumbar stenosis is difficult, certain facts have been established. Sunderland (39) believes that ischemia of a nerve root must accompany any compression that is great enough to alter its nerve function. Such compression produces nerve sheath constriction, axonal narrowing, and partial obstruction of the vasa nervorum. Nerve roots are more vulnerable to stretch than are peripheral nerves (40). The pain of neurogenic claudication is that of paresthesias and numbness in the legs due to the mechanical compression of the nerve roots. While documenting this phenomenon, Ehni (38) found simultaneous impairment of the perceptions of touch, pressure, and pain stimuli applied to the area supplied by the affected nerves. He believes that this may explain the imprecise and puzzling complaint of the patient who reports that his painful legs "go dead" or "go out" when he walks or stands.

Sebolt and Elies (41) report that 28 patients in the neurology department of the University of Tubingen who underwent disc surgery were found to have a 25% increase of blood supply to the lower extremities within 2 to 3 weeks following surgical root decompression. An explanation for the relief of leg pain and for the increased blood flow in the lower extremity is that the irritation of the cauda equina by disc protrusion or a narrowed canal also creates a relative ischemia of the involved nerve roots. This results in hypoxia, which is further aggravated by exercise and the increased oxygen consumption in the activated nerves (42). Evans (43) found that his patients could walk farther before claudication symptoms appeared when they breathed 100% pure oxygen. Experimental studies have demonstrated that oxygen uptake in nerves increases proportionately with an increase in frequency of fiber stimulation (44).

Therefore, in summary, true intermittent claudication due to arterial blockage, as in atheroscleromatous plaqueing of the femoral arteries, results in lower extremity pain at exercise, which is relieved by rest. Hyperextension of the lumbar spine does not aggravate the pain associated with true intermittent claudication. In neurogenic intermittent claudication, the pain not only is brought about by walking but also is brought about by hyperextension of the lumbar spine and by standing and is not relieved by rest. Always remember that the patient with neurogenic intermittent claudication tends to stand in a bent-forward posture, so as to relieve the pressure on the cauda equina. This is not true of the patient with true intermittent claudication.

Warren (as discussed in Ref. 45) set forth three criteria that define what he called true claudication. First, the pain must begin as a muscle cramp in the calf or thigh after the patient has walked a predictable distance. Second, it must be relieved by rest in the standing position after a predictable period of time. Finally, the pain must occur again after the patient walks a similar distance, and the pain must be relieved again by rest in the standing position after the same period of time as before. Exertional leg pain that does not satisfy all of these criteria must be suspected of being neuromuscular in origin. Pain of neuromuscular or skeletal etiology is generally much less consistent than arterial claudication. In contrast to true vascular claudication, the pain may begin in the lower back with radiation into the thigh, calf, and foot. The pain may begin after walking an unpredictable distance or may even occur with the patient in a standing or a sitting position. The history of pain that occurs with standing or sitting should alert the astute clinician to a diagnosis other than vascular claudication. The patient often states that he has good and bad days. He may give a history of being able to walk a prolonged distance on one day and only a few steps on a subsequent day. This pattern of inconsistency argues strongly against a vascular etiology. The pain of musculoskeletal etiology is also relieved if the patient assumes a supine or specific sitting position. Again, this is very uncharacteristic of vascular pain.

Vascular Claudication

The patient with advanced peripheral vascular insufficiency shows evidence of hair loss and skin atrophy. Transcutaneous flow detection based on the principle of the Doppler effect uses blood pressure determination as a standard part of the physical examination for vascular disease. This is routinely measured in both upper extremities. A differential blood pressure between the upper extremities suggests vascular disease in the large branches of the aorta. Doppler testing has made it possible to determine the blood pressure at the ankle level in both the dorsalis pedis and the posterior tibialis artery. Pressure at the ankle should be equal to or slightly greater than arm pressure with the patient in the supine position. A systolic pressure in the ankle less than the systolic pressure in the arm suggests peripheral arterial disease. Comparison of the systolic pressures obtained at the ankle with those in the arm provides the ankle-to-arm index. This index is used to define the presence of hemodynamically significant vascular disease. An index of 0.6 or less has been determined to be diagnostic of vascular insufficiency significant enough to cause intermittent claudication. The index may be as low as 0.26 in the presence of rest, pain, and gangrene. Once it has been established that there is an abnormal index, the next step in this noninvasive evaluation is to measure the postexercise ankle pressure. The normal physiological response to moderate exercise is a slight increase in the ankle pressure. In the presence of occlusive disease to the lower extremities, the major inflow vessels are unable to accommodate the increased demand to the lower extremities. The increased demand results in a lower peripheral resistance, opening of the collateral vascular beds, and a subsequent drop in perfusion pressure in the ankle. As a result of a limited inflow secondary to hemodynamically significant disease, the ankle pressure in patients with claudication falls after a period of exercise. This allows a documentation of the physiological events causing claudication. Exertional leg pain that occurs with walking but does not occur on the exercise bicycle is most characteristic of spinal stenosis. Verbiest (46) in 1954 described a leg pain that was similar to that in the patient with true claudication and was associated with developmental narrowing of the lumbar spinal canal and called it spinal stenosis. Patients with leg pain due to spinal stenosis often experience the onset of symptoms while walking. These patients obtain relief by sitting down or bending at the waist. It is for this reason that these patients do not experience leg pain while pedaling the exercise bicycle.

The lateral recess syndrome (LRS) represents stenosis of the lateral subarticular gutter that will often lead to nerve root compression. The most common etiology is hypertrophy of the superior articular facets, which is associated with lumbar instability and arthrosis of the posterior joint complex. The diagnosis may be made clinically with a routine lumbosacral x-ray series but is not definitive without the use of CT scanning. Recent studies show that spinal manipulation can provide relief and should be considered before surgical referral for decompression is made (47).

STOOP TEST

Dyck (48) states that in claudication patients, stooping increases the sagittal diameter of the vertebral canal and relieves back and leg pain.

It was found that there is a trend toward a narrower-than-normal canal in patients with a prolapsed disc (49). Thus, it has been concluded that, in patients with a prolapsed lumbar intervertebral disc, such narrowing enhances the effect of any disc protrusion, leading to severe symptoms of back and leg pain. Plain film lateral radiographs were made to measure the anteroposterior diameter of the spinal canal from the midline of the back of the vertebral body to the base of the opposing spinous process. Ratios of body to canal were made, with 1:2.5 being normal and 1:4.5 being narrow.

CT scanning has shown that the smallest normal anteroposterior diameters of the lumbar spinal canal occur between the posterior wall of the vertebral body and the anterosuperior margin of the spinous process and that the largest diameters occur at a level at which the inferior margin of the spinous process is opposite the posterosuperior margin of the next lower vertebral body. The smallest anteroposterior diameter that was normal was 11.5 mm (50).

Porter (as discussed in Ref. 51) found that 10% of the healthy population had lumbar spinal canals less than 1.4 cm wide. Of 154 patients with sciatica, 56% had spinal canals less than 1.4 cm wide. The implication is that individuals with narrow canals are more prone to back pain, since the main cause of severe back pain is intervertebral disc damage.

PLAIN RADIOGRAPHIC EVALUATION FOR STENOSIS

Figures 7.8 and 7.9 are photographs of two lumbar vertebrae. Figure 7.8 shows the typical round vertebral canal with fairly well-developed pedicles, whereas Figure 7.9 shows a trefoil canal with underdeveloped pedicles.

Various clinicians have measured the interpedicular and sagittal diameters of the canal. Epstein et al. (52) found the sagittal diameter normally to be 15 to 23 mm, with a measurement of less than 13 mm clinically significant of narrowing. He further noted that accompanying the shortened pedicles are thickened neural arches and prominent facets which further narrow the diameter. Paine and Haung (29) report that the sagittal diameter of canals in patients with stenosis is 8 mm. The pioneer and perhaps the best authority on stenosis of the canal is Verbiest (46), who states that a sagittal diameter of less than 12 mm is definitely too short. His conclusion is based on the measurements of the vertebrae of American (53), Dutch (54), Norwegian and Lapp (55), and White and Zulu skeletons (56). According to Verbiest (46), absolute stenosis is indicated when the sagittal diameter is 10 mm or less, and which may produce signs of radicular compression in the absence of any additional compressive agent, such as disc protrusion, ligamentum flavum hypertyrophy, and lamina hypertrophy. Midsagittal diameters between 10 and 12 mm are classified as relative stenosis and serve as warnings of possible future disturbances caused by the

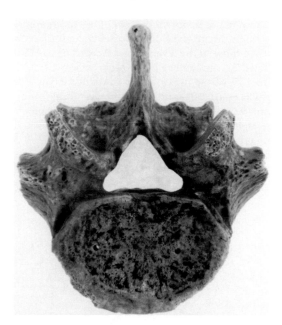

Figure 7.9. Photograph of a trefoil-shaped vertebral canal with underdeveloped pedicles.

development of spondylosis and its accompanying arthritic changes in the facets. According to Verbiest, the narrow canal in the presence of mild disc protrusion or minimal ventral osteophytosis produces symptoms which could be well tolerated in a lumbar canal of normal size.

Stenosis Plain Film Markings

In our clinical investigation, we used the technique of Eisenstein (56), which is illustrated in Figures 7.10, 7.11, and 7.12, and demonstrates the use of this technique on actual x-rays. Figure 7.11 reveals the sagittal diameter of a well-formed canal. According to Epstein et al. (52), the sagittal diameter of a good-sized canal is equal to one-half of the diameter of the vertebral body. Application of the Eisenstein technique in Figure 7.12 reveals stenosis of the L5 level, since the sagittal diameter of the canal measures less than 12 mm; this underdevelopment can be seen by scanning the radiograph even if one does not measure the diameter. It is well to remember that the L5-S1 intervertebral foramina are the smallest in the lumbar spine and that the size of the L5 nerve root exiting through them is the largest of the lumbar cauda equina. Rabinovitch (57) observed that the L3 through S5 nerve roots are less mobile than those above these levels, making

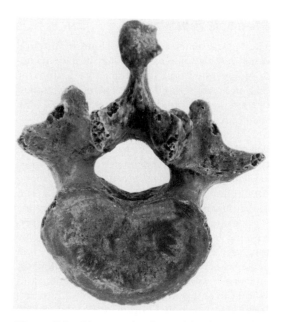

Figure 7.8. Photograph of actual lumbar vertebra showing a rounded vertebral canal with well-developed pedicles.

these nerve roots more susceptible to compression by disc protrusion and osteophyte formation than those in the levels above. According to Hadley (58), the lumbar nerve roots occupy from 17 to 25% of the upper aspect of the foramina. Epstein et al. (52) found that intervertebral foramina in normal cadavers have a sagittal diameter roughly equal to that of both the foramen and neural canal but that they are consistently 2 to 3 mm less in the lower three lumbar segments, where the nerve roots are larger.

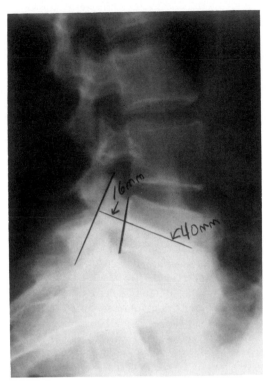

Figure 7.11. Radiograph demonstrating a well-developed sagittal diameter of the vertebral canal.

Accuracy of Plain Film Stenosis Markings

The sagittal dimensions of five lumbar vertebral canals tended to be more shallow in patients undergoing operation for lumbar radiculopathy than in a group of controls. The more frequent occurrence of radiculopathy in patients with small canals can be explained by the fact that for only a small protrusion of intervertebral disc, or any other structural abnormality, can impinge on the nerve. The sagittal diameter can be obtained easily from the lateral roentgenogram and, therefore, requires no invasive or expensive tests. This measurement can be quite helpful in interpreting myelographic defects and in planning and performing operations on patients with radiculopathy (59).

An association between lumbar radiculopathy and a narrow sagittal diameter of the lumbar vertebral canals is noted. Abnormalities of intervertebral discs, vertebrae, ligaments, blood vessels, and nerves have been incriminated—individually and in combinations—in lumbar radiculopathy, but attempts to understand the pathophysiology

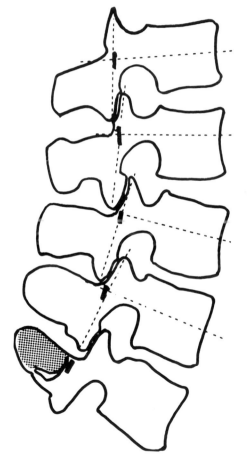

Figure 7.10. Tracing of radiograph showing the method of locating the posterior border of the spinal canal. The posterior border of the canal at the 5th lumbar vertebra is consistently more posterior than is expected. (Reproduced with permission from Eisenstein S: Measurements of the lumbar spinal canal in 2 racial groups. *Clin Orthop* 115:43, 1976.)

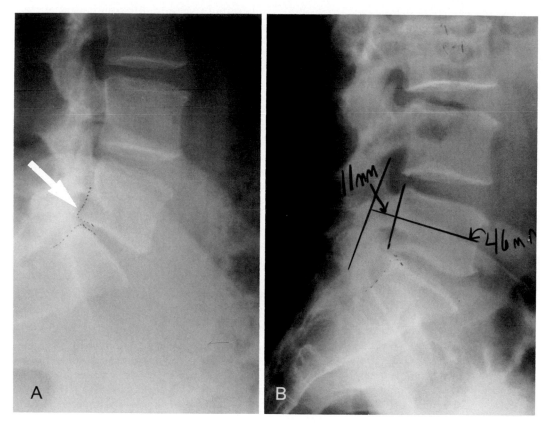

Figure 7.12. Radiographs of a stenotic vertebral canal in a patient with symptoms of intermittent neurogenic claudication. **A**, retrolisthesis of L5 on the sacrum (*arrow*); **B**, stenosis measurements.

and to improve the results of treatment have concentrated heavily upon the intervertebral discs. Many pathological, psychological, occupational, and anatomical factors that may be important in patients with lumbar radiculopathy have not been addressed.

Although often used interchangeably, the terms *spinal canal* and *vertebral canal* are not synonymous. Each person has one spinal canal bounded by bone and ligaments but many vertebral canals, one in each vertebra. Therefore, measurements based on bony landmarks apparent on radiographs are, accurately speaking, measurements of the vertebral canals (59).

ACCURACY OF PLAIN FILM STENOSIS MEASUREMENT WITHIN 1 MILLIMETER

The role of the narrow lumbar spinal canal in back and sciatic pain is well established. The accu-

racy of measurements obtained from lumbar radiographs was therefore analyzed in lumbar spine specimens taken from 132 male cadavers. After removal of soft tissues, the same distances were measured on the bones of 80 specimens. Comparisons were made after correction for magnification, the radiographic measurements of interpedicular distances being, on average, 2 mm greater than the osteological ones at L3, and 4 cm greater at L5. Interarticular distances, midsagittal diameters, and pedicular lengths were, on average, 1 mm greater, and foraminal anteroposterior measurements 1 mm less than the osteological ones. *These results confirm and amplify preliminary observations and indicate the potential value of simple measurements on lumbar spine films as an alternative to more sophisticated and expensive radiological investigations (60).*

Midsagittal diameter (MSD) and interpedicular distance (IPD) in the thoracolumbar junctional region (T10-L1) of 24 male cadaveric spines were measured both from radiographs and directly from bones after removal of the soft tissues in order to assess the accuracy of plain radiographs. It was found that the mean difference between bone and radiographic measurements in the IPD on different vertebral levels was 1.0 mm ($r = 0.98$) (61).

The measurements of the size and shape of the lumbar spinal canal obtained from survey lumbar radiographs have been shown to be valid as compared with bony specimens from cadavers (62).

Borderline Depth for Stenotic Canal

Radiographs of the lumbosacral spine from 29 patients (15 men and 14 women) who had undergone lumbar laminectomy on the neurosurgical service of the Peter Bent Brigham Hospital for radiculopathy due to protrusion of one or more lumbar intervertebral discs were reviewed (59).

The age and sex of each patient were recorded, along with the following measurements from each of the five lumbar vertebrae: (*a*) sagittal diameter of the vertebral canal at the midpoint of the vertebral body; (*b*) interpediculate diameter of the vertebral canal; (*c*) the sagittal diameter; and (*d*) the transverse diameter of the middle of the vertebral body. Measurements of the sagittal diameter of the vertebral canals were made in a manner similar to that described by Eisenstein. All radiographs were made using the standard 40-inch target-film distance. Measurements were made without knowledge of which patients were the controls and which had undergone operation (59).

None of the controls had a vertebral canal that was less than 15 mm in depth—the commonly accepted lower limit of normal depths for all lumbar vertebrae—and two were exactly 15 mm. Nine of the surgical patients had a total of 10 vertebrae measuring less than 15 mm and 11 vertebrae exactly at that value.

Results showed that the mean sagittal diameters of the lumbar canals (all five are significantly more shallow in patients operated for "lumbar disc disease" than in a control group, although nearly all are within the normal range. This was determined from simple measurements taken from lateral roentgenograms of lumbar spines. In relatively large vertebral canals, a prolapsed or protruding disc may displace epidural fat or dura, or even alter slightly the course of a nerve root

but without significantly compressing it. In a small vertebral canal, there is little or no "extra" space, and therefore a small encroachment into the canal can cause the nerve to impinge against the bone. Thus, an association between the size of the canal and the occurrence of radiculopathy can help in understanding asymptomatic patients with myelographic evidence of protruding discs and symptomatic patients with small protrusions. This interpretation of the data supports Verbiest's opinion that, "in the presence of a narrow, although not normally narrow, lumbar vertebral canal, additional slight deformities, such as posterior lipping or small disc protrusion can produce symptoms of compression (63). In summary, less anatomical change is required to impinge upon a nerve root in a small canal (59).

CLINICAL RELEVANCE OF STENOSIS

Two hundred fourteen patients with spinal spondylosis were reviewed with clinical and radiographic records. Sixty-three patients (29%) were symptomatic with cervical spondylosis, 123 patients (58%) presented with symptoms of lumbar spondylosis, and 28 patients (13%) presented with complaints referable to both the cervical and lumbar spondylotic changes. The segmental sagittal diameters of the spinal canals of the symptomatic areas were measured (64).

A narrow spinal canal was present in 64% of patients with cervical spondylosis, in 71% of patients with lumbar spondylosis, and in 64% of patients with combined degenerative disease of the cervical and lumbar spine.

In the cervical area, myelopathy will likely occur when the midcervical diameters approach 10 mm. A premyelopathic group may be predicted with developmental midcervical diameters of 10 to 13 mm. From 13 to 17 mm, patients may be prone to develop symptomatic cervical spondylosis, but few will be prone to myelopathy. Above 17 mm, patients may be less prone to symptomatic disease.

In the lumbar area, patients with small developmental sagittal diameters seem prone to refractory disease and the occurrence of spinal stenosis with *neurogenic claudication* when the canal is narrowed *below 15 mm* radiographically. Patients with canal diameters of 15 to 20 mm comprise a large group of clinically symptomatic patients who may require more surgical treatment. Conversely, when the lumbar sagittal diameters are

20 mm or more radiographically, patients require more spondylotic change for the expression of the same clinical symptoms (64).

The degree of concavity (i.e., the scalloping) on the posterior surface of the lumbar vertebral bodies has been evaluated quantitatively by means of a simple measuring device. The scalloping in the median sagittal plane was found to differ from that in the lateral plane, near the pedicular attachments. In the medial plane, an increase in scalloping from L1 to L4 is noted, with a subsequent decrease at L5 (65). Laterally, the concavity deepens from L1 to L5, the values here being larger than those medially at all levels. Scalloping in the lateral sagittal plane is, especially at the fourth and fifth lumbar levels, presumed to be caused mainly by pressure exerted by the spinal nerves. The medial scalloping is presumed to be partially due to hydrostatic pressure of the cerebrospinal fluid in the dural sac. This pressure will, at the edges of the superior and inferior end plates, be counteracted by the tractional stresses of the fibers of the discal annulus fibrosus which are inserted at the vertebral surface that constitutes part of the anterior wall of the spinal canal. Therefore, its shape has relevance in cases of spinal stenosis (65).

Figure 7.13 schematically shows how the posterior vertebral surface is modeled by tractive and pressure forces. Figure 7.14 shows myelographic changes induced in the cauda equina by these pressure forces as flexion and extension occur.

Herniated lumbar disc or definite sciatica was diagnosed in 16 of 195 men and women who had reported a history of low back pain in a health survey. Measurements relating the size and shape of the lumbar spinal canal were subsequently made from the survey radiographs and compared between various types of back syndrome. Age, body height, body mass index, occupation, and parity of women were controlled as potential confounders using analysis of covariance. Several dimensions of lumbar vertebral canals appeared more shallow in the subjects who had a herniated disc or definite sciatica than in the others. In particular, the interarticular distance of the first sacral vertebra was found to be narrowed in the presence of sciatica, the difference of the adjusted distances to the back pain category being, in men, 30.5 mm versus 35.1 mm (p=0.02), and in women, 23.8 mm versus 30.3 mm (p=0.002), respectively (67).

Herniated lumbar intervertebral disc is often symptomless (12).

The measurements of the size and shape of the lumbar spinal canal obtained from survey lumbar radiographs have been shown to be valid as compared with bony specimens from cadavers. The radiological measurements performed in the present series have proved repeatable, as described in previous reports (62).

The results of Hellovaara et al. (62), in general, accord with the hypothesis that a shallow spinal canal contributes to lumbar radiculopathy. This is consistent with the findings of Ramani (49), Porter et al. (66), and Winston et al. (59), except for the fact that, unlike their data, in this series there was no significant difference in the midsagittal diameter.

Plain films are of great usefulness in the diagnosis of lumbar spinal stenosis, contrary to the opinions of some authorities who feel that plain films are of little value. In a large number of cases, the clinical presentation and the careful analysis of plain films is sufficient to provide an almost certain diagnosis (67).

Root Entrapment Signs

Four criteria are used for recognition of entrapment of the lumbar root within the root canal: (*a*) severe, constant root pain to the lower leg, (*b*) pain unrelieved by bed rest, (*c*) minimal tension signs, and (*d*) patients over 40 years of age. In one study (68), two hundred forty-nine patients ful-

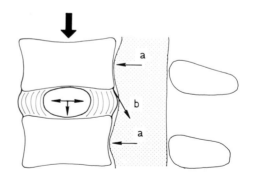

Figure 7.13. Modelling forces on the posterior vertebral surface (PVS). The body weight (*thick arrow*) is transmitted to the nucleus pulposus. This gives rise to a tractional force (*b*) mediated by the annulus fibrosus, which counteracts that due to the cerebrospinal fluid (CSF) pressure (*a*). There is no such opposing force at the midvertebral level. (Reproduced with permission from Larsen JL: The posterior surface of the lumbar vertebral bodies. Part I. *Spine* 10(1):55, 1985.)

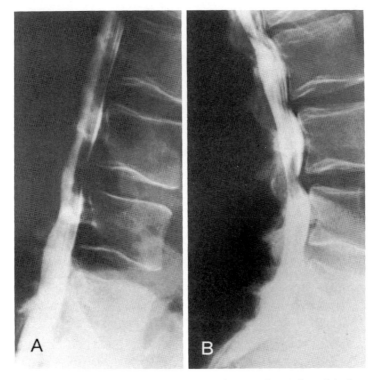

Figure 7.14. **A**, *left.* In ventral flexion, the dural sac is closer to the posterior surface of the intervertebral discs; **B**, *right*, in extension, it is closer to the central parts of the PVS as shown in these lateral myelograms. (Reproduced with permission from Larsen JL: The posterior surface of the lumbar vertebral bodies. Part I. *Spine* 10(1):54, 1985.)

filled the criteria, representing 11% of patients attending a back pain clinic. Most had restricted spinal extension, but few had abnormal neurological signs. Degenerative change was common, especially disc space reduction. Central canal size measured by ultrasound was normal, compatible with a variable past history of back pain. Patients with a long history of back pain numbered 80%, and 90.4% were managed by nonoperative means. Although 78% of these still had some root pain between 1 and 4 years after first attendance, most of them were not troubled sufficiently to have sought alternative help (68).

The disc has enjoyed an era of popularity over several decades; at one time, root pain was almost synonymous with a diagnosis of disc lesion. It is now recognized that a lumbar root can be affected by other pathology and at a different site from the acute disc lesion.

Patients with a root canal lesion are identified by four criteria: *severe root pain, in the older patient, unrelieved by bed rest, and yet without gross limitation of straight leg raising.*

Root canal pathology can occur from spondyl-olysis, from congenital facet hypertrophy at L5-S1, and from previous trauma to the apophyseal joint, but the high incidence of *disc space resorption* suggests that previous disc pathology *is a major cause of this syndrome.* Radiographs of the lumbar spine showed a greater incidence of disc space narrowing than would be expected (69).

Intraosseous pressure (IOP) and cerebrospinal fluid pressure (CSFP) in the lumbar region were measured simultaneously in two groups of patients with either spinal canal stenosis or disc herniation, to compare dynamic changes with positional changes, and to learn whether these pressure changes may have some role in the onset of claudication. IOP and CSFP showed almost the same change patterns with positional changes in two groups. They were lowest in the prone position and highest in the standing position. In standing with flexion, they were almost the same as in the prone position, but *in extension, they increased above the standing pressure.* The dynamic pressure changes could act as a compression force to the cauda equina in the patient with spinal canal stenosis (70).

Concluding Comments Regarding Stenosis Determination and Treatment Influence

The existence of the stenotic lumbar canal is another factor to be considered in the effectiveness of manipulation of the lumbar spine. Certainly, the congenital presence of this abnormality cannot be reversed without surgical relief. Yet the best of manipulation may well render a measure of relief for the patients without providing 100% relief from symptoms. The changes occurring with the stenotic changes, namely, ligamentum flavum hypertrophy and disc degeneration, may not be reversible. Ehni, Weinstein (37), and others have had a 70% success rate with surgery in decompression laminotomy of patients with a stenotic lumbar spine. Thus, clinical investigation and statistic keeping eventually will provide an answer to the effectiveness of manipulation versus that of surgery in the treatment of patients with this condition.

With the techniques of measurement outlined in this chapter, it certainly is possible to determine the existence of lumbar canal stenosis and the prevalence of spondylotic canal radiculopathy by clinical investigation. Clinically, follow-up will show the effectiveness of manipulation. In a report in the *Journal of the Canadian Chiropractic Association* (71), 744 patients with neck and back pain were treated with spinal manipulation. These patients were referred from the Orthopedic Clinic at the University Hospital in Saskatoon. The reports covered only those suffering with low back and leg pain and the effects of manipulation. It was found that 70% of the patients did well and that spinal manipulation now receives top priority in the conservative management of back problems at the University center. One of the main points that I wish to stress is that the postsurgical patient did very well under chiropractic care and that center patients were routinely referred back 3 months after surgery for manipulative care. Spinal surgery was regarded not as the end but rather as the beginning of manipulative involvement. Thus, there is the strong possibility that in the treatment of the patient with a stenotic lumbar canal, the combination of surgical decompression and manipulation may render the greatest benefit.

A sophisticated study (72) of various methods of measuring the inner diameter of the lumbar vertebral canal was presented in the June 1978 issue of the *Journal of Manipulative and Physiologi-cal Therapeutics* by Michael T. Buehler, D.C., Chief of Radiology, National College of Chiropractic. You are urged to read it for an excellent study of lumbar canal mensuration.

Figure 7.15 shows various stenotic formations. X-ray may reveal the osteoarthritic involvement of facets that enter and reduce the lateral recess of the vertebral canal. Myelographic studies to define it are performed by injecting 30 ml of dye into the subarachnoid space and taking films with the patient upright. An anteroposterior diameter of less than 14 mm is suggestive of stenosis (73). The lumbar spinal canal usually becomes progressively wider from L1 to L5 (74), and is shallowest at L5.

Figure 7.16 illustrates the formula of Jones and Thomson (75) for measuring the ratio of the canal to the vertebral body, which is an accurate radiographic indicator of lumbar stenosis. This

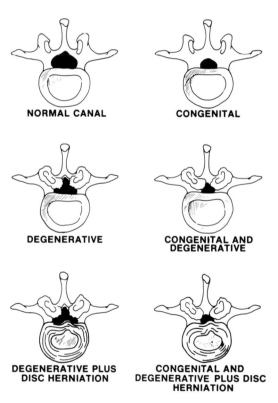

Figure 7.15. This diagram shows the normal canal and various combinations of conditions that may cause spinal stenosis. Congenital stenosis with disc herniation alone, not pictured here, is another possibility. (Reproduced with permission from White AA, Panjabi MM: *Clinical Biomechanics of the Spine.* Philadelphia, JB Lippincott, 1978, p 293.)

technique eliminated misinterpretation of the plain radiographs due to patient size, magnification, and rotation and provided good clinical correlation in 12 of 13 patients. Ratios of 1:2 to 1:4 (small normal) were considered normal, and ratios of 1:4 to 1:6 were considered stenotic. Of course, this technique does not provide as accurate a measurement as does CT scan, but it is a good indicator that more detailed tests such as CT or myelography are needed.

According to Epstein et al. (76), an anteroposterior spinal canal diameter of less than 13 mm (from the posterior margin of the intervertebral foramen to the posterior surface of the vertebral body) indicates stenosis. Hypertrophic osteoarthritic spurs may be tolerated in a normal canal but create severe compression of nerve roots in stenosis. Considerably more spurring can be tolerated at L5-S1 than at L4-L5 because of a "snug" bony confine at L4-L5 and a "great" amount of space at L5-S1 between neural elements and bone.

Figures 7.17 and 7.18 reveal why patients with stenosis stand in a flexed posture: i.e., to maximize the sagittal diameter of the spinal canal.

Thecal Sac Pressure in Stenosis

Different morphological measurements were studied in the evaluation of patients with lumbar spinal stenosis (18). Preoperative CT scans from 24 patients who underwent surgery for central lumbar stenosis were analyzed.

In the majority of patients, the common tissues causing stenosis appeared to be protrusion of soft tissues, including the disc and ligamentum flavum.

It was concluded that: (a) Bony measurements alone do not reliably identify patients with spinal stenosis. (b) The size of the dural sac is a more reliable measure of stenosis than bony measurements. Measurement of the transverse area of the dural sac on CT scans, enhanced by contrast in the sac, is the most accurate method for identifying stenosis. (c) Myelography is still considered to have an important role in the evaluation of a patient with stenosis, because the size of the dural sac can be estimated from myelographic data. (d) Degenerative changes within the facet joints and intervertebral discs, as well as encroachment upon the canal by the ligamentum flavum, were the most common abnormalities associated with spinal stenosis. (e) Further investigation is needed to determine the critical size of the dural sac.

In order to register pressure changes within the cauda equina, a highly sensitive pressure-measuring catheter was inserted through a hole in the dural sac (Fig. 7.19) (19). Then, by circumferentially restricting the transverse area of the intact cauda equina, Schonstrom et al. found that pressure started to build up in it at a cross-sectional area of the dural sac ranging from 60 to 80 mm². Once this critical size was reached, even a

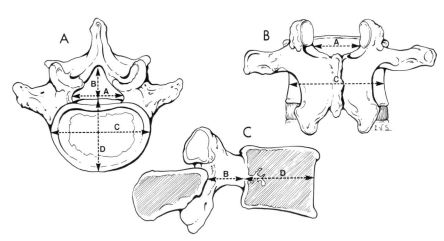

Figure 7.16. **A**, Axial section showing anteroposterior diameter of a fifth lumbar vertebra; **B**, superior view; **C**, median sagittal view. *A*, interpedicular distance; *B*, anteroposterior diameter of spinal canal; *C*, transverse diameter of vertebral body; *D*, anteroposterior diameter of vertebral body. The products *AB* and *CD* are compared. (Reproduced with permission from DL McRae: Radiology of the Lumbar Spinal Canal. In PR Weinstein et al.: *Lumbar Spondylosis: Diagnosis, Management and Surgical Treatment.* Year Book Medical Publishers, © Chicago, 1977.)

minimal further reduction of the area caused a distinct pressure increase among the nerve roots (19).

INCIDENCE OF SPINAL STENOSIS

Eisenstein (77) measured the sagittal diameters of 2166 lumbar vertebrae of 433 adult Negro and white skeletons and found the overall lower limit of normal sagittal diameter to be 15 mm. Of the 2166 vertebrae, 6.3% showed midsagittal stenosis, with none less than 11 mm. Midsagittal stenosis was twice as frequent as other types. Eisenstein felt the structural reason to be an increase in the interlaminar angle (shortening of the laminae) rather than a shortening of the pedicle.

To evaluate the width of the spinal canal when diagnosing spinal stenosis, 91 patients who were older than 59 years of age when undergoing myelography were studied. Using a sagittal diameter

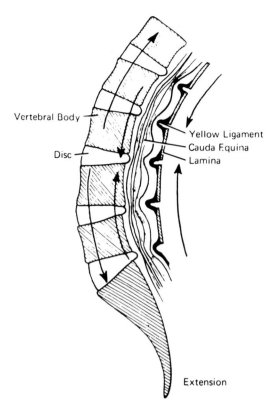

Figure 7.18. Decreased spinal canal volume and increased nerve root bulk with extension. (Reproduced with permission from Finneson BE: *Low Back Pain,* ed 2. Philadelphia, JB Lippincott, 1980, p 432.)

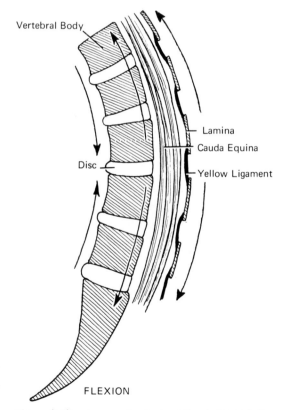

Figure 7.17. Increased spinal canal volume and decreased nerve root (cauda equina) bulk with flexion. (Reproduced with permission from Finneson BE: *Low Back Pain,* ed 2. Philadelphia, JB Lippincott, 1980, p 432.)

of 11 mm as the borderline value for the diagnosis of spinal stenosis, it was found that 31 of the 66 patients with spinal claudication, suspicion of spinal claudication, and sciatic pain fulfilled this criterion, and that $^3/_{25}$ of the control group and those with atypical symptoms had a sagittal diameter of 11 mm or less. Five patients showed a complete block on the myelogram, and all of them had a typical spinal claudication. The spinal canal will narrow with age in asymptomatic patients as well, and the myelographic finding of stenosis in elderly patients is not always indicative of a clinical diagnosis of spinal stenosis (78).

In a prospective study, the incidence, causes, and management of atypical claudication were investigated. All patients had a clinical assessment, Doppler ultrasound studies, and x-rays of the lumbosacral spine; some had epidural injections, myelography with computerized axial tomography, and arteriography. The incidence of atypical claudication was low, 13% of all claudicants, and

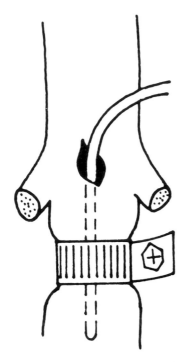

Figure 7.19. The pressure-recording catheter inserted through a hole in the dural sac. The hose clamp was applied around the sac around 5 mm below the exit of the nerve roots. (Reproduced with permission from Schonstrom N, Bolender NF, Spengler DM, Hansson TH: Pressure changes within the cauda equina following constriction of the dural sac: an in vitro experimental study. *Spine* 9(6):605, 1984.)

although difficulties in diagnosis were encountered, spinal and arterial causes were found to have an approximately equal incidence. Only one patient had a definite central spinal stenosis. The need for invasive investigations was low (18%) and the need for surgery was even lower (7%); *the majority of the patients' symptoms responded to conservative management* (79).

OPERATIVE TREATMENT MORE COMMON IN CANALS UNDER 18 MILLIMETERS

Interpedicular distance, interfacet distance, midsagittal diameter, and cross-sectional area at the upper aspect of the fifth lumbar spinal canal were measured from the CT scans of the spine performed during a period of 1 year (Fig. 7.20) (80). The patients were divided into four groups. Group 1 (25 patients) was the normal control group. Group 2 comprised 29 symptomatic patients who were thought to have an L4-L5 herniated nucleus pulposus (HNP) by CT and did not undergo surgery. Group 3A was made up of 24 patients who underwent an L4-L5 discectomy and had favorable results, and group 3B (three patients) included those who failed to improve following surgery.

The patients who are likely to undergo operative treatment have a midsagittal diameter that is <1.6 cm and a cross-sectional area that is >2.5 cm².

Surgical treatment is not advocated on the basis of canal size; however, a small canal size should suggest to the physician that the prognosis for resolution of symptoms is less than favorable (80).

ASYMPTOMATIC PERSONS HAVE ABNORMAL CT SCANS IN ONE-THIRD OF CASES

Fifty-two CT studies from a control population with no history of back trouble were mixed randomly with six scans from patients with surgically proven spinal disease, and all were interpreted by three neuroradiologists in a blind study (12).

Over 35% of asymptomatic people were found to have abnormal computed axial tomograms, and over 19% of those study subjects under the age of 40 were diagnosed as having herniated nucleus pulposus. The patients over 40 years of age showed a 50% abnormal rate, with the most common diagnoses being canal stenosis and facet degeneration. It thus seems apparent that the credibility of the CT scan of the lumbar spine as a diagnostic tool is by and large dependent on its correlation with the clinical picture (12).

One hundred twenty-two patients with surgically confirmed pathology consisting of either herniated lumbar disc, spinal stenosis, or both were included in an investigation (81). For each of these patients, preoperative metrizamide myelography and computed tomography were performed. Each myelogram and CT scan was read blind, so that the neuroradiologist interpreting the study had no knowledge of the patient's surgical pathology, the clinical examination, or the interpretation of the other preoperative test. Myelography was found to be more accurate than computed tomography (83% vs. 72%). In the diagnosis of spinal stenosis, myelography was slightly more accurate than computed tomography (93% vs. 89%). Based upon the results of this study, the authors conclude that metrizamide myelography is more accurate than computed tomography in the diagnosis of both herniated lumbar disc and spinal stenosis and remains the diagnostic study of choice for these conditions (81).

Much has been written regarding the natural history, preferred treatment, and ultimate prognosis of patients with sciatica. Fundamental to any clinical study of mechanical sciatica is the ability to diagnose accurately the exact pathology in question. Hakelius (82) reported a 63% correlation between clinical neurological signs and operatively proven pathology. Similar data was reported by Hirsch and Nachemson (83), who reported a 55% correlation between neurological signs and the presence of herniated lumbar disc. They found that the presence of both a positive straight leg raising sign and positive neurological signs produces the correct diagnosis in 86% of their patients. When a positive myelogram, however, was correlated with the positive neurological examination and positive leg raising sign, the accuracy increased to 95% (81).

Correlation of Clinical with Imaging Findings

These findings further reinforce the futility of basing major surgical decisions on diagnostic tests in isolation from the clinical picture. Inasmuch as an asymptomatic individual has better than one chance in three of having an abnormal CT scan, the test can be given little credibility in the absence of clinical confirmation. A CT scan diagnosis that does not correlate with the objective clinical findings may not be the cause of the patient's pain, and any attempt at surgical correction could very well be the first step toward a failed back syndrome. In fact, the mere performance of the test in the absence of appropriate indications often leads to so-called exploratory back surgery, with all its disastrous implications (12).

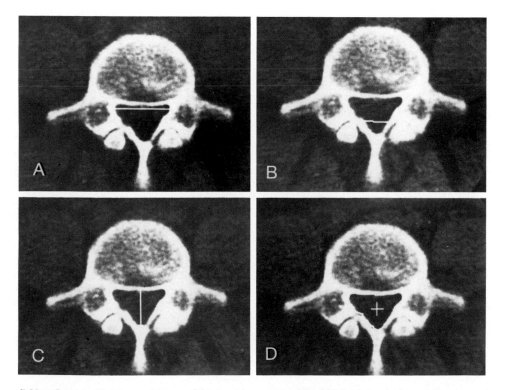

Figure 7.20. Computed tomography scan of the superior aspect of the fifth lumbar spinal canal demonstrating the measurements of: **A**, interpedicular distance, **B**, interfacet distance, **C**, midsagittal diameter, and **D**, cross-sectional area. (Reproduced with permission from Kornberg M, Rechtine GR: Quantitative assessment of the fifth lumbar spinal canal by computed tomography in symptomatic L4-L5 disc disease. *Spine* 10(4):329, 1985.)

STENOSIS INCIDENCE IN DISC HERNIATION

Computed tomography (CT) and transverse axial tomography (TAT) were used to study the lumbar spines of 164 patients with persistent or recurrent low back pain and/or radiculopathy. Of those patients with previous spinal fusion and of those with previous discectomy, 43% and 28%, respectively, demonstrated bony stenosis of the lumbar spinal canal. Of the patients who underwent surgery for this narrowed canal, 91% showed clinical improvement (84).

The case histories are reported of four brothers with lumbosciatic syndrome due to acute disc herniations, and associated spinal stenosis. Hereditary factors, although not hitherto reported, may be implicated for these spinal lesions, as the parents had also undergone spinal operations previously (85).

Midsagittal diameter as measured by diagnostic ultrasound was smaller in patients with symptomatic disc lesions than in asymptomatic subjects, and the narrowest canals were reported in the patients who required surgical treatment (80).

Coxhead et al. (86) measured radiographs from a series of 158 patients undergoing conservative treatment for sciatic symptoms. They found an association between neurological signs and narrowing of the interarticular distance at L4 and L5 and narrowing of the midsagittal diameter at L5.

Baddeley (87) found narrowing of the interarticular distance, pedicular length, and midsagittal diameter in the groups of patients with disc prolapse and with the cauda equina syndrome.

Kornberg (80) found, in comparing normal patients with those having symptoms of herniated disc, that symptomatic patients with an L4-L5 herniated nucleus pulposus seen on CT who did not undergo operative treatment had smaller canals than did the control group. Patients requiring discectomy were found to have smaller canals when compared with the nonoperative group. Failed surgical cases were found to have smaller canals than successfully operated cases. Finally, Kornberg stated that smaller canal size should suggest a poor prognosis for resolution of symptoms.

Ramani (49) found a trend toward a narrower-than-normal canal in patients with prolapsed discs. He concluded that, in patients with prolapsed lumbar discs, the canal tends to be narrower than normal, and that such narrowing enhances the effect of any disc protrusion, leading to severe symptoms of back and leg pain. He used plain film lateral radiographs to measure the anteroposterior diameter of the spinal canal from the midline of the back of the vertebral body to the base of the opposing spinous process. Ratios of body to canal were calculated, with 1:2.5 being normal and 1:4.5 being stenotic.

One-Sixth of Cadavers Reveal Free Fragments as Stenosis Etiology

Schmorl examined, in detail, the spines from 10,000 autopsies, and Andrae further examined some of Schmorl's material (368 spines). They found that 11.5% of the male and 19.7% of the female spines had a posterior prolapse of intervertebral disc beneath the posterior longitudinal ligament, and over one-half of the spines with such a prolapse had more than one. What percentage was symptomatic was not known, but if the results can be extrapolated to current, living populations, then relatively few herniations become symptomatic—or, at least, sufficiently symptomatic to require surgical attention (59).

PERIPHERAL VASCULAR OR NEUROGENIC DISEASE

Nonvascular Conditions That Mimic Intermittent Claudication

One neurological condition that can be difficult to differentiate from intermittent claudication is appropriately called *pseudoclaudication*, a symptom complex produced by spinal stenosis that has an anatomical basis. A helpful point in identifying spinal stenosis is that the discomfort in the limb or limbs is more paresthetic than painful and is produced by activities that cause lumbar extension. Standing or holding a heavy object may bring on the symptoms; if these are related to walking, the distance is generally much more variable than in true claudication. Since increased lumbar lordosis aggravates spinal stenosis, relief of symptoms requires the patient to sit down or lean against something, often for 15 minutes or more (88).

When pseudoclaudication is the problem, CT of the lumbar spine demonstrates the region of stenosis of the spinal canal, and electromyography often demonstrates the multiple nerve root involvement. When pseudoclaudication and occlusive arterial disease coexist, noninvasive testing of the arterial circulation before and after exercise is extremely useful in distinguishing the relative role of each.

Peripheral and Cardiovascular Signs Coexist

PHYSICAL EXAMINATION

Evaluation of the carotid artery pulses is recommended because atherosclerosis, the most prevalent cause of occlusive peripheral arterial disease, commonly affects the carotids as well as the peripheral arteries (88).

After examination of the peripheral arterial pulses is completed, auscultation over the carotids, abdominal aorta, and femoral and popliteal arteries is useful in detecting mild occlusive arterial disease. A systolic bruit is indicative of turbulence, most often due to atherosclerosis proximally; a bruit extending into diastole is heard when the arterial narrowing proximally is severe enough to produce a gradient (and therefore flow) in diastole—a very useful sign of significant occlusive arterial disease.

Determination of Degree of Occlusive Arterial Disease by Grading of Pallor of Elevated Extremity (88)

Grade of Pallor	Appearance at Designated Duration of Elevation
0	No pallor in 60 seconds
1	Definite pallor in 60 seconds
2	Definite pallor in <60 seconds
3	Definite pallor in <30 seconds
4	Pallor with no elevation of extremity

RELATIONSHIP OF LUMBAR CANAL SIZE TO BACK MOBILITY

A study was done to test the relationship between measurements of the shape and size of the spinal canal and the restriction of back mobility (20). Anteroposterior foraminal distances and pedicu-

lar lengths were less in men with restricted extension and sidebending, although not in women. Interarticular distance and the ratio between interarticular and interpedicular distances were significantly less in women with restriction of lumbar extension, sidebending, and rotation; this was not the case in men. The radiographic differences between men and women with restricted back mobility arise partly from the sexual differences in interarticular and anteroposterior foraminal distance, the former being less in women, the latter in men.

Clinical Significance of Intermittent Claudication in Arteriosclerosis

Physicians often reassure their patients that intermittent claudication caused by arteriosclerosis obliterans is not a fatal disease and usually has a benign course (89). However, physicians and patients must realize that atherosclerosis of the aortoiliac or limb vessels usually indicates the presence of disease in other blood vessels, such as the coronary and extracranial cerebral arteries. Patients with intermittent claudication have an overall decrease in life expectancy of 10 years. Survival rates are approximately 70 to 80% for 5 years, 40% for 10 years, and only 26% for 15 years. The overwhelming causes of death are coronary artery disease and diabetes mellitus (89).

Significant coronary artery disease has been documented by coronary arteriography in 30 to 50% of patients with intermittent claudication, and many of these patients were without cardiac symptoms (89).

EFFECT OF STENOSIS ON INTRAOSSEOUS BLOOD FLOW

In recent years, investigations by means of intraosseous phlebography have provided evidence of disturbed venous outflow from juxtachondral bone marrow of osteoarthritic joints (90).

Intraosseous stasis is accompanied by a rise of intramedullary pressure. Aching pain at rest, a typical symptom of advanced osteoarthritis, seems to be provoked by high pressure in the bone marrow, and release of intraosseous hypertension by osteotomy or critical fenestration is followed by prompt disappearance of these pains.

Intraosseous pressures in the lumbar vertebrae of patients with low back pain show that low back pain seems very similar in quality to the aching rest pain experienced by patients with severe osteoarthritis, and the x-ray changes observed in spondylosis deformans are indicative of processes similar to osteoarthritis. Arnoldi (90) reported on intervertebral pressure measurements in patients with various types of lumbar pain. The pressures were measured in the spinous processes, and at least three vertebrae were examined simultaneously in each patient. In roentgenologically normal vertebrae, the intraosseous pressures varied within narrow limits (2 to 13 mm Hg), with a mean value of 8.3 mm Hg. In vertebrae with spondylotic changes in the radiogram, the pressure was significantly higher (28.1 mm Hg mean, 14 to 49 mm Hg range). All pressures are referred to heart level. There was no relationship between the degree of spondylotic changes in the radiogram and the elevation of intraosseous pressure. As far as this author (J.M.C.) is aware, this is as yet the only report on intraosseous pressures in patients with lumbar pain. As mentioned before, it is a preliminary report and its value is limited. It contains no data from healthy subjects, and no measurements were performed on patients with asymptomatic spondylosis deformans. Phlebography was not done in this study (90).

NEUROPHYSIOLOGY OF DORSAL ROOT GANGLION

We will look at the compression changes of the dorsal root ganglion, which lies in the intervertebral foramen of the lumbar spine and is susceptible to stenotic changes.

The dorsal root ganglion is a vital link between the internal and external environment and the spinal cord. The primary sensory role of the spinal cord is to receive afferent stimuli in the form of action potentials and to relay the information transmitted to and from the brain (91).

The cells in the dorsal root ganglion were originally divided into two classes according to their diameters. The large cells give rise to large myelinated fibers and the small cells to the unmyelinated (C) and finely myelinated (A) fibers. The central terminations of these primary afferent fibers, derived from the small cells, end mainly in the substantia gelatinosa, lamina 2 of the spinal cord. Several peptides, including calcitonin gene-related peptide and substance P, have been localized to a subpopulation of small dorsal root ganglion cells. To date, calcitonin gene-related peptide is the most abundant peptide in the dorsal root ganglion.

In 1983, Wall (91) also demonstrated the dorsal root ganglion to have ongoing activity and mechanical sensitivity that could be a source of pain-producing impulses and could contribute to pain in those conditions of peripheral nerve damage where pain persists after peripheral anesthesia.

NONDISCAL CAUSES OF STENOSIS

In a consecutive series of 600 patients scanned by CT for various spinal diseases, those with low back and sciatic pain without disc herniation were selected for study. The causes proved to be joint facet degeneration (32 cases), stenosis of the neural foramina (13 cases), stenosis of the spinal canal (13 cases), lateral recess stenosis (six cases), and spondylolisthesis (six cases). The predominance of joint facet pathology as the underlying cause of low back and sciatic pain in the absence of disc herniation is confirmed. CT scanning of the soft tissues as well as of the skeletal structures is crucial to the etiological diagnosis of the condition under study and hence to the proper planning of treatment (92).

Pagetoid spinal stenoses may occur in three stages as a progressive clinical syndrome. Several diagnostic procedures, including CT, are analyzed to introduce the concept of spinal reserve capacity (SRC). Treatment with calcitonin is recommended at the appropriate stages of the syndrome (93).

Ossification of Posterior Longitudinal Ligament in Stenosis

An enlarged and ossified posterior longitudinal ligament, a rare cause of spinal stenosis syndrome, can occupy up to 80% of the cervical spinal canal, resulting in severe, sometimes permanent, myelopathy.

Ossification of the posterior longitudinal ligaments (OPLL) has also been found in the thoracic and lumbar spine. Minorv found major differences between the clinical presentation of thoracic and lumbar OPLL and those of cervical OPLL. Thoracic OPLL is nearly always asymptomatic and affects women three times more often than men, whereas cervical OPLL occurs predominantly in men. The upper thoracic and midthoracic spine is affected most often in thoracic OPLL (94).

STENOSIS AS A CAUSE OF CAUDA EQUINA COMPROMISE

Although partial or complete cauda equina compromise due to lumbar stenosis is extremely uncommon, a patient with a 3-week history of right thigh and buttock pain, who developed right scrotal and buttock numbness, urinary retention, and difficulty with bowel evacuation, is cited. The patient had diminished sensation to right buttock and anus pinprick with decreased anal sphincter tone and absent bulbocavernosus reflex. Lumbosacral spine films revealed only minimal degenerative changes, while a lumbar myelogram showed L4-L5 and L5-S1 ventral extradural defects. Only a drop of Pantopaque descended caudally below the level of the L5-S1 interspace. Operatively, significant stenosis and thickening of the posterior sacrum with compromise of the lower sacral nerve roots was noted. Bilateral sacral laminectomy was performed, and the symptoms resolved postoperatively. This case illustrated an unusual clinical entity: partial cauda equina compromise due to sacral stenosis (95).

Reflex Sympathetic Dystrophy

Reflex sympathetic dystrophy is a syndrome of burning pain, hyperesthesia, swelling, hyperhidrosis, and trophic changes in the skin and bone of the affected extremity. It is precipitated by a wide variety of factors in addition to nerve injury. It occurs outside of dermatomal distributions and can spread to involve other extremities without new injury. The diagnosis is primarily clinical, but roentgenography, scintigraphy, and sympathetic blockade can help to confirm the diagnosis. The most successful therapies are directed toward blocking the sympathetic innervation to the affected extremity, in conjunction with physical therapy. The theories proposed to explain the pathophysiology of reflex sympathetic dystrophy include "reverberating circuits" in the spinal cord which are triggered by intense pain, ephaptic transmission between sympathetic efferents and sensory afferents, and the presence of ectopic pacemakers in an injured nerve (22).

Causalgia was an old designation for this condition, named after soldiers who showed persistent burning pain and progressive trophic changes in a limb following gunshot injuries. Today, all such manifestations of sympathetic overactivity are termed *reflex sympathetic dystrophy*.

Reflex sympathetic dystrophy can be associated with lumbar disc herniations. Both central and peripheral neuroanatomical pathways can be implicated in the development of this syndrome. Clinical findings of (*a*) vasomotor instability in the leg, supported by plain roentgenograms showing osteopenia; (*b*) bone scan showing increased uptake; and (*c*) a favorable response with sympathetic blocks suggest the diagnosis. Symptoms should be relieved with appropriate nerve root decompression but may require, in addition, a therapeutic lumbar sympathetic blockade (96).

DIAGNOSIS OF STENOSIS

A new technique has been designed to improve myelographic examinations of the entire lumbar spinal canal in patients with severe spinal stenosis using a single needle puncture. When a high-grade obstruction to the caudal flow of contrast material is encountered, the patient is placed in a flexed sitting position for 1 minute. This technique was performed in eight patients with severe lumbar spinal stenosis. It successfully helped depict the lower lumbosacral canal below an apparently complete block in four patients and resulted in improved visualization of the lower sac in four patients with partial block (97).

Doppler ultrasound flowmeter measurement of the arm and ankle systolic arterial pressures before and immediately after walking exercise can detect even the smallest element of arterial disease contributing to claudication (98).

Thermography in Stenosis

The role of liquid crystal thermography (LCT) in the investigation of nerve root compression due to lumbosacral lateral spinal stenosis was evaluated using a quantitative analysis technique. In 28 healthy volunteers, normal lower limb dermatomal asymmetry was found to follow a gaussian distribution, with a normal range of $< 1.0\,°C$ for the lower limbs and $< 1.9\,°C$ for the feet. The results of LCT from a patient group were compared to those from other investigations, with the following results: clinical assessment (107 patients), 53% agreement; myelography (60 patients), 45% agreement; computed tomography (35% patients), 46% agreement; electromyography (27 patients), 41% agreement; and surgical findings (19 patients), 53% agreement. Each method of investigation was compared against the surgeon's final overall assessment. Clinical assessment agreed in 76%, myelography in 71%, computed tomography in 71%, and electromyography in 70%. However, agreement could be demonstrated in only 48% of cases using LCT; therefore, it would appear that LCT is by far the least reliable of these techniques in the diagnosis of nerve root compression (99).

Ultrasonographic Study of Stenosis

In the course of reviewing ultrasound scans of the lumbar spine in 67 symptomatic patients, focal stenosis, either as an isolated finding or in conjunction with diffuse stenosis, was noted in 44 patients. The results of ultrasonograms are compared with findings at myelography and surgery. In addition, using gray-scale technique, we found it possible to examine areas of focal stenosis and to visualize herniated discs with a high degree of accuracy. The finding of focal stenosis alone was associated with disc herniation in 53% of patients who came to surgery. Where ultrasound identified a "triple density" representing soft-tissue protrusion between two bony landmarks within the extradural space resulting in focal stenosis, the sensitivity for indicating disc disease was 89% (100).

Somatosensory Evoked Potential Examination for Stenosis

Cortical somatosensory evoked potential (CSEP) examinations were performed on 20 patients with lumbar spinal stenosis 1 day prior to surgery and 10 to 12 days after spinal decompression and bilateral lateral fusion (101). CSEPs were recorded following stimulation of 32 tibial, peroneal, and sural nerves and 16 saphenous nerves. A total of 110 nerves were examined. Using CSEP P1 latency as criteria for inclusion in the study, 21 tibial, 20 peroneal, and 17 sural nerves were subjected to paired two-tailed t tests to determine whether the CSEP changes that occurred postoperatively were statistically significant ($P < 0.005$). Postoperative P1 latencies of tibial, peroneal, and sural nerves changed significantly, as did N1 latencies and P1-N1 amplitudes of tibial and peroneal nerves. Ten patients improved clinically. It was postulated that pathogenic narrowing of the spinal canal in spinal stenosis leads to nerve root compression and ischemia, with resultant dysfunction primarily affecting large-diameter myelinated fibers, and that a decompression procedure may adequately relieve the underlying pathological processes. Improvement in CSEPs may be due to an increase in available numbers of functioning large-diameter myelinated fibers, conversion to normal from a conduction block, and perhaps, improved axoplasmic flow (101).

Keim et al. (102) described the use of somatosensory evoked potentials (SEPs) in localizing the level, extent, and laterality of nerve root entrapment. The results confirm a high incidence of fourth and fifth lumbar and first sacral nerve root involvement. The posterior tibial nerve was abnormal in 95% of cases, the peroneal in 90%, and the sural in 60% in the symptomatic lower extremity.

Significant stenosis may cause compression of the nerve roots of the cauda equina in the lateral recess or in one or more foramina. Patients with symptomatic lumbar stenosis with or without neurogenic claudication may report pain, paresthesia, or lower extremity weakness, usually patchy in distribution. Different roots may be involved unilaterally or bilaterally. The condition is much more common than has been suspected in the past and is probably present to some extent in most persons over the age of 60 years.

Anatomically, spinal stenosis may have the following variations: (a) lateral, due to hypertrophy of the superior articular process; (b) medial, due to hypertrophy of the inferior articular process; (c) central, due to bony projection (diastematomyelia) or hypertrophic spurs, thickening of ligamentum flavum or superior edge of the lamina of the inferior vertebra; (c) fleur-de-lis (cloverleaf), due to posterolateral bulging caused by thickening of laminae.

Patients with spinal stenosis often present with vague, patchy clinical findings that are usually misleading. The majority of patients present with symptoms of pain because the sensory, not the motor, fibers are primarily affected. It is not uncommon that the usual electrodiagnostic procedures such as electromyography (EMG), motor nerve conduction, and F waves are unrevealing. The "H" reflex can be utilized to evaluate sensory fibers, but its value is limited to the S1 function of primary afferent pathways.

SEPs are technically easy to perform, noninvasive, and painless. The technique has proven to be a reliable diagnostic tool with a high yield of accuracy in delineating the extent and laterality of nerve root involvement in spinal stenosis (102).

GRADING SYSTEM FOR STENOSIS

Rothman and Glenn (103) use a grading system to evaluate pathology of the intervertebral disc, intervertebral foramen, facet joints, and vertebral canal (Figs. 7.21–7.27).

Figure 7.21 shows that this grading system is based on foraminal stenosis, disc protrusion size, and facet hypertrophy. This system allows optimal understanding of the stage of pathological degeneration. The foraminal sagittal view demonstrates the foraminal opening and the entrapment of the nerve root by soft tissue or bony stenosis. Disc protrusion is graded by how many millimeters of bulge enters the vertebral canal. For example, a 5-mm protrusion is grade 4. It is pointed out by Rothman and Glenn that a grade 4 disc/annulus protrusion has greater significance in a congenitally small spinal canal than in a very large spinal canal.

The fourth row reveals the progression of facet joint abnormality.

The fifth row determines the vertebral canal shape and size and its lateral recesses. Bone or soft tissue can be responsible for the stenosis.

Disc Bulge into Vertebral Canal

Figure 7.22 shows the slight physiological bulge of the disc, with the annulus fibrosus extending some millimeters beyond the bony end plates.

Degenerative Osteophytic Changes in the Foramen

Figure 7.23 shows marked foraminal narrowing due to degenerative osteophytic ridging arising from the vertebral end plate.

Facet Syndrome Subluxation Changes

Figure 7.24 shows us a typical facet syndrome in which the superior facet below creates foraminal encroachment as it telescopes upward. This sagittal reformation shows the marked narrowing of the L4-L5 intervertebral disc space allowing the upward subluxation of the superior L5 facet into the neural foramen. Note how widened the facet joint space appears.

Disc Herniation

Figure 7.25 shows a grade 4 (5-mm) disc herniation at L4-L5 and a 3-mm bulge of the annulus at L5-S1.

Stenosis

Absolute stenosis of the central canal exists when it measures 10 mm or less in its midsagittal diameter. Here, cauda equina syndrome can occur with no other evidence of soft tissue or bony encroachment. Relative stenosis is present when the midsagittal diameter is 10 to 12 mm (103). In that case, slight degenerative change can cause further stenosis because the reserve capacity is so reduced within the vertebral canal. Very little further encroachment is required to cause symptoms.

Developmental Stenosis

Figure 7.26 shows developmental central stenosis of a 9-mm canal with a 6-mm L4-L5 disc protrusion into it. This could be very symptom-producing, as there is potential for great nerve compression.

Acquired Lateral Recess Stenosis

Lateral recess stenosis due to facet hypertrophy is seen in Figure 7.27. Here, the superior articular process has subluxated upward into the neural foramen and entraps the exiting nerve root.

CLINICAL PICTURE OF INTERMITTENT CLAUDICATION

Morris (69) reported on 13 patients referred with claudication thought by the referring doctor to be vascular in origin. A careful history and physical examination followed by contrast radiculography showed their symptoms to be due to spinal nerve compression. The clinical picture was presented and the main pitfalls in diagnosis considered. It was stressed that the taking of a careful history is the most important factor in arriving at a correct diagnosis.

A good detailed history is of greatest importance in making the diagnosis. There are many differences between arterial claudication and claudication due to spinal nerve compression (69).

In arterial claudication, the claudication walking distance tends to be fairly constant, whereas in spinal claudication, the claudication distance is

Schematic Diagram	14" x 17" Film Layout	Film Quadrant	Detailed Blow-Up

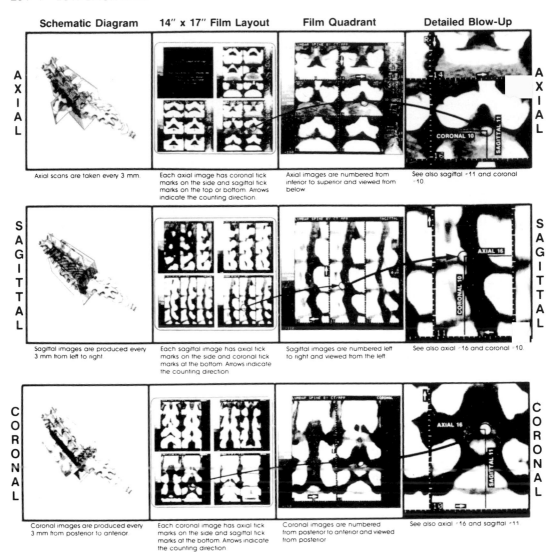

A X I A L

Axial scans are taken every 3 mm.

Each axial image has coronal tick marks on the side and sagittal tick marks on the top or bottom. Arrows indicate the counting direction.

Axial images are numbered from inferior to superior and viewed from below.

See also sagittal #11 and coronal #10.

S A G I T T A L

Sagittal images are produced every 3 mm from left to right.

Each sagittal image has axial tick marks on the side and coronal tick marks at the bottom. Arrows indicate the counting direction.

Sagittal images are numbered left to right and viewed from the left.

See also axial #16 and coronal #10.

C O R O N A L

Coronal images are produced every 3 mm from posterior to anterior.

Each coronal image has axial tick marks on the side and sagittal tick marks at the bottom. Arrows indicate the counting direction.

Coronal images are numbered from posterior to anterior and viewed from posterior.

See also axial #16 and sagittal #11.

Figure 7.21. Grading system used by Rothman and Glenn to evaluate pathology of the intervertebral disc, intervertebral foramen, facet joints, and vertebral canal. (From Rothman SLG, Glenn WV: *Multiplanar CT of the Spine.* Rockville, MD, Aspen, 1985, pp 28, 29. Reprinted with permission of Aspen Publishers, Inc.)

quite irregular. In claudication of arterial origin, the pain comes on more quickly when walking uphill, whereas in spinal claudication this is not always so, and it may be worse walking downhill or worse over rough ground. In arterial claudication, the spine is always relieved by standing still, whereas in spinal claudication this is not so. The patient has to assume some other position in order to relieve the pain, and it takes quite a long time for relief to occur. This is an important point in the differential diagnosis. In arterial claudication, the pain does not occur at rest, but with spinal nerve compression, the pain may occur on prolonged sitting, standing, or lying, and it sometimes occurs on straining during defecation or micturation. Patients with spinal claudication also often have paresthesia, whereas this is uncommon in arterial claudication. Straight leg raising is often restricted and may reproduce the pain of which they complain, but sometimes straight leg raising may be very free and produce no pain whatsoever. The changes can usually be enhanced by exercising the patient to the point of pain before examination (69).

GRADING SYSTEM EXAMPLES

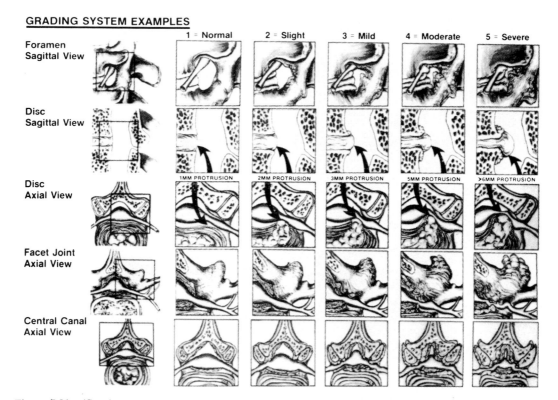

Figure 7.21—*(Cont.)*

Degenerative spinal stenosis occurs most commonly at the third and fourth and the fourth and fifth motion segments of the lumbar spine. Symptoms usually do not develop until the 7th decade of life, and they occur more frequently in men. As degenerative changes develop in the aging lumbar spine, the structures that are responsible for stenosis include the zygapophyseal joints, ligamentum flavum, intervertebral discs, epidural venous structures, laminae, and pedicles. The degeneration of these structures causes encroachment on the spinal canal, both directly and as a result of narrowing of the disc space (104).

The most common physical findings in patients who have spinal stenosis include an increase in pain with extension of the lumbar spine, weakness of the extensor hallucis longus, and sensory changes that follow a specific dermatomal distribution. Signs of tension on the sciatic nerve are found only occasionally, and they usually indicate lateral entrapment of the nerve root. Neurological findings may be more readily detected if the patient is examined shortly after performing any exercise such as climbing stairs. However, as pain in the lower part of the back and changes in

the lumbar spine that are associated with aging are almost universal, all elderly patients who have these symptoms must undergo a thorough evaluation to ensure that they are indeed caused by the observed degenerative changes (104).

Pseudospondylolisthesis is a subluxation of the lumbar vertebrae due to incompetent facet joints. The resulting stenosis of the lumbar spinal canal may impinge on the nerve roots of the cauda equina and induce neurogenic claudication. This syndrome is difficult to distinguish clinically from lower extremity claudication of vascular etiology. Accurate diagnosis requires radiographic examination of the spine (105).

TREATMENT OF STENOSIS

Conservative versus Surgical Care of Stenosis

Surgical treatment of lumbar stenosis should be considered only after an adequate trial of conservative therapy has failed. This includes exercises, supports, medications, and manipulation. Conservative therapy should be continued indefi-

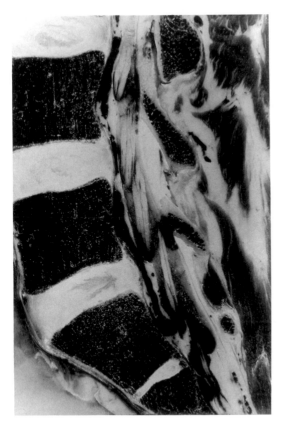

Figure 7.22. Disc bulge into vertebral canal. (From Rothman SLG, Glenn WV: *Multiplanar CT of the Spine.* Rockville, MD, Aspen, 1985, p 77. Reprinted with permission of Aspen Publishers, Inc.)

nitely as long as pain is tolerated (106). According to Wiltse et al. (107), neurological changes alone are rarely indications for surgery.

Ben-Eliyahu (47) states that recent studies show that spinal manipulation can provide relief and should be considered before surgical referral is made for decompression.

Drug Treatment of Stenosis

Pentoxifylline is approved by the Food and Drug Administration for the treatment of patients with intermittent claudication on the basis of chronic occlusive arterial disease of the limbs. It is not a substitute for surgical bypass or removal of arterial obstructions, but it will improve function and symptoms of the disease state. The mechanism by which pentoxifylline works is not well known but appears to be related to erythrocyte adenosine triphosphate (ATP) concentrations and the phos-

phorylation of erythrocyte membrane proteins, both mechanisms resulting in an improvement in erythrocyte flexibility. Efficacy studies indicate that pentoxifylline is significantly more effective than placebo or nylidrin hydrochloride therapy. Adverse reactions are mainly of the gastrointesti-

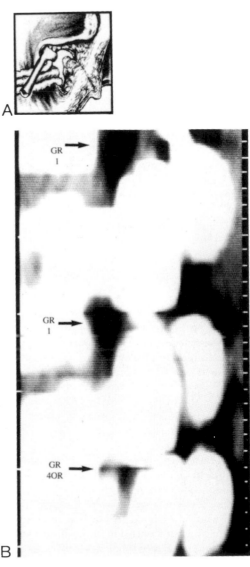

Figure 7.23. Grade 4 moderate foraminal narrowing. **A,** Diagram. **B,** Sagittal reformation on a patient with a grade 4 neural foramen. Note the degenerative osteophytic ridging arising from the vertebral end plate. The coded diagnosis is 4OR (osteophytic ridging). (From Rothman SLG, Glenn WV: *Multiplanar CT of the Spine.* Rockville, MD, Aspen, 1985, p 91. Reprinted with permission of Aspen Publishers, Inc.)

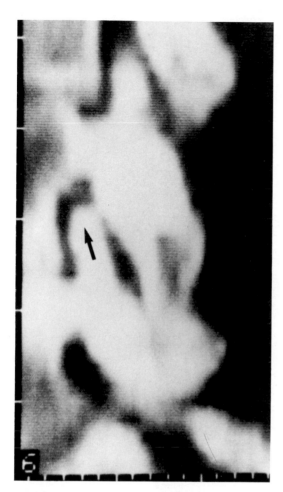

Figure 7.24. Foraminal encroachment due to upward subluxation of a facet. Sagittal reformation reveals a narrowed L4-L5 intervertebral disc space. The superior facet of L5 is herniated upward into the neural foramen. The facet joint space is abnormally widened as well. (From Rothman SLG, Glenn WV: *Multiplanar CT of the Spine.* Rockville, MD, Aspen, 1985, p 93. Reprinted with permission of Aspen Publishers, Inc.)

nal type and are minimized by the use of controlled release dosage form (108).

Mesoinositol hexanicotinate (Hexopal), a derivative of nicotinic acid, has been employed for some years in the symptomatic treatment of various vascular disorders including intermittent claudication.

It may therefore be concluded that in this double-blind, placebo-controlled study, Hexopal was shown to be effective, confirming previously published reports (109).

Long-term treatment produced no significant

changes in intermittent claudication (IC) (140±50 meters), and clinical deterioration occurred in three patients. The rise in hyperemic venous resistance (VR) implies an adverse effect on blood flow properties in the ischemic limb. These findings do not support a beneficial effect upon exercise tolerance, hemodynamics, or hyperemic perfusion during maintenance therapy with pentoxifylline and suggest a detrimental effect in some patients (110).

Side Effects of Surgery for Stenosis

Anterior vertebral body slip after decompression for myelographically verified spinal stenosis (AP diameter < 11 mm) was studied in 45 patients (32 men and 13 women). Mean age at the time of operation was 64 years. Degenerative spondylolisthesis was found in 20 patients and acquired spinal stenosis in 25. Postoperative slipping was seen in 18 patients. An enhanced risk of further slipping was seen in degenerative spondylolisthesis, but it did not influence the result of the operation (111).

Six cases of acute postdiscectomy cauda equina syndrome (CES) following lumbar discectomy were reviewed retrospectively in a series of 2842 lumbar discectomies over a 10-year period. Five cases had coexisting bony spinal stenosis at the level of the disc protrusion. The bony spinal stenosis was not decompressed at the time of discectomy. Inadequate decompression played a role in the postoperative neurological deterioration. The cause of the sixth case is unknown. Bowel and bladder recovery was good when the cauda equina was decompressed early; sensory recovery was universally good, and motor recovery was poor if a severe deficit had developed before decompression. Careful review of the preoperative myelogram to rule out spinal stenosis and decompression of bony stenosis at discectomy is recommended for prevention of postoperative CES. Urgent decompression of postoperative CES is advisable if compression of the cauda equina is confirmed radiographically (112).

PATHOLOGICAL SEQUENCE OF LUMBAR DYSFUNCTION

Understanding the pathological process and making a concise and precise diagnosis of which nerve or nerves are affected are important steps in the formation of a logical plan of treatment (113).

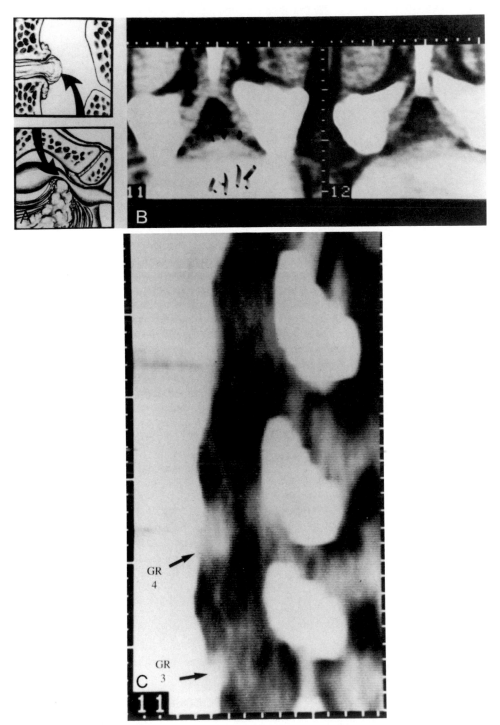

Figure 7.25. Grade 4 disc herniation. **A,** Sagittal and axial diagrams of a 5-mm disc herniation. **B,** Axial scan demonstrates a 5-mm central herniated disc. **C,** Sagittal reformation demonstrates a 5-mm L4-L5 disc herniation and a 3-mm bulge of the annulus at L5-S1. (From Rothman SLG, Glenn WV: *Multiplanar CT of the Spine.* Rockville, MD, Aspen, 1985, p 97. Reprinted with permission of Aspen Publishers, Inc.)

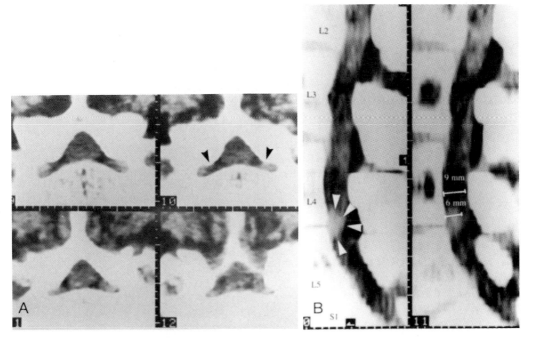

Figure 7.26. Developmental central stenosis. **A,** A sequence of axial scans demonstrate congenitally short pedicles and lateral canal indentation (*arrowheads*) by prominent superior articular processes and lamina. **B,** Midsagittal reformation demonstrates a narrow spinal canal and an L4-L5 disc (*arrowheads*). (From Rothman SLG, Glenn WV: *Multiplanar CT of the Spine*. Rockville, MD, Aspen, 1985, p 199. Reprinted with permission of Aspen Publishers, Inc.)

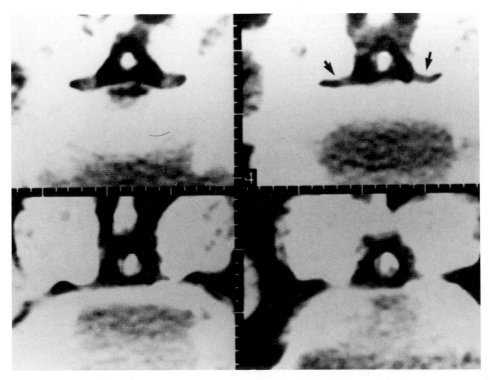

Figure 7.27. Lateral canal stenosis (subarticular recess stenosis). Axial soft-tissue views demonstrate prominent lateral subarticular stenosis. The descending roots are compressed between the superior articular process and the disc space (*arrows*). (From Rothman SLG, Glenn WV: *Multiplanar CT of the Spine*. Rockville, MD, Aspen, 1985, p 205. Reprinted with permission of Aspen Publishers, Inc.)

The pathological process of low back pain comprises:

1. Dysfunction. This can nearly always be relieved by nonoperative measures. Ninety percent of patients with low back pain have this symptom. Attendance at a spine education program, a light elastic garment, manipulations, or posterior joint injections relieve most patients of their symptoms.

2. Disc Herniation. Seventy-five percent of patients with a first herniation respond well to the measures outlined immediately above, together with a period of rest in bed. The other 25% may require chemonucleolysis or discectomy.

3. Lateral Entrapment (Stenosis). Approximately 50% of patients with this type of lesion respond to nonoperative measures. *Manipulation is an effective method of treatment.* The other 50% in most cases require operative decompression with enlargement of the narrow lateral canal.

4. Central Stenosis. Combining a clinical assessment with EMG studies, radiographic and CT scan examination, and sometimes a selective nerve block, it is not usually difficult to identify the entrapped nerve or nerves. A few patients respond to nonoperative measures. Many require decompression.

5. Instability. Patients with a minor degree of instability often require no more than decompression. Those with major instability require fusion of the affected level following decompression and at the same operation (113).

DISCAL DEHYDRATION DECOMPRESSES THE NERVE ROOT

An instrumented probe mounted on the anterior surface of the lumbar spine over an excised lumbar intervertebral disc was used to simulate a disc protrusion in 12 fresh cadavers (114). The contact force between probe and nerve root was measured as a function of two independent variables: probe protrusion depth and disc space height. The contact force on the nerve root was found to increase with increasing probe depth. Widening the disc space increased the contact force, while narrowing the disc space decreased it. A simple mechanical model analysis confirmed that the force exerted on the nerve root by the probe is the result of tension produced in the nerve root as it is deformed by the probe. The mechanical principle that disc narrowing can reduce the pressure on a nerve root produced by

root protrusion may be an explanation of how chemonucleolysis relieves sciatic pain (114).

CASE PRESENTATIONS ON STENOSIS

CASE 1

Figures 7.28, 7.29, and 7.30 show the lumbar spine and pelvis x-rays of a 73-year-old white male whose chief complaints were aching and cramp-like pain in both legs, worse in the left leg, upon walking. Orthopedic examination revealed the Kemp's signs to be bilaterally positive, the Valsalva maneuver to be negative, and the straight leg raise to be positive at 75° bilaterally, with positive Braggard's sign creating pain through the ankle. The deep reflexes were +2 bilaterally at the patella and ankle.

Atherosclerosis of the abdominal aorta and iliac common arteries into the pelvis were seen. Also noted was

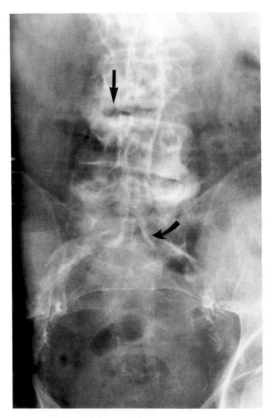

Figure 7.28. Anteroposterior lumbar spine x-ray shows dextrorotatory scoliosis with advanced degenerative disc disease and left unequal weight-bearing of the articular facets (*straight arrow*). Arteriosclerosis of the abdominal aorta and common iliac arteries is seen (*curved arrow*).

marked degenerative disc disease throughout the lumbar spine with a dextrorotatory scoliosis of the lumbar vertebrae. L5 is anterior on the sacrum, representing degenerative spondylolisthesis.

Due to the symptoms of intermittent claudication, a Doppler examination was performed. The blood pressure of the upper extremity was 180/90, while that of the right leg at the posterior tibialis artery was 140 mm Hg and that of the left leg was 150 mm Hg. We therefore had a definite diminished blood flow into the lower extremities.

Treatment in this case consisted of flexion distraction manipulation with range of motion applied to each facet throughout the lumbar spine. After 1 week of treatment, the patient stated he could walk further without leg pain, and in 2 weeks he was walking 5 blocks without discomfort. After 6 weeks of treatment, he stated he could walk 23 blocks, only stopping once to rest.

Obviously, the relief was not due to alleviation of the vascular insufficiency, but was in the treatment of the

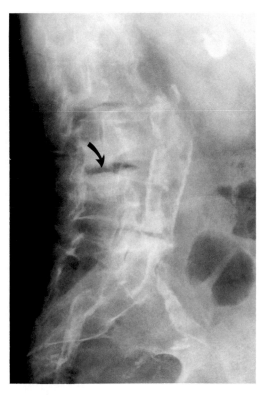

Figure 7.30. An oblique view shows the same findings as the last two figures in a different profile. In all the cases, note the osteochondrosis of the disc as evidenced by the vacuum phenomenon of gas within the nucleus pulposus (*curved arrow*).

neurogenic type of intermittent claudication, which is assisted through spinal manipulation.

CASE 2

This case was contributed from the practice of David Taylor, D.C. Figures 7.31, 7.32, 7.33, 7.34, 7.35, and 7.36 show a patient with degenerative spondylolisthesis at the L4 level. The patient's symptoms did not respond to conservative chiropractic care, so the myelogram was performed. Flexion and extension studies, as compared to neutral views, allow comparison of the stenotic changes of the dye-filled subarachnoid space. Flexion (Fig. 7.32) reveals increased stenosis of the dye-filled subarachnoid space, and there is an apparent reduction of the stenosis in extension (Fig. 7.33). The posteroanterior view further reveals the defect at the L4-L5 segment by the tractioning effect of the anterior slippage of L4 creating compressive stenosis of the dye-filled subarachnoid space.

Figures 7.35 and 7.36 reveal the decompression laminectomy at the L4 level with the placement of the Har-

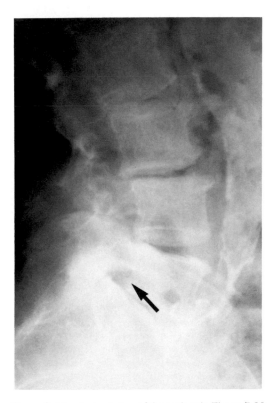

Figure 7.29. Lateral view of the patient in Figure 7.28 demonstrates degenerative spondylolisthesis of L5 on the sacrum (*straight arrow*) with extensive L5-S1 degenerative disc disease. The same findings to a lesser degree are noted at the mid lumbar areas. Abdominal aorta arteriosclerosis is observed.

rington instruments between the lamina of L3 and L5 to create stability of the L4 segment.

This case is presented to demonstrate the changes within the cauda equina brought about by degenerative spondylolisthesis, as well as motion study alteration of the cauda equina during flexion and extension.

Chapter 13, "Spondylolisthesis," will discuss the clinical findings of degenerative spondylolisthesis, and the reader is urged to read that chapter with this case presentation.

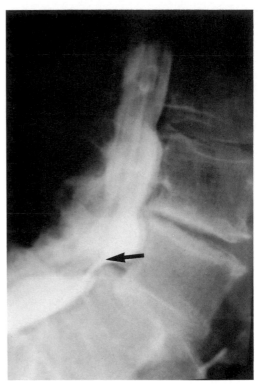

Figure 7.32. Flexion shows the increased stenosis of the dye-filled subarachnoid space (*arrow*).

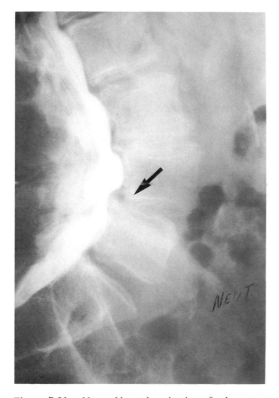

Figure 7.31. Neutral lateral projection of a degenerative spondylolisthesis at L4 (*arrow*). Note the narrowed subarachnoid space behind the L4-L5 disc interspace and the concavity formed by the dye-filled column behind the vertebral bodies. Swenson (105) points out that such pseudospondylolisthesis is a subluxation of the lumbar vertebra due to incompetent facet joints. This stenosis may impinge on the nerve roots of the cauda equina and induce neurogenic claudication. This syndrome is difficult to distinguish from lower extremity claudication of vascular etiology. Accurate diagnosis depends on radiographic examination of the spine. (This case was submitted by David Taylor, D.C.)

CASE 3

A 60-year-old female complaining of low back and neck pain was seen. Her surgical history was a decompression laminectomy at the L2-L5 levels, as seen in Figure 7.37. Figures 7.38, 7.39, and 7.40 reveal a cervical spine surgical fusion of the fifth, sixth, and seventh cervical vertebral bodies. The neutrolateral, flexion, and extension views reveal instability of the C4-C5 disc space, especially the anterolisthesis subluxation on flexion. You will note that extension shows a complete reversal of this subluxation, and a neutral view reveals a partial hyperflexion subluxation of C4 on C5. The flexion and extension that used to occur at the C5-C7 levels must now occur at the C4-C5 segment. This patient came to us because of neck and shoulder discomfort without radiation into the brachial plexus. She did have a positive Déjérine triad in the cervical spine, creating pain in the neck and shoulder area but nothing into the upper extremities.

Treatment of this case consisted of isometric exercises of the cervical spine and mild range-of-motion distraction at the C1-C4 segments. She received spinal manipulation to the thoracic area and wore a soft cervical collar during treatment. The treatment result was 75% relief of subjective pain, to the point that she could now do her household duties, gardening, and other usual activities of daily living.

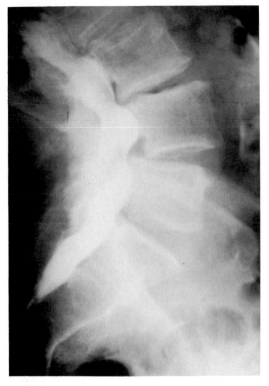

Figure 7.33. Extension shows some increased sagittal diameter of the vertebral canal as evidenced by decompression of the cauda equina.

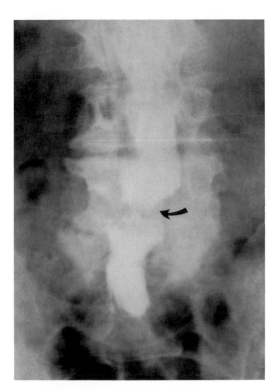

Figure 7.34. Posteroanterior projection again reveals stenosis of the subarachnoid dye-filled space at the L4-L5 level due to anterior slippage of L4 on L5 (*arrow*).

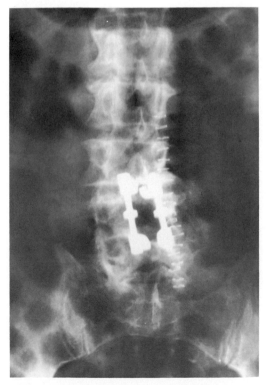

Figure 7.35. Surgical decompression with fusion of the arches by rods has been performed.

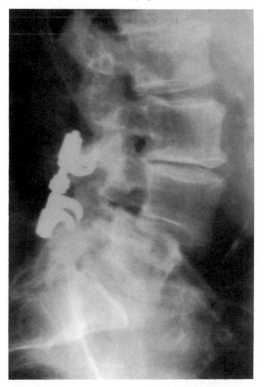

Figure 7.36. Lateral view of the surgical fusion. Note that the slippage is unchanged. This treatment is only undertaken in patients exhibiting cauda equina syndrome symptoms, motor weakness, or intolerable pain.

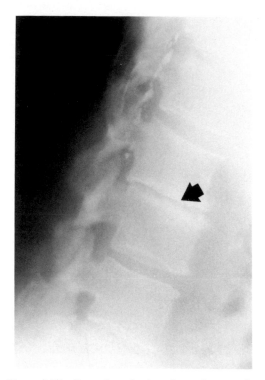

Figure 7.37. Lateral projection shows degenerative disc disease at the L2-L3 level (*arrow*) with decompression laminectomy having been performed in the past. Note the Pantopaque dye present in the subarachnoid space from prior myelography.

This is an interesting case of a patient who had both cervical and lumbar spine surgery followed by decompression laminectomy of the lumbar spine. She subsequently suffered from instability of the disc above the fusion of C5-C7. A surgeon wanted to perform another surgery to carry out fusion further cephalad in the cervical spine, probably into at least the C4-C5 and perhaps the C3-C4 level. This patient received adequate relief through chiropractic manipulation to avoid another surgery.

CASE 4

Case 4 was of a 50-year-old white man who had had low back pain for 12 days. His history revealed that he had had low back and leg pain 10 years previously.

Straight leg raising was negative except for the hamstrings, which were extremely short. Déjérine's triad was negative. Kemp's sign was negative. Range of motion was 80° on flexion and 20° on extension. All other movements were normal.

X-rays reveal:

1. The intercrestal line cuts the L4 body (Fig. 7.41). This means that maximum mobility is at the L4-L5 disc level, based on the work of Macgibbon and Farfan (115). Interestingly, the L4-L5 and L3-L4 discs show more degenerative changes than does the L5-S1 disc. Note the sagittal facet facings at L4-L5 and L5-S1.

2. Discogenic spondyloarthrosis can be seen at the L3-L4 and L4-L5 levels (Fig. 7.42). The lumbar angle is 37°, and the sacral angle is 38°. The lumbar angle is the angle formed by drawing two lines perpendicular to the superior plate of L1 and the inferior plate of L5 to their intersection.

3. Stenosis is evident, as measurement shows (Fig. 7.43). The ratio of body to canal at L4 and L5 is 5:1, with the L5 sagittal diameter being 8 mm (80% of 10 mm) and the L4 sagittal diameter being 10 mm (80% of 12 mm).

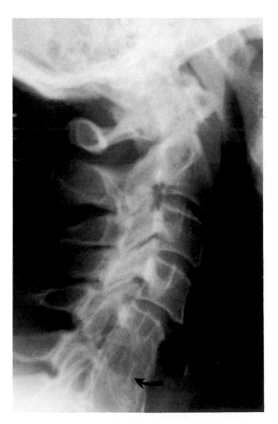

Figure 7.38. Neutral lateral cervical spine reveals interbody fusion at the C5 to C7 levels (*arrow*).

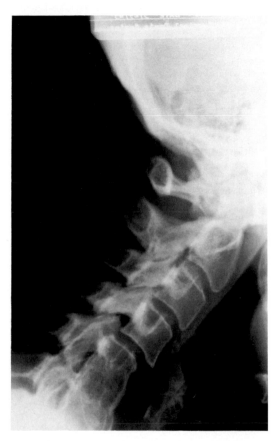

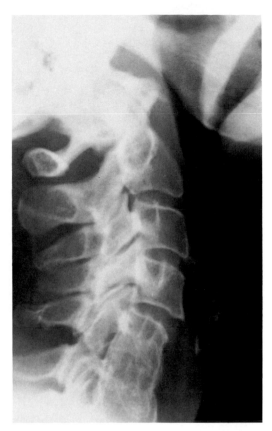

Figure 7.39. Flexion shows excessive motion of C4 on C5 on flexion. All the motion that normally would have occurred at the lower cervical curve now takes place at the C4-C5 level, and this disc becomes unstable.

Figure 7.40. Extension is shown here. Note that the C4 body translates posteriorly to align with the C5 posterior body margin and creates a normal George's line.

4. Osteophytic changes of the anterolateral body plates can be seen at L3-L4 and L4-L5, as can reduction in the facet joint space at L5-S1 and telescoping of the superior S1 facet into the intervertebral foramen at L5-S1 (Fig. 7.44).

This patient has discogenic spondyloarthrosis at L2-L3, L3-L4, L4-L5, and L5-S1 and stenosis of the vertebral canal at the L4 and L5 levels and sagittal facet facings at the L5-S1 and L4-L5 levels. Thus, he has a combination of mechanical faults—stenosis, sagittal facets, and degenerative discs.

Cox flexion distraction was applied to each level of the lumbar and lower thoracic spine. Positive galvanism and tetanizing current was applied to the L4-L5 and L5-S1 discs and the paravertebral muscles, respectively. Exercises were prescribed, especially hamstring stretching exercises. The patient was sent to low back school to learn ergonomics of the lumbar spine. He obtained ex-

cellent relief from pain and was able to learn to prevent irritation of his low back.

CASE 5

Case 5 is of a 55-year-old white man who had low back and bilateral leg pain that was worse on the left than on the right. He also described numbness made worse on walking, leg pain aggravated by sitting, and pain in the testicles. He had been to chiropractors and was referred to us by his last doctor.

Straight leg raise was bilaterally positive at 45°, creating low back pain. Range of motion was normal. Kemp's sign was negative. Muscle strengths were normal in the lower extremities. Right ankle jerk was absent. Atrophy of the right thigh and calf were present, with the circumference being 30 mm less in the right thigh than in the left thigh and 17 mm less in the right calf than in the left calf. Milgram's sign was positive bilaterally. Nachlas', Yeoman's, and Ely's maneuvers and prone lumbar flexion all increased low back pain. Doppler

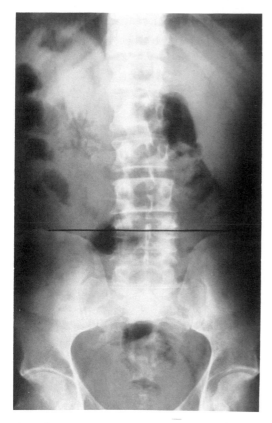

Figure 7.41. Neutral anteroposterior view. The intercrestal line cuts the L4 vertebral body.

testing revealed a reading of 110 mm at the left posterior tibialis (upper arm, 130 systolic) and a 50 mm reading at the right posterior tibialis. Varicose veins of the left leg were noted. Laboratory tests (CBC, sedimentation rate, and SMAC) were normal. Triglycerides were 291 mg/dl (normal is 30 to 175). The prostate was normal. There were external hemorrhoids. X-rays reveal:

1. Over 50% reduction in L5-S1 disc space height can be seen, with retrolisthesis of L5 and lipping and spurring of the anterolateral body plates at L3-L4, L4-L5, and L5-S1 (Fig. 7.45).

2. Stenosis as determined by Eisenstein's measurement is evident, with the sagittal canal being 11 mm, and the body being 46 mm, the body-to-canal ratio being 4:1 (Fig. 7.45).

3. Lateral bending is normal (Figs. 7.46–7.48).

This patient had:

1. L5 stenosis with retrolisthesis subluxation of L5 on S1.

2. Discogenic spondyloarthrosis at L3-L4, L4-L5, and L5-S1.
3. An old, healed L5 disc rupture, as evidenced by an absent right ankle reflex, and past untreated leg pain.
4. Intermittent claudication pain in both legs, with a marked insufficiency in the right leg where blood pressure was greatly reduced at the posterior tibialis artery. The stenosis may cause neurogenic claudication in both legs.
5. Left L5-S1 medial disc protrusion causing S1 dermatome sciatica.

Following the above diagnosis, it was decided to apply treatment four times daily at the outset, for 3 weeks. If 50% relief was obtained, both subjectively as evidenced by patient response and objectively as evidenced, by tests for Kemp's sign, Déjérine's triad, range of motion, and straight leg raising, 2 more months of treatment would be given. If there was no relief, a vascular surgeon and, possibly, a neurosurgeon would be consulted.

Cox distraction manipulation was given, followed by therapy four times daily for 3 weeks. The result was a

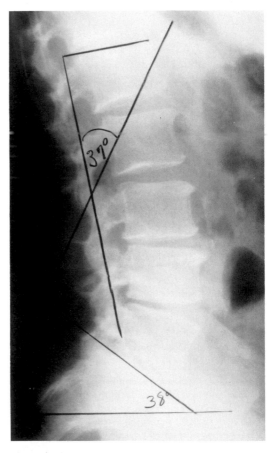

Figure 7.42. Lateral projection.

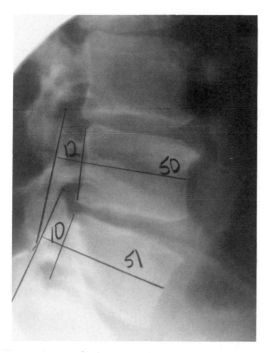

Figure 7.43. Lateral spot view. Note the stenosis at the L4 and L5 vertebral canals.

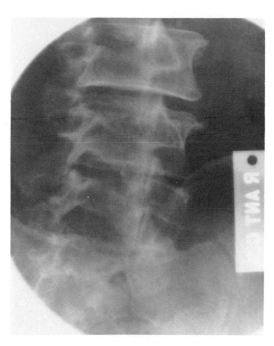

Figure 7.44. Oblique view. Note the loss of the L5-S1 facet joint space and telescoping of the first sacral facet superiorly into the intervertebral foramen at L5-S1.

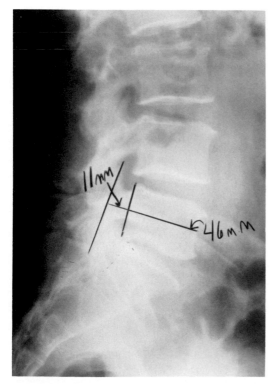

Figure 7.45. Lateral lumbar view. Retrolisthesis subluxation of L5 on the sacrum, with stenosis of the vertebral canal at L5 determined by Eisenstein's measurement.

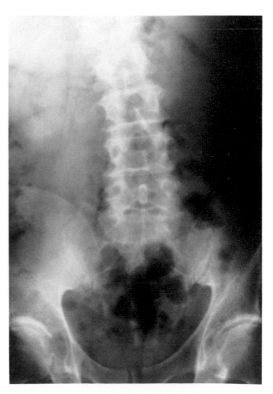

Figure 7.46. Posteroanterior left lateral bending view. Normal lateral bending is shown.

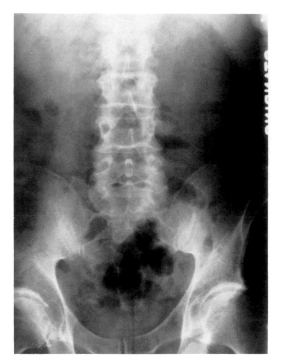

Figure 7.47. Neutral posteroanterior view.

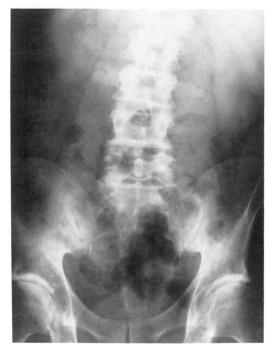

Figure 7.48. Posteroanterior right lateral bending view. Normal lateral bending is shown.

right lower extremity blood pressure of 90 mm, which was approximately 80% the blood pressure of the left leg. The leg pain ceased and the back pain localized in the gluteus maximus muscle.

Treatment consisted of three or four distractions daily with positive galvanic current to the L5-S1 disc and B54. Tetanizing current was applied to the adductor and gluteus medius muscles. Acupressure points B24 through B31 were goaded. A belt was worn on the low back 24 hours daily. Sitting was prohibited, and exercises for the low back were given.

The patient was sent home to be treated by his family chiropractor.

Prior to returning to work 3 months after the onset of treatment, the patient went through our low back pain school, where he was taught the movements dangerous to the low back, how to lift and bend, how to pick up objects from the floor or from shelves, and how to protect the back in activities of daily living.

At the end of 3 months, the patient had obtained 75% relief from pain. The major symptom was left hip and buttock stiffness on standing or walking.

CASE 6

Case 6 is of a 32-year-old woman who had low back pain for 6 years following delivery of triplets. She also expe-

rienced painful menstruation and an increase of back pain at menstruation. Treatments by two chiropractors had previously rendered some relief. She was a mesomorph, was 70 inches tall, and weighed 142 lb.

Range of motion was 90° on flexion, 20° on extension, 10° on right lateral flexion, 10° on left lateral flexion, 20° on right rotation, and 20° on left rotation. Straight leg raise was positive on the right at 80°. Kemp's sign is bilaterally positive. Déjérine's triad is positive for low back pain. No motor or sensory changes are noted.

X-rays reveal:

1. Left inferior hemipelvis with 20-mm-short left femoral head (Fig. 7.49).
2. Levoscoliosis of the lumbar spine (Fig. 7.49).
3. A 15-mm heel and sole lift to the left shoe (Fig. 7.50).
4. Spondylolisthesis at L5 and a 25% slippage with a pars interarticularis separation (Fig. 7.51).

This patient has true spondylolisthesis at L5 and a 20-mm short left lower extremity with concomitant levoscoliosis of the lumbar spine.

Treatment consisted of Cox flexion distraction for spondylolisthesis. Acupressure points B24 to B54 were goaded. A 15-mm heel and sole lift was added to the left shoe, and the patient was advised not to wear high heel shoes. Cox exercises 1 to 4 were advised. The patient was given Discat supplement. She was advised to use hot and cold alternating packs in acute stage and was sent to our low back pain school to learn to lift, bend, and carry out activities of normal daily life.

This patient obtained complete relief from pain after 7 office visits over 22 days.

CASE 7

Figure 7.52 reveals a calcification projecting bilaterally from the pedicles into the vertebral canal. Helms and Sims (116) feel that these spurs most likely represent ossification of the ligamentum flavum at its point of insertion and contend that they should not be mistaken for osteophytes, free disc fragments, or fracture fragments. You will see these ossifications occasionally on CT scan, and it is noted that they are usually asymptomatic. You will note that a disc protrusion is present on this CT scan.

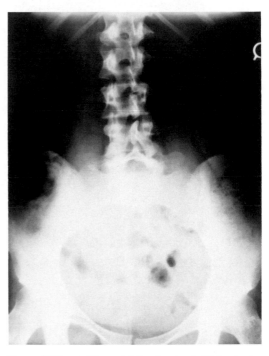

Figure 7.50. A 15-mm left heel and sole lift levels the pelvis and partially corrects the levoscoliosis.

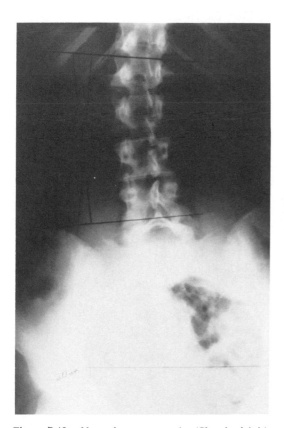

Figure 7.49. Neutral posteroanterior (Chamberlain's) view of the lumbar spine and pelvis reveals a 20-mm inferior left hemipelvis and femoral head with levoscoliosis of the lumbar spine.

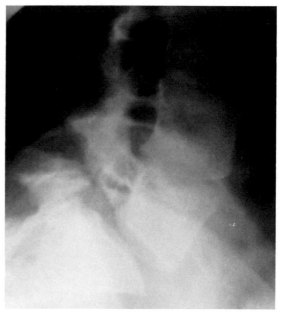

Figure 7.51. Lateral view reveals a 25% spondylolisthesis of L5 on the sacrum. A 20-mm short leg could add to this instability.

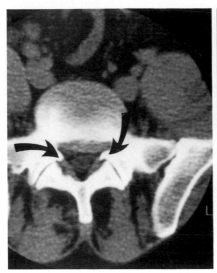
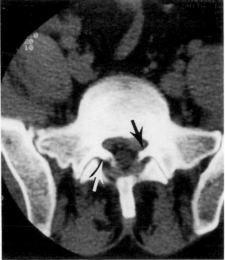

Figure 7.52. Superior facet calcifications at the attachment of the ligamentum flavum at the insertion into the facet (*arrows*).

CASE 8

Figure 7.53 is a lateral radiograph showing an approximately 60% loss of vertical height of the T9 vertebral body. This occurred in this 59-year-old female following a fall. Her pain continued, and Figure 7.54 represents the same x-ray taken 3 months following Figure 7.53. You can see that the compression fracture has continued to deteriorate. Proper blood tests did not suggest any evidence of pathological fracture. This patient became asymptomatic under conservative extension-type manipulation and physiological rest.

This case is shown to you to represent the progressive collapse of a vertebral compression fracture in the months following the original injury. One must be aware of this in clinical practice, as it can explain the further pain the patient may experience within weeks following the original compression fracture. Such flexion deformity can cause narrowing (stenosis) of the vertebral canal to the point of obstructing dye flow in the subarachnoid space on myelography.

CASE 9

A 70-year-old male fell from a tree and sustained approximately 75% compression fracture of the L1 vertebral body. He was taken to the hospital and was catheterized because he could not urinate. He wore this catheter for 2 months when he had prostate surgery. However, the reason for the catheter was that he could not urinate due to cauda equina compression by the narrowing of the vertebral canal following the compression fracture shown in Figure 7.55. This can be compared with the adjacent vertebra (Fig. 7.56).

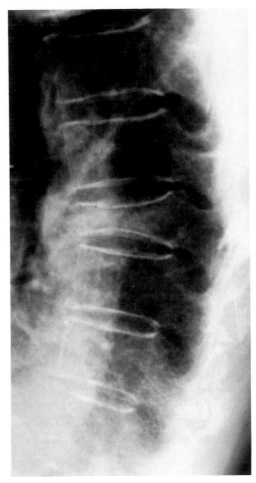

Figure 7.53. There is approximately a 60% loss of height of the T9 vertebral body in a 59-year-old female following a fall. This x-ray was made the day of the fall.

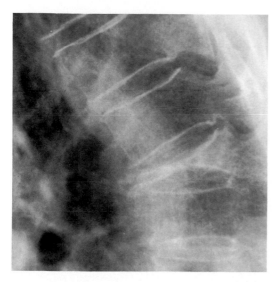

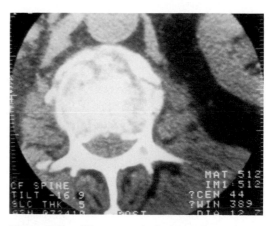

Figure 7.55. CT scan reveals the impaction compression deformity of the L1 vertebral body with invasion of the vertebral canal to create stenosis of the canal and spinal cord.

Figure 7.54. Three months later, following persistent back pain, another radiograph shows progressive compression deformity of the T9 body.

When we first saw this patient, his purpose in coming was to find out whether any treatment other than a Harrington rod fusion could be given.

Examination of this patient revealed both ankle jerks absent, while the patellar reflexes were +2 bilaterally. We observe in Figure 7.57 that there is degenerative disc disease at the L5-S1 level and that this may be creating stenosis with possible compression of the S1 nerve roots resulting in the absent ankle jerks. The leg and foot discomfort that this patient complained of may not have been due to the L1 fracture. At this time, the pa-

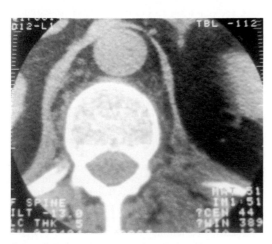

Figure 7.56. Normal vertebral body and canal of the adjacent segment for comparison with Figure 7.55.

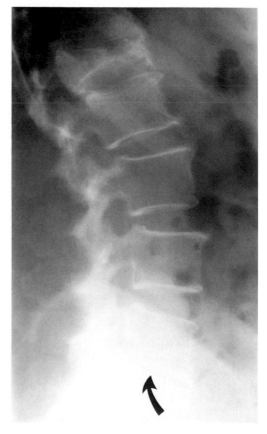

Figure 7.57. Note the degenerative L5-S1 disc disease (*arrow*) as well as the fracture of L1.

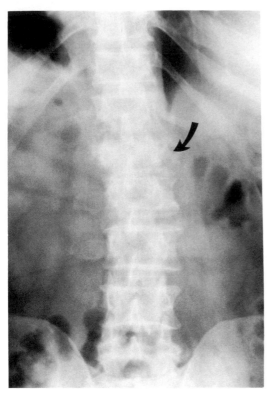

Figure 7.58. Anteroposterior lumbar spine shows the compression defect at L1 (*arrow*) but no extensive degenerative changes.

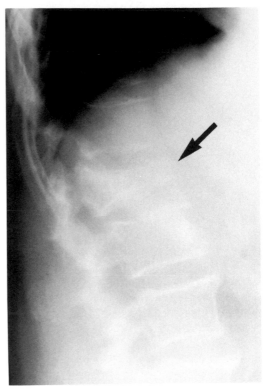

Figure 7.59. Lateral projection shows neither anterior degenerative change at L1, L2, or L3 nor ankylosis at the level of the L1 compression fracture (*arrow*).

tient was having normal urination and no other signs of cauda equina syndrome.

The cremasteric and Babinski reflexes were normal. There was weakness on contraction of the anal sphincter muscles to some degree, but the patient had no problem with control of the bowels. There was hypesthesia of the S1 dermatomes bilaterally. Please note that in Figures 7.58 and 7.59, taken at the time of the fracture, there is no anterolateral lipping and spurring; but on Figure 7.60, taken 7 months later, there is now extensive ankylosis of the anterolateral vertebral body plate by hypertrophy and calcification. This would represent the body's own attempt to fuse this area into stability.

In considering a surgical fusion versus the body's own attempt to fuse, we consider the work of Taylor et al. (117), who stated that compression fractures of the dorsolumbar spine without neurological involvement were studied. A long-term follow-up study was carried out on 216 patients with fractures of the dorsolumbar spine. None of these patients had neurological impairment. The average period of follow-up was 9 years, and it was found that the functional results were no different for

patients with a single fracture and those with multiple fractures, nor could statistical clinical differences be established between patients whose fractures went on to spontaneous fusion and those whose fractures did not. Correlations could not be established for residual symptoms, reduction in vertebral height, encroachment upon the spinal canal, and persistent kyphotic deformities. It was concluded that the nonoperative treatment of these fractures was a sound method and that attempts at reduction were not justifiable. No patient in this series had undergone a surgical procedure because of persistent symptoms.

With these thoughts in mind, we suggested to the patient that, since fusion was occurring and it had been 6 months now since his initial fracture, he should question strongly what could be guaranteed to him through the use of a Harrington strut and fusion. He did not want the surgery. In fact, he stated that he would rather die than have the surgery done. Therefore, we treated this man, as we have other compression fracture cases, with mild flexion and extension manipulation followed by tetanizing current applied paravertebrally over the fracture site. The results of this care were persistent loss of pain in the dorsal lumbar spine and regaining of

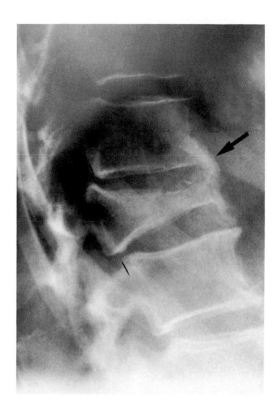

Figure 7.60. Three months after the film in Figures 7.58 and 7.59, there is extensive anterior ankylosis by calcification of the anterior longitudinal ligament and hypertrophic changes (*arrow*). The body has provided its own natural fusion at the site of instability.

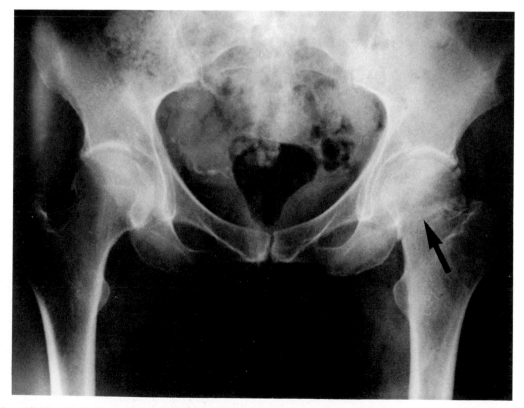

Figure 7.61. An impaction fracture of the left femoral cervical area is noted (*arrow*).

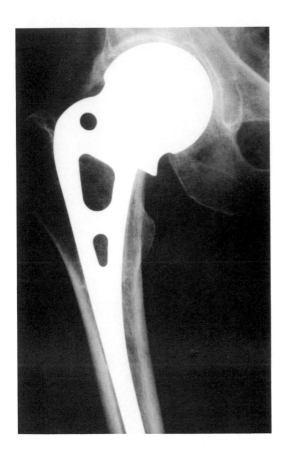

Figure 7.62. A hip arthroplasty is performed on the hip joint in Figure 7.61.

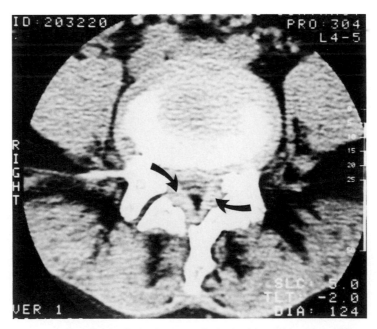

Figure 7.63. CT scan reveals ligamentum flavum hypertrophy (*arrows*) creating stenosis of the vertebral canal felt to have been responsible for the persistent pain in the left hip which was relieved by spinal flexion distraction manipulation.

enough physiological range of motion to be compatible with his everyday living. In the past 3 years that we have followed this case, this patient has been comfortable without cauda equina symptoms.

CASE 10

Figure 7.61 reveals an impaction-type fracture within the cervical area of the left femur. Figure 7.62 shows an eventual hip arthroplasty that was performed.

Chiropractic involvement with this case came about due to the persistent pain in the left buttock and hip area.

Figure 7.63 is a CT scan showing ligamentum flavum hypertrophy at the L4-L5 level. Clinically it was felt that perhaps this ligamentum flavum hypertrophy was creating some degree of stenosis at this level. Flexion distraction manipulation was given to this patient. She also attended low back wellness school and was instructed in how to prevent hyperextension motions that could further aggravate her stenotic condition. Accompanying exercises in flexion mode to strengthen abdominal muscles, stretch hamstring muscles, and maintain a slight flexion of the lumbar spine resulted in gradual relief of this patient's pain of approximately 50%.

This case is presented to show the possibility of ligamentum flavum hypertrophy as a cause of persistent hip and buttock pain that perhaps was masked by the fact that this patient had a hip arthroplasty. Further, the effects of manipulation in this type of case are demonstrated.

References

1. Huffnagle FT: Lumbar spinal stenosis: diagnosis and treatment. *J Neurol Orthop Med Surg* 6(1): 63–69, 1985.
2. Verbiest H: Primaire stenose can het lumbale werveelkanaal bej volwassenen. *Ned Tijdschr Geneeskd* 94:2415–2433, 1950.
3. Ciric I, Mikhael MA: Lumbar spinal-lateral recess stenosis. *Neurol Clin* 3(2):417–423, 1985.
4. Kavanaugh GJ, Svien HJ, Holman CB, et al.: Pseudoclaudication syndrome produced by compression of the cauda equina. *JAMA* 206: 2477–2481, 1983.
5. Hood SA, Weigl K: Lumbar spinal stenosis: surgical intervention for the older person. *Isr J Med Sci* 19:169–172, 1983.
6. Clark GA, Panjabi MM, Wetzel FT: Can infant malnutrition cause adult vertebral stenosis?. *Spine* 10(2):165–170, 1985.
7. Roaf R: Vertebral growth and its mechanical control *J Bone Joint Surg* 42B:40–59, 1960.
8. Porter RW, Hibbert C, Wellman P: Backache and the lumbar spinal canal. *Spine* 5:99–105, 1980.
9. Eisenstein S: Lumbar vertebral canal morphometry for computerized tomography in spinal stenosis. *Spine* 8:187–191, 1983.
10. Hinck VC, Clark WM, Hopkins CE: Normal interpediculate distances (minimum and maximum) in children and adults. *Radiology* 97:141–153, 1966.
11. Burton C, Heithoff K, Kirkaldy-Willis W, Ray C: Computed tomographic scanning and the lumbar spine. *Spine* 4:356–368, 1979.
12. Weisel S, Tsourmas N, Feffer H, Citrin C, Patronas N: A study of computer-assisted tomography: the incidence of positive CT scans in an asymptomatic group of patients. *Spine* 9(6): 549–551, 1984.
13. Rydevik B, Brown MD, Lundborg G: Pathoanatomy and pathophysiology of nerve root compression. *Spine* 9(1):7–15, 1984.
14. Dahlin LB, Danielson N, McLean WG, Rydevik B, Sjostrand J: Critical pressure level for impairment of fast axonal transport during experimental compression of rabbit vagus nerve. *J Physiol* 84P, 1981.
15. Rydevik B, Lundborg G: Permeability of intraneural microvessels and perineurium following acute, graded experimental nerve compression. *Scand J Plast Reconstr Surg* 11:179–189, 1977.
16. Rydevik B, Lundborg G, Nordborg C: Intraneural tissue reactions induced by internal neurolysis. *Scand J Plast Reconstr Surg* 10:3–8, 1976.
17. Rydevik B, McLean WG, Sjostrand J, Lundborg G: Blockage of axonal transport induced by acute, graded compression of the rabbit vagus nerve. *J Neurol Neurosurg Psychiatry* 43:690–698, 1980.
18. Schonstrom NSR, Bolender NF, Spengler DM: The pathomorphology of spinal stenosis as seen on CT scan of the lumbar spine. *Spine* 10(9): 806–811, 1985.
19. Schonstrom N, Bolender NF, Spengler DM, Hansson TH: Pressure changes within the cauda equina following constriction of the dural sac: an in vitro experimental study. *Spine* 9(6):604–607, 1984.
20. Vanharanta H, Korpi J, Heliovarra M, Troup JDG: Radiographic measurements of lumbar spinal canal size and their relation to back mobility. *Spine* 10(5):461–466, 1985.
21. Kirkaldy-Willis WH, Paine KWE, Couch-Oix J, et al.: Lumbar spinal stenosis. *Clin Orthop* 99:30–50, 1974.
22. Schwartzman RJ, McLellan TL: Reflex sympathetic dystrophy: a review. *Arch Neurol* 44(May): 555–559, 1987.
23. Weinstein PR: Diagnosis and management of lumbar spinal stenosis. *Clin Neurosurg* 30:677–697, 1983.
24. Dorwart RH, Vogler III JB, Helms CA: Spinal stenosis. *Radiol Clin North Am* 21:301–325, 1983.
25. Brodsky AE: Iatrogenic spinal stenosis and poste-

rior compression of the cauda equina. Paper read at S.I.C.O.T., Tel Aviv, October 1972.

26. Choudhury AR, Taylor JC: Occult lumbar spinal stenosis. *J Neurol Neurosurg Psychiatry* 40: 506–570, 1977.

27. Yong-Hing K, Kirkaldy-Willis WH: The pathophysiology of degenerative disease of the lumbar spine. *Orthop Clin North Am* 14:491–504, 1983.

28. Panjabi MM, Krag MH, Chung TQ: Effects of disc injury on mechanical behavior of the human spine. *Spine* 9(7):707–713, 1984.

29. Paine K, Haung P: Lumbar disc syndrome. *J Neurosurg* 37:75, 1972.

30. Sarpyener MA: Congenital stricture of that canal. *J Bone Joint Surg* 27:70, 1945.

31. Verbiest H: A radicular syndrome from developmental narrowing of the lumbar vertebral canal. *J Bone Joint Surg* 36B:230, 1954.

32. Vernon-Roberts B, Pirie C: Degenerative changes in the invertebral discs of the lumbar spine and their sequelae. *Rheumatol Rehabil* 16:13, 1977.

33. Collins DH: Degenerative diseases. In Nassim R, Burrows JH (eds): *Modern Trends in Diseases of the Vertebral Column.* London, Butterworth & Co., 1959.

34. Schmorl C, Junghanns H: *The Human Spine in Health and Disease.* New York, Grune & Stratton, 1959.

35. Dyck P, Pheasant HC, Doyle JB, Rieder JJ: Intermittent cauda equina compression syndrome. *Spine* 2(1):75, 1977.

36. Goldthwaite JE: The lumbosacral articulation: an explanation of many cases of "lumbago," "sciatica" and paraplegia. *Bost Med Surg J* 164: 365–372, 1911.

37. Weinstein P, Ehni G, Wilson C: *Lumbar Spondylosis.* Chicago, *Year Book*, 1977, p 119.

38. Ehni G: Spondylitic cauda equina radiculopathy. *Tex J Med* 61:746, 1965.

39. Sunderland S: *Nerves and Nerve Injuries.* Baltimore, Williams & Wilkins, 1968.

40. Sunderland S, Bradley KC: Stress-strain phenomena in human spinal nerve roots. *Brain* 94:120, 1971.

41. Sebolt H, Elies W: The method of surgical root decompression on patients with unilateral lumbar disc prolapse and muscle blood flow of the lower extremities. *VASA,* Band 5, Heft 3, 1976.

42. Wilson CB: Significance of the small lumbar spinal canal: cauda equina syndromes due to spondylosis, Part III, Intermittent claudication. *J Neurosurg* 31:499, 1969.

43. Evans JG: Neurologic intermittent claudication. *Br Med J* 2:985, 1964.

44. Blau JN, Rushworth G: Observation on the blood vessels of the spinal cord and their responses to motor activity. *Brain* 81:354, 1958.

45. Greenfield GQ, Anderson CA: Evaluation of the exertional leg pain—claudication or neuromuscular pain. *Orthopedics* 5(11):34, 1982.

46. Verbiest H: Fallacies of the present definition, nomenclature, and classification of the stenoses of the lumbar vertebral canal. *Spine* 1(4):217–225, 1976.

47. Ben-Eliyahu DJ, Rutili MM, Przbysz JA: Leteral recess syndrome: diagnosis and chiropractic management. *J Manipulative Physiol Ther* 6:25, 1983.

48. Dyck P: The stoop test in lumbar entrapment radiculopathy. *Spine* 4:89, 1979.

49. Ramani P: Variations in the size of the bony lumbar canal in patients with prolapse of lumbar intervertebral discs. *Clin Radiol* 27:301–307, 1976.

50. Ullrich CG, Binet ER, Sanecki MG, Kieffer SA: Quantitative assessment of the lumbar spinal canal by computed tomography. *Radiology* 134: 137–143, 1980.

51. Eagle R: A pain in the back. *New Scientist* (October 18):170–173, 1979.

52. Epstein BS, Epstein JA, Lavine L: The effect of anatomic variations in the lumbar vertebrae and spinal canal on cauda equina nerve root syndromes. *Am J Roetgenol Radium Ther Nucl Med* 91: 105, 1964.

53. Elsberg CA, Dyke CG: The diagnosis and localization of tumors of the spinal cord by means of measurements made on x-ray films of the vertebrae, and the correlation of the clinical and x-ray findings. *Bull Neural Inst NY* 3:359–394, 1934.

54. Huizinga J, Heiden JA vd. Vinken PJG: The human vertebral canal: a biometric study. *Proc R Netherlands Acad Sci C* 55:22–33, 1952.

55. Sand PG: The human lumbo-sacral vertebral column: an osteometric study. Oslo Universitets forlaget Trynkningssentral, 1970.

56. Eisenstein S: Measurements of the lumbar spinal canal in 2 racial groups. *Clin Orthop* 115:42–45, 1976.

57. Rabinovitch R: *Diseases of the Intervertebral Disc and Its Surrounding Tissues.* Springfield, IL, Charles C. Thomas, 1961.

58. Hadley LA: *Anatomico-Roentgenographic Studies of the Spine.* Springfield, IL, Charles C. Thomas, 1964.

59. Winston K, Rumbaugh C, Colucci V: The vertebral canals in lumbar disc disease. *Spine* 9(4): 414–417, 1984.

60. Leiviska T, Videman T, Nurminen T, Troup JDG: Radiographic versus direct measurements of the spinal canal at lumbar vertebrae L3-L5 and their relations to age and body stature. *Acta Radiol Diag* 26(4):403–411, 1985.

61. Malmivaara A, Videman T, Kuosma E, Troup J: Radiographic vs. direct measurements of the spinal canal of the thoracolumbar junctional region (T10-L1) of the spine. *Spine* 11(6):574, 1986.

62. Hellovaara M, Vanharanta H, Korpi J, Troup

JDG: Herniated lumbar disc syndrome and vertebral canals. *Spine* 11(5):433–435, 1986.

63. Verbiest H: Further experiences on the pathological influence of a developmental narrowness of bony lumbar vertebral canal. *J Bone Joint Surg* 37B:576–583, 1955.

64. Edwards WC, LaRocca SH: The developmental segmental sagittal diameter in combined cervical and lumbar spondylosis. *Spine* 10(1):42–49, 1985.

65. Larsen JL: The posterior surface of the lumbar vertebral bodies. Part I. *Spine* 10(1):50–58, 1985.

66. Porter RV, Hibbert CS, Wicks M: The spinal canal in symptomatic lumbar disc lesions. *J Bone Joint Surg* 60B:485–487, 1978.

67. Chynn KY, Altman WI, Finby N: The roentgenographic manifestations and clinical features of lumbar spinal stenosis with special emphasis on the superior articular facet. *Neuroradiology* 16:378–380, 1978.

68. Porter RW, Hibbert C, Evans C: The natural history of root entrapment syndrome. *Spine* 9(4), 1984.

69. Morris WT: Spinal nerve compression: a cause of claudication. *New Zealand Med Journal* 88:101–103, 1978.

70. Hanai K, Kawai K, Itoh Y, Satake T, Fujiyoshi F, Abematsu N: Simultaneous measurement of intraosseous and cerebrospinal fluid pressures in lumbar region. *Spine* 10(1):64–68, 1985.

71. Potter G: A story of 744 cases of neck and back pain treated with spinal manipulation. *J Can Chiropractic Assn* 154(December), 1977.

72. Buehler MT: Spinal stenosis. *J Manipulative Physiol Ther* 2:103–112, 1978.

73. White AA, Panjabi MM: *Basic Biomechanics*. Philadelphia, JB Lippincott, 1978, p 292.

74. Helms CA: CT of the lumbar spine stenosis and arthrosis. *Comput Radiol* 6:359–369, 1982.

75. Jones RAC, Thomson JLG: The narrow lumbar canal, a clinical and radiological review. *J Bone Joint Surg* 50B:595, 1968.

76. Epstein JA, Epstein BS, Levine L: Nerve root compression associated with narrowing of the lumbar spinal canal. *J Neurol Neurosurg Psychiatry* 25:165, 1962.

77. Eisenstein S: The morphometry and pathological anatomy of the lumbar spine in South African Negroes and Caucasoids with specific reference to spinal stenosis. *J Bone Joint Surg* 59B:166, 1977.

78. Uden A, Johnsson K-E, Jonsson K, Pettersson H: Myelography in the elderly and the diagnosis of spinal stenosis. *Spine* 10(2):171–174, 1985.

79. Tait WF, Charlesworth D, Lemon JG: Atypical claudication. *Br J Surg* 72(4):315–316, 1985.

80. Kornberg M, Rechtine GR: Quantitative assessment of the fifth lumbar spinal canal by computed tomography in symptomatic L4-L5 disc disease. *Spine* 10(4):328–330, 1985.

81. Bell G, Rothman R, Booth R, Cuckler J, Garfin S,

Herkowitz H, Simeone F, Doninskas C, Han S: A study of computer-assisted tomography. II. Comparison of metrizamide myelography and computed tomography in the diagnosis of herniated lumbar disc and spinal stenosis. *Spine* 9(6):552–556, 1984.

82. Hakelius A: Prognosis in sciatica. *Acta Orchop Scand* 129(Suppl):1–76, 1970.

83. Hirsch C, Nachemson A: The reliability of lumbar disc surgery. *Clin Orthop (Can)* 189–195, 1963.

84. Quencer RM, Murtagh FR, Post JD, Rosomoff HL, Stokes NA: Postoperative bony stenosis of the lumbar spinal canal: evaluation of 164 symptomatic patients with axial radiography. *Am J Roentgenol* 131(December):1059–1064, 1978.

85. Varughese G, Quartey GRC: Familial lumbar spinal stenosis with acute disc herniations: case reports of four brothers. *J Neurosurg* 51:234–236, 1979.

86. Coxhead CE, Franklin S, Troup JDG: Radiographic variables in patients with sciatic symptoms. Paper presented at the annual meeting of the Society for Back Pain Research, London, November 1981.

87. Baddeley H: Radiology of the lumbar spine. In Jayson M (ed):*The Lumbar Spine and Back Pain*. London, Sector Publishing, 1976, pp 151–171.

88. Spittel JA: Evaluation of the patient with intermittent claudication. *Postgrad Med* 78(2):163–168, 1985.

89. Coffman JD: Intermittent claudication: not so benign. *Am Heart J* (November), 1986.

90. Arnoldi CC: Intraosseous hypertension: a possible cause of low back pain? *Clin Orthop* 115:30–34, 1976.

91. Weinstein J: Mechanisms of spinal pain: the dorsal root ganglion and its role as a mediator of low-back pain. *Spine* 11(10):999–1001, 1986.

92. Rosa M, Capellini C, Canevari MA, Prosetti D, Schivoni S: CT in low back and sciatic pain due to lumbar canal osseous changes. *Neuroradiology* 28:237–240, 1986.

93. Weisz G: Lumbar canal stenosis in Paget's disease. *Clin Orthop* 206(May):223–227, 1986.

94. Foreman SM: Ossification of the posterior longitudinal ligaments: a cause of spinal stenosis syndrome. *J Manipulative Physiol Ther* 8:251–255, 1985.

95. Buszek MC, Ellenberg M, Friedman P: Partial cauda equina compression: result of sacral stenosis. *Arch Phys Med Rehabil* 66:825–826, 1985.

96. Bernini PM, Simeone F: Reflex sympathetic dystrophy associated with low lumbar disc herniation. *Spine* 6(2):180–184, 1981.

97. Kapila A, Chakeres DW: Flexed sitting maneuver for complete lumbar myelography in patients with severe spinal stenosis and apparent block. *Radiology* 160(1):265–267, 1986.

98. Walker MA, Spence VA, Walker WF: Diagnosis of

neurospinous claudication. *Lancet* (November 9): 1077, 1985.

99. Mills GH, Davies GK, Getty CJM, Conway J: The evaluation of liquid crystal thermography in the investigation of nerve root compression due to lumbosacral lateral spinal stenosis. *Spine* 11(5): 427–432, 1986.

100. Engel JM, Engel GM, Gunn DR: Ultrasound of the spine in focal stenosis and disc disease. *Spine* 10(10):928–931, 1985.

101. Gonzalez EG, Hajdu M, Bruno R, et al.: Lumbar spinal stenosis: analysis of pre and postoperative somatosensory evoked potentials. *Arch Phys Med Rehabil* 66:11–14, 1985.

102. Keim HA, Hajdu M, Gonzalez EG, Brand L, Balasubramanian E: Somatosensory evoked potentials as an aid in the diagnosis and intraoperative management of spinal stenosis. *Spine* 10(4): 338–344, 1985.

103. Rothman SLG, Glenn Jr WV: *Multiplanar CT of the Spine*. Baltimore, University Park Press, 1985, p 29.

104. Spengler DM: Current concepts review: degenerative stenosis of the lumbar spine. *J Bone Joint Surg* 69A:305, 1987.

105. Swenson MR: Neurogenic claudication due to pseudospondylolisthesis. *Am Fam Physician* 28(4): 250, 1983.

106. Echeverria T, Lockwood R: Lumbar spinal stenosis. *NY J Med* (May):872–873, 1979.

107. Wiltse LL, Kirkaldy-Willis WH, McIvor GW: The treatment of spinal stenosis. *Clin Orthop* 115:483, 1976.

108. Baker DE, Campbell RK: Pentoxifylline: a new agent for intermittent claudication. *Drug Intell Clin Pharm* 19(5):345–348, 1985.

109. O'Hara J: A double-blind placebo-controlled study of Hexopal in the treatment of intermittent claudication. *J Int Med Res* 13:322, 1985.

110. Halaperin JL, Rothlauf EB, Stern A: Potential adverse effects of pentoxifylline on limb hemodynamics in patients with intermittent claudication. *J Am Coll Cardiol* 7(2):A177, 1977.

111. Johnsson K, Willner S, Johnsson K: Postoperative instability after decompression for lumbar stenosis. *Spine* 11(2):107–110, 1986.

112. McLaren AC, Bailey SI: Cauda equina syndrome: a complication of lumbar discectomy. *Clin Orthop* 204:143–149, 1986.

113. Kirkaldy-Willis WH: The relationship of structural pathology to the nerve root. *Spine* 9(1): 49–52, 1984.

114. Spencer DL, Miller JAA, Bertolini JE: The effect of intervertebral disc space narrowing on the contact force between the nerve root and a simulated disc protrusion. *Spine* 9(1):23–30, 1984.

115. Macgibbon B, Farfan H: A radiologic survey of various configurations of the lumbar spine. *Spine* 4(3):258–266, 1979.

116. Helms CA, Sims R: Foraminal spurs: a normal variant in the lumbar spine. *Radiology* 160:153–154, 1986.

117. Taylor TKF, Roff SJ, Alglietti PL, DiMiria GV, Macucci M, Novenbri A, Innocenti M: The long term results of wedge and compression fractures of the dorsolumbar spine without neurological involvement. *J Bone Joint Surg* 69A:334, 1987.

8

Scoliosis

Donald D. Aspegren, D.C.

Our life is what our thoughts make it

—**M. Aurelius**

INTRODUCTION AND HISTORY

Scoliosis has mystified and intrigued chiropractors for years. In its adolescent form, children who are otherwise healthy are adversely affected by a gradual deterioration causing spinal and truncal deformity. Adult forms may result from previous adolescent malformation or may be the result of de novo development. The elements of pain or cosmetic concern can affect the adult group with equal severity. Having a sound knowledge of scoliosis is fundamental to all chiropractors.

Scoliosis is defined by *Stedman's* as a lateral curvature of the spine (1). As the magnitude of the lateral deformity increases, so does the accompanying rotation. The rotation of the vertebral column promotes prominence of the rib heads and transverse processes. The resultant truncal asymmetry, commonly seen on observation, is fundamental for early detection of the condition (Figs. 8.1 and 8.2). The normal spine has anterior-to-posterior curves when the patient is viewed from the side and no lateral deviation when observed from behind.

The term *scoliosis* is derived from the Greek word meaning curvature. The term was first used by Galen (131–201 AD). However, Hippocrates is credited with the first description of the disorder. Treatment was crude during this time in history. Attempts to straighten the spine included the use of horizontal traction, and underarm and leg distraction while the patient was suspended. Later, braces were produced by blacksmiths who normally made armor (2).

People afflicted with scoliosis, like those with many other physically disabling disorders, have been scorned by the public for centuries. Even in

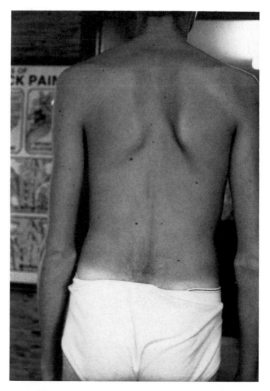

Figure 8.1. Posterior view of a male patient with adolescent idiopathic scoliosis. Note the lack of fullness of the interscapular region. The patient has a hypokyphosis as well.

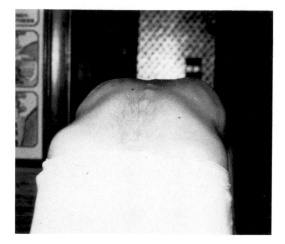

Figure 8.2. Forward bending view of patient observed in Figure 8.1. A right rib hump is visualized.

today's society, it is recognized that one of the most concerning aspects of scoliosis may be the psychological disturbances patients develop due to observable trunk imbalances.

During the 20th century, and in particular during the last 2 decades, a tremendous amount of research has been directed toward understanding and treating scoliosis. Guerin has been credited with the first surgery for scoliosis in 1839. Volkman resected rib deformities in 1889 (3). Stevens (2) writes of Wilhelm Konrad Roentgen, who first utilized roentgen rays and opened new doors to our understanding of scoliosis in 1895.

During the early 1900s, tuberculosis was much more widespread than studies report today, and spinal fusion was used to control the spinal involvement of tuberculosis (3). Hibbs devised a modification of this technique, with which he performed the first spinal fusion for scoliosis in 1914. Since that time, tremendous change has occurred in the treatment of the more serious curves. Bone grafting, either auto- or allogenous, may be employed. Bracing after surgery may or may not be utilized. The use of different forms of instrumentation also has been introduced. The Harrington, Luque, and most recently, Cotrel-Dubousset systems are the most popular.

For less severe curves, bracing has been popular. In 1946, Blount and Schmidt introduced the Milwaukee brace. The brace used counterpressure on the side of the patient, as well as distraction, to control the deformity. Ironically, the brace was first introduced for postsurgical care; it was later modified for use in what is today its prevalent application: advanced conservative care in an attempt to avoid surgery. The modern version of the Milwaukee brace is generally used for thoracic curves with apices from about T7 upward. Lower apical curves are treated with braces such as the Wilmington or Boston brace by practitioners who prefer external truncal orthosis (4).

In the later 1970s, electrical stimulation was introduced. Initially, this form of care used implanted electrodes (5). Recently, transcutaneous stimulation has become the accepted mode of treatment (6).

The majority of recorded studies focus on the case of idiopathic scoliosis. This is believed to represent the largest classification group, reportedly approaching 80 to 90% of all cases. The role of chiropractors treating all forms of skeletally immature scolioses remains vague (7). With adult patients whose most common complaints are pain caused by facet, discal, and related pathology, chiropractors are quite successful. However, when dealing with younger patients at risk of demonstrating curve progression, the role of a chiropractor is not as well defined.

SCHOOL SCREENING AND INCIDENCE

One of the major avenues that directs a young, skeletally immature patient with a suggested spinal deformity to a doctor's office is the school screening. These screenings are commonly performed by nurses; however, other divisions of the health care team are found to be involved.

Torell et al. (8) demonstrated success in performing school screening and effectively reducing the number of children who progress to a protocol indicating surgical stabilization. The study had early detection and treatment of idiopathic scoliosis as its primary focus; it covered 10 years in a stable Swedish population of 1.56 million people. Seven hundred twenty-five patients less than 20 years of age and with scoliosis greater than 20° were followed during this period. Although treatment was essentially the same, Torell et al. found that the percentage of patients requiring an operation decreased each year (Fig. 8.3). There was a general decrease in severe curve magnitude, from 64° to 44°. Though the heightened efforts had resulted in a threefold increase in the number of patients treated for scoliosis, the number requiring surgery had declined.

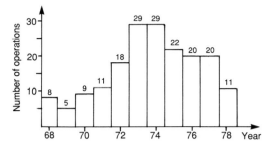

Figure 8.3. The graph shows a decrease in the number of scoliosis surgeries performed on children, believed to be a direct result of early screening and bracing. (Reproduced with permission from Torell G, Norwall A, Nachemson A: The changing patterns of scoliosis treatment due to effective treatment. *J Bone Joint Surg* 63A:340, 1981.)

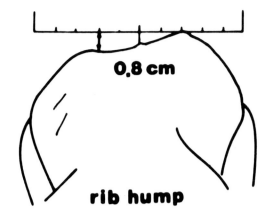

Figure 8.4. A rib hump is shown. A measurement of 8 mm is significant. (Reproduced with permission from Vercautern M, et al.: Trunk asymmetries in a Belgian school population. *Spine* 7(6):556, 1982.)

Their study is considered one of the few in the literature reflecting the actual positive effect of early detection and early conservative care.

Currently, three methods of assessing spinal deformity are employed throughout the world. The first is to have the patient flex forward while standing and to observe the horizon created by the thoracic and lumbar region. This general visual technique has been used by the majority of screeners for years. Unfortunately, this system is extremely subjective and offers no quantitative findings by which one screening or exam can be compared to the next. Consequently, investigators have continued their attempts to better this method.

The second system, which was popularized by a Belgian school study (9), utilizes the same forward flexion; however, this time, the rib hump and lumbar prominence are measured with a ruler and spirit level (Fig. 8.4). The purpose of measuring for an increase in the rib and lumbar region is to reduce the large number of insignificant and false positive curves that were previously detected (Fig. 8.5). In addition to the rib hump and lumbar prominence, considered to be the most significant landmarks measured, the height of the shoulder, the scapula, the iliac crest, and the axillary gaps are also assessed (Fig. 8.6).

The third system utilizes an inclinometer to detect significant trunk asymmetries for referral and advanced evaluation. The most popular inclinometer was developed by William Bunnel (10) and is named the *Scoliometer* (Fig. 8.7). The Scoliometer is placed on the dorsal region of the forward-bending patient in the thoracic or lumbar region at the apices of the curves. Investigators may waiver several vertebral segments and still find measurements that are acceptable for screening procedures. The suggested minimal angle of trunk rotation (ATR) is 5°. At 5° of ATR, Bunnell believes that the student should be referred for possible radiographic assessment. To avoid further radiation, the Scoliometer may be used on subsequent follow-up visits to monitor for progression. For example, if an ATR measurement of 7° had been found 3 months previously on a patient, and currently the patient has the

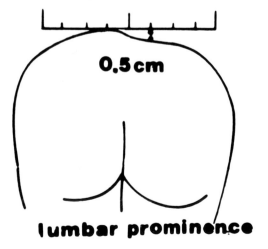

Figure 8.5. A lumbar prominence is shown. Here a 5-mm asymmetry is significant. (Reproduced with permission from Vercautern M, et al.: Trunk asymmetries in a Belgian school population. *Spine* 7(6):556, 1982.)

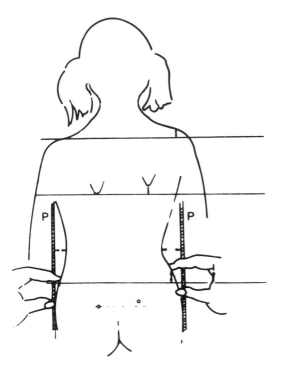

Figure 8.6. Measurements while the patient is standing. (Reproduced with permission from Vercautern M, et al.: Trunk asymmetries in a Belgian school population. *Spine* 7(6):556, 1982.)

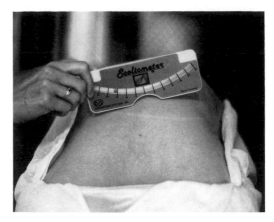

Figure 8.7. Use of Scoliometer for angle of trunk rotation (ATR) measurement.

year (14). The reported worldwide prevalence of scoliosis varies. The results of various studies range from a prevalence of 0.35% to a prevalence of 31.5% reported in Australia (15). One reason for this wide range lies in the definition of scolio-

same measurement recorded, the patient should not need radiographic study. However, if the angle of trunk rotation had increased by 3°, to 10°, an additional study would be performed. Results thus far using the Scoliometer have ranged from very good (11) to marginal (12).

As stated, all three studies utilized the forward-bending posture. Some texts suggest that the adolescent bend forward and touch the fingertips together. However, Stirling and colleagues (13) recently presented a report on how common arm length discrepancies may artificially camouflage or induce rib or lumbar deformities. They believe that the influence of arm asymmetry on trunk deformity may be eliminated by adopting a standard position in the forward-bending test and allowing the arms to hang freely (Figs. 8.8–8.10).

When discussing the occurrence of scoliosis in a population, the proper term to use is *prevalence*. Prevalence describes the proportion of a population afflicted by the disorder. Many authors use the term *incidence*; however, this refers to the rate of occurrence of new cases of the disorder per

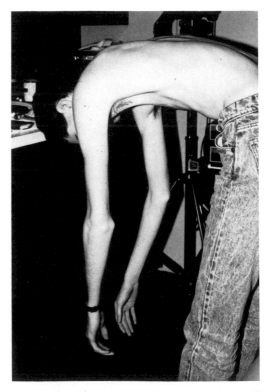

Figure 8.8. The proper method of performing the forward bending test. Allow the arms to hang freely.

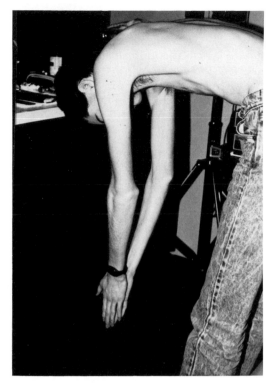

Figure 8.9. The improper method of performing the forward bending test.

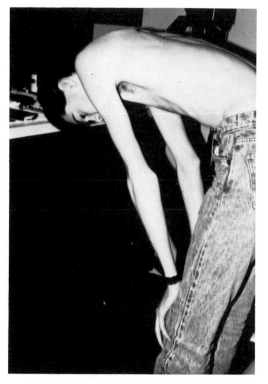

Figure 8.10. If the patient leans forward too long during observation and measurement of the rib hump, he may become fatigued and assume an incorrect position.

sis, or the amount of curvature necessary to be considered a scoliosis. Some studies require 10°, while others require only 5°.

Most studies report relatively similar proportions of mild curves in the 5° to 10° range in males and females. However, as the curvatures increase in magnitude, the balance quickly swings to favor the female gender. Rogala et al. (16) reported an equal balance in small curves, finding a female-to-male ratio of 1.25:1.0 overall in 26,947 screened students. The ratio varied directly with the severity of the curve. Curves of 6° to 10° showed a 1:1 ratio, and curves greater than 20° showed a 5.4:1 ratio (Table 8.1). Curvature requiring advanced care, such as bracing or surgical stabilization, showed a 7:1 female-to-male ratio.

In a recent study performed by Morais et al. (17) on a group of 29,195 children in a community health district in the province of Quebec, 11.4% were referred for additional evaluation after their positive screen. Of the 11.4%, 9.7% refused further evaluation, 7.8% elected to consult their family physicians for their condition, and 1.6% consulted a chiropractor. The remaining 86% were examined by an orthopedic surgeon.

EXAMINATION OF THE SCOLIOSIS PATIENT

One of the most important aspects of scoliosis care is the performance of a proper and thorough examination of the patient. A diagnosis is first achieved. Then, prognostic indicators are accumulated to arrive at a proper decision as to what form of therapy should be implemented.

Table 8.1.
Sex Incidence of Idiopathic Scoliosis According to Severity of the Curve[a]

| Curve | No of Students | | Girls:Boys |
	Girls	Boys	
6–10°	316	322	1:1
11–20°	299	208	1.4:1
21° or more	65	12	5.4:1
Total	680	542	

[a]Reprinted with permission from Rogala E, Drummond D, Gurr J: Scoliosis: incidence and natural history. *J Bone Joint Surg* 60A:173–176, 1978.

The accumulated data, combined with knowledge of the natural history of the condition, are used for each individual case. No two cases are alike; therefore, the therapy for each case differs. A special examination form specifically directed to scoliosis patients has been developed by the author (Figs. 8.11–8.14). This form has obvious similarities to other examination forms; however, it concentrates on seeking out certain prognostic indicators that are utilized in the care of spinal deformities. Much of the first page of the examination involves the history and general recording of past illnesses. Chiropractic assistants should be trained to record an initial history covering information such as chronological age and chief complaint. Most patients will simply state that they have been referred for a scoliosis exam, but occasionally they will report other symptoms, such as back pain.

A history of scoliosis in the family is important not only to determine its genetic link, but also to seek out the potential for scoliosis within the siblings. Ruth Wynne-Davies (18) reports that first-degree siblings of scoliosis patients have a 40-fold increased risk of developing spinal deformities as compared to the general population. Many times, scoliotic deformities are quite advanced by the time they are referred to an office that specializes in scoliosis. This leaves the practitioner feeling somewhat helpless; however, an alert physician may investigate the possibility of the siblings having a deformity and may possibly prevent the remaining members of the family from developing a large curve.

The secondary sex characteristics and menarche play an important part in determining approximately how much growth the female has remaining. Breast formation and the growth of axillary and pubic hair will begin approximately 2 years before menarche. The onset of menses is very important when working with spinal deformities in females, as it signifies the termination of the rapid growth experienced during the adolescent growth spurt (Fig. 8.15). It is this adolescent growth spurt which many times causes the small, relatively dormant spinal deformities to accelerate into larger, very aggressive advancing curves. Prognostically, if a female with a 30° curve has only recently developed pubic and axillary hair and has not started her menstrual periods, she is in much greater danger of experiencing curve progression than a female with a 30° curve who experienced menarche 1 year to 1½ years previously.

In male patients, voice change may be used to identify puberty and a consequential slowing of growth rate. Males generally experience this slowing of growth approximately 2 years later than females.

General examination procedures, such as measurement of blood pressure and other vital signs, with particular emphasis upon the observation of skin markings, should always be performed. Small birthmarks, particularly in the axillary region, may signify a possible neurofibromatosis patient.

After the history has been elicited, the doctors will examine the gowned patient with one of the parents present. It is preferable to have the mother present, particularly when discussing menarche and the other discussed secondary sex characteristics. During the physical exam, measurements such as leg lengths are performed to assess for asymmetry. The standing procedure tested by Aspegren et al. (19) is reasonably accurate during this physical examination. Further, a plumb line is lowered from C7 to find its relationship with the gluteal crease and to determine if the curve is balanced. The shoulder height is measured at the acromioclavicular joint, and the difference and high side are recorded. The inferior pole of the scapula is measured while the patient stands, and the doctor records which is higher. The rib hump and lumbar prominence are further measured to determine if they are significant. The axillary gap is also measured while the patient stands. At this time, the angle of trunk rotation is measured, utilizing the Scoliometer, to determine whether further assessment is indicated. If the measurements are not significant and the angle of trunk rotation falls below 5°, the patient will be categorized in an observation group and asked to return in approximately 6 months for follow-up. Without significant findings in this portion of the exam, additional exam time and radiographic studies are not indicated.

If the recordings are considered significant, examination would advance into the assessment of the integrity of the neuromuscular system for both the upper and lower extremities. This portion of the exam would include deep tendon reflex assessment for the upper and lower extremity, as well as assessment of muscular strengths in these areas. Several reports point to an involved neurological pathology of asymmetry that may be integral to the development of spinal deformities. The patient should be assessed for

PHYSICAL EXAMINATION FORM FOR SCOLIOSIS

Name: _____ Employer: _____

Age: Sex: S.M.W.D.   Ht.   Wt.

Chief Complaint:

History of Scoliosis in Family:

History:
If Accident   D/A   H/A   W/A

Surgical:

Past Illness: TB: Cancer:

Heart & Blood Vessels: Rheumatic Fever:

Smoker: Alcohol:

M: F:

Drugs:
Bowels:
Urination: Digestion:

Menstrual: Date of Menarche:
Date Developed Axillary Hair   —
               Pubic Hair   —
               Breast Formation —

Other Doctors Treating Patient Now:

Present or Past Therapy for Scoliosis:

EXAMINATION
B/P   Pulse: Resp: Temp: Lungs:

Thyroid: Heart Sounds: Skin:

Abdomen: EENT:

Pelvic:

Other:

Figure 8.11. First page of scoliosis examination form is shown. This includes general health questions as well as those specific for scoliotic patients, such as menarche.

upper motor neuron lesions and for dysfunction in the cerebellum and mid-brain region.

Thumb extension is measured to assess for possible connective tissue disorders (20) (Fig. 8.16). Marfan's syndrome and Ehlers-Danlos syndrome have been implicated as playing a role in

	Date				
	Difference				
Leg Length					
Plumbline Through C7 Gluteal Crease					
Differences of Inclination _____High					
– Shoulder at A.C. Jt. – R or L					
– Scapulae – R or L					
– Iliac Crest – R or L					
– Rib Hump – R or L					
– Lumbar Prominence – R or L					
– Axillary Gap – R L					

Figure 8.12. Second page of scoliosis examination form is for recording physical measurements.

the pathogenesis of idiopathic scoliosis. Binns quantified joint laxity in 500 normal Chinese women and in 109 individuals with adolescent idiopathic scoliosis (AIS). His results demonstrated that those with AIS had significantly more laxity, thus suggesting that the two conditions (joint laxity and AIS) are associated. Measurements were recorded by observing the distance from the middle of the thumb to the forearm during passive wrist flexion and thumb apposition. Of the 109 AIS patients reviewed, two groups were formed. Sixty-one patients (56%) demonstrated complete thumb apposition to the forearm, while the remaining 48 patients (44%) had an average thumb-to-forearm distance of 2.0 cm. These measurements were significantly less than those in the normal population, which averaged 4.25 cm.

Beighton et al. (21) and Wynne-Davies (22) have described five criteria to be used in assessment for joint laxity:

1. Knee hyperextension of more than 10°;
2. Elbow hyperextension of more than 10°;
3. Hyperextension of the wrist with the fingers parallel to the forearm;
4. Dorsiflexion of the ankle beyond 45°;
5. Passive apposition of the thumb to the forearm.

If three or more paired joints demonstrated this degree of laxity, the patient was considered positive for a "hyperlaxity syndrome." This appears to correlate to Binn's group of 61 patients with total approximation of the thumb and forearm.

At this stage of the examination, if the findings are significant, a radiographic study would be performed.

THE RADIOGRAPHIC EXAM

The radiographic evaluation is one of the most valuable diagnostic tools available for the physician's use. Only patients having significant asymmetries, found during the physical exam, will warrant radiographic assessment. Not all curves should be radiographed. Many children find themselves in doctors' offices after a positive school screening. A large number of these cases are false positives. Under the well-trained eye of a physician, it should be found that a large majority of curves are trivial. Unfortunately, it has been

Table 1 — Neurology of the Upper Extremity

Reflex	Muscles
Biceps Reflex	Deltoid Biceps
Brachioradialis Reflex (Biceps Reflex)	Wrist Extension Biceps
Triceps Reflex	Wrist Flexors Finger Extension Triceps
	Finger Flexion Hand Intrinsics
	Hand Intrinsics

Table 2 — Neurology of the Lower Extremity

Reflex	Muscles
Patellar	Gluteals
Hamstring	Quads
Achilles	Planter Flexors
	Dorsiflexors

General Neurology	Lumbar ROM	Thumb Extension
– Babinski	– Flex	
– Proprioception	– Ext	
– Rapit Pronation and Supination	– LLB	
	– RLB	
	– LR	
	– RR	

Figure 8.13. Third page of scoliosis examination form covers many areas of the neuromuscular system.

found that a majority of the curves referred for physician assessment are radiographed (11).

The primary purpose of the radiographic procedure is to assist in the determination of etiology and diagnosis. In addition, radiographs are taken to determine the therapeutic and clinical significance of the scoliosis and to obtain information regarding curve magnitude, skeletal age, vertebral rotation, or vertebral body wedging.

The most routine study should include a posterior-to-anterior (PA) and a lateral view of the spine (Figs. 8.17 and 8.18). In addition, a view of the left wrist should be obtained to determine skeletal age (SA) for patients less than 20 years of age (Fig. 8.19) (23). PA views have been found to be effective in reducing radiation to the visceral organs and particularly to the breasts, as compared to AP views when a shield is not used. Many

```
X-RAY                  Date
                       |        |       |       |       |       |       |
---------------------------------------------------------------------------------
Curve 1      Degrees   |        |       |       |       |       |       |
 - Levels              |        |       |       |       |       |       |
 - Measurement         |        |       |       |       |       |       |
 - Apex With Degree    |        |       |       |       |       |       |
     Rotation          |        |       |       |       |       |       |
---------------------------------------------------------------------------------
Curve 2      Degrees   |        |       |       |       |       |       |
 - Levels              |        |       |       |       |       |       |
 - Measurement         |        |       |       |       |       |       |
 - Apex With Degree    |        |       |       |       |       |       |
     Rotation          |        |       |       |       |       |       |
---------------------------------------------------------------------------------
Curve 3      Degrees   |        |       |       |       |       |       |
 - Levels              |        |       |       |       |       |       |
 - Measurement         |        |       |       |       |       |       |
 - Apex With Degree    |        |       |       |       |       |       |
     Rotation          |        |       |       |       |       |       |
---------------------------------------------------------------------------------
Kyphosis               |        |       |       |       |       |       |
---------------------------------------------------------------------------------
Risser Sign            |        |       |       |       |       |       |
---------------------------------------------------------------------------------
Vertebral Ring         |        |       |       |       |       |       |
 Apophysis             |        |       |       |       |       |       |
---------------------------------------------------------------------------------
Hazy Endplates         |        |       |       |       |       |       |
---------------------------------------------------------------------------------
Metha Angle Diff.      |        |       |       |       |       |       |
---------------------------------------------------------------------------------
Flexibility            |        |       |       |       |       |       |
 - Lat.                |        |       |       |       |       |       |
---------------------------------------------------------------------------------
```

Other Findings:

Diagnosis:

Figure 8.14. Last page of scoliosis examination form allows for comparing information from serial x-ray studies.

primary care physicians do not equip their offices with the special shielding equipment necessary to perform AP views properly. Therefore, we recommend utilization of the PA patient positioning to assist in patient safety (24, 25). Rare earth screens should also be utilized to minimize radiation in these adolescent patients. These patients may need serial studies over the course of years while a curve is being observed and/or treated. Rare earth screens and PA views will significantly reduce radiation.

Skeletal age is far more important than chron-

ological age when dealing with the skeletally immature scoliosis patient. The skeletal age may vary by months or years from the chronological age. This variance will be of extreme importance when determining the prognosis. The standard method for determining skeletal age is to compare a view of the left wrist and hand of a patient with the standardized atlas of Greulich and Pyle (26). Although there are other methods and tests available, the Greulich and Pyle atlas is the most accurate method (27).

Lateral flexion views may be necessary to pro-

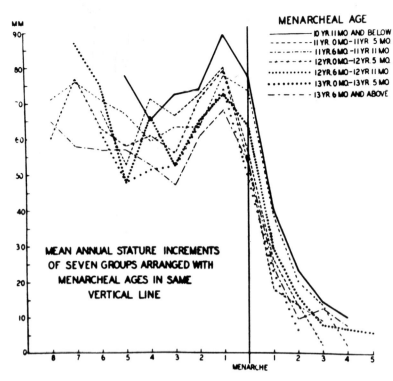

Figure 8.15. This chart depicts the relationship between rate of growth and menarche. When menarche starts, the growth rate quickly decreases. (Reprinted from *Radiographic Atlas of Skeletal Development of the Hand and Wrist*, ed 2, by William Walter Greulich and S. Idell Pyle with the permission of the publishers, Stanford University Press. © 1950 and 1959 by the Board of Trustees of the Leland Stanford Junior University.)

vide information regarding the structural development of the curves. For instance, if nighttime stimulation were about to be implemented, it would be necessary to understand which is the major curve that requires treatment, or whether both curves require control. In cases found in the observation stage which have not yet reached the magnitude for advanced care, lateral bending would not be recommended. Lateral flexion studies are usually performed in a recumbent position and may be done prone or supine.

The most widely utilized method of curve measurement is the Cobb method. In Cobb's (28) teaching, he gives credit to Robert Lippman, who suggested using a particular measuring system in 1935. Cobb later used this system in his teachings, and, over time, this most accurate system of curve magnitude measuring took on Cobb's name.

The Cobb measurements are performed by locating the maximally tilted vertebral bodies of a curvature in the AP or PA projection. A line is drawn through the top end plate of the most su-

perior vertebral body, and a perpendicular line is then drawn downward. Next, a line is drawn through the inferior end plate of the bottom maximally tilted vertebral body and a perpendicular line is drawn cephalad from this line. An angle will be formed at the intersection of these lines and represents the curve magnitude (Fig. 8.20).

Another prognostic sign that can be harvested from the radiographs is vertebral body rotation. Initially, rotation was assessed by observing the spinous process and its migration through the vertebral body during the common rotation accompanying a scoliotic deformity. However, the spinous process is not always easily observed, and a new system has been devised to utilize the observation of the pedicle across the vertebral body. One system commonly used employs a grading scale of 0 to +4. A system slightly easier to remember than the grading procedure is based on subdividing the vertebral body into percentages, as is done with grading a spondylolisthesis slippage. As the pedicle migrates across the vertebral

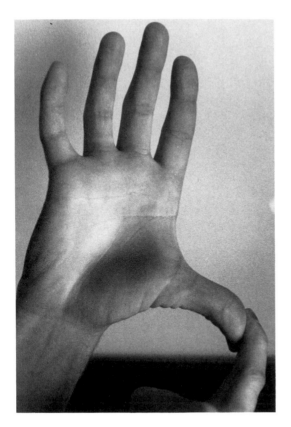

Figure 8.16. Testing for thumb extension used as a screen for joint laxity seen in certain connective tissue disorders.

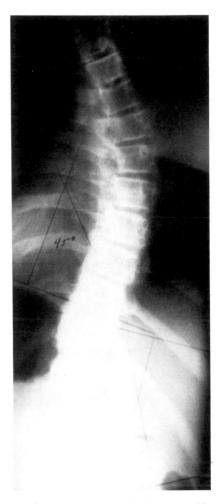

Figure 8.17. Routine x-rays for frontal Cobb measurement are performed PA.

body, it is given a percentage value based upon the amount of migration (Fig. 8.21).

The AP or PA view may be used also to observe the Risser sign. This is the secondary ring apophysis that develops over the top of each iliac crest. The apophysis will appear at the most lateral aspects of the crest near the anterior superior iliac spine (ASIS) and migrate medially toward the sacral ala. As the apophysis migrates medially, it is graded from 1 to 4 (Fig. 8.22). A grading of 4 (for females) and 5 (for males) signifies that growth has stopped. As the apophysis fuses to the iliac crest, it is given a grade of 5 (Fig. 8.23). The Risser sign can also be used as a prognostic indicator. A child with a low-grade Risser sign (i.e., 1) and a scoliotic deformity of significant magnitude has a poorer prognosis than one who has a high-grade Risser sign (i.e., 4) and equal curve magnitude. The low-grade Risser sign suggests more growth potential and associated curve progression than the higher-grade Risser sign. The pa-

tient with a high-grade Risser sign has less growth remaining and is less likely to demonstrate curve progression.

The lateral spine view is assessed initially to rule out any pathological condition capable of causing a scoliotic deformity. The lateral projection is also utilized for prognostic purposes as the vertebral body ring apophyses are also assessed. Some authors feel that this might be one of the most important prognostic signs (29). As long as the end plate is not fused, it remains very impressionable by gravitational forces unevenly distributed across a vertebral body. These uneven pressures may result in permanent vertebral body wedging, consequently adding to structural spinal deformity.

The lateral projections of the lumbar and tho-

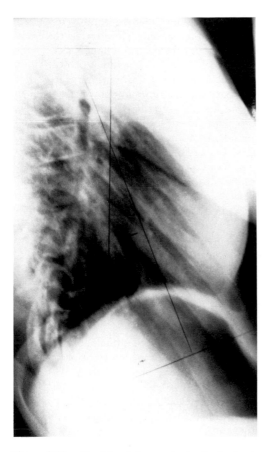

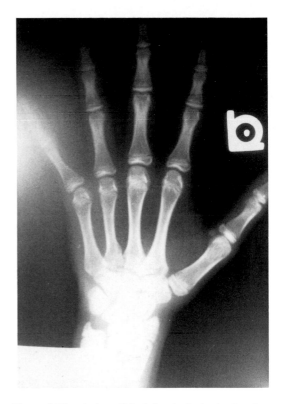

Figure 8.19. A view of the left wrist is obtained to determine skeletal age.

Figure 8.18. The lateral view evaluates for kyphosis.

racic region may also offer a better understanding of the three-dimensional aspects of the case. Shufflebarger and King (30) recently demonstrated their combination procedure using a frontal Cobb measurement as well as a lateral projection measurement to arrive at a better understanding of the true effect the scoliotic deformity was having on the patient.

In skeletally immature patients (boys with a skeletal age of 18 years or less, and girls with a skeletal age of 16 years or less), the most common type of scoliosis is caused by unknown factors. This type of scoliosis is referred to as *idiopathic*. Though we will discuss some of the suggested theories and probable explanations for idiopathic curves, we must admit that the majority of deformities seen in our offices are caused by mechanisms not yet totally understood. The second major type of scoliotic deformity is caused by the short leg. Authors such as Dickson (31) report that approximately 40% of the curves detected on

school screening may be attributed to leg length inequality during adolescence.

SCOLIOSIS CLASSIFICATION

In an attempt to classify cases of scoliosis according to cause, it becomes apparent that there is an overlap between structural and nonstructural causes. A nonstructural curve is described as a nonprogressive scoliosis, possessing symmetrical side-bending movements on clinical and radiographic examination. The curve is generally mild and is found in the lumbar and thoracolumbar regions. The major cause of these curves is the short leg, and is quite commonly found in practice. The structural scoliosis deformity is characterized as being more likely to progress, having fixed vertebral body rotation, and a prominence viewed in the thoracic or lumbar region. This prominence, referred to as a rib hump or lumbar prominence, persists through side bending on clinical exam. On side-bending radiographic studies, the curvature will reduce; however, it will persist, and the symmetrical side-bending appear-

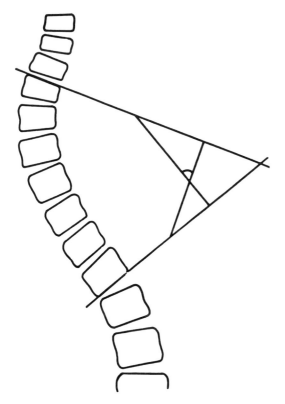

Figure 8.20. Cobb's measurement is shown.

ance found in nonstructural, or functional, curves will not be present.

The distinction between the two major subdi-

visions, functional and structural deformities, seems relatively clearcut. However, as Goldstein and Waugh (29) believe, the importance of the nonstructural curve lies in its ability to evolve into a structural deformity. Once the curve has taken on a structural manifestation, it is more likely to progress and darkens the prognostic outlook for the patient. If curves caused by leg length inequality are found in these early functional stages, they can be corrected by such mechanisms as a heel or shoe lift and be prevented from transforming into structural deformities. As a result, the patient may be spared a tremendous amount of work and anxiety. Once a structural deformity has been allowed to entrench itself in the patient's spine, the altered biomechanical forces may promote further asymmetrical growth and motion. A prime example of this altered growth pattern is explained by the Heuter-Volkman law. As the law suggests, altered end plate pressure may retard normal vertebral body development, resulting in body wedging.

The transformation of a functional to a structural progressive curvature has been produced (with animals) in a laboratory setting. Within this lab setting, studies have been performed to promote asymmetrical growth in previously normal spines, thus producing progressive spinal deformities (32, 33).

Though there will be some overlap between different classification categories, a basic fundamental breakdown for the initial understanding and categorization of the patient is offered be-

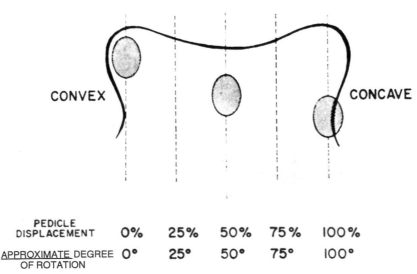

PEDICLE DISPLACEMENT	0%	25%	50%	75%	100%
APPROXIMATE DEGREE OF ROTATION	0°	25°	50°	75°	100°

Figure 8.21. Shown is a method for recording rotation. (Reproduced with permission from Nash CL Jr, Moe J: A study of vertebral rotation. *J Bone Joint Surg* 51A:228, 1969.)

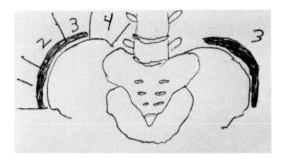

Figure 8.22. The grading of the Risser sign.

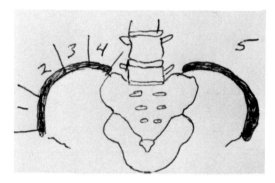

Figure 8.23. A Risser sign of 5.

low, with the intention of developing a more universal dialogue between physicians.

Classification

NONSTRUCTURAL SCOLIOSIS

I. Postural scoliosis
II. Scoliosis due to leg length discrepancy
III. Sciatic scoliosis
  A. Herniated nucleus pulposus
  B. Tumors
  C. Other space-occupying lesion with pressure on nerve roots
IV. Inflammatory scoliosis
  A. Appendicitis
  B. Perinephric abscess
  C. Other infectious disorders

STRUCTURAL SCOLIOSIS

I. Idiopathic scoliosis
  A. Infantile (0 to 3 years)
  B. Juvenile (3 to 10 years)
  C. Adolescent (10 years to skeletal maturity; skeletal maturity for boys, 18 years; for girls, 16 years)

II. Congenital scoliosis
  A. Failure of formation
    1. Hemivertebra
    2. Wedge vertebra
  B. Failure of segmentation
    1. Partial or unilateral bar
    2. Complete or bilateral "block"
    3. Mixed
III. Neuromuscular scoliosis
  A. Neuropathic
    1. Lower motor neuron
      a. Poliomyelitis
      b. Traumatic
      c. Spinal muscular atrophy
      d. Myelomeningocele
    2. Upper motor neuron
      a. Cerebral palsy
      b. Spinocerebellar degeneration
    3. Other
      a. Central nervous system trauma
      b. Syringomyelia
  B. Myopathic
    1. Muscular dystrophy
      a. Duchenne's
      b. Limb-girdle
      c. Fascioscapulohumeral
    2. Amyotonia congenita
    3. Other
IV. Scoliosis due to neurofibromatosis
V. Scoliosis due to mesenchymal disorders
  A. Congenital
    1. Marfan's syndrome
    2. Morquio's disease
    3. Others
  B. Acquired
    1. Rheumatoid arthritis
VI. Traumatic scoliosis
  A. Fracture
  B. Surgery
    1. Vertebral
    2. Thorax
  C. Irradiation
VII. Scoliosis due to metabolic disorders
  A. Rickets
  B. Drug induced
  C. Osteogenesis imperfecta
VIII. Scoliosis due to lumbosacral joint anomalies
  A. Congenital
    1. Transitional segments
    2. Others
  B. Acquired
    1. Spondylolysis and spondylolisthesis
    2. Others

TREATMENT

Manipulation

Manipulation may be used for those patients categorized in the advanced observation stage and the advanced conservative care stage. Goals of the manipulation of the scoliotic patient include the following:

1. Alleviation of facet subluxations of the spine. White (34) theorizes that malalignment of spinal facets may be the initial precipitating condition in the development of an adolescent deformity. Facet fixations may set off a chain of events leading to asymmetrical loading on the epiphyseal plates and to muscle and ligamentous imbalance, ultimately resulting in curve progression. This evolution of events, compounded with an adolescent growth spurt, may demonstrate how a benign flexible functional curve is transformed into a malignant progressive spinal deformity. Manipulation may be used to help restore normal facet orientation and intersegmental motion.

2. Increased spinal flexibility is regarded as a positive prognostic sign. A rigid curve lacking flexibility is more likely to progress, and it is more difficult to control its progressive nature. A rigid curve is also not as responsive to bracing or nighttime stimulation and is not as easily straightened during surgery. The literature includes several reports of attempts to increase the amount of spinal flexibility to assist the orthosis or surgery. Dickson and Leatherman (35) were able to increase flexibility by the use of physical exercise performed for 1 to 2 hours over 8 consecutive days. They used lateral flexion exercises to increase flexibility. A major contribution of chiropractic care for structural idiopathic adolescent curves will be to help increase spinal flexibility. Chiropractic therapy may address the specific region of the curve. Manipulation is used to derotate the spine and to stretch shortened concave structures such as discs, muscle, and ligaments (Figs. 8.24–8.26). The advantage of manipulation over general lateral exercises is that manipulation is more specific and concentrates reducing forces at the needed levels. Lateral flexion and other traditional scoliosis exercises have difficulty directing force to the rigid part of the curve. These exercises allow much of the correcting motion to occur in the flexible, functional compensatory levels that do not need correction.

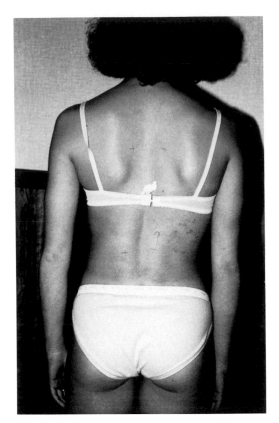

Figure 8.24. A posterior view of an AIS patient. Note the right scapular elevation.

Neuromuscular Nighttime Stimulation

For years, physicians treating scoliosis have traditionally turned to the Milwaukee, Wilmington, or Boston braces as the accepted means of controlling those curves which are beyond the observation stage but not yet advanced far enough for surgery. With the use of these external trunk orthoses came concern about the adverse psychological effects they might have (36), concern about noncompliance by patients who were reluctant to wear the devices (37), and, more recently, concern about their effectiveness in controlling spinal deformities (38, 39). Consequently, other forms of care have been sought. The most accepted alternative to bracing has been to offer the patient in this category neuromuscular nighttime stimulation.

Some of the most preliminary studies in this field were performed on animals (5, 32, 40). Walter P. Bobechko, M.D. (5), from Toronto, On-

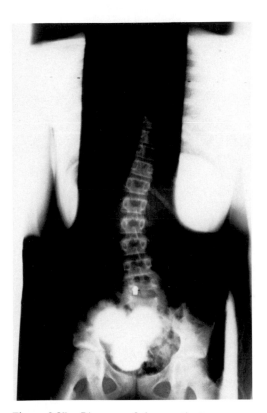

Figure 8.25. PA x-rays of above patient.

tario, reported how he was able to successfully induce and reduce a scoliosis in younger animals by implanting electrodes in the paraspinal muscles. The electrodes were powered with an intermittent cyclic current of about 1-second duration at 10-second intervals. Muscle fatigue was encountered if stimulation was continuous, and the inducive advantage was lost. This curve-reducing ability proved valuable in more recent clinical work with human curves. Bobechko later described how he was able to reduce thoracolumbar curves measuring from 45° to 10° by much the same method.

The earliest forms of electrical stimulation in the treatment of idiopathic scoliosis used implanted electrodes. Herbert and Bobechko (41) recently cited the advantages and disadvantages of using implanted electrodes, referred to as electrospinal instrumentation (ESI). ESI requires surgical insertion of a receiver and requires a short hospital stay. However, the procedure is considered relatively safe, simple, and fast. An advantage with ESI is that no skin irritation is en-

countered, as is found in surface electrical spinal orthosis (ESO).

Of the 90 patients Herbert and Bobechko have treated with ESI, 75 (84%) have been successful to or past skeletal maturity. The doctors believe that ESI is best suited for younger patients in whom treatment may be required for more than a few years.

The more widely used form of electrical stimulation to control scoliosis is via placement of surface electrodes (Fig. 8.27). Several names may be used to describe this form of care, e.g., electrical spinal orthosis (ESO), lateral electrical surface stimulation (LESS), and transcutaneous neuromuscular stimulation (TNS).

The introduction of electrical spinal orthosis has not been without controversy. Some believe that the device is quite successful in controlling progressive adolescent idiopathic scoliosis (AIS) (41–48), while others have found it to be not as successful (49–51).

In support of LESS therapy are John Brown, M.D., and Jens Axelgaard, Ph.D., from the Rancho Los Amigos Rehabilitation Engineering Center in Downey, California. These researchers have pioneered much of the development of the TNS unit named Scolitron, currently manufactured by EBI Medical Systems, Inc., Fairfield, New Jersey. In one of the largest, most highly quoted studies in favor of LESS (48), 548 patients were treated by 54 principal investigators in North America and Western Europe. Patient selection was limited to those individuals with a rapidly progressing scoliosis and at least 1 year of growth remaining. With a mean follow-up time of 12 months, analysis reports stated that 72% of the patients had either reduced or stabilized their curves. Thirteen percent of the patients experienced temporary progression with eventual stabilization. Progression was noted in 15% of the children. This latter group was terminated from the study.

Fisher, Rapp, and Emkes (45) recently reported their results of a 3-year study comparing the ESO with the Milwaukee brace for treatment of AIS. Fifty patients were assigned to each group. One group received the ESO and the other the Milwaukee brace. Members of each group were comparable in age, sex, Risser sign, and curve morphology. Seventy percent of each group had their curves successfully controlled over the course of 3 years. The test concluded that electrical stimulation is comparable to the

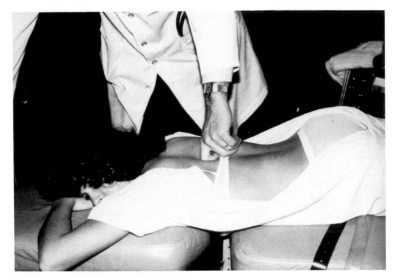

Figure 8.26. Manipulation of the thoracic curve is demonstrated. Note that the patient is turned end-for-end with her head now on the caudal section.

Milwaukee brace, finding no significant differences in rate of curve progression or failure.

McCullough (46) published a recent study involving several of the top researchers in the field of scoliosis. ESO was utilized on 379 patients by 42 surgeons from 28 different centers. The results offered a 90% success rate for curves below 30° and 78% for curves measuring 30° to 40°.

Also found in the literature were several reports of the unsuccessful use of neuromuscular stimulation in the control of AIS. One of the most recent reports is from Goldbert et al. (49) of the Lady's Hospital for Sick Children, Dublin, Ireland. The Scolitron device, then produced by Neuromedics, and the Orthatron device, from Raymar, were used. Forty-one patients with adolescent or juvenile idiopathic scoliosis were treated. Nineteen were removed from the study due to curve progression or unacceptable deformity. Sixteen required surgery, while 13 report-

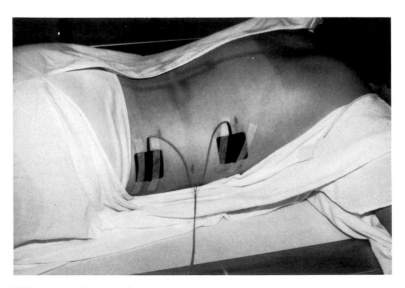

Figure 8.27. LESS being used on a scoliosis patient.

edly reached skeletal maturity without significant curve deterioration. The patients who did well were from the lower risk groups and had more positive prognostic indicators. As a consequence of the above results, Lady's Hospital has stopped using TNS for their conservative care of progressive juvenile or adolescent idiopathic scoliotic deformities.

Bylund and colleagues (51) also offer disappointing results from their use of LESS via the Scolitron stimulator. In their paper, the results of 18 cases were offered. Of the children who discontinued care because of discomfort, five did not carry through an adequate treatment program. Nine (50%) followed through properly. Of the nine in the latter group, five showed progression of their scoliosis during treatment. Bylund et al. believed that LESS had not proven to be an effective treatment for scoliosis. Of interest were the results of muscle biopsies taken before and after treatment. The results suggested a "spilling over" of the stimulation to the concave aspect of the curve, thus promoting curve progression rather than preventing it as intended.

COMPLIANCE

Compliance of the patient is always of concern when prescribing any form of patient-involved activity. Brace therapy has encountered a notable degree of resistance from adolescents, primarily due to the concern for social stigma arising from wearing an external orthosis readily observable by one's peers. Kahanovitz and Weiser (37) compared patient compliance in LESS therapy and bracing. Their retrospective study involved interviews with 40 mothers of females with AIS. Fifty percent of these patients reportedly showed good or total compliance, 10% fair, and 5% poor, while 35% were classified as failures. Skin irritation was the most frequent excuse for discontinuation. Interestingly, the longer the patients used LESS, the more compliant they became. Conversely, braced patients were just the opposite. Kahanovitz and Weiser concluded by stating, "overall compliance appears to be somewhat better for electrical stimulation programs than for bracing" (37).

In this author's own practice, compliance has not been a definitive problem when using LESS and the Scolitron device. Perhaps this is due to a slightly different approach taken by chiropractors. This will be further discussed in the case studies.

Kahanovitz, Snow, and Pinter (36) address the psychological concerns of bracing versus LESS. They reported that LESS patients had a significantly higher level of self esteem than the brace group, and that brace patients demonstrated a much greater perception of hostility than the LESS group. Brace patients focused more on their emotional problems than on the physical problems of their disease. LESS patients were found to be more physically active, vigorous, and outgoing, and much less anxious and depressed than brace patients.

INDICATIONS FOR USE OF LESS

The clinician's manual for the Scolitron neuromuscular stimulator (52), published by EBI Medical Systems, lists the following parameters: "The stimulator is to be used in conjunction with the prescribed electrode placement technique of lateral electrical surface stimulation for treatment of scoliosis. Its use is indicated to arrest or retard curve progression in juvenile or adolescent single or double major idiopathic scoliosis. Those patients with single major curves should be selected on a basis of being at risk for curve progression. The major curve should have an apex at or caudal to T5 with a magnitude not greater than 45 degrees. Curves less than 20 degrees may be treated only if prognostic factors place the patient at high risk of curve progression."[a]

Patients undergoing LESS are maintained under care until reaching skeletal maturity, which is indicated by:

1. No vertical growth for 18 months;
2. Risser's sign of 4+ or 5+;
3. Closure of distal radius;
4. Closure of all ring apophyses.

In the writings of several authors using an ESO, it has been suggested that patients with curves in the 20° to 30° range have demonstrated curve progression of 5° or more within the preceding 12 months. Curves that have demonstrated a progressive tendency are more likely to continue to advance than those which have not. Curves 30° or greater in skeletally immature patients are considered progressive and do not re-

---

[a] Reproduced with permission from *Clinician's Manual and Operating Instructions.* Fairfield, NJ, EBI Medical Systems.

quire past films for progression documentation. Further, at least 1 year's growth should be remaining in those patients being considered for stimulation. This is calculated by determining the skeletal age by comparing the left wrist of the patient with the standards from the Gruelich-Pyle atlas and by Risser's iliac crest evaluation.

In neuromuscular stimulation, unlike brace therapy, no weaning period is utilized. However, in consideration of the literature regarding disc maturation, continued use for a short period of time may benefit the patient.

Case Presentations

CASE 1

The first case to be offered involves an adolescent female with a 27° thoracolumbar dextrorotatory scoliosis (Fig. 8.28). She had a chronological age of 14 years and 4 months (CA, 14+4) and, more importantly, a skeletal age of 14 years, 0 months (SA, 14+0). A hip hump of 12 mm was present on the right. The patient brought past

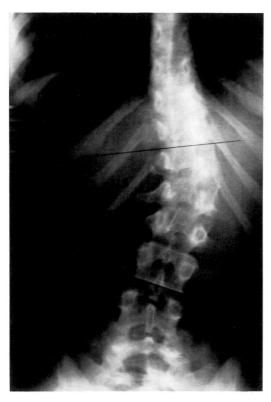

Figure 8.28. A 27° curve was present when therapy began on this patient's progressive AIS. Her curve had been progressing at approximately 1° per month.

films demonstrating 9° of progression within the last 9 months. Menarche had begun approximately 2 months previously.

Nighttime stimulation was initiated with the Scolitron unit, in conjunction with manipulation. The patient was seen three times a week for the first 3 weeks for manipulation. This time is known as a "warm-up" period. During this phase, stimulation amplitude is gradually increased to the prescribed 70 mA required for therapeutic stimulation and correction. During these visits, the patient and parents are counseled on whatever problems they may be confronting. Skin irritation, appearing in the form of a rash, is by far the most frequent complaint. To control this rash, the prescribed region of pad placement is kept clean. The conducting element, Tac Gel (Pharmaceutical Innovators, Inc., Newark, New Jersey), a hypoallergenic conductive element, has proven to be useful in reducing skin irritation.

During this warm-up period, the patient received manipulation to reduce mechanical problems such as facet subluxations. Further, manipulation was used to increase flexibility of the concave structures, i.e., ligaments and muscle tissues, to further potentiate the effect of the stimulator.

After the end of the warm-up period, permanent pad placement was obtained by placing the patient prone and taking films of the patient without the stimulator, then again while wearing it. Five degrees of reduced angulation is required to identify proper placement. (A more thorough description of this procedure may be found in Reference 53.)

At the time of this writing, it is 1 year after skeletal maturity was reached in this patient, at which time stimulation was terminated. We did not use a weaning period for this patient. The patient has stabilized at 30° (Fig. 8.29). An initial reduction had been experienced, similar to the initial rapid reduction commonly observed in bracing; however, a slow, gradual return plus 3° of lateral curvature was experienced.

CASE 2

A young girl with a chronological age of 14+5 was referred to our clinic. Her height was 59¾ inches and her weight 91 lb. Her chief complaint was a scoliosis, initially found during a school screening. There was no past history of scoliosis in her family. No significant past illnesses were reported, nor were genetic disorders known.

Secondary sex characteristics such as breast formation and growth of axillary and pubic hair had begun approximately 2 years previously. Menarche had occurred 6 months prior to the initial exam.

The physical examination demonstrated no skin lesions. The right acromioclavicular (AC) joint was 20 mm

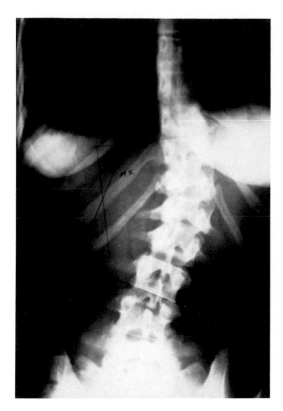

Figure 8.29. A 30° curvature after skeletal maturity.

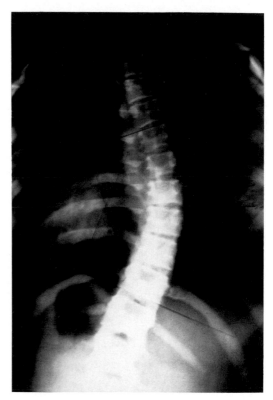

Figure 8.30. A 40° curve is observed at the onset of care for a progressive single major thoracic AIS deformity.

higher than the left. The right scapula was elevated 15 mm compared to the left. A right rib hump of 30 mm with an ATR of 12° was found. The left leg appeared short by ½ inch. Normal muscle strength and deep tendon reflex patterns were observed. Thumb extension was limited to 90°.

The patient brought x-rays from her referring chiropractor. The major curve was from T5 to T11, measuring 40° (Fig. 8.30). The apex was observed at T8 with a 20% rotation. A minor curve from T12 to L1 measured 28°. A skeletal age of 14+0 was observed by comparison of the patient's left wrist with standards from the Greulich and Pyle atlas. The vertebral ring apophysis was unfused, with the end plates from T5 to T10 observed as being hazy. Also observed was a pars defect at the L5 level. An impression of progressive adolescent idiopathic scoliosis with spondylolysis of L5 was recorded.

Nighttime stimulation was initiated with the Scolitron stimulator. A single-channel unit was prescribed.

Follow-up radiographic studies to evaluate for progression were performed. The first was 4 months after the end of the warm-up phase and the determination of permanent pad placement. Frontal Cobb measurement

of the major curve showed a reduction to 31° from the previously recorded 40° (Fig. 8.31). The compensatory lower curve also decreased several degrees.

Films obtained 3 months later confirmed further improvement, with reduction of the curve to 29°. At that time, the patient's skeletal age was 14+9 (Fig. 8.32).

Currently, the patient is treated every 2 weeks with manipulation. In this case, a technique in which the patient is turned end-for-end is used. The patient's head is placed on the caudal section and turned to derotate the spine. Placing the patient in this manner allows the chiropractor to use the more mobile caudal section on the upper, larger, major thoracic curve. In this case, the upper curve had more structural changes.

Minimal skin irritation and no sleep disturbances have been reported in this case.

Bracing

During the last 40 years, bracing has been the most common form of therapy for patients with curves ranging from 20° to 45°. The traditional

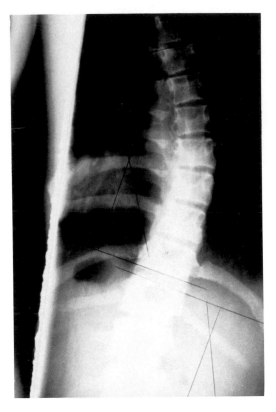

Figure 8.31. The above patient is shown 9 months into care, still skeletally immature and continuing to use nighttime stimulation.

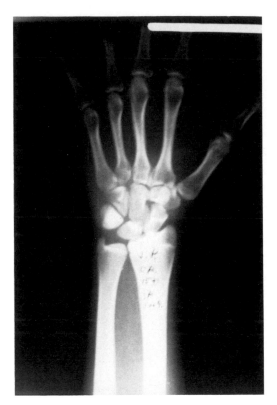

Figure 8.32. Left wrist showing a skeletal age of 14 years and 9 months (SA, 14+9).

form of bracing, to which all others are compared, is the use of the Milwaukee brace. The other two braces commonly used are the Boston and Wilmington braces.

Braces used in the treatment of scoliosis patients include two basic categories (54), the first of which is the CTLSO (cervical-thoracic-lumbar-sacral orthosis), also known as the Milwaukee brace. The CTLSO was originally developed in 1944 by Drs. Blount and Schmidt, and was designed for postsurgical care of scoliosis patients. Researchers such as Moe became so impressed with its use that it was incorporated into the care of presurgical patients or those needing advanced conservative care. The Milwaukee brace is generally indicated for thoracic curves, with some authors suggesting only primary thoracic curves with an apex of T8 or higher.

The second category of braces commonly used in scoliosis care is the TLSO (thoracic-lumbar-sacral orthosis) or "underarm" type of orthosis.

The Wilmington and Boston braces are found in this group. The TLSO will be used for double major curve patterns or those curves with an apex of T8 or lower.

As recently as the 1970s, brace therapy was considered to be indicated in skeletally immature patients with a curve magnitude of 20° to 45°. Taken into consideration were physiological signs of maturity and growth in the preceding months. Since this time, greater emphasis has been placed on documenting curve progression prior to prescribing an external trunk orthosis (54).

Current indications for brace therapy include documentation of 5° or more of curve advancement in the previous year for curves in the 20° to 30° range. Those patients with curves above 30° need not demonstrate progression, as they are considered progressive. Brace therapy may also be used in large curves, ranging to 50° or 60°, with the purpose of controlling the spinal deformity until skeletal maturity, and then performing spinal instrumentation and fusion.

High thoracic curves (Figs. 8.33 and 8.34) or

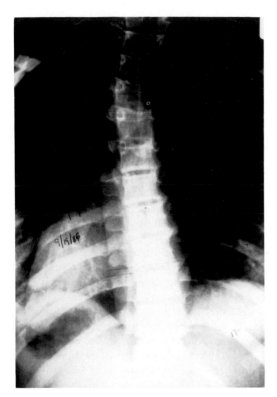

Figure 8.33. High apical curves offer a poor prognosis.

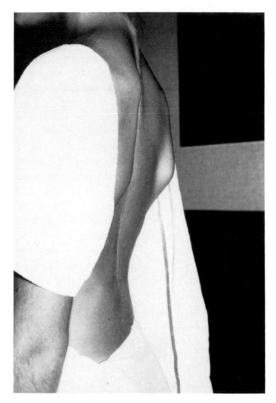

Figure 8.34. Lateral view demonstrating the loss in kyphosis. These curves tend to be very progressive in skeletally immature patients.

thoracic curves with a lordosis have been found to have a poor clinical outlook and likely will proceed unaltered even with brace therapy (55). The effectiveness of brace therapy may be predicted by observing the degree of initial correctedness induced by wearing the brace. If the brace causes the curve to decrease by 50%, a favorable outlook is suggested. However, if the curve does not decrease by 50%, and seems rigid, the prognosis is poorer and the brace will likely be less effective in controlling the curve's progressiveness (56).

Weaning the patient from the brace can be a long and difficult process. The patient may be allowed to advance to part-time wear from the previous schedule (23 of 24 hours) used during full-time wear. During this part-time wear, the clinician will monitor the curve magnitude. From the time of skeletal maturity (when part-time wear or weaning may begin), to the early twenties, the intervertebral disc will be maturing. Different patients mature at different rates; thus, there is a need for continued monitoring after skeletal maturity. As a general rule, the more flexible the

curve, the longer the follow-up time will be, as these cases tend to be more immature in disc and related connective tissue (57).

Surgery

Surgery is considered in only a small number of scoliosis cases. Most cases are only observed, or receive one of the advanced conservative care devices, i.e., bracing or LESS. However, every clinician dealing with spinal deformity should have an awareness of surgeries for the advanced forms of this disorder.

As in many areas of health care, controversy surrounds the question of when surgery is or is not indicated. To address this important topic, one must first consider what harm a spinal deformity offers the patient. Pertinent questions each clinician must address are as follows: Will pain be the major problem later in life? Will the patient's life be adversely affected by the curve? If the patient's life is affected, at what degree of curve magnitude did this occur? These questions demand answers before any form of care is offered. One must weigh the disadvantages of allowing a spinal deformity to run its natural course against the benefits that may be gained by offering spinal surgery. The cure must not be worse than the disease.

A discussion is presented here of two significant papers considered by many to be useful in deciding on therapy for a scoliosis patient. First, Nachemsor (58) addressed the effect of severe lateral curvature on the patient's ability to work and maintain health, and on the survival rate. His follow-up study of 117 adult patients with severe scoliosis (80° or more) indicated grave disturbances in the heart and lung functions, irrespective of the curve etiology. The results showed that this group of patients suffered from nearly a 100% increased mortality as compared to the general population. The paper also reported that the mortality rate of a population with severe scoliosis was well above that of an average population. In this retrospective study of 117 patients, 20 died; this was compared to the 11.4 deaths predicted in a group of equal size by the national average death rate for the general population. Sixteen of the scoliosis patients died from hyposcoliotic cardiopathy with cor pulmonale. Decrease in work capacity was also much higher in this group of survivors.

The second paper to address this area was written by Nilsonne and Lundgren (59), who followed 102 patients. The mortality rate was reported to be 2.2 times higher than in the general population. Deaths most frequently occurred after the age of 45. Cardiac and pulmonary disease was the cause of 60% of the deaths. Physical work capacity was also reportedly decreased in this group, with only half the patients able to work. Interestingly, the psychological problems resulting from the cosmetic deformity were suggested to be the cause of an extremely high proportion of unmarried women in this group.

With the above information in mind, the clinician may utilize the available natural history studies to draw a conclusion as to whether the patient will likely reach these levels of curve magnitude.

NATURAL HISTORY

Natural history studies (60, 61) are essential in determining the treatment mode for any group of patients, i.e., observation, advanced conservative care, or surgery in the juvenile, adolescent, or adult. Many of the prognostic indicators, such as the Risser sign age at diagnosis, growth, and the timing of menarche, are useful for predicting curve progression. However, future growth potential and curve severity remain the most reliable indicators in predicting curve progression.

At one time, it was believed that once the patient reached skeletal maturity, no further curve progression would occur. However, over the last 2 decades, we have come to understand that this is not true. Certain curves do progress after skeletal maturity.

One of the most frequently quoted studies involves the work of Weinstein and Ponseti (60, 61). In 1978, these authors located 219 patients with untreated adolescent idiopathic scoliosis seen at the University of Iowa between 1932 and 1948. Eighty-four percent were women; 16% were men. The average follow-up age was 40 years. Current x-rays were obtained for comparison. These revealed that 68% of the curves progressed more than 5° after skeletal maturity. Curves measuring less than 30° at skeletal maturity did not progress in adult life. Curves greater than 30° did progress, though to a variable degree depending on pattern, magnitude, rotation and Mehta angle (Table 8.2).

Unfortunately, all clinicians are confronted with patients in the "gray zone." It is a struggle to decide what treatment is best for these patients. The studies from the University of Iowa are helpful, yet each case comes down to an individual decision. What is best for the patient?

RESPIRATORY FUNCTION

Researchers such as Chong et al. (62), and more recently, DiRocco and Vaccaro (63) have attempted to identify patients who may be experiencing increased cardiopulmonary restriction that could render them susceptible to cardiopathy later in life.

As Chong et al. (62) describe, it is well recognized that scoliosis in excess of 65° results in cardiorespiratory impairment. Patients with curves of lesser magnitude have been noted to have nearly normal resting respiratory function. Because of a great cardiorespiratory reserve, decreases in pulmonary function secondary to scoliosis may be masked in studies conducted while the patient is at rest. In the experiment conducted by Chong et al., 30 adolescents with idio-

Table 8.2.
Curve Progression After Maturity (Average 40-Year Follow-Up)[a]

	Curve at Maturity (°)	Average Progression at Follow-Up (°)
Thoracic	<30	2.6
	30–50	10.2
	50–75	29.4
	75–100	12.6
	>100	10.3
Lumbar	<30	0
	30–50	15.4
	>50	18.5
Thoracolumbar	<30	14
	30–50	11
	>50	22.3
Combined	<30	3
		5.6
Thoracic	30–50	10.1
Lumbar		12.7
	50–75	18.3
		23.1
	>75	11
		15.4

[a]Adapted from Weinstein SL, Ponseti IV: Curve progression in idiopathic scoliosis. *J Bone Joint Surg* 65A:447, 1983.

pathic scoliosis of varying degrees were tested for work capacity. Maximum oxygen capacity and endurance time were measured and compared with those of a group of normal controls. A significant negative correlation was found between percentile endurance time and degree of spinal curvature. A 10% reduction in endurance time was noted with every 20% increase in spinal curvature. The application of the "exercise capacity test" as an investigative tool for scoliosis was reported to be practical, since endurance time is a reliable index of cardiopulmonary status.

DiRocco and Vaccaro (63) tested adolescent patients with mild idiopathic scoliosis. Nineteen of the adolescents, ages 10 to 17 years, had idiopathic thoracic scoliosis. The mean scoliotic curve was 21.5°. Resting vital capacity and forced expiratory volume were evaluated with a standardized clinical spirometry technique. Work capacity was measured using a graded incremental exercise tolerance test employing a treadmill. Twelve of the 19 subjects had vital capacity measuring 1 standard deviation or more below normal and had maximum volume of oxygen utilization (VO_2 max) scores below 40 ml/kg/min. Patients with curves of 25° or greater had a mean VO_2

max of 32.6 ml/kg/min, whereas those with curves less than 25° recorded a mean VO_2 max of 42.6 ml/kg/min. The study indicated that pulmonary limitations begin with mild curves, and that those individuals with curves measuring 25° or more will have some adverse affect on work capacity.

From these studies, we begin to understand the major indication for surgery in adolescents. The major concern is pulmonary function with secondary cardiopathies. A more distant concern is the issue of cosmesis and resultant psychogenic disorders (64). This varies slightly for adults, as the most common reason for adult scoliosis surgery is pain, followed by curve progression, and lastly cosmesis (65).

When to refer a patient for surgical stabilization has been debated by surgeons and nonsurgeons alike. One of the classic debates on this subject was between John Hall, M.D., and Alf Nachemson, M.D. (66). Hall took the position that all curves of 45° or greater require surgical stabilization. However, Nachemson countered with opinions recommending the use of prognostic signs to differentiate those curves likely to progress and confront significant cardiopulmonary complications from those not so likely.

Scoliosis surgery is a long and difficult operation, not without risk. Possible serious complications include neurological damage, even death. Yet advanced curves will increase mortality and morbidity, and adversely affect work performance. Nachemson stated that 90% of the curves in the 45° to 50° range after growth was completed would not require surgery. However, smaller curves of 30° or more prior to puberty, with a larger amount of growth potential remaining and hormonal fluctuation occurring, were more likely to demonstrate a serious curve progression and also were more likely to require surgery.

DIFFERENT FORMS OF SURGERY

Many variations of surgical stabilization are implemented today by orthopedic surgeons. Though many variations exist, general similarities may also be identified. The goal in most cases is to reduce the lateral curvature, stop progression, and obtain a solid spinal arthrodesis resulting in loss of spinal mobility.

Solid arthrodesis is achieved by arduous debridement of the posterior spinal lamina segments of muscle and ligaments. Bony decortication is then performed, followed by bone grafting, spinal implantation with one of several rods, and lastly, postoperative immobilization. Usually facet joint excision has been performed; however, some surgeons recently have attempted to leave the joint intact.

The most commonly used stabilizing rods are the Harrington rod, the Luque or L rod, and, more recently, a rod receiving a great deal of attention, the Cotrel-Dubousset rod.

Bone grafting utilizes copious amounts of autogenous or allogenous cortical cancellous bone placed over the decorticated region to ensure a solid long-term spinal fusion. The term *autogenous bone* refers to bone material removed from the patient, generally from the iliac crest, for spinal fusion. *Allogenous* indicates that the bone is from a bone bank supplied by prior harvesting of bone from a cadaver. The bone allografts are usually preserved by either freezing or freeze-drying. One reason many surgeons elect to use autogenous bone first is the difference in healing behavior. New bone will form faster, with greater vascular penetration (67).

One advantage of using allogenous bone is that it involves less surgical time, less blood loss, and consequently less stress on the patient. The success of fusion, or "take-rate," is reportedly equal for both sources of osseous material; it is, however, slower for allogenous grafts. Failure to use large amounts of bone jeopardizes adequate fusion and increases the risk of future pseudoarthrosis and rod failure. Instrumentation alone is not sufficient to achieve a stable spine.

Of the various forms of instrumentation used today, the Harrington rod is the standard with which new operative procedures for scoliosis are usually compared (68). When Harrington first developed his instrument in the late 1950s, he did not perform a spinal fusion. His results quickly directed him to use bone grafting to maintain stabilization and correction. The Harrington rod system may employ one or both of two basic forms of force—distraction and compression—on the spine. Distractive force via a distraction Harrington rod is the major correcting force on the spinal deformity and is applied on the concave aspect of the curve. The compression rod is not as strong as the distractive rod and is applied on the convex side of the curve. Compression rods may be bent and will aid in correction, offering an additional 20° of reduction (69); however, compression rods are contraindicated in thoracic hypokyphosis. Correction of the curvature in the frontal plane is generally 50%. Loss of 5° to 10° over the next 2 postoperative years is not unusual (68).

Though the Harrington system has been the most widely used instrumentation technique over the years, it is not without flaws. For example, the stronger distractive rod is straight. This is satisfactory for the correction of a lateral curve in the frontal plane; however, the ability to regain a normal lordosis or kyphosis in the lumbar or thoracic regions, respectively, is severely limited (69). As a result, the development of bent rods that address these sagittal curves has received attention.

The first of the contoured shaping rods to be discussed is the Luque or L rod. The term *segmental spinal instrumentation* (SSI) was first advocated by Luque and Cordosa in 1976, and may be used in conjunction with this system. SSI describes fixing, usually by wire, each spinal level to the instrument. This is unlike the Harrington instrument, which only attaches at the ends by using hooks.

The Luque system uses one or two smooth rods bent on the ends into an "L" shape to prevent rotation and migration. The concave and convex rods were designed to connect the lamina end with the intervertebral disc, creating a three-point fixation to resist lateral and rotation strains. Dove (70) contests tightening the wires, reporting that drawing the rods closer to the midline gives poor control of rotation.

SSI is generally used with arthrodesis to ensure long-lasting stability. Attempts to use SSI without spinal fusion in children with large progressive curves and an anticipated large amount of growth remaining has not been encouraging (71). Further, Luque instrumentation also offers an increased risk of neurological injury (72).

Over the last several years, increased emphasis has been placed on the three-dimensional component of a scoliotic deformity. One reason for the increased concern is the documented deleterious effect that lordosis in the thoracic spine has on pulmonary function (73, 74). Restoration of the thoracic kyphosis is not a strong suit of the Harrington instrument.

Cotrel and Dubousset (75) have made an attempt to address the concerns of pulmonary function and possible neurological damage. Recently, they have introduced instrumentation, tagged with their names, designed to take these variables into consideration.

Shufflebarger and King (30) recently offered a composite measurement system to address the three-dimensional component, offering strong support for the Cotrel-Dubousset (CD) rod over the Luque and the Harrington systems. The CD and the Luque rods outperformed the Harrington instrumentation in the ability to restore a normal thoracic kyphosis.

Birch et al. (76) also offered strong support to the Cotrel-Dubousset instrument, offering promising preliminary results for 37 AIS patients. They also reported significant rib deformity improvement. This is achieved by the rotational correction initiated with CD instrumentation. This has not been the case with Harrington rod utilization.

Gaines et al. (77) reported that attempts to use the Harrington system for decreasing the rib hump were not successful. However, the "valley" could be elevated to help with some of the asymmetry when using compression rods. Jefferson et al. (78) recommend a costoplasty to address the cosmetic problem of back shape when using Harrington rods.

Birch et al. (76) report that no rib resection has been recorded, nor is it necessary when implementing the CD rod. They also reportedly did not use postoperative external immobilization. Ambulation began 2 days postoperatively. Normal activities were resumed in 6 weeks and full activities after 3 months.

The reduced need for postoperative external orthosis is due to the increased stabilization found with the CD system, attributed in part to the large number of hook sites (79).

Regardless of the type of instrumentation used, solid arthrodesis is essential for long-term spinal stabilization. Occasionally, patients will present with failure of their instruments. Generally, this is attributed not to a fault in the rod but to a fault in the fusion itself, as will be discussed in the following case presentation.

CASE 3

A 34-year-old white married female presented with mild mid-thoracic tenderness. She had recently been involved in a car accident. Eleven years previously, she had received Harrington instrumentation with fusion for a 70° idiopathic scoliosis she had had since adolescence.

A posteroanterior film demonstrates rod failure at the junction of the rod and ratchets (Fig. 8.35).

SPINAL INSTRUMENTATION FAILURE

Dove (80) reports on 25 surgeons, members of the British Scoliosis Society, who operated on 1116 patients during 1983 and 1984. The most common form of instrumentation was Harrington distraction (331 patients), with Luque "L" rods (275 patients), Harriluque rods (135 patients), and Harrington rods with distraction and compression (146 patients) following. The study reported that 55 (4.9%) complications occurred. Breakage of the instrumentation was the most common complication, accounting for 33 (3%) of the cases.

The breakage of a rod is usually a result of inadequate fusion and is considered a sign of weakness in the fusion until proven otherwise (81). Seldom does a rod fail when the fusion is solid. Lonstein (14) reports that, when failure of the Harrington distractive instrument does occur, it is usually at the junction of the solid portion of the rod and ratchets.

Instrument failure generally signifies that a pseudoarthrosis has formed at the vertebral level

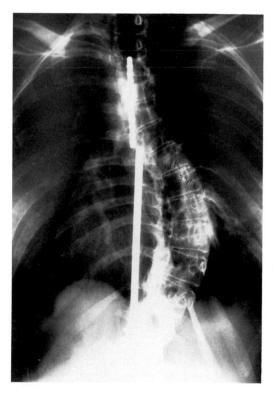

Figure 8.35. Lateral view showing Harrington rod breakage.

corresponding to the failure. The surrounding cutaneous tissue may become painful and very sensitive to touch. Further, the spine may become unstable due to the failure of the fusion and instrument. The amount of instability or loss of curve correction is pertinent to whether further surgical intervention is needed. Proper instrument apposition and adequate spinal stability may be maintained by the influence of the strengthened surrounding fibrotic tissue.

CONCLUSION

The field of scoliosis is very complex, and extensive study and thought are demanded prior to treating any patient with this disorder. A thorough clinical exam and knowledge of the natural history assist all clinicians in determining the prescribed course of treatment. Though advances in therapy have been made, much exploration remains ahead for pioneering researchers and clinicians.

Manipulation, exercises, bracing, neuromuscular stimulation, and surgery are not to be accepted as the definitive solution to scoliotic disorders. Further research will, it is to be hoped, take us in a direction that addresses the etiology of scoliosis and works more in line with chiropractic care by controlling the disorder before it starts. Attempting to work with the secondary manifestations of any pathogenic disorder is always much more difficult, and some day we are likely to look back on our approach to scoliosis and think how crude we were. But today we are afforded the luxury of only implementing that of which we know.

ACKNOWLEDGMENT

The author wishes to express his sincere gratitude to Beth Mouch, literary consultant, for her untiring efforts in the completion of this chapter.

References

1. *Stedman's Medical Dictionary*, ed 24. Baltimore, Williams & Wilkins, 1982.
2. Cox J: *Low Back Pain: Mechanism, Diagnosis and Treatment*, ed 4. Baltimore, Williams & Wilkins, 1985.
3. Moe J, Bradford D, Lonstein J, Ogilvie J, Winter R: *Moe's Textbook of Scoliosis and Other Spinal Deformities*, ed 2. Philadelphia, WB Saunders, 1987.
4. Winter R, Carlson J: Modern orthotics for spinal deformities. *Clin Orthop* 126:74–86, 1977.
5. Bobechko W: Scoliosis spinal pacemakers. *J Bone Joint Surg* 56A:442, 1974.
6. Aspegren D, Cox J: Correction of progressive idiopathic scoliosis utilizing neuromuscular stimulation and manipulation: a case report. *J Manipulative Physiol Ther* 10:147–156, 1987.
7. Nykoliation J, Cassidy J, Arther B, Wedge J: An algorithm for the management of scoliosis. *J Manipulative Physiol Ther* 9:1–13, 1986.
8. Torell G, Nordwall A, Nachemson A: The changing pattern of scoliosis treatment due to effective screening. *J Bone Joint Surg* 63A:337–341, 1981.
9. Vercautern M, et al.: Trunk asymmetries in a Belgian school population. *Spine* 7:555–562, 1982.
10. Bunnell W: When does scoliosis need referral? *Patient Care* (September):53–60, 1987.
11. Bunnell W: *The Angle of Trunk Rotation: Use in Scoliosis Screening and Follow-up.* Haywood, CA, OSI Orthopedic Systems.
12. Murbarak S, Wyatt M, Leach J: Evaluation of the intra-examiner and inter-examiner reliability of the scoliometer in measuring trunk rotation. *Orthop Trans* 9:113–114, 1983.
13. Stirling A, Smith R, Dickson R: Screening for scoliosis: the problem of arm length. *Br Med J* 292:1305–1306, 1986.
14. Lonstein J: Risk of progression of idiopathic scoliosis in skeletally immature patients. *Spine:* State of the Art Review 1:181–193, 1987.
15. Chan A, Moller J, et al.: Scoliosis screening: a needs study. *J Bone Joint Surg* 69B:167, 1987.
16. Rogala E, Drummond D, Gurr J: Scoliosis: incidence and natural history. *J Bone Joint Surg* 60A:173–176, 1978.
17. Morais T, Bernier M, Turcotte F: Age- and sex-specific prevalence of scoliosis and the value of school screening programs. *Am J Public Health* 75:1377–1380, 1985.
18. Wynne-Davies R: Familial (idiopathic) scoliosis: a family survey. *J Bone Joint Surg* 50B:24–30, 1968.
19. Aspegren D, Cox J, Trier L: Short leg correction: a clinical trial of radiographic vs. non-radiographic procedures. *J Manipulative Physiol Ther* 10:232–238, 1987.
20. Binns M: Joint laxity in idiopathic adolescent scoliosis. *J Bone Joint Surg* 70B:420–422, 1988.
21. Beighton P, Solomon L, Soskalne C: Articular mobility in an African population. *Ann Rheum Dis* 32:413–418, 1973.
22. Wynne-Davies R: *Heritable Disorders in Orthopaedic Practice.* Oxford, Blackwell Scientific, 1973.
23. Farren J: Routine radiographic assessment of the scoliotic spine. *Radiography* 47:92–96, 1981.
24. Nash C, Gregg E, Brown R, Pillai K: Risk of exposure to x-rays in patients undergoing long-term treatment for scoliosis. *J Bone Joint Surg* 61A:372–374, 1979.
25. Hellstrom G, Irstran L, Nachemson A: Reduction

of radiation dose in radiologic examination of patients with scoliosis. *Spine* 8:28, 1983.

26. Greulich W, Pyle S: *Radiographic Atlas of Skeletal Development of the Hand and Wrist,* ed 2. Stanford, Stanford University Press, 1959.

27. Edeiken J: *Roentgen Diagnosis of Diseases of Bone,* ed 3. Baltimore, Williams & Wilkins, 1981.

28. Cobb J: *Outline for the Study of Scoliosis,* vol 5 of *Instructional Course Lectures, the American Academy of Orthopedic Surgeons.* JW Edwards, 1948, pp 261–275.

29. Goldstien L, Waugh T: Classification and terminology of scoliosis. *Clin Orthop* 93:10–22, 1973.

30. Shufflebarger H, King W: Composite measurement of scoliosis: a new method of analysis of the deformity. *Spine* 12:228–232, 1987.

31. Dickson R: Scoliosis in the community. *Br Med J* 286:615–618, 1983.

32. Olsen G, Rosen H, Stoll S, Brown G: The use of muscle stimulation for inducing scoliotic curves: a preliminary report. *Clin Orthop* 113:198–211, 1975.

33. Agadir M, Sevastik B, Sevastik J, Persson A, Isberg B: Induction of scoliosis in the growing rabbit by unilateral rib-growth stimulation. *Spine* 13: 1065–1069, 1988.

34. White A, Panjabi M: *Clinical Biomechanics of the Spine.* Philadelphia, JB Lippincott, 1978.

35. Dickson R, Leatherman K: Cotrel traction, exercises, casting in the treatment of idiopathic scoliosis. *Acta Orthop Scand* 49:46–48, 1978.

36. Kahanovitz N, Snow B, Pinter I: The comparative results of psychologic testing in scoliosis patients treated with electrical stimulation or bracing. *Spine* 7:76–77, 1983.

37. Kahanovitz N, Weiser S: Lateral electrical surface stimulation (LESS) compliance in adolescent female scoliosis patients. *Spine* 11:753–755, 1986.

38. Miller J, Nachemson A, Schultz A: Effectiveness of braces in mild idiopathic scoliosis. *Spine* 9: 632–635, 1984.

39. Dickson R: Conservative treatment for idiopathic scoliosis. *J Bone Joint Surg* 67B:176–181, 1985.

40. Monticelli G, Ascani E, Salsano V, Salsano A: Experimental scoliosis induced by prolonged minimal electrical stimulation of the paravertebral muscles. *Ital J Orthop Traumatol* 1:39–54, 1975.

41. Herbert M, Bobechko W: Paraspinal muscle stimulation for the treatment of idiopathic scoliosis in children. *Adv Orthop Surg* 11:174–175, 1988.

42. Bradford D, Tanguy A, Vanselow J: Surface electrical stimulation in the treatment of idiopathic scoliosis: preliminary results in 30 patients. *Spine* 8: 757–764, 1983.

43. Axelgaard J, Brown J: Lateral electrical surface stimulation for the treatment of progressive idiopathic scoliosis. *Spine* 8:242–260, 1983.

44. Schultz A, Haderspeck K, Takashima S: Correction

45. of scoliosis by muscle stimulation: biomechanical analysis. *Spine* 6:468–476, 1981.

45. Fisher D, Rapp G, Emkes M: Idiopathic scoliosis: transcutaneous muscle stimulation versus the Milwaukee brace. *Spine* 12:987–991, 1987.

46. McCullough N, III: Nonoperative treatment of idiopathic scoliosis using surface electrical stimulation. *Spine* 11:802–804, 1986.

47. Herbert M, Bobechko W: Paraspinal muscle stimulation for the treatment of idiopathic scoliosis in children. *Orthopedics* 10:1125–1132, 1987.

48. Brown J, Axelgaard J, Howson D: Multicenter trial of a noninvasive stimulation method of idiopathic scoliosis: a summary of early treatment results. *Spine* 9:382–387, 1984.

49. Goldberg C, et al.: Electro-spinal stimulation in children with adolescent and juvenile scoliosis. *Spine* 13:482–484, 1988.

50. O'Donnell C, et al.: Electrical stimulation in the treatment of idiopathic scoliosis. *Clin Orthop* 229: 107–113, 1988.

51. Bylund P. Aaro S, Gottfries B, Jansson E: Is lateral electrical surface stimulation an effective treatment for scoliosis? *J Pediatr Orthop* 7:298–300, 1987.

52. *Clinician's Manual and Operating Instructions.* Fairfield, NJ, EBI Medical Systems.

53. Aspergren D, Cox J: Correction of progressive idiopathic scoliosis utilizing neuromuscular stimulation and manipulation: a case report. *J Manipulative Physiol Ther* 10:147–156, 1987.

54. Nash C: Scoliosis Dancing. *J Bone Joint Surg* 62A: 848–852, 1980.

55. Andriacci T, Schultz A, Belytschko T, Dewald R: Milwaukee brace correction of idiopathic scoliosis. *J Bone Joint Surg* 58A:806–815, 1976.

56. Emans J, Kaelin A, Bancel P, Hall J, Miller M: The Boston bracing system for idiopathic scoliosis: follow-up results in 295 patients. *Spine* 11:792–801, 1986.

57. Mellencamp D, Blount W, Anderson A: Milwaukee brace treatment of idiopathic scoliosis. *Clin Orthop* 126:47–57, 1977.

58. Nachemson A: A long term follow-up study of nontreated scoliosis. *Acta Orthop Scand* 39:466–476, 1968.

59. Nilsonne V, Lundgren K: Long-term prognosis in idiopathic scoliosis. *Acta Orthop Scand* 39:456–465, 1968.

60. Weinstein S, Ponseti I: Curve progression in idiopathic scoliosis. *J Bone Joint Surg* 65A:447–455, 1983.

61. Collins DK, Ponseti I: Long-term follow-up of patients with idiopathic scoliosis not treated surgically. *J Bone Joint Surg* 51A:425–445, 1969.

62. Chong K, Letts R, Cumming G: Influence of spinal curvature on exercise capacity. *J Pediatr Orthop* 1: 251–254, 1981.

63. DiRocco P, Vaccaro P: Cardiopulmonary function-

ing in adolescent patients with mild idiopathic scoliosis. *Arch Phys Med Rehabil* 69:198–201, 1988.

64. Sponseller P, Cohen M, Nachemson A, Hall J, Wohl M: Results of surgical treatment of adults with idiopathic scoliosis. *J Bone Joint Surg* 69A:667–675, 1987.

65. Bradford D: Adult scoliosis: current concepts of treatment. *Clin Orthop* 227:70, 1988.

66. Hall J, Nachemson A: Debate: scoliosis. *Spine* 2: 318–324, 1977.

67. Dunsker S, Schmidak H, Frymoyer J, Kahn A III: *The Unstable Spine (Thoracic, Lumbar, and Sacral Regions)*. Orlando, FL, Grune & Stratton, 1986.

68. Erwin W, Dickson J: Harrington spine instrumentation and fusion for scoliosis. *Spine:* State of the Art Reviews 1:227–237, 1987.

69. Harrington P, Dickson J: An eleven-year clinical investigation of Harrington instrumentation: a preliminary report on 578 cases. *Clin Orthop* 93: 113–130, 1973.

70. Dove J: Luque segmental spinal instrumentation: the use of the Hartshill rectable. *Adv Orthop Surg* 11:182–183, 1988.

71. Rinsky L, Gamble J, Bleck E: Segmental instrumentation without fusion in children with progressive scoliosis. *J Pediatr Orthop* 5:687–690, 1985.

72. Wilber R, Thompson G, Shaffer J, Brown R, Nash C: Postoperative neurological deficits in segmental spinal instrumentation. *J Bone Joint Surg* 66A:1178, 1984.

73. Aaro S, Ohlund G: Scoliosis and pulmonary function. *Spine* 9:220–222, 1984.

74. Cochran T, Irstram L, Nachemson A: Long-term anatomic and functional changes in patients with adolescent idiopathic scoliosis treated by Harrington rod fusion. *Spine* 9:576, 1983.

75. Cotrel Y, Dubousset J: Nouvelle techniques d'osteosynthèse rachidienne segmentaire par voie postérieur. *Rev Chir Orthop* 70:489, 1984.

76. Birch J, Herring J, Roach J, Johnston C: Cotrel-Dubousset instrumentation in idiopathic scoliosis: a preliminary report. *Clin Orthop* 227:24–29, 1988.

77. Gaines R, McKinley M, Leatherman K: Effect of the Harrington compression system on the correction of the rib hump in spinal instrumentation for idiopathic scoliosis. *Spine* 6:489, 1981.

78. Jefferson R, Weisz I, Smith A, Harris J, Houghton G: Scoliosis surgery and its effects on back shape. *J Bone Joint Surg* 70B:261, 1988.

79. Bergoin M, Bollini G, Hornung H, Tallet J, Gennari J: Is the Cotrel-Dubousset really universal in the surgical treatment of idiopathic scoliosis? *J Pediatr Orthop* 8:45–48, 1988.

80. Dove J: Segmental spinal instrumentation: British Scoliosis Society morbidity report. *J Bone Joint Surg* 68B:680, 1986.

81. Erwin W, Dickson J, Harrington P: Clinical review of patients with broken Harrington rods. *J Bone Joint Surg* 62A:1302–1307, 1980.

9

Diagnosis of the Patient with Low Back Pain

James M. Cox, D.C., D.A.C.B.R.

I Keep Six Honest Serving Men,

(They Taught Me All I Knew);

Their Names Are What and Why and

When and How and Where and Who.

—Rudyard Kipling

In the United States, 6.8% of the adult population has been found to have back pain at any given time. Twelve percent of those with low back pain will have sciatica. The prevalence of low back pain rises after age 25 to a peak in the 55- to 64-year-old range, with a falling prevalence after age 65. For sciatica-like pain, the prevalence peaks at the 45- to 54-year-old range. Consideration of the specific age of onset shows that 11% of persons are afflicted at less than 20 years of age; 28% at 20 to 29 years, 25% at 30 to 39 years, 20% at 40 to 49 years, 11% at 50 to 59 years, and 5% at more than 60 years of age (1).

The demographic prevalence shows regionally that the northeastern United States has a 38% higher rate of low back pain than the western states. Men and women are afflicted similarly, with white men having the highest prevalence and black men the lowest. Less educated persons have a 50% increased incidence over better educated persons (1).

SOURCES OF LOW BACK COMPLAINTS

As with all human disease, the diagnosis and treatment of low back problems begin with the history, followed by clinical work-up, selected imaging modalities for confirmation, and establishment of a treatment protocol. Questioning of the patient allows concepts to form as to the involved anatomy. For example, low back pain alone is more common in annular tears and facet degenerative and subluxation syndromes, whereas sciatica leads to consideration of disc protrusion or stenosis within the vertebral canal. We feel that serious disc lesions are preceded by numerous and worsening bouts of low back pain. Low back pain that suddenly is transformed into only leg pain probably represents a contained disc that becomes a noncontained disc.

Five common causes of sciatica have been suggested (2):

1. Herniated disc;
2. Annular tears;
3. Myogenic, or muscle-related, disease;
4. Spinal stenosis;
5. Facet joint arthropathy.

Table 9.1 outlines the key differential diagnostic points of these five common causes of sciatica.

Table 9.1.
Key Diagnostic Tips for Distinguishing among Five Causes of Sciatica[a]

Herniated nucleus pulposus
—History of specific trauma
—Leg pain greater than back pain
—Neurologic deficit present; nerve tension signs present
—Pain increases with sitting and leaning forward, coughing, sneezing, and straining; pain reproduced with ipsilateral straight leg raising and sciatic stretch tests; contralateral straight leg raising test may also reproduce pain
—Radiologic evidence of nerve root impingement (metrizamide myelography, CT)
Annular tears
—History of significant trauma
—Back pain is usually greater than leg pain; leg pain bilateral or unilateral
—Nerve tension signs present (but no radiologic evidence of impingement)
—Pain increases with sitting and leaning forward, coughing, sneezing, and straining
—Back pain is exacerbated with straight leg raising and sciatic-stretch tests (perform straight leg raising test bilaterally)
—Diskography is diagnostic (neither CT scan nor myelogram show abnormality)
Myogenic or muscle-related disease
—History of injury to muscle, recurrent pain symptoms related to its use
—Lumbar paravertebral myositis produces back pain; gluteus maximus myositis causes buttock and thigh pain
—Pain is unilateral or bilateral, rather than midline; does not extend past knee
—Soreness or stiffness present on arising in the morning and after resting; is worse when muscles are chilled or when the weather changes (arthritis-like symptoms)
—Pain increases with prolonged muscle use; is most intense after cessation of muscle use (directly afterward and on following day)
—Symptom intensity reflects daily cumulative muscle use
—Local tenderness palpable in the belly of the involved muscle
—Pain reproduced with sustained muscle contraction against resistance, and by passive stretch of the muscle
—Contralateral pain present with side bending
—No radiologic evidence
Spinal stenosis
—Back and/or leg (bilateral or unilateral) pain develops after patient walks a limited distance; symptoms worsen with continued walking
—Leg weakness or numbness present, with or without sciatica
—Flexion relieves symptoms
—No neurologic deficit present
—Pain not reproduced on straight leg raising; pain reproduced with prolonged spinal extension and relieved afterward when spine flexed
—Radiologic evidence: Hypertrophic changes, disc narrowing, interlaminar space narrowing, facet hypertrophy, degenerative spondylolisthesis (L4-L5)
Facet-joint arthropathy
—History of injury
—Localized tenderness present unilaterally over joint
—Pain occurs immediately on spinal extension
—Pain is exacerbated with ipsilateral side-bending
—Pain blocked by intrajoint injection of local anesthetic or corticosteroid

[a]Reproduced with permission from McCarron RF, Laros GS: What is the cause of your patient's sciatica? *Journal of Musculoskeletal Medicine* (June):65, 1987.

Does Annular Tearing Cause Low Back or Leg Pain?

Devanny (3) states that the classic low back syndrome referred to as "muscle spasm" or a "strained back" usually has the disc as the source of pain. If there is only back pain without leg pain, most likely a weakened annulus fibrosus with a disc bulge, not a disc herniation, is the cause of the pain.

Macnab (4), by placing a catheter under inflamed nerve roots at laminectomy and inflating them later, found that previously irritated nerve roots reproduced the patients' sciatic symptoms. Normal nerve roots only produced feelings of numbness. He deduced that there was both chemical and mechanical irritation of the nerve root analogous to the pain produced by a sunburn of the skin—there might be sunburn, but pain is produced only if it is touched. Similarly, a nerve root might be chemically inflamed but only painful upon mechanical compression.

Vanharanta et al. (5) found that, in 225 discs injected for discography, painful discs had higher degeneration and disruption scores than painless discs. The annular disruption was likely to be the source of exact pain production. The pain was not always similar to the patient's clinical back pain, but exact reproduction or similar pain was found to increase consistently with the amount of disc deterioration. These results suggested that increasing deterioration of lumbar discs was associated with increasing clinical pain. Even small amounts of deterioration may be the cause of a disc being painful on discography.

Saal (6) reported that anatomical studies have demonstrated the presence of nociceptive nerve endings in the annulus fibrosus of the lumbar discs and that annular tears can therefore cause pain referral of purely discogenic origin into the low back, buttock, sacroiliac joint region, and lower extremities even in the absence of neural compression.

Marshall (7) found that extract of glycoprotein from the human nucleus pulposus releases considerable quantities of histamine, another protein, and amine components that he considered a local irritant of the nerve root, producing edema and pain.

Crock (2) described "internal disc disruption" as being the annular fiber tearing and felt it to be another discogenic cause of sciatic pain. Sciatica results when a tear in the annulus fibrosus leaks nuclear material posteriorly, and the escaped nuclear material irritates the dural sac and nerve sleeves.

Rothman and Simeone (8) state that radiating cracks in the annulus fibrosus develop in the most centrally situated lamellae and extend outward to the periphery. These radiating clefts in the annulus weaken its resistance to nuclear herniation. Herniation is a greater threat to a younger individual between the ages of 30 and 50 having good nuclear turgor than it is to the elderly in whom the nucleus is fibrotic. Falconer (9) states that myelographic defects are seen unchanged after successful conservative treatment of sciatica and that this is due not to mechanical factors but to clinical nerve root symptoms created by the biochemical irritation of the nerve root degeneration and its resultant irritants on the nerve root. Rothman and Simeone (8) discuss variations of the spinal canal in detail. The trefoil canal, which Finneson

(10) discussed also, is common at the L4 and L5 level. The trefoil canal has lateral recesses that render the canal narrower and thereby more vulnerable to compression by extruded disc material. We discuss the finding on x-ray of underdeveloped pedicles which would result in a decreased anteroposterior measurement of the vertebral canal and thus create a stenotic vertebral canal. This would result in more pronounced symptoms of disc protrusion. Imagine the combination of a trefoil canal with lateral recesses, underdeveloped pedicles, and articular facet degenerative arthrosis, all of which are narrowing the vertebral canal and, when coupled with disc protrusion, result in an exceptionally painful condition. It is well to remember that the lumbar nerve roots lie in the superior part of the intervertebral foramen in a relatively protected position and that it is only in disc narrowing that the superior articular facet of the vertebra below might subluxate in a position to create nerve root pressure. Rothman and Simeone (8) also state that a small nuclear herniation of only 1 to 2-mm in height can cause marked nerve root compression in a patient with a small lumbar spinal canal and particularly with a narrow lateral recess that makes the patient susceptible to degenerative changes of the intervertebral disc (8).

How Does Nuclear Degeneration Start and Progress?

Figure 9.1 shows a classification scheme for degenerative disc disease (11). Annular disruption, "leaking/protrusion/annular fissuring," is graphically shown in Figure 9.1. A numerical code indicates how far the contrast material has escaped into the periphery through tears in the annulus: *0* represents a normal disc, and *1* to *3* represent progression of contrast medium into the annulus fibrosus. As the contrast medium advances into the annular periphery, the pain response of the patient is recorded. Table 9.2 shows a code for classifying the pain response according to whether the patient described it as similar or dissimilar to the pain experienced prior to the examination.

Figure 9.2 shows Videman et al.'s (12) classification of discographic appearances, from the normal contained disc to the bulging contained disc and leaking, noncontained fragmentation of the disc.

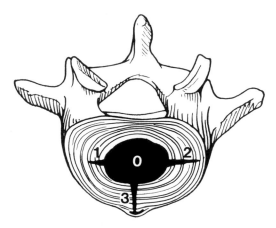

Figure 9.1. The concentric circumferential areas of the annulus used for grading annular disruption as contrast material progressively moves away from the center of the nuclear injection. Areas *0, 1, 2,* and *3* are noted. (Reproduced with permission from Sachs BL, Vanharanta H, Spivey MA, Guyer RD, Videman T, Rashbaum RF, Johnson RG, Hochschuler SH, Mooney V: Dallas discogram description: a new classification of CT/discography in low-back disorders. *Spine* 12(3):288, 1987.)

Pathway of Nuclear Entrance into the Vertebral Canal

We commonly recognize nuclear disc posterolateral prolapse, as shown in Figure 9.3, but we must realize that the nuclear material may find its way into the lateral recesses and vertebral canal through a lateral route to "enter through the side door" into the canal. This is shown so well in Figure 9.4.

The value of discography with CT is shown in Figure 9.5, in which a large free fragment of disc is not seen on a myelographic enhanced CT scan but is seen on a discographically enhanced CT scan.

Another interesting study of 441 surgical and autopsy specimens of disc tissue found that the annulus fibrosus was more commonly degenerated than the nuclear material, suggesting that the pathomechanism of disc protrusion is predominantly one of annular protrusion as opposed to nuclear protrusion (13).

DIAGNOSTIC BIOMECHANICS

The most important spinal component is the intervertebral disc. It is the key structure in the movable segment (or, as Schmorl calls it, the "motor segment"), and its lesions (tears, prolapses, and degeneration) affect the rest of the movable segment (14). The axis of sagittal movement of the spine passes through the middle to the posterior portion of the disc, and as the axis pivots around the nucleus pulposus, which acts as a fulcrum, it may shift slightly. In horizontally rotatory movement, the annular fibers in the lumbar region undergo shearing stress leading to tears or rupture, even in younger people, since the vertical axis of rotation is posterior to the vertebral bodies.

Both rupture of annular fibers, or the dissect-

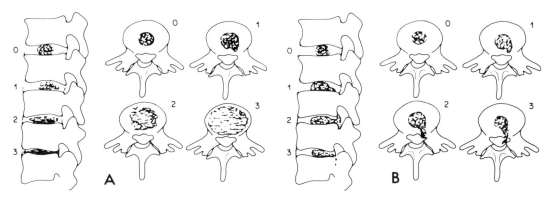

Figure 9.2. **A,** The general appearance of discograms was classified using the following scale: 0 = normal, 1 = slight, 2 = moderate, and 3 = severe degeneration. **B,** The annular ruptures were classified using the following scale: 0 = none; 1 = "annular fissure," where dye goes through annulus but is not outside the contour of the normal disc; 2 = "protrusion," where dye can be seen bulging outside the contour of the normal disc; and 3 = "leaking," where dye can be seen in spinal canal coming through the annulus. (Reproduced with permission from Videman T, Malmivaara A, Mooney V: The value of the axial view in assessing discograms: an experimental study with cadavers. *Spine* 12(3): 300, 1987.)

ing prolapse of the nucleus pulposus through the annulus fibrosus, and fracture and destruction of the basal cartilaginous and bony apophyseal plate may allow prolapse of the nucleus pulposus. This

happens especially in young people with high intradiscal pressures sustained on loading in flexion and on high shearing stress in rotation, either into the posterior lateral extradural space

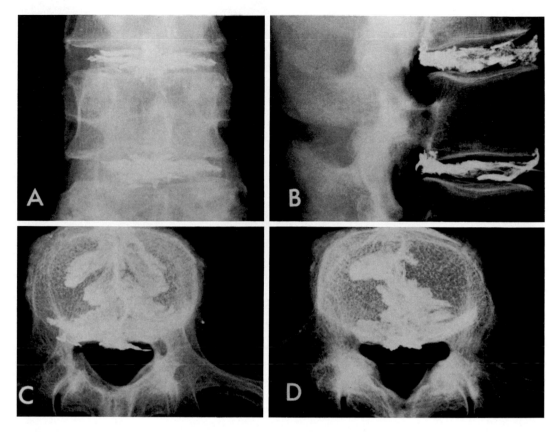

Figure 9.3. **A**, View of two lumbar discograms from levels L3-L4 and L4-L5 using barium sulfate. General degeneration is severe with associated protrusions. **B**, In a lateral view, the degeneration is moderate. **C**, In the axial view at level L3-L4, the nature of degeneration is clear and two separate protrusions can be seen. **D**, In the axial view of level L4-L5, an anterior annular fissure can be seen. (Reproduced with permission from Videman T, Malmivaara A, Mooney V: The value of the axial view in assessing discograms: an experimental study with cadavers. *Spine* 12(3):302, 1987.)

Table 9.2.
Dallas Discogram Description[a]

Degeneration (Annulus)	Annular Disruption (Contrast Extension)	Pain
0—No change	0—None	P—Pressure
1—Local (<10%)	1—Into inner annulus	D—Dissimilar
2—Partial (<50%)	2—Into outer annulus	S—Similar
3—Total (>50%)	3—Beyond outer annulus	R—Exact reproduction

[a]Reproduced with permission from Sachs BL, Vanharanta H, Spivey MA, Guyer RD, Videman T, Rashbaum RF, Johnson RG, Hochschuler SH, Mooney V: Dallas discogram description: a new classification of CT/discography in low-back disorders. *Spine* 12(3):287, 1987.

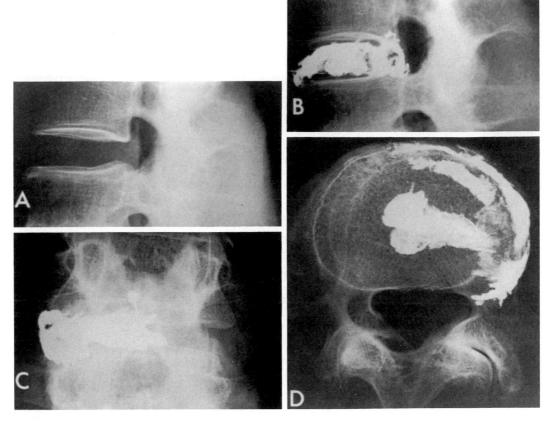

Figure 9.4. **A,** In the plain roentgenogram, the L3-L4 level looks quite normal, but the lateral discogram (**B**) shows severe degeneration. PA view again (**C**) shows marked asymmetry. The axial view (**D**) gives a more exact picture of the nature of the disc lesion degeneration. (Reproduced with permission from Videman T, Malmivaara A, Mooney V: The value of the axial view in assessing discograms: an experimental study with cadavers. *Spine* 12(3):300, 1987.)

(with the middle being protected somewhat by the posterior longitudinal ligament in most instances) or vertically into the bone through gaps, weak places, or fractures of the bony cartilaginous plate (14).

Clinical and experimental observations suggest that the disc may be one of the sources of idiopathic low back pain (15). In patients who develop definite disc herniation, one or more episodes of back pain frequently precede the herniation. These episodes of pain may be very similar to the pain experienced by patients who do not develop disc herniation. Hirsch (16) and Lindblom (17) increased the intradiscal pressure in patients with a history of back pain by injecting saline into the discs. They found that increased intradiscal pressure reproduced the patient's pain. If the disc was injected with a local anesthetic prior to the increases in intradiscal pres-

sure, pain did not develop. If Hypaque was injected into a disc and the dye extended into the annulus, severe pain was sometimes produced. If the dye remained in the nucleus, pain did not occur. Direct mechanical stimulation of the annulus and cartilage plate may also produce pain. These findings indicate that irritation or abnormalities of the disc may cause pain, but even if the disc is not the primary source of pain in some syndromes, alterations in the disc may produce symptoms by changing the loads on other structures, including facet joints, spinal ligaments, paraspinal muscles, and nerve roots.

Discal Back Pain and Sciatica

Patients present with back pain and sciatica, with back pain and no sciatica, and with sciatica and no back pain. The most overlooked diagnosis of disc

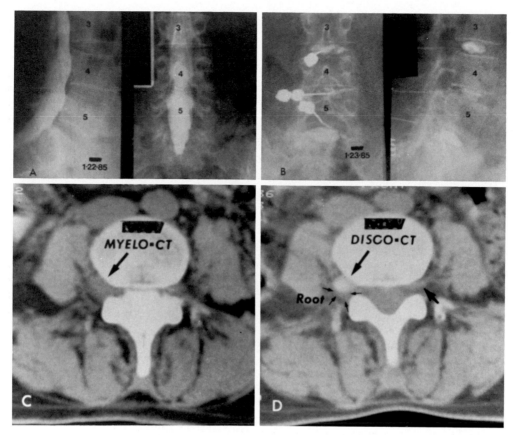

Figure 9.5. **A,** Negative myelogram with slight annular bulging at L4-L5 on lateral view. **B,** Discogram with only minimal degenerative changes. **C,** Myelo-CT interpreted as negative, suggests asymmetry in soft tissues lateral to foramen on right (*arrow*). **D,** Positive disco-CT with large extraforaminal disc fragment (*largest arrow*) and displaced right L4 nerve root (*small arrows*). (Reproduced with permission from Jackson RP, Glah JJ: Foraminal and extraforaminal lumbar disc herniation: diagnosis and treatment. *Spine* 12(6):581, 1987.)

protrusion in clinical practice probably involves the patient with back pain without sciatica. Early nuclear protrusion into the annular fibers often involves the patient with acute back pain and perhaps an antalgic lean to one side. It is well documented that the annulus fibrosus is well innervated by the sinuvertebral nerve, becoming more so from the central portion to the peripheral portion of the disc (8). Radiating cracks in the annulus fibrosus develop in the most centrally situated lamellae and extend outward toward the periphery (18). Turek (19) states that this cracking and fissuring begins as early as the 15th year and may take place silently over many years. The annulus, under the pressure of nuclear protrusion, becomes progressively weaker and thinner. As this pathological state develops, the intensity of pain and the antalgic lean of the patient increase.

As the annular fibers progressively thin and the protruding nuclear material makes mild contact with the nerve root, the manifestations of sciatica are first observed. If the annular fibers completely tear and the protruding material bursts forth, the intensity of the sciatica proportionately increases.

The pressure on protruding nuclear material is greater in the young person with a turgid nucleus, which contains up to 80% water, than in the older person in whom the nucleus pulposus has become dehydrated and converted into a hardened mass. Therefore, a patient may have a nuclear bulge creating low back pain resulting from aggravation of the annular fibers, he may have back pain and sciatica as the protruding disc material contacts the nerve root, or he may have only sciatica if the disc protrudes through the annulus and contacts only the nerve root, with no other structures innervated by the recurrent meningeal nerve being irritated.

Equally important is the fact that the nucleus that bulges through the annulus fibrosus and comes to lie free under the posterior longitudinal ligament may migrate cephalad and caudally along the posterior vertebral body. Nuclear material that breaks continuity with the remaining nucleus is called a free fragment or prolapsed disc.

White and Panjabi (20) prepared an update of Charnley's (21) hypothesis on low back pain.[a] The following are the classifications of back pain from White and Panjabi (20).

ACUTE BACK SPRAIN (TYPE I)

Acute back sprain (type I) characteristically occurs when a laborer attempts to sustain a sudden additional load. There is immediate severe pain that may last for several weeks. The pain is primarily in the low back, without sciatica, and may be due to several factors. Charnley suggested the possibility of rupture of some of the deep layers of the annulus. We believe that, while this rupture is possible, the inner fibers are not innervated, and there is relatively less loading and deformation of the deeper fibers than of the periphery. There are other possibilities, however. One is that peripheral annular fibers may be injured or ruptured along with any of the other posterior ligaments or musculotendinous structures; another is that some of these injuries may involve rupture of muscle fibers or be associated with nondisplaced or minimally displaced vertebral end-plate fractures (Fig. 9.6). Whatever the cause, these conditions should respond to a period of rest, followed by a gradual resumption of normal activities.

ORGANIC OR IDIOPATHIC FLUID INGESTION (TYPE II)

An attack of low back pain and muscle spasm may be produced by the sudden passage of fluid into the nucleus pulposus for some unknown reason (21, 22), (Fig. 9.7). Charnley suggested that this passage of fluid irritated the peripheral annular fibers, causing the characteristic pain. There is little to discredit the hypothesis 20 years later. Naylor (22) suggests that increased fluid uptake in the nucleus is a precipitating factor in the biochemical chain of events that can lead to disc disease.[b] Very indirect evidence, however, suggests that increases in fluid in the disc structure may not cause spine pain. This evidence is based on the observation that astronauts returning from outer space have heightened disc space but no back pain according to Kazarian (23). On the other hand, there is evidence, although inconsistent, that suggests that fluid injection into the normal disc causes low back pain (24). This discrepancy may be partially explained by the differences in the rate of change in fluid pressure. The hypothesis of fluid ingestion is consistent with the clinical data because it is compatible with the characteristic clinical course of exacerbations and remissions, with or without progression to other clinical syndromes. In other words, movement of fluid in and out of the disc can explain the onset and resolution of the clinical symptoms. We suggest that this may be the explanation for spontaneous idiopathic organic spine pain (cervical, thoracic, or lumbar) unrelated to trauma, which accounts for a significant number of the many cases of spine pain.

POSTEROLATERAL ANNULUS DISRUPTION (TYPE III)

If there is failure or disruption of some of the annular fibers, posterolateral irritation in this region may cause back pain with referral into the sacroiliac region, the buttock, or the back of the thigh (Fig. 9.8). This referred pain is due to stimulation of the sensory innervation by mechanical, chemical, or inflammatory irritants. Thus, "referred sciatica," as Charnley called it, is distinguished from true sciatica by a negative straight leg raising test and a lack of neuromuscular deficit. As suggested previously, this referred pain may be explained by the "gate" control theory. This referred sciatica may resolve itself through reabsorption or neutralization of the irritants and/or phagocytosis and painless healing of the disrupted annular fibers.

---

[a] Charnley's article (21) is a classic exposition on the topic. There is a clear theoretical presentation of the mechanism, diagnosis, and treatment of the various combinations of back pain and sciatica. It is highly recommended for both the primary care physician and the specialist.

---

[b] Naylor's article (22) provides a superb, comprehensive review of this hypothesis.

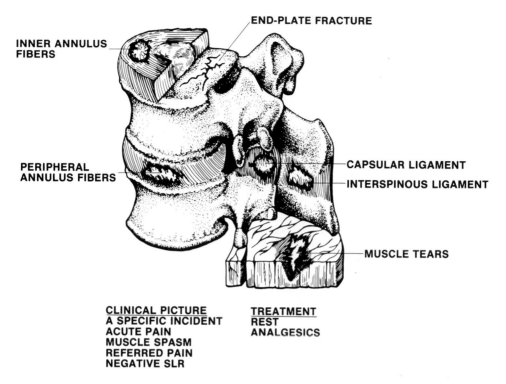

INNER ANNULUS FIBERS

END-PLATE FRACTURE

PERIPHERAL ANNULUS FIBERS

CAPSULAR LIGAMENT

INTERSPINOUS LIGAMENT

MUSCLE TEARS

CLINICAL PICTURE
A SPECIFIC INCIDENT
ACUTE PAIN
MUSCLE SPASM
REFERRED PAIN
NEGATIVE SLR

TREATMENT
REST
ANALGESICS

Figure 9.6. A clinical picture of acute back sprain (type I) may involve damage to any number of ligamentous structures, the muscle, or even vertebral end-plate fracture. *SLR*, straight leg raising test. (Reproduced with permission from White AA, Panjabi MM: *Clinical Biomechanics of the Spine*. Philadelphia, JB Lippincott, 1978, p 286.)

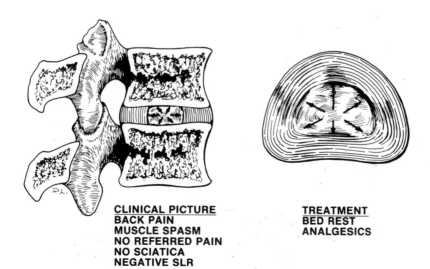

CLINICAL PICTURE
BACK PAIN
MUSCLE SPASM
NO REFERRED PAIN
NO SCIATICA
NEGATIVE SLR

TREATMENT
BED REST
ANALGESICS

Figure 9.7. Organic or idiopathic fluid ingestion (type II). This mechanism may account for a large portion of back pain for which no distinct diagnosis nor etiology has been determined. (Reproduced with permission from White AA, Panjabi MM: *Clinical Biomechanics of the Spine*. Philadelphia, JB Lippincott, 1978, p 286.)

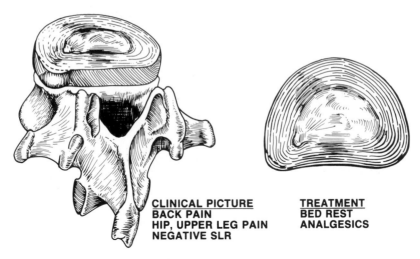

CLINICAL PICTURE
BACK PAIN
HIP, UPPER LEG PAIN
NEGATIVE SLR

TREATMENT
BED REST
ANALGESICS

Figure 9.8. Posterolateral annulus disruption (type III). The *dotted line* represents the original normal contour of the disc. Hip and thigh pain are referred pain rather than true sciatica. (Reproduced with permission from White AA, Panjabi MM: *Clinical Biomechanics of the Spine.* Philadelphia, JB Lippincott, 1978, p 287.)

BULGING DISC (TYPE IV)

Another proposed mechanism of low back pain and sciatica involves protrusion of the nucleus pulposus, which remains covered with some annular fibers and, possibly, the posterior longitudinal ligament (Fig. 9.9). There may be "true acute sciatica" with mechanical and, possibly, chemical and/or inflammatory irritation of the nerve roots. The pain may include the back, buttock, thigh, lower leg, and even the foot and may be increased with coughing and sneezing; the straight leg raising test is positive. In this situation, radiographs usually do not indicate narrowing. It is feasible that traction or spinal manipulation may alter the mechanics and possibly may be therapeutic. With rest, the irritation

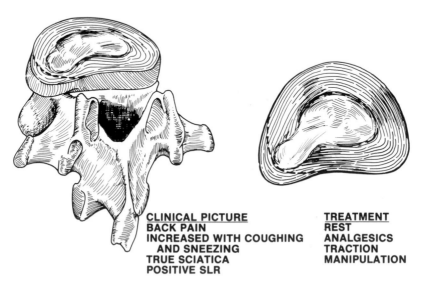

CLINICAL PICTURE
BACK PAIN
INCREASED WITH COUGHING
AND SNEEZING
TRUE SCIATICA
POSITIVE SLR

TREATMENT
REST
ANALGESICS
TRACTION
MANIPULATION

Figure 9.9. Bulging disc (type IV). In the patient with a bulging disc, the annulus is bulging to such an extent that nerve root irritation has caused sciatica. The *dotted line* shows the normal position of the annulus rim. (Reproduced with permission from White AA, Panjabi MM: *Clinical Biomechanics of the Spine.* Philadelphia, JB Lippincott, 1978, p 287.)

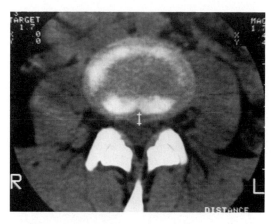

Figure 9.10. CT scan at the L3-L4 level performed in October 1986 shows a 4.2-mm disc protrusion.

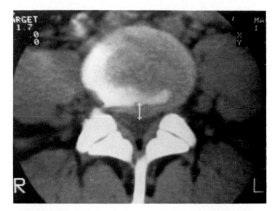

Figure 9.11. L4-L5 level performed in October 1986 shows a 6.1-mm central disc protrusion, and the vertebral canal, by CT, measures 10.7-mm sagittal diameter.

may subside and remain stable or may return spontaneously after mobilization.

A good example of type III and IV annular disruption and disc bulging, seen at our clinic, is presented below.

CASE 1

A 38-year-old white married female was seen at the referral of another chiropractor for the chief complaint of low back, left buttock, and left upper thigh pain. This had started approximately 1 year prior to our first seeing the patient, following bending, lifting, and twisting at the waist while picking up a 30-pound dog. She felt a sharp pain at the time and could not stand upright. She saw a chiropractor the following day, who treated her and gave some relief. She continued to feel a nagging ache in her low back despite a home exercise program, and 9 months after the initial injury again sought chiropractic relief. At that time, a lesion on the left leg was diagnosed as malignant melanoma and was surgically removed.

A CT scan was performed in October 1986; it is shown in Figures 9.10, 9.11, and 9.12. This CT was interpreted as showing a 4.2-mm L3-L4 bulging disc (Fig. 9.10), an L4-L5 central disc protrusion measuring 6.1-mm with a 10.7-mm sagittal diameter of the vertebral canal (Fig. 9.11), and a 3.8-mm L5-S1 bulging disc with a vertebral canal at L5-S1 measuring 10.7-mm in its sagittal diameter (Fig. 9.12). This was interpreted as representing anteroposterior stenosis at the L4-S1 levels, since the lower limit of normal is given as 11.5-mm. Therefore, the final diagnosis from the October 1986 CT scan was a protruding L4-L5 disc and bulging L3-L4 and L5-S1 discs, with stenosis present at the lower two levels.

This patient underwent physical therapy while confined to her home. Due to persistent pain, she had a repeat

CT scan performed in April 1987, which is seen in Figures 9.13, 9.14, and 9.15. Figure 9.13 shows the L3-L4 scan, which demonstrates a small central herniated nucleus pulposus with no evidence of free fragment or sequestration. The central canal is measured at 16-mm at the lower aspect of L3 and 14-mm at the superior aspect of L4.

The L4-L5 scan (Fig. 9.14) reveals a central and left-sided herniated nucleus pulposus with no indication of free fragment or sequestration. The central canal anteroposterior dimension is 1.5 cm at the inferior aspect of L4 and 1.3 cm at the superior aspect of L5.

The CT at the L5-S1 level (Fig. 9.15) reveals a small left herniated nucleus pulposus with no free fragment or sequestration. Mild degenerative changes are seen at the zygapophyseal joints (Fig. 9.16), with hypertrophy causing encroachment upon the intervertebral foramen bi-

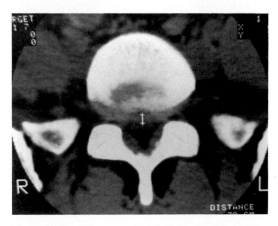

Figure 9.12. CT scan at the L5-S1 level performed in October 1986 shows a 3.8-mm L5-S1 disc bulge, and a sagittal vertebral canal CT measurement of 10.7-mm.

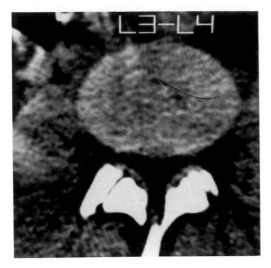

Figure 9.13. Repeat CT scan of Figure 9.10 at L3-L4 in April 1987 still shows a left central disc bulge but no evidence of disc herniation or free fragmentation.

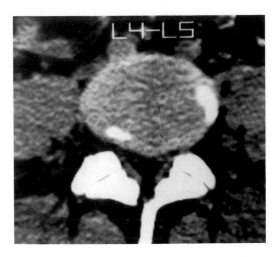

Figure 9.14. Repeat CT scan of Figure 9.11 in April 1987 at the L4-L5 level still shows a left central contained disc protrusion without the presence of a free fragment. Stenosis was not reported by the radiologist reading the CT scan.

laterally. The central canal anteroposterior distance measures 1.4 cm at the inferior aspect of L5 and 1.4 cm at the superior aspect of S1.

Interestingly, the first CT scan diagnosed 10.7-mm canals at the L4-L5 level and the L5-S1 level, whereas the second CT scan found them to be approximately 1.4 to 1.5 cm in diameter. This is almost ½ of a centimeter

difference and would mean the difference between stenosis or no stenosis being present. It raises the question of accuracy of the measurement of the sagittal vertebral canal dimension on the CT scan.

Figure 9.16 does reveal the ossification of the facet capsule that is causing encroachment into the lateral recess of the vertebral canal. This is at the L5-S1 level.

Following the second CT study, surgery was recommended to remove the L4-L5 disc and fuse L4 through the sacrum. At this point, the patient sought consultation at our clinic.

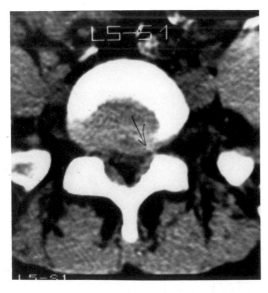

Figure 9.15. Repeat CT scan at the L5-S1 level in April 1987 shows a small left posterolateral contained disc protrusion with no fragmentation noted. Stenosis was not reported.

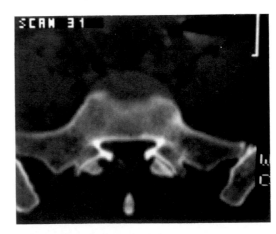

Figure 9.16. Mild degenerative changes are seen at the L5-S1 zygapophyseal joints, with probable ossification of the facet capsule at the attachment of the ligamentum flavum.

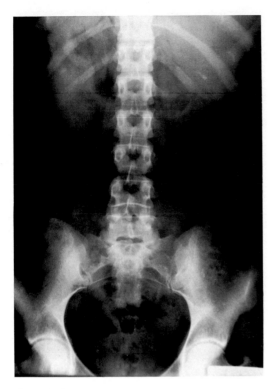

Figure 9.17. Posteroanterior plain x-ray study of the patient seen in CT in Figures 9.10 to 9.16.

Our examination revealed tenderness to palpation at the left L5-S1 joint, into the left buttock and upper thigh. The straight leg raises were negative. The deep reflexes were +2 bilaterally at the hamstring, patella, and ankle, and no sensory findings were present to pinwheel examination. The ranges of motion were all normal except that 25° of extension created low back pain. The Kemp's sign was positive to the left, creating low back and left buttock pain. The Déjérine triad was negative. No sign of hip disease was present. Again, the patient stated that very rarely did the pain ever extend to the knee and even more rarely did it extend below the knee.

Prone examination revealed that the Nachlas, Elys, and prone lumbar flexion exacerbated the patient's low back and left buttock pain. The left leg measured longer than the right on prone mensuration. Plain x-ray examination in the posteroanterior, lateral flexion, and lateral views (Figs. 9.17 to 9.21) reveals left lateral flexion subluxation of L4 on L5 and L5 on the sacrum in neutral posteroanterior view (Fig. 9.18). Left lateral flexion (Fig. 9.19) is a Lovett reverse rotation in that the spinous processes rotate into the convexity on the right instead of into the concavity on the left. Figure 9.20, right lateral flexion, reveals that L4 maintains its left lateral flexion and does not lateral flex to the right. We note that the spinous processes do stop at the midline

but again fail to rotate to the right concavity, which would be a normal rotational finding on right lateral flexion. Therefore, we see a left lateral flexion subluxation that is maintained in lateral bending. Figure 9.21 is a lateral projection that reveals L5 to be posterior on the sacrum. No stenosis is present. The sacral angle is 41°, and the lumbar lordotic angle 51°.

This case so well meets the criteria of Charnley's type III to type IV disc classes. We found no true sciatica. Certainly there were no motor, sensory, or reflex findings compatible with a marked compression of a lumbar or sacral nerve root by a disc protrusion or prolapse. We have CT evidence of disc protrusion at the lower three lumbar disc levels, L4-L5 being the most marked disc protrusion.

A dilemma is created by CT or MRI scans that show numerous discs to be bulging. Obviously, all of these are not causing nerve root compression compatible with sciatica. We know from the work of Wiesel et al. (25) that fully 36% of normal people, those having never had leg pain, will show these disc bulges on routine CT or myelographic examinations. Therefore, we are confronted with a diagnostic challenge when we have multiple-level disc lesions identified by an imaging modality.

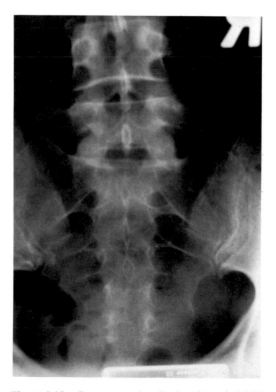

Figure 9.18. Posteroanterior tilt view through L4-L5 and L5-S1 shows left lateral flexion of L4 on L5 and L5 on the sacrum.

A careful clinical examination is still very necessary to determine the proper level of disc involvement. Without the CT and MRI, we are often devoid of information, whereas with them we oftentimes have more information, or at least information that needs further classification. There is never an ideal situation in diagnosing a disc lesion. Good diagnosis still starts with a careful clinical, neurological, and orthopedic examination. Putting this information into a proper diagnostic flow chart helps the doctor to arrive at the proper diagnosis; CT or MRI should then hopefully confirm the clinical diagnosis.

In this case, we did not feel that surgery was necessary. Our treatment program included the following: (a) flexion distraction manipulation applied at the three lower disc levels, with range of motion of the articular facets at each of these areas applied as the patient showed 50% improvement of the low back and upper left thigh pain; (b) low back wellness school to teach this patient the hazards of sitting and how to bend and lift in daily living with creation of minimum stress to the lumbar spine; (c) a strong exercise program of Cox exercises to correct the weakness of the abdominal, low back, and gluteal muscles; (d) adjustment, in side posture, of an anterior innominate subluxation that accompanied the long left leg, followed by the wearing of a

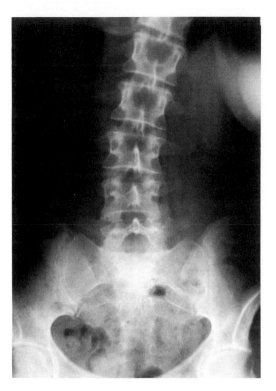

Figure 9.20. On right lateral flexion, L4 fails to right lateral flex on L5. The spinous processes of L1 through L5 rotate only to the midline when this patient lateral flexes to the right side. This is restricted rotation, since normally we would see the spinous processes rotate to the concavity on the right.

trochanter belt to support this left sacroiliac joint during healing; (e) appropriate home instructions to apply hot and cold alternating packs to the low back, left buttock, and upper thigh; (f) Nautilus extension exercises, started on the third day of treatment.

During treatment, this patient's pain actually settled into the sacrum and sacrococcygeal articulation. Rectal adjustment of the coccyx to check its alignment with the sacrum was done.

This patient was treated in our clinic for 30 days and returned home with a letter of referral to her referring chiropractor. Her remaining complaint on dismissal was left L5-S1 pain.

SEQUESTERED FRAGMENT (WANDERING DISC MATERIAL) (TYPE V)

A sequestered nucleus pulposus and/or annulus fibrosus (Fig. 9.22) associated with the normal degenerative processes of the disc and/or other

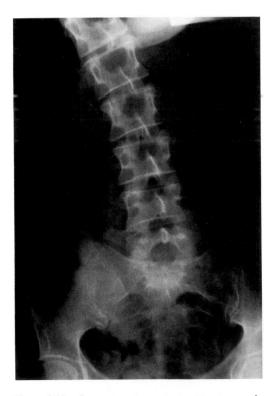

Figure 9.19. Lovett reverse rotatory curve seen as the spinous processes of the lumbar spine rotate right (the convex side of the curve) during left lateral flexion.

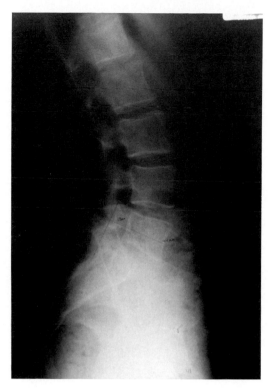

Figure 9.21. A lateral view of the patient in Figures 9.10 through 9.20 shows good disc spaces without degenerative disc disease changes. L5 shows retrolisthesis on the sacrum.

presently unknown pathologic changes may develop with time. This sequestrum may move about in a random fashion in response to the directions and magnitude of forces produced at the motion segment by the activity of the individual. This movement may permit the sequestrum to irritate the annular fibers (by physical presence and/or chemical breakdown products) and to produce low back pain with or without sciatica. It may also produce a bulge in an area in which it can cause true sciatica. The sequestration may move about, so that it either may be asymptomatic or may cause some combination of spine pain, referred pain, and true radiculopathy. Because of the movement of the sequestered fragment in response to forces at the motion segment, it may be possible, through axial traction or spinal manipulation of the motion segment, to move the sequestrum temporarily or permanently from a location in which it stimulates a nerve to one in which it causes no irritation. Subsequent motion of the disc fragment into areas of

pain insensitivity or subsequent scarring may result in no recurrence. On the other hand, if there is no scarring, the random movement of the sequestered portion of the disc may include positions of subsequent nerve root irritation.

DISPLACED SEQUESTERED FRAGMENT (ANCHORED) (TYPE VI)

Another clinical and mechanical cause of low back pain and sciatica is displacement of a sequestrum of the annulus and/or nucleus into the spinal canal or intervertebral foramen (Fig. 9.23). The fragment is to some degree fixed in position. The nerve root irritation results from inflammation due to mechanical pressure, chemical irritation, an autoimmune response, or some combination of the three. There is true sciatica with the positive straight leg raising sign. In association with a displaced portion of the intervertebral disc (sequestration), there may be narrowing of the interspace at the involved level. Axial traction, manipulation, and random movement are unlikely to help. Chymopapain injected into the disc space may never reach or affect the sequestrum, especially if there has been scarring or blockage of the hole in the disc structure. We hypothesize that, when this situation subsides spontaneously, it is the result of phagocytosis and/or some physiological adjustment of the neural structures to the irritation. Patients with a displaced sequestered fragment show the best results when treated with surgery, as suggested by Charnley and subsequently confirmed by Sprangfort (21, 25a).[c]

Examples of Charnley's type V and VI disc lesions from our clinic are presented below.

CASE 2

A 30-year-old white married female developed low back pain following delivery approximately 7 to 8 weeks prior to seeing us. The start of low back pain felt like a pinching and then eventually continued down the left lower extremity. The history revealed lower back pain 3 years previously, which was relieved with exercise.

Figure 9.24 reveals the marked sciatic scoliosis of this patient. Note the flexed left knee to relieve stretch on the sciatic nerve. This patient's low back and leg pain were aggravated by the Déjérine triad. Straight leg rais-

[c] Spangfort's article (25) is an excellent discussion of the significance of various physical findings in the evaluation and interpretation of low back pain and sciatica.

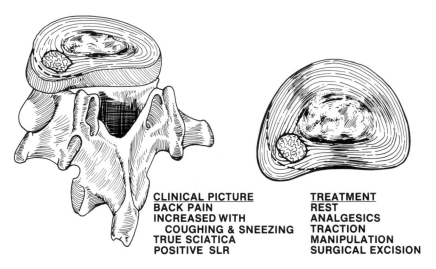

CLINICAL PICTURE
BACK PAIN
INCREASED WITH
    COUGHING & SNEEZING
TRUE SCIATICA
POSITIVE SLR

TREATMENT
REST
ANALGESICS
TRACTION
MANIPULATION
SURGICAL EXCISION

Figure 9.22. Sequestered fragment (the wandering disc) (type V). The results of treatment with surgery are better in the type V patient than in the type I to type IV patient, but they are probably not as good in the type V patient as they are in the type VI and type VII patient. The wandering disc is a possible explanation for the clinical picture of exacerbations and remissions which is so frequently encountered. It may also be a partial explanation of why some patients show a good response to traction or manipulation. (Reproduced with permission of White AA, Panjabi MM: *Clinical Biomechanics of the Spine.* Philadelphia, JB Lippincott, 1978, p 288.)

ing was positive sitting and recumbent at 10°, creating low back and leg pain. Marked reduction of her ranges of motion was noted. The deep reflexes and sensory examination were within normal limits. Circulation of the lower extremity was normal. The hamstring reflexes were +2 bilaterally. No atrophy was noted.

Figures 9.25, 9.26, and 9.27 are neutral, right, and left lateral flexion studies of this patient. You note the strong right lateral flexion subluxation of L4 on L5 and the inability of this patient to laterally flex to the left. Figure 9.28 shows the PA film taken at the time of myelography; you will note the large filling defect at the L4-

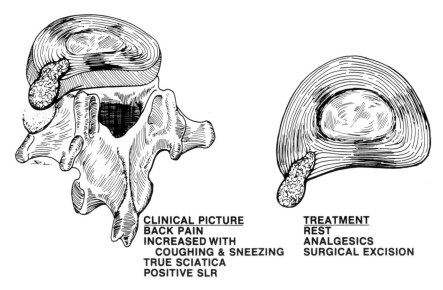

CLINICAL PICTURE
BACK PAIN
INCREASED WITH
    COUGHING & SNEEZING
TRUE SCIATICA
POSITIVE SLR

TREATMENT
REST
ANALGESICS
SURGICAL EXCISION

Figure 9.23. With type VI, there is sequestration and displacement, but there is some anchoring of the ligament, so that it cannot move about. This is likely to be helped by traction or manipulation. (Reproduced with permission from White AA, Panjabi MM: *Clinical Biomechanics of the Spine.* Philadelphia, JB Lippincott, 1978, p 289.)

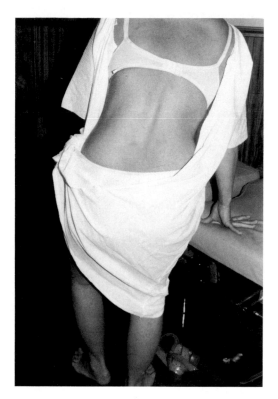

Figure 9.24. Severe right sciatic scoliosis in a patient with left fifth lumbar nerve root paresthesia. Note that the left knee is held flexed to prevent stretch on the sciatic nerve (Neri's bow sign).

L5 segment. The same is shown on Figure 9.29, the lateral projection. Figure 9.30 is the oblique view, revealing the filling defect due to the intervertebral disc protrusion compressing the dye-filled subarachnoid space. Figure 9.31 is the CT scan, revealing an extremely large left central intervertebral disc protrusion.

This was surgically removed, and the patient had 100% relief of symptoms. Treatment was attempted with flexion distraction, but due to the extreme size of this disc lesion the patient could not tolerate any attempt at therapy or spinal manipulation. This is a good case of surgical necessity.

DEGENERATIVE DISC (TYPE VII)

Disc degeneration (Fig. 9.32) involves a disruption of the normal annular fibers of the disc to such an extent that the disc is no longer able to serve an adequate mechanical function. This disruption may be associated with degenerative arthritic processes of the vertebral bodies and/or the intervertebral joints. There may be chronic pain, intermittent pain, or no pain.

Charnley's type VII degenerative disc is shown in a case from our clinic:

CASE 3

This case was a 52-year-old white female who had had back surgery 1 year prior to her first visit to our clinic. She had had low back and leg pain prior to the surgery; and 1 year following surgery, she was in greater low back pain and the pain was radiating into her right lower extremity fifth lumbar dermatome.

Figure 9.33 shows an x-ray taken prior to her back surgery. Here we see a pseudosacralization at L5 on the right with marked loss of the L4-L5 disc space and discogenic spondyloarthrotic changes. The left L4 inferior articular facet is hyperplastic, creating a pseudoarticulation with the laminae of L5. L3 is in right lateral flexion subluxation, and tropism at this level is noted, the facet on the right being sagittal and the left coronal. You will also note that there are arthrotic changes of the pseudosacralization between L5 and the sacrum and ilium on the right. Figure 9.34 shows a repeat x-ray of

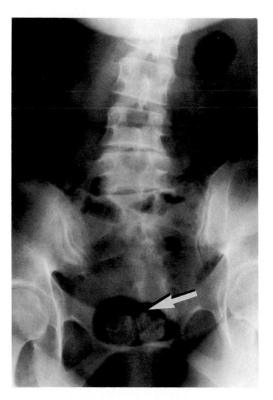

Figure 9.25. Right lateral list of the lumbar spine is seen in the patient in Figure 9.24. Note how the pelvis is posterior as evidenced by the loss of height of the pelvic ring and how high the symphysis pubes lies over the sacrum (*arrow*).

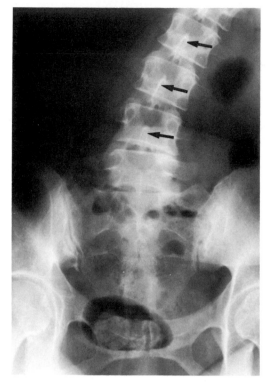

Figure 9.26. On right lateral flexion, minimal motion occurs, and we see how the spinous processes (*arrows*) fail to rotate to the right concavity and instead rotate to the left convexity of the curve.

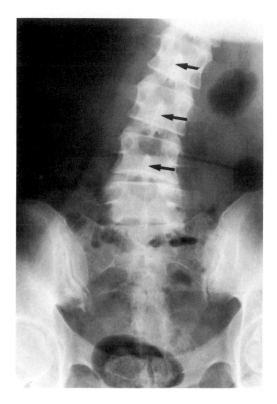

Figure 9.27. On attempted left lateral flexion, the spinous processes (*arrows*) are in the midline and actually represent the only motion seen in the lumbar segments in attempted left lateral flexion. There just is no movement into the left, painful, side of this lumbar spine and left lower extremity.

her spine 1 year following her back surgery. You will note that there is further degenerative change in the L4-L5 disc and also at the L3-L4 disc, where there is a marked loss of disc space and bone periosteal reaction on contact with the vertebral bodies. This represents the concept of moving the ranges of motion up one segment cephalad following degeneration of a disc.

As we know in Bertolotti's syndrome, due to the transitional segment at L5 on the sacrum, the motion takes place at the L4-L5 level. As the L4-L5 disc degenerates and is surgically operated on, as in this case, the motion shifts to the L3 level, and as can be seen, this disc, when asked to take up 95% of the flexion and extension motion of the lumbar spine, soon deteriorates. Normally L5-S1 makes up 75% of the flexion and extension motion, and L4-L5 20%, with only 5% of the flexion and extension occurring in the upper lumbar segments. As you ask each succeeding lumbar disc to assume more mobility as the one below degenerates, that disc is less capable of maintaining that motion, and the disc undergoes degenerative change.

Figure 9.35 is a lateral view of the lumbar spine prior to surgery. Here you see the L4-L5 disc degenerated and

L3 posteriorly subluxated on L4 but still maintaining a rather good disc space.

Figure 9.36 was taken 1 year following surgery, and here you can see that the L4-L5 disc has increased its degenerative change; however the L3-L4 disc is markedly degenerated, with marked anterolateral lipping and spurring and subchondrosclerosis of the opposing vertebral body plates.

This is a good case which reveals a Bertolotti's syndrome at L5 with an L4-L5 disc protrusion. Following surgery at L4-L5, the movement shifted to the L3 segment, which now became the level of maximum mobility and also the level of maximum degenerative change—a good example of a "domino" effect of disc degeneration moving from caudal to cephalic disc levels. This is a good example of the Charnley type VII disc classification.

ORGANIC IDIOPATHIC SPINE PAIN

Organic idiopathic spine pain is the type of pain present in patients who are diagnosed clinically as

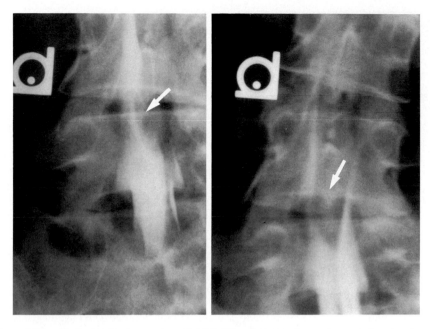

Figure 9.28. Myelography shows a large L4-L5 filling defect in the posteroanterior view (*arrow*).

having organic spine pain without sciatica for which there is no known etiology. Pain may emanate from the disc, or it may be caused by increased fluid uptake by the disc (type II), any combination of the previously described etiological factors, or some mechanism yet to be discovered.

CONTAINED (PROTRUDED) AND NON-CONTAINED (PROLAPSED) DISCS

Definition and Principles

We classified the change within the nucleus pulposus, when it escaped the confines of the annulus, as either a protrusion or prolapse. Protrusion of nuclear material occurs when the protruding nucleus is contiguous with the remaining nucleus and the annulus fibrosus is stretched, thinned, and under pressure. The protrusion may cause only back pain if the outer nerve-innervated annulus is irritated, or it may cause both back and leg pain if the annulus bulge contacts the dural lined nerve root within the lateral recess of the vertebral column. Keep in mind that the pressure within the nucleus is 30 psi (26) and that Nachemson and Morris (27) have found this pressure to be 30% less in the standing position than in the sitting position, with 50% less pressure in the reclining position than in the sit-

ting position. The cerebrospinal fluid pressure is 100-mm of water in the recumbent posture and 400-mm in the sitting posture (28). This is important in treating the disc lesion, as sitting is to be avoided. An epidemiological study (29) conducted in Baltimore, Maryland, demonstrated that suburban dwellers who drive to work have twice the incidence of severe back pain than do those who do not drive, and that those workers who drive during most of their working day, such as truck drivers, have three times the incidence. Fahrni (30) surveyed a jungle people in India who squat rather than sit and found that they had a zero incidence of back pain and a greatly diminished incidence of disc degeneration on x-ray.

Gresham and Miller (31) carried out postmortem discograms on 63 fresh autopsies; these patients who came to autopsy were between 14 and 80 years old and had had relatively asymptomatic backs. Gresham and Miller found that all of the specimens that came from patients between 46 and 59 years old revealed evidence of disc degeneration at L5-S1.

Prolapse exists when the extruded nucleus loses continuity with the remaining nuclear material and forms a free fragment, or what in Europe is termed a sequestered disc fragment, within the spinal canal. Arns et al. (32) state that the first stage of disc lesion is nuclear bulge which causes lumbago and symptoms of Déjérine's triad. The

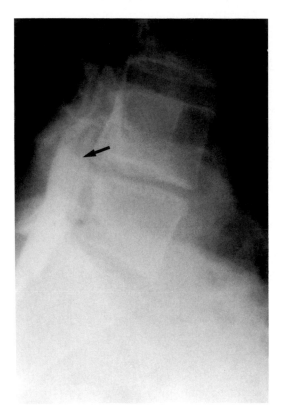

Figure 9.29. Lateral projection of Figure 9.28 shows the flexion of L4 on L5 and the bulging of the L4-L5 disc into the dye-filled subarachnoid space (*arrow*).

Pelvic Disease and Disc Compression of Nerve Roots

A connection between lumbar disc degeneration and pelvic disease has been documented by Herlin, who says that it has been suspected for years and that painful and chronic infectious conditions of the urogenital organs have been associated with compression of one or several of the lower sacral nerve roots. He further states that endometriosis sometimes is combined with sciatica, and that it seems justifiable to investigate the relationship between sacral nerve root compression and the development of endometriosis. He believes that, in males, lower sacral nerve root compression as a cause of chronic prostatovesiculitis ought to be considered (34). He has documented that, in one patient, two miscarriages were due to sacral nerve root compression which caused most of the patient's sciatica later (34). In another patient, he believes that there is a probable connection between chronic urogenital infection due to disc compression of sacral nerve roots

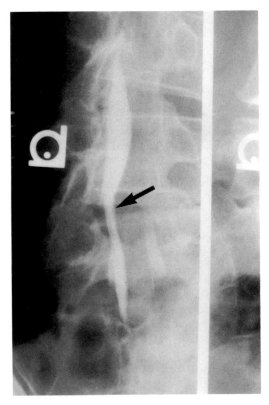

Figure 9.30. The oblique view shows the filling defect at L4-L5 due to the massive L4-L5 disc prolapse (*arrow*).

second stage is the onset of sciatica as the nuclear bulge contacts the nerve root, and the third and final stage is prolapse.

Opinions as to the efficacy of myelography, electromyography, and discography in the diagnosis of disc protrusions have varied. Semmes (33) states that because nearly one-third of myelograms are not definitive or are misleading, the history and clinical findings have proved more reliable. He states that myelography is used too frequently for diagnosis and indication for surgery and that he has used it in less than 3% of his last 350 surgeries. In the Scandinavian countries, the use of oil-based media in myelography has been banned due to the risk of arachnoiditis (29). Herlin states that myelography is not a sufficiently reliable method of investigation in the diagnosis of sciatica (34) and has utilized myelography in only 10% of his cases (34).

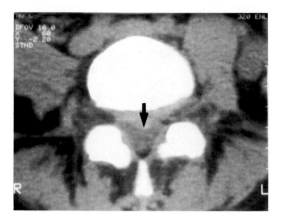

Figure 9.31. CT shows a very large left central disc prolapse at the L4-L5 level (*arrow*).

and rheumatoid arthritis (34). Herlin has also documented a connection between sacral nerve root compression and chronic prostatitis (34). He also believes that, although there is no definite proof as yet, the possibility of sacral nerve root compression as a cause of sterility must be considered (34). He presents a case of pain originating bilaterally in the medial region of the gluteal muscles and radiating into the minor pudendal labiae and clitoris, with a decrease to loss of the duration of intensity of orgasm. Following surgery for the removal of a medial fifth lumbar disc lesion,

the patient's sexual function normalized within 2 months (34).

Emmett and Love (35) and Ross and Jackson (36) believe that disc disease should be ruled out in young and middle-aged patients who develop problems of urinary retention, vesicle irritability, or incontinence. Amelar and Dubin (37), however, link lumbar disc disorders with sexual impotence and bladder function disturbances through organic parasympathetic involvement rather than psychological causes.

PUDENDAL PLEXUS

Understanding the neurovisceral connection between the disc lesion and disease of the pelvic organs requires understanding of the pudendal plexus. The pudendal plexus is formed from the second, third, and fourth sacral nerves and is the innervation of certain pelvic organs (38). Parasympathetic fibers innervate the urinary bladder, prostate gland, and seminal vesicles. The uterus and external genitalia also are innervated by nerve fibers from this plexus, and the alimentary tract is controlled by the pudendal plexus as well. The pudendal nerve, a branch of the pudendal plexus, gives rise to the inferior hemorrhoidal nerve, the perineal nerve to the transversus perinei profundus, the sphincter urethrae membranacea, bulbocavernosus, ischiocavernosus,

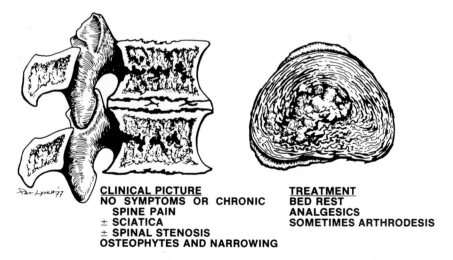

CLINICAL PICTURE
NO SYMPTOMS OR CHRONIC SPINE PAIN
± SCIATICA
± SPINAL STENOSIS
OSTEOPHYTES AND NARROWING

TREATMENT
BED REST
ANALGESICS
SOMETIMES ARTHRODESIS

Figure 9.32. A degenerated disc (type VII) either may be the end process of the mechanical and biological effects of normal functioning or may be associated with considerable pain and disability. There may also be arthritis in the intervertebral joints. It is important to emphasize that these various stages are a continuum. A given disc may move or decelerate, stop, or, in some instances, even reverse. (Reproduced with permission from White AA, Panjabi MM: *Clinical Biomechanics of the Spine.* Philadelphia, JB Lippincott, 1978, p 290.)

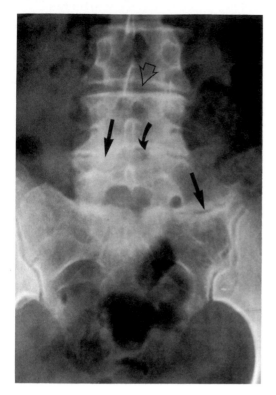

Figure 9.33. Pseudosacralization of the right L5 transverse process (*straight arrow*), with marked degenerative changes at the L4-L5 disc level (*curved arrow*) and to a lesser degree at the L3-L4 level (*open arrow*). L3 is in right lateral flexion on L4. The left L4 inferior facet is hyperplastic and creates a pseudoarticulation with the lamina of L5 (*long arrow*). Also note the degenerative change at the pseudoarticulation of the overdeveloped right L5 transverse process with the sacrum.

Occurrence and Onset of Back and Leg Pain

The onset of sciatica or back pain represents a starting point for diagnosis. It is possible for a disc to protrude and contact a nerve root, resulting in the sudden onset of sciatica without accompanying back pain. This protrusion may result in isolated pain in an area of specific nerve innervation such as the heel, calf, great toe, or posterior thigh. Back pain preceding sciatica indicates irritation of the annulus fibrosus, ligaments, and dura mater innervated by the recurrent meningeal nerve prior to contact with the involved

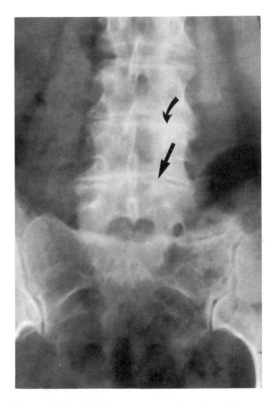

Figure 9.34. This is a posteroanterior view of the patient seen in Figure 9.33, 1 year after surgery for removal of an L4-L5 disc protrusion, and we can see the further disc degeneration at the L4-L5 (*straight arrow*) and L3-L4 (*curved arrow*) levels. Remember that the combination of a transitional segment and disc degenerative or protrusion changes above it is called Bertolotti's syndrome. The transitional segment has a rudimentary disc and places the movement that normally occurred at that level on the disc above. Thus, the increased stress causes the disc to become unstable and undergo degeneration. This is a good example of type VII disc degeneration by Charnley's classification.

transversus perinei superficialis, the corpus cavernosum urethrae, the urethra, the mucous membrane of the urethra, the urogenital diaphragm, and a scrotal branch to the scrotum and labiae. Another branch of the pudendal nerve, the dorsal nerve of the penis, innervates the urogenital diaphragm, the corpus cavernosum penis, and dorsum of the penis ending in the glans. The clitoris is innervated similarly in the female.

Neuroanatomically, the pressure on the sacral nerve roots by disc lesion can create aberrant nerve supply to the organs described and resultant disease. On this neurological basis, one can see the reason many authorities state that disc lesion should be considered in the etiology of any condition of the urogenital system or reproductive system.

nerve root. The sudden onset of leg pain without back pain indicates extrusion (prolapse) of the disc (8).

A differential diagnosis between protrusion and prolapse may include the findings shown in Table 9.3.

The cauda equina symptoms caused by large midline disc protrusions contacting several roots of the cauda equina present a particular problem in diagnosis. Difficulty with urination, incontinence, rectal difficulties, difficulty in walking, or symptoms of abdominal viscera are indicative of the diagnosis of a large midline disc protrusion. These represent true surgical emergencies and must be handled as such.

The delay in the onset of pain in disc injuries can be the key to diagnosis. The cartilage of the spine has a poor blood supply and reacts to injuries slowly. Therefore, it may be 2 or 3 days after

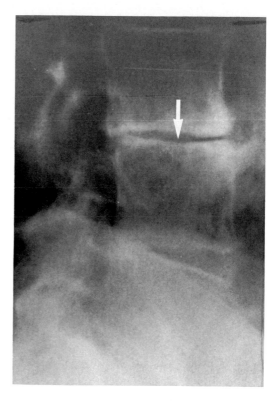

Figure 9.36. One year postsurgically, the same patient seen in Figure 9.35, and shown in posteroanterior view in Figure 9.34, shows extreme L3-L4 discal degeneration (*straight arrow*), as evidenced by loss of joint space and subchondral sclerosis and anterolateral hypertrophic spurring. The vacuum phenomenon is seen in the anterior L3-L4 disc area. The L4-L5 disc shows the same degenerative changes as prior to surgery.

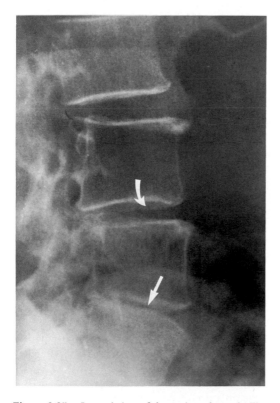

Figure 9.35. Lateral view of the patient shown in Figure 9.33, prior to surgery, shows advanced loss of joint space at the L4-L5 disc level (*straight arrow*), with vertebral plate sclerosis and anterolateral hypertrophic traction spurring. The L3-L4 disc (*curved arrow*) also shows, to a lesser extent, the same findings as L4-L5.

injury that the oozing of the nuclear material and the slow swelling of the disc result in the pain that follows an injury and protrusion of a disc (39).

Table 9.3.
Clinical Differentiation Findings in Protrusion and Prolapse

Differential Diagnosis	Protrusion	Prolapse
Pain on compression and distraction	Yes, usually	Not as frequently
Flexion and extension	Yes	Only on flexion
Cough, sneeze, and strain	Yes	Not always
Onset of pain	Gradual	Sudden, intense

Specific Diagnostic Criteria of Disc Lesions

L3-L4 DISC PROTRUSION (L4 NERVE ROOT COMPRESSION) FINDINGS

Weakness of the quadriceps muscle (Fig. 9.37). Diminished or absent patellar reflex (Fig. 9.38).

The test for the straight leg raising sign may be negative in lesions of the L3-L4 disc. Pinwheel examination may reveal hyperesthesia or hypoesthesia of the L4 dermatome.

L4-L5 DISC PROTRUSION (L5 NERVE ROOT COMPRESSION) FINDINGS

Weakness of tibialis anterior muscle, extensor digitorum and hallucis longus muscles (Fig. 9.39).

Weakness of the extensor hallucis muscle (Fig. 9.40).

Weakness of the peroneus longus and brevis muscles. Weakness in these muscles also occurs when an L5-S1 disc protrusion compresses the S1 nerve root (Fig. 9.41).

Dysesthesia of the L5 dermatome is determined by simultaneous testing of the sensation of the extremities (Fig. 9.42).

Foot and great toe dorsiflexion (ankle eversion) strengths depend upon the nerve supply of the peroneal nerve to the anterior tibialis and extensor muscles. The SLR will be positive in proportion to nerve compression by the disc.

L5-S1 DISC PROTRUSION (S1 NERVE ROOT COMPRESSION) FINDINGS

Several muscles are tested for L5-S1 compression of the first and second sacral nerve roots.

Weakness of the biceps femoris, semimembranosus, or semitendinosus muscles (Fig. 9.43).

Weakness of the gluteus maximus is found by comparison of contralateral sides. The opposite pelvis should be stabilized while the thigh on the side to be tested is compressed (Fig. 9.44). The gluteus maximus muscle is innervated by the inferior gluteal nerve whose origin is in the roots of L5-S1-S2.

The gluteal skyline sign was present in 60% of patients with disc lesions of the lower lumbar spine. This sign is second only to the straight leg raising sign in frequency and was the only finding except for pain in 13% of the patients with disc protrusion (40). The patient is asked to contract his buttocks. Flaccidity is found on the side of the disc protrusion (Fig. 9.45).

Diminished or absent ankle jerks (Achilles reflexes) may be noted (Fig. 9.46).

Weakness of the calf muscles (Fig. 9.47).

Weakness of the flexor muscle of the great toe (Fig. 9.48).

Dysesthesia of the S1 dermatome by comparing the sensation of each extremity simultaneously (Fig. 9.49).

The SLR will be positive, the severity depending upon the pressure of the disc bulge or protrusion on the compressed nerve root.

It must be stated that these tests are strong indicators for disc level involvement, but there is some overlap of innervation to those muscles suppled by all three nerve roots—L4, L5, and S1.

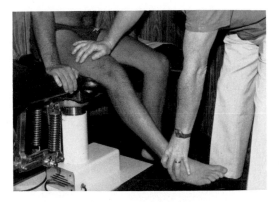

Figure 9.37. Quadriceps muscle testing.

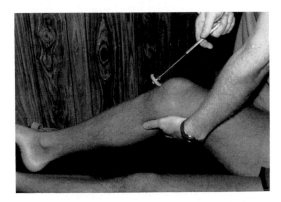

Figure 9.38. Patellar reflex testing.

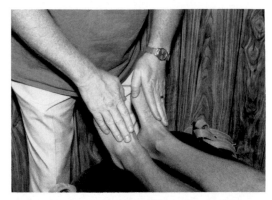

Figure 9.39. Dorsiflexion (ankle eversion) of the foot.

Motor Changes in Discal Lesions

Special mention of motor changes in these radicular compressions is needed, since they represent perhaps the most serious side effects of disc protrusion. Disc lesions can cripple, and motor

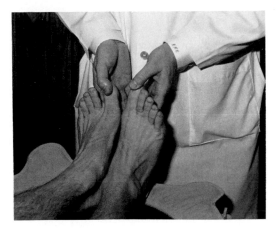

Figure 9.40. Dorsiflexion of the great toe.

changes are the most serious side effects for the patient and the most serious potential medicolegal problems for the physician, whether the approach be conservative or surgical.

Occasionally, muscle weakness due to neurapraxia or degeneration may be present with little or no pain. Of course, muscle weakness usually follows sensory changes of the lower extremity. Nevertheless, regardless of the pain in a patient complaining of low back pain, leg pain, or an inability to walk on the toes or heels the clinician must always do kinesiological muscle testing.

Depending on the muscle involved, patients may complain of falling, having equilibrium problems (which really means they tend to limp due to weak muscles), or having the knee "give out" under them. Gait changes, such as limping due to calf muscle weakness and inability to lift the heel, or

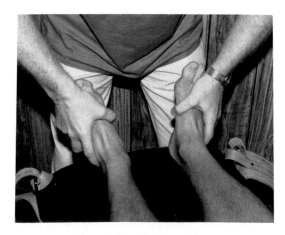

Figure 9.41. Eversion of foot.

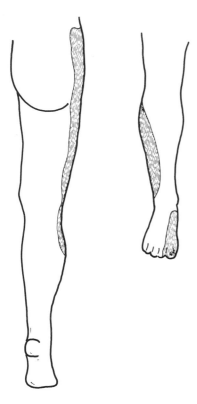

Figure 9.42. Dysesthesia and pain distribution of the L5 dermatome.

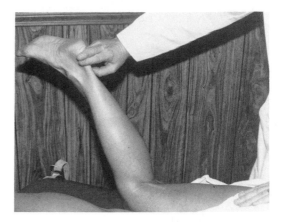

Figure 9.43. Hamstring muscle strength testing.

"stubbing" the great toe on carpet or steps due to weak anterior tibialis muscles or peroneal muscles, may be present. Patients may walk with the knee flexed so as to prevent "stretching" of the swollen or inflamed sciatic nerve. This would be a "walking" Néri bowing sign.

Validity of Determination of L4, L5, S1 Dermatome Innervation

Ninety percent of patients with disc protrusion or degeneration will have L5 or S1 nerve root involvement. Five percent of people have congenital failures of segmentation of these nerve roots which may present problems in localization of the involved nerve root. Electronic stimulation of 50 patients' L5 and S1 nerve roots proved that segmental innervation is essentially reliable in identifying the dominant nerve root. Sixteen percent of these patients did exhibit significant departure from the usual dermatome innervation (41).

First sacral nerve projection pain is most common. Four hundred and three patients had their clinical test results compared with myelographic and operative findings to determine the accuracy of the clinical examination in diagnosing the involved disc and nerve root (42). L5 dermatome involvement had the same accuracy for localizing an L4-L5 disc lesion as myelography, 80% of the time finding an L5 dermatome distribution due to an L4-L5 disc lesion. S1 nerve root involvement was due to an L4-L5 disc 34% of the time and an L5-S1 disc 63% of the time. Associated L5 and S1 dermatome pain was found in L4-L5 disc involvement 75% of the time.

Kortelainen et al. (42) concluded that, in single nerve root involvement with motor, reflex, and sensory disturbances, the accuracy of clinical investigation was equal to that of myelography. With two nerve roots involved, clinical diagnosis is not completely reliable in lower lumbar herniated discs, necessitating CT or myelography prior to surgery in order to avoid unnecessary explorations.

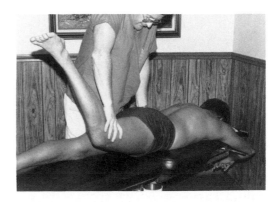

Figure 9.44. Gluteus maximus muscle testing.

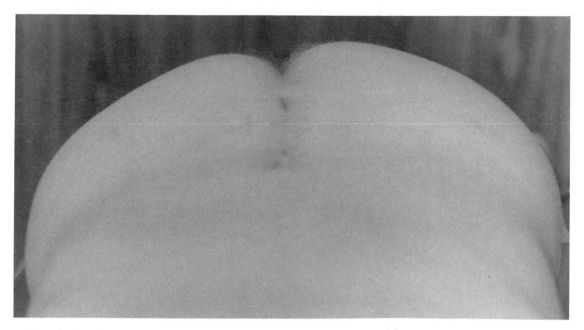

Figure 9.45. Gluteal skyline sign in a 36-year-old man with a history of 3½ months of right low back and first sacral nerve root sciatica. The ankle jerk reflex is absent, and there is marked loss of the tone of the gluteus maximus muscle, as noted by the flattened contour of the right gluteus maximus muscle. The CT scan and myelogram were positive for a prolapse of the L5-S1 disc on the right. Surgery was necessary to remove the fragment.

Initial Treatment Based on Clinical Investigative Impression

This author (J.M.C.) points out that in our diagnostic approach to the intervertebral disc lesion, we rely on the clinical workup to give us the impression of the disc level and type. If the patient is not at least 50% improved within 3 to 4 weeks of manipulative care based on this impression, more invasive testing, such as MRI, CT, EMG, or perhaps myelography, is ordered. Of course, if serious findings such as cauda equina signs, increased motor weakness, or unbearable pain set in, we will move quickly to the more definitive diagnostic imaging modalities. However, based on our clinical impression, we will successfully re-

Figure 9.46. Ankle jerk testing.

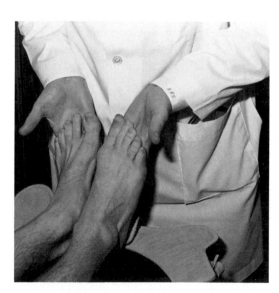

Figure 9.47. Plantar flexion of foot.

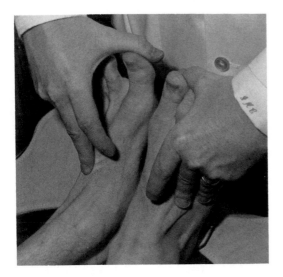

Figure 9.48. Plantar flexion of the great toe.

lieve well over 90% of our low back pain patients and avoid the more invasive and costly imaging modalities.

Schoedinger (43) states that a detailed history and physical examination, in combination with a positive diagnostic imaging tool such as CT or myelography, are sufficient to establish the diagnosis of disc rupture.

Semmes (33) states that the clinical findings and history are more reliable than myelograms, since nearly one-third of myelograms are uncertain or misleading. He even stated that myelography was wholly unnecessary in the diagnosis of the average patient requiring surgery for a ruptured disc. I would assume that his concept would be altered by modern imaging modalities such as CT and MRI.

Gainer and Nugent (44) stated that lumbar disc herniation is one of the most common causes of back pain and leg pain and is usually easily diagnosed by a history and physical examination.

Accuracy in Diagnosing Disc Lesion from Clinical Findings

Bell et al. (45) reported that Hakelius reported a 63% correlation between clinical neurological signs and operatively proven pathology. Furthermore, Hirsch and Nachemson were claimed to have reported a 55% correlation between neurological signs and the presence of herniated lumbar disc; they found that the presence of a

positive straight leg raising sign in addition to positive neurological signs produced the correct diagnosis in 86% of their patients. The same positive neurological examination and positive straight leg raising sign, coupled with a positive myelogram, increased the accuracy to 95%. This author (J.M.C.) would suggest that the 86% accuracy, in the absence of cauda equina syndrome signs or worsening motor deficit, is strong enough clinical indication to justify 3 weeks of conservative care before utilizing the more invasive and institutionally necessitated CT or MRI.

S2 and S3 Nerve Root Compression Signs

White and Leslie (46) reported that the posterior two-thirds of the scrotum is supplied by the second and third sacral nerves. They urge the value of examination of the lumbar spine in cases of unexplained scrotal pain.

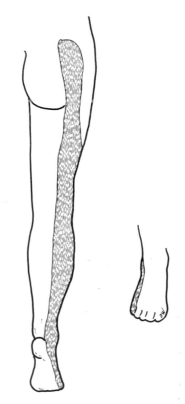

Figure 9.49. Dysesthesia and pain distribution of S1 dermatome.

Summary of Diagnosis of Disc Lesions

The steps in diagnosis of disc lesions are as follows:

1. Note the specific distribution of pain into the lower extremity and whether it involves the L4, L5, or S1 nerve root.

2. Note whether there is any lean of the lumbar spine.

3. Do x-rays reveal any right or left lateral flexion of the vertebrae at the level of disc involvement ascertained from dermatome evaluation? That is, if an L5 dermatome sensitivity is found, does the L4 vertebra have a right or left lateral flexion subluxation? If it is the S1 dermatome, does the L5 vertebra have a left or right lateral flexion?

4. Correlate the findings from above to differentiate protrusion from prolapse. Statistically, prolapses are much more difficult to treat than are protrusions.

5. Correlate the straight leg raising sign with a medial or lateral disc. That is, is it positive on the side of sciatica, indicating lateral disc or medial disc, or is it positive on the well leg raising sign, indicating a medial disc on the side of sciatica?

6. Investigate the site of original pain, i.e., whether it was back or leg, to rule out tumor, infection, or other organic disease as a probable etiology. Refer to Table 9.4 to aid in the differential diagnosis between a tumor and a disc lesion.

7. If a disc involvement truly seems probable, after the site has been determined to be either medial or lateral, explain to the patient that manipulative therapy may not be adequate and that surgical intervention may be necessary.

EXAMINATION

Gleis and Johnson (47) recommend a preprinted pro forma examination form for recording the findings of a physical examination for lumbar pain. They recommend that the examination be done in a logical sequence that helps the examiner to reach a working diagnosis and treatment plan. We present such an approach at this time.

History

Table 9.5 shows the low back pain examination form that we use. A history of the patient usually is compiled by an assistant. The patient's chief complaint should be recorded as exactly as possi-

Table 9.4.
Differential Diagnostic Findings of Discal versus Tumor Etiology

Differential Diagnosis	Neoplasm	Protrusion
Sitting and standing	No change	Aggravates
Bilateral	Often	Seldom
Night pain	Yes	Less
Character of pain	Unrelenting	Intermittent
Cauda equina symptoms	More	Less
Onset first leg or back pain	Back usually	Either

ble; e.g., pain in the low back radiating into the calf of the right leg, or pain in the side of the leg with numbness of the great toe. The history of the complaint should include specific details as to how the pain began, i.e., whether the pain in the back started with or without leg pain, or whether the leg pain started sometime after the pain in the back. *A chronological sequence of back or leg pain from its first incidence in life to the present should be recorded by month and year and should include the present symptoms.* Note that on this form the date of pain onset and the date of first examination are requested. These dates allow the doctor to notice the time lapse between the onset of symptoms and the consultation. If this lapse has been long, the patient may have sought other care, and a careful screening of past procedures and diagnosis is necessary.

The history of the patient should include any surgical interventions. Be particularly alert to any disease that could metastasize to the spine and mimic a disc lesion. Any symptoms of gastrointestinal, genitourinary, and menstrual problems should be listed. These allow for documentation of any pudendal plexus symptoms for evaluation following the mechanical relief of back pain. Thus, it is possible to evaluate the effects of chiropractic treatment not only on biomechanical faults but also on organic disease.

The family incidence of back pain also is recorded. This record should include whether the father, mother, or siblings have had low back pain, leg pain, or surgery, whether the back pain or leg pain started first or both began simultaneously, whether the pain is aggravated by coughing, sneezing, straining at the stool, bending and lifting, or sitting, and how far down the lower extremity the pain radiates.

Table 9.5.
Low Back Pain Examination Form

LOW BACK EXAMINATION FORM FOR CLINICAL EVALUATION
AND STATISTICAL RESEARCH OF LOW BACK AND DISC DISORDERS

Name _____ Age _____ Sex _____ S.M.W.D.

Occupation _____

Date of Pain Onset _____ Date of First Examination _____

Chief Complaint:

History of Complaint:

PHYSICAL EXAMINATION

Surgical History:

Bowel Habits:

Urinary Habits:

Menstrual Periods:

Digestion:
Drugs:
Past Illnesses:
B/P: Heart Rate: Rhythm: Sounds: Lung:

Abdomen: Prostate:
Testicle Pain: Impotency:

FAMILY HISTORY OF BACK PROBLEMS:

Sciatica	Low Back Pain	Surgery for Disc
____ None	____ None	____ None
____ Father	____ Father	____ Father
____ Mother	____ Mother	____ Mother
____ Brother	____ Brother	____ Brother
____ Sister	____ Sister	____ Sister
____ Other	____ Other	____ Other
____ Unknown	____ Unknown	____ Unknown

Location of Pain	Pain Aggravated by	Extent of Pain
____ Right Leg		____ Buttock
____ Left Leg		____ Thigh
____ Both Legs	____ Coughing	____ Knee
____ Alternating	____ Sneezing	____ Calf
____ Leg Pain Came	____ Straining at stool	____ Ankle
____ Before Back Pain	____ Bending & Lifting	____ Foot
____ Simultaneous with	____ Sitting	____ Toes
back pain		____ Unknown
____ After Back Pain		

Table 9.5—*Continued*
Low Back Pain Examination Form

Prone Examination

Nachlas'	Yeoman's	Ely's	Prone Lumbar Flexion	Popliteal Fossa Pain
___ Positive ___ Rt ___ Lt ___ Negative	___ Positive ___ Rt ___ Lt ___ Negative	___ Positive ___ Rt ___ Lt ___ Negative	___ No Change ___ Change	___ Positive ___ Rt. ___ Lt. ___ Negative

NONORGANIC PHYSICAL SIGNS

Libman's	Tenderness to Skin Pinch	Mannkopf's	Burns' Bench	Flip Test	Plantar Flexion	Flexed Hip Test
___ Positive ___ Negative	___ Specific ___ Nonanatomic	___ Positive ___ Negative	___ Positive ___ Negative	___ Positive ___ Negative	___ Positive ___ Negative	___ Positive ___ Negative

Axial Loading	Rotation of Shoulders & Pelvis
___ L.B.P. ___ Negative	___ L.B.P. ___ Negative

X-RAYS STANDING OR RECUMBENT

SPINAL MECHANICS

Spinal Tilt	Scoliosis	Sacral Angle	Facet Asymmetry	Facet Syndrome	Van Ankerveeken Stability
___ No ___ Rt ___ Lt ___ L1 ___ L2 ___ L3 ___ L4 ___ L5	___ No ___ Rt ___ Lt ___ L1 ___ L2 ___ L3 ___ L4 ___ L5 ___ Mild ___ Moderate ___ Severe	Lumbar Lordosis Angle	S Sagittal C Coronal Lt Rt L1-L2 L2-L3 L3-L4 L4-L5 L5-S1	___ Present ___ L5-S1 ___ L4-L5 ___ Not Present	___ Stable ___ Unstable

CONGENITAL ABNORMALITIES					Intercrestal Line Cuts	L5 Transverse Processes
Spina Bifida	Spondylolysis	Spondylolisthesis	Transitional Vertebra	Stenosis		
___ None ___ L1 ___ L2 ___ L3 ___ L4 ___ L5 ___ S1 ___ S2 ___ S3	___ None ___ L1 ___ L2 ___ L3 ___ L4 ___ L5 ___ S1	___ No ___ L1 ___ L3 ___ L4 ___ L5 Per Cent	Sacralization ___ Right ___ Left Lumbarization ___ Right ___ Left ___ True ___ False	Sagittal Diameter Spinal Canal L1-L2 L2-L3 L3-L4 L4-L5 L5-S1 Sagittal Diameter Vertebral Body L1-L2 L2-L3 L3-L4 L4-L5 L5-S1	___ L4 Body ___ L5 Body	___ Less ___ Greater Than L3
Other						

ACQUIRED ABNORMALITIES

Schmorl's Nodes	Narrowed Disc Space	Spondylosis	Articular Facet Arthrosis	Retrolisthesis	Other
___ No ___ L1 ___ L2 ___ L3 ___ L4 ___ L5	___ No ___ L1-L2 ___ L2-L3 ___ L3-L4 ___ L4-L5 ___ L5-S1	___ None or Slight BODY L1-L2 L2-L3 L3-L4 L4-L5 L5-S1	___ None or Slight Rt Lt ___ L1-L2 ___ L1-L2 ___ L2-L3 ___ L2-L3 ___ L3-L4 ___ L3-L4 ___ L4-L5 ___ L4-L5 ___ L5-S1 ___ L5-S1	___ None ___ L1 ___ L2 ___ L3 ___ L4 ___ L5	

Table 9.5—Continued
Low Back Pain Examination Form

Examination · Sitting / Examination · Standing

Minor's Sign	Bechterew's Sign	Valsalva	Valsalva with Bechterew's	Neri's Bow	Lewin's Standing
___ Positive ___ Negative	___ Positive ___ L.B.P. ___ L.P. ___ Negative	___ Positive ___ L.B.P. ___ L.P. ___ Negative	___ Positive ___ L.B.P. ___ L.P. ___ Negative	___ Negative ___ Positive ___ Rt. ___ Lt	___ Positive ___ L.B.P ___ S.I. ___ Negative

Examination · Standing Cont.

Gait	Spine Tilt	Pain on Palpation	Percussion	Kemp's	Motion	Toe Walk	Heel Walk
___ Normal ___ Rt Limp ___ Lt Limp ___ Other	___ None ___ Right ___ Left **Lordosis** ___ Normal ___ Loss ___ Increased	___ Negative **Paravertebral** Rt. ___ Lt ___ L1 ___ L1 ___ L2 ___ L2 ___ L3 ___ L3 ___ L4 ___ L4 ___ L5 ___ L5 ___ S1 ___ S1	___ Negative ___ L1 ___ L2 ___ L3 ___ L4 ___ L5 ___ S1	Right ___ Negative ___ Positive Left ___ Negative ___ Positive	Pain Present Flexion ___/90 ___ Extension ___/30 ___ Lateral Flexion Rt ___/20 ___ Left ___/20 ___ Rotation Rt ___/30 ___ Lt ___/30 ___	___ Positive ___ Rt ___ Lt ___ Negative	___ Positive ___ Rt ___ Lt ___ Negative

Examination · Supine

Lindner's	Straight Leg Raise			Patrick's	Gaenslen's
___ Positive ___ L.B.P. ___ L.P. ___ Negative	Right ___ Negative o ___ Positive at ___ L.B.P ___ L.P ___ Both Left ___ Negative o ___ Positive at ___ L.B.P. ___ L.P. ___ Both	**Braggard's** ___ Negative ___ Positive **Braggard's** ___ Negative ___ Positive	Well Leg Raising ___ Positive ___ Negative Medial Hip Rotation ___ L.B.P. ___ L.P. ___ Negative	Right ___ Negative ___ Positive Left ___ Negative ___ Positive	Right ___ Negative ___ Positive Left ___ Negative ___ Positive

Muscle Strength

Cox's Sign	Amoss'		Dorsi-Flexion		Plantar-Flexion		Great Toe Flexion		Great Toe Extension		Foot Eversion	
			Rt.	Lt.	Rt.	Lt.	Rt.	Lt.	Rt.	Lt.	Rt.	Lt.
___ Positive ___ Negative	___ Positive ___ Negative	Normal										
		Weakness										

Thigh & Calf / Milgram's / Tendon Reflexes / Sensory Examination

Thigh & Calf Circumference	Milgram's	Tendon Reflexes			Sensory Examination	
					Hyperesthesia	Hypoesthesia
Rt Thigh _____ Lt Thigh _____ Rt Calf _____ Lt Calf _____	Positive ___ Rt ___ Lt Negative	0 Active & Equal 1 Increased 2 Decreased 3 Absent 4 Unknown	Ankle Rt. ___ Lt.	Knee Rt. ___ Lt.	Rt ___ Lt ___ None ___ None Dermatome ___ L3 ___ L3 ___ L4 ___ L4 ___ L5 ___ L5 ___ S1 ___ S1 ___ S2 ___ S2 ___ Other ___ Other	Rt. ___ Lt. ___ None ___ None Dermatome ___ L3 ___ L3 ___ L4 ___ L4 ___ L5 ___ L5 ___ S1 ___ S1 ___ S2 ___ S2 ___ Other ___ Other

Circulation

Circulation	Normal	Diminished	Moses'
Femoral Artery			Positive
Popliteal Artery			Rt.
Post. Tibial Artery			Lt.
Dorsalis Pedis Artery			Negative

Table 9.5—*Continued*
Low Back Pain Examination Form

FLOW CHART FOR CORRELATIVE DIAGNOSIS
LOW BACK AND/OR LEG PAIN (BELOW KNEE DIAGNOSIS)

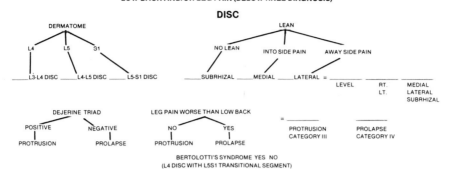

DISC

DERMATOME

L4   L5   S1

____ L3-L4 DISC   ____ L4-L5 DISC   ____ L5-S1 DISC

LEAN

NO LEAN   INTO SIDE PAIN   AWAY SIDE PAIN

____ SUBRHIZAL   ____ MEDIAL   ____ LATERAL = ____ ____ ____

LEVEL   RT.   MEDIAL
LT.   LATERAL
SUBRHIZAL

DEJERINE TRIAD

POSITIVE   NEGATIVE
| |
PROTRUSION   PROLAPSE

LEG PAIN WORSE THAN LOW BACK

NO   YES
| |
PROTRUSION   PROLAPSE

= ____

PROTRUSION   PROLAPSE
CATEGORY III   CATEGORY IV

BERTOLOTTI'S SYNDROME YES NO
(L4 DISC WITH L5S1 TRANSITIONAL SEGMENT)

LOW BACK PAIN (NO LEG PAIN BELOW KNEE) DIAGNOSIS

CATEGORY I
ANNULAR TEAR
-Low Back Pain

Clinical Judgement - No hard objective findings - rotation and flexion injury.

CATEGORY II
Nuclear Bulge
-Low Back Pain
-Buttock Pain into thigh to knee

CATEGORY V
Discogenic Spondyloarthrosis
____ L1-L2
____ L2-L3
____ L3-L4
____ L4-L5
____ L5-S1

CATEGORY VI
Facet Syndrome

Stable (◄ 3MM)	Unstable (► 3MM)
____ L1-L2	____ L1-L2
____ L2-L3	____ L2-L3
____ L3-L4	____ L3-L4
____ L4-L5	____ L4-L5
____ L5-S1	____ L5-S1

CATEGORY VII
Spondylolisthesis

True	False
(Pars Defect)	(Degenerative)

L1 ____ L2 ____ L3 ____ L4 ____ L5 ____
% ____

CATEGORY VIII
Stenosis
(Eisenstein ◄ 12MM or Body Canal Ratio ► 4:1)

____ L1 ____ L2 ____ L3 ____ L4
____ L5
Pedicogenic (◄ 12MM)
Acquired (Degenerative Facets)

CATEGORY IX
F.B.S.S.
(Failed Back Surgical Syndrome) **Level**

Fusion ____
Microsurgery ____
Laminectomy ____
Chemonucleolysis ____
Epidural Steroid ____
Rhizotomy ____

CATEGORY XI
Sprain ____
Strain ____
____ L1-L2
____ L2-L3
____ L3-L4
____ L4-L5
____ L5-S1

CATEGORY XII - SUBLUXATION
Sacroiliac

RT ____	L1	Retrolisthesis
LT ____	L2	Anterolisthesis
POST ____	L3	Right Lateral Flexion
ANT ____	L4	Left Lateral Flexion
Short Legs	L5	Right Rotation
RT ____		Left Rotation
LT ____		Hyperflexion
		Hyperextension

CATEGORY XIII
Tropism

CATEGORY XIII
L1-L2 ____
L2-L3 ____
L3-L4 ____
L4-L5 ____
L5 S1 ____

CATEGORY XIV
Transitional Segment Yes ____
No ____

RT ____ L5 ____ True ____
LT ____ L6 ____ False ____
Sacralization ____
Lumbarization ____

CATEGORY XV
Scoliosis and other Pathologies

Levo   Dextro

Thoracic L1 L2 L3 L4 L5
Sacrum

CORRELATIVE DIAGNOSIS OF LOW BACK PAIN AND LEG PAIN

RT	L3-L4	Lateral	Discal Protrusion	**WITH**
LT	L4-L5	Medial	Discal Prolapse	
	L5-S1	Subrhizal		
		Central		

CORRELATIVE DIAGNOSIS OF LOW BACK PAIN

		L1 L2	L2 L3	L3 L4	L4 L5	L5 S1
CATEGORY V	Discogenic Spondyloarthrosis					
CATEGORY VI	Stable or Unstable Facet Syndrome					
CATEGORY VII	Spondylolisthesis (True or False)					
CATEGORY VIII	Stenosis (Pedicogenic or Degenerative)					
CATEGORY IX	Post Surgical Spine					
CATEGORY XI	Sprain or Strain					
CATEGORY XII	Subluxation					
CATEGORY XIII	Tropism					
CATEGORY XIV	Transitional Segment					
CATEGORY XIV	Scoliosis					
	or Other Pathology					

Physical Examination

As you proceed through the examination, mark the proper answer on the examination form and keep in mind the findings indicative of intervertebral disc protrusion (contained disc) and prolapse (noncontained disc) as shown in Table 9.6.

EXAMINATION WITH THE PATIENT SITTING

Minor's Sign (Fig. 9.50). Minor's sign is manifest when the patient, in rising from sitting, lifts his body weight with his arms and places his body weight on the unaffected leg. He may place his hand on his low back. The painful lower extremity is spared of weight bearing.

Bechterew's Sign (Fig. 9.51). The test for Bechterew's sign is performed by having the patient extend the knee while in a sitting position. This sitting straight leg raise again stretches the sciatica nerve root and creates either back or leg pain or both if there is a disc lesion.

The straight leg raising sign is a more positive sign of disc lesion in younger people; i.e., under age 40, than it is in older people. This is because,

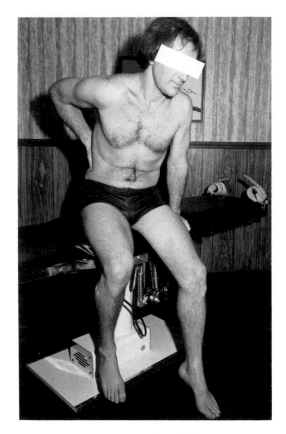

Figure 9.50. Minor's sign.

Table 9.6.
Criteria for Diagnosis of Sciatica Due to a Herniated Intervertebral Disc[a]

1. Leg pain is the dominant symptom when compared with back pain. It affects one leg only and follows a typical sciatic (or femoral) nerve distribution.
2. Paresthesiae are localized to a dermatomal distribution.
3. Straight leg raising is reduced by 50% of normal, and/or pain crosses over to the symptomatic leg when the unaffected leg is elevated, and/or pain radiates proximally or distally with digital pressure on the tibial nerve in the popliteal fossa.
4. Two of four neurologic signs (wasting, motor weakness, diminished sensory appreciation, and diminution of reflex activity) are present.
5. A contrast study is positive and corresponds to the clinical level.

[a]Based on McCullough JA: Chemonucleolysis. *J Bone Joint Surg* 159B: 45–52; 1977.

as the intradiscal pressure decreases with age, the turgor of the nucleus becomes less, and the nucleus is less likely to compress severely against the nerve root during such maneuvers as straight leg raising, Valsalva, or Bechterew's.

The sitting straight leg raising sign often is positive, whereas the supine recumbent straight leg raising sign is negative. This author feels that the reason for this difference is that the higher intradiscal pressure with the patient sitting adds to the nerve root compression; this, when coupled with the stretching of the nerve root during leg raising, creates a much more positive sign of nerve root compression. Remember that Fisk (48) states that the hip joint acts as a pulley and tractions the sciatic nerve going from 15° to 30°

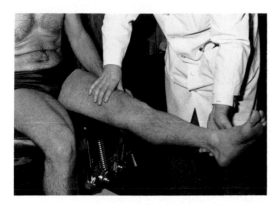

Figure 9.51. Bechterew's sign.

literates the disc bulge and, assuming that motion of an irritated nerve root over a bulging disc is often the source of the patient's back and leg pain, thus could be the explanation for relief of pain with flexion treatment. He demonstrated that both the Valsalva maneuver and abdominal compression obliterate the myelographic defect. Again, if it is assumed that motion of an irritated nerve root over a disc bulge is one of the causes of pain, the findings here could explain how abdominal compression or Valsalva maneuver done abruptly increases the patient's pain as the defect appears and disappears and thereby moves the nerve root over the disc.

Bechterew's Test, Lindner's Sign, and Valsalva Maneuver (Fig. 9.53). If Bechterew's test is added to the Valsalva maneuver, further stretching the nerve roots behind the intervertebral disc space, this increased stretching accentuates the patient's pain in nuclear escape. The combination of the Valsalva maneuver, Bechterew's test, and Lindner's sign indicates the presence of a disc lesion. One test alone might not be positive.

of leg raising. Between L4 and L5, the L5 nerve root normally moves 2.5 cm during the full range of straight leg raising.

Always perform the straight leg raising test, whether sitting or recumbent, slowly, as it can create much pain in the low back or lower extremity for the patient and negatively affect the results of other testing.

Valsalva Maneuver and Lindner's Sign (Fig. 9.52). For the Valsalva maneuver, the patient attempts to expel air against a closed glottis. This movement can be described to the patient as straining to move the bowel. During this maneuver, the intradiscal pressure increases, and the increased force against the anterior dura lining of the nerve root accentuates the patient's back and/or leg pain. Note also that the patient is asked to flex the head upon the chest, which increases the traction of the nerve root against the disc bulge (Lindner's sign).

Raney (49) has stated that with a contained disc, i.e., the posterior annulus is not ruptured, flexion or maintenance of the flexed position ob-

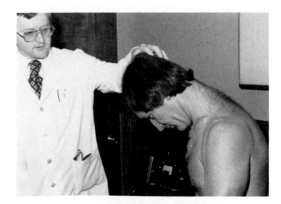

Figure 9.52. Valsalva maneuver and Lindner's sign.

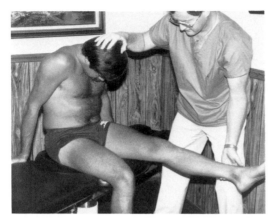

Figure 9.53. Bechterew's test, Lindner's sign, and the Valsalva maneuver.

EXAMINATION WITH THE PATIENT STANDING

Néri's Bowing Sign (Fig. 9.54). With Néri's sign, as the patient bows forward, the affected leg flexes, as in a curtsey, as the sciatic nerve is irritated. Flexion of the knee removes the tractive irritation from the inflamed sciatic nerve.

Lewin's Standing Sign (Fig. 9.55). Lewin's standing sign is manifested with the patient's knees placed in extension. Increased pain in the low back or leg can cause the knee to snap back into flexion. If this is observed, a disc, gluteal, or sacroiliac disturbance is indicated.

Gait (Fig. 9.56). Note whether the patient limps while walking and the extremity affected.

Patient Lean (Fig. 9.57). Note whether the patient leans to the right or the left. Later, correlation of this antalgia with the side of pain will aid in determining whether the nuclear bulge is medial, lateral, or subrhizal.

In detailing the meaning of the sciatic scoliotic

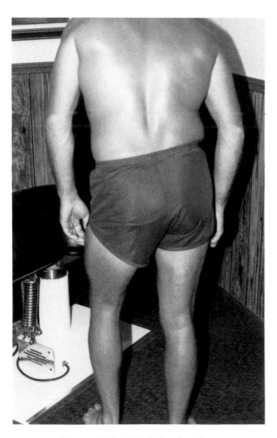

Figure 9.54. Néri's bowing sign.

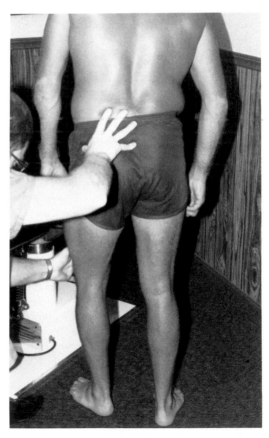

Figure 9.55. Lewin's sign.

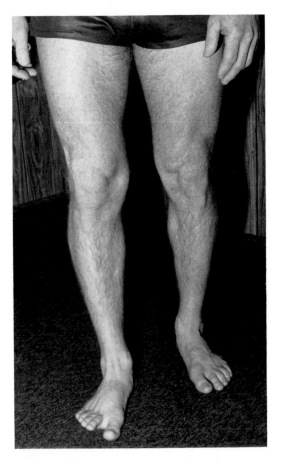

Figure 9.56. Gait.

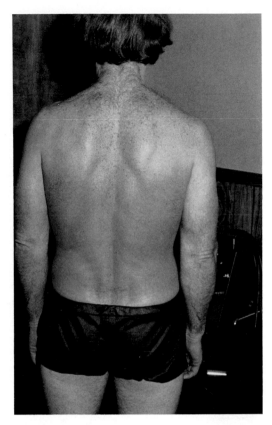

Figure 9.57. Lean of patient.

antalgic lean of a patient, that is, whether the patient leans away from the side of pain for a lateral disc lesion or into the side of pain for a medial one, please remember two important references. First, Lindblom (50) enhanced our thinking on the importance of the lateral bending significance of disc protrusion by his finding that, in rat tails tied into "U" shapes, degeneration and rupture occurred on the concave side of the spine while the convex side remained normal. Second, Porter and Miller (51) stated that 20 patients they studied did not indicate the side of the list to be related to the side of the sciatica or to the topographic position of the disc in relation to the nerve root. It is, therefore, up to the clinician to carefully integrate lateral flexion lists with other findings to arrive at the correct clinical impression.

Lumbar Lordosis (Fig. 9.58). Note whether the patient while standing reveals increased, decreased, or normal lumbar lordosis. The typical disc patient will have a loss of lumbar lordosis because this posture opens the dorsal intervertebral disc space, thus relieving the pressure of nuclear bulge on the involved nerve root and/or cauda equina.

Pain on Palpation (Fig. 9.59). Note the levels of pain that the patient experiences upon deep digital pressure. Sometimes, not only the back pain but also a radiating sciatic discomfort can be elicited.

Percussion (Fig. 9.60). Tapping over the involved paraspinal and spinous process levels creates pain if there are inflammatory changes around the involved nerve roots.

Kemp's Sign (Fig. 9.61). The test for Kemp's sign can be performed with the patient in either the standing or the sitting position. Sitting increases intradiscal pressure and, therefore, maximizes stress to the disc, whereas standing increases weight bearing and maximizes stress to the facets. The test for Kemp's sign should be per-

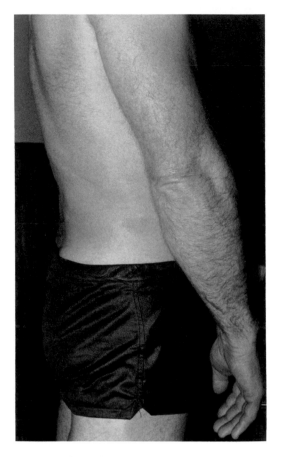

Figure 9.58. Lumbar lordosis.

formed in both positions. Kemp's sign can be positive for facet irritation or compression of a bulging nucleus against a nerve root. If both are

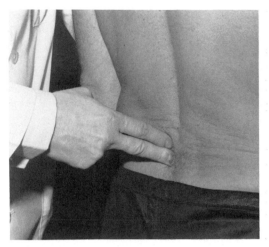

Figure 9.59. Pain on palpation.

present, low back pain is elicited. With a disc bulge, accentuation of the lower extremity radiculopathy is increased. Some patients with disc lesion experience only back pain with Kemp's sign. With a medial disc, Kemp's sign is usually positive when the patient is flexed either to the right or to

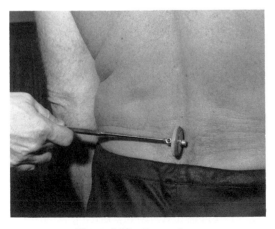

Figure 9.60. Percussion.

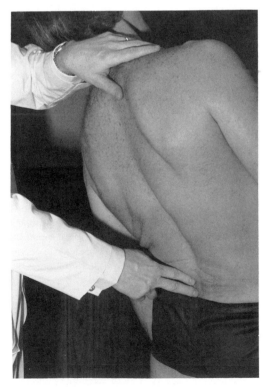

Figure 9.61. Kemp's sign.

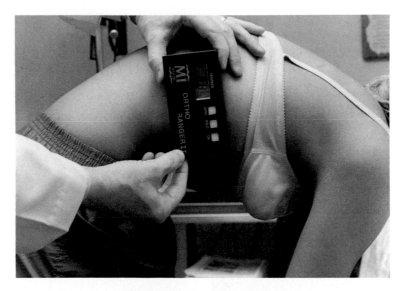

Figure 9.62. Flexion measured.

the left in extension. Pain occurs because a medial disc can irritate a nerve root regardless of the direction in which the patient is posteriorly and laterally flexed. It is to be expected that, in medial disc protrusion, the patient will experience greater pain when flexed away from the side of pain or disc lesion, whereas in lateral disc protrusion, the patient will experience greater pain when flexed into the side of low back and lower extremity pain.

Goniometric Measurements (Figs. 9.62 to 9.65). Goniometric measurements should be taken with the patient in flexion, extension, lateral bending, and rotation of the lumbar spine. These measurements provide a record of the ranges of motion for comparison with future measurements and for verification of patient response or failure to treatment.

Digital computerized goniometers have shown greater accuracy than older-style, hand-held metal or plastic goniometers. The goniometer shown in Figures 9.62 through 9.64 is made by Medical Instruments Technology, Daytona Beach, Florida, and serves this author in clinical practice. The accuracy of goniometric measurement is critical, since range of motion status, coupled with improvement of the straight leg raising sign, are the two tests used to determine the progress of a patient under care. Specifically, in our clinical practice, we feel that a patient must show at least 50% improvement within 3 to 4 weeks of conservative manipulative care or we change our

treatment protocol and perform more diagnostic tests and entertain surgical consultation. Million

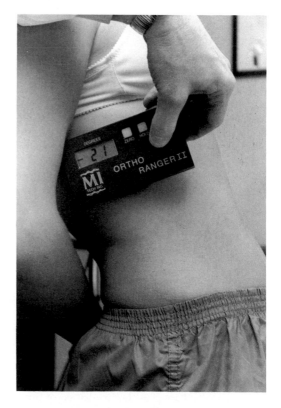

Figure 9.63. Extension measured.

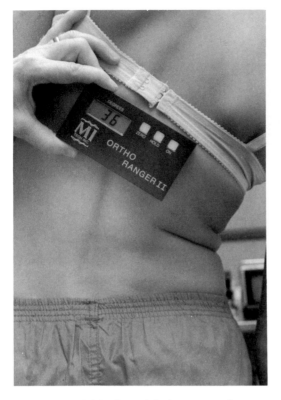

Figure 9.64. Lateral flexion measured.

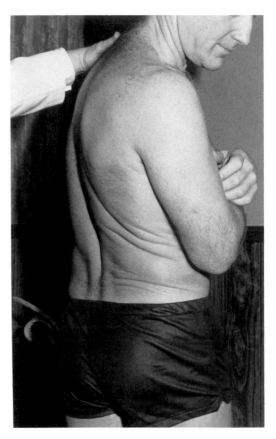

Figure 9.65. Rotation measured.

and Hall et al. (52) found objective assessments of spinal motion and straight leg raising to show a high degree of intraobserver reproducibility, thereby emphasizing their importance in evaluating the progress of the low back pain patient.

Toe Walk (Fig. 9.66). The inability to walk on the toes indicates an L5-S1 disc problem due to weakness of the calf muscles supplied by the tibial nerve

Heel Walk (Fig. 9.67). The inability to walk on the heels indicates an L4-L5 disc problem due to weakness of the anterior leg muscles supplied by the common peroneal nerve.

EXAMINATION WITH THE PATIENT IN THE SUPINE POSITION

Some of these tests may be done with the patient in the prone position, depending on which position is more comfortable for the doctor and/or patient.

Lindner's Sign (Fig. 9.68). The test for Lindner's sign (also known as the Brudzinski or Soto-Hall sign) is often performed in conjunction with the straight leg raising test or the Valsalva maneuver for maximum effect. Lindner's sign refers to stretching of the dural linings of the nerve roots

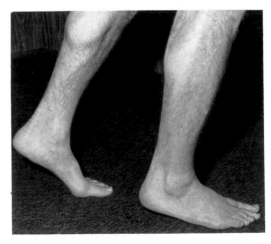

Figure 9.66. Toe walk.

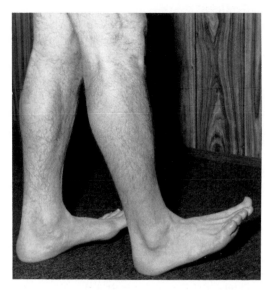

Figure 9.67. Heel walk.

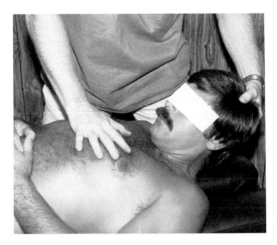

Figure 9.68. Lindner's sign.

behind the bulging disc material, which causes pain when performed.

Straight Leg Raising Sign (Figs. 9.69A and B, and 9.70). During straight leg raising (SLR), the lumbosacral nerve roots move through their intervertebral foramina up to several millimeters, depending upon the author quoted (53). Fisk states that the nerve roots move 2.5 cm (48). There is a great deal of traction of the sciatic nerve at the sacral ala and the sciatic notch, with movement first seen at the sciatic notch and later

at the roots. If the patient feels pain soon after initiating the straight leg raising maneuver, it can indicate either a large disc protrusion or sensitivity of the nerve at the sacral ala or sciatic notch. Movement of the sciatic nerve diminishes with age and proximity to the spinal cord.

Laségue (54) described the painful effect in patients with sciatica of stretching the sciatic nerve by extending the knee with the hip flexed; he also described the relief from pain when the knee was then flexed. This is the classic leg raising sign. Variations of this sign, along with interpretations of its meaning, lend much more knowledge to the examining physician than merely noting that at a certain degree of leg raise the pa-

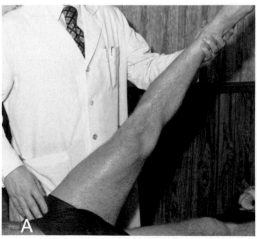

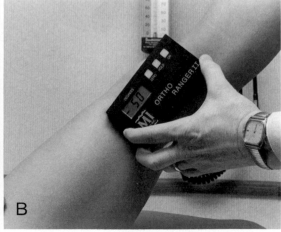

Figure 9.69. **A,** Straight leg raising and medial hip rotation performed simultaneously. **B,** Goniometer measurement of angle at which SLR is positive.

tient experiences either back or leg pain or both back and leg pain. On the examination form, record whether the leg raising sign is positive and, if so, at what degree of elevation (Fig. 9.69**B**).

Breig and Troup (55) add a degree of sophistication to this test. After noting the level of pain on straight leg raising, lower the extremity a few degrees to relieve the pain and then dorsiflex the ankle while medially rotating the hip. Medial hip rotation places greater stretch upon the lumbar and sacral nerve roots and accentuates the straight leg raising sign. These authors state that if the pain which limits straight leg raising is elicited by such dorsiflexion and medial hip rotation, increased root tension is indicated and the site of pain may help in locating the level of the disc causing the pain. Figure 9.69**A** shows medial hip rotation and Figure 9.70**B** shows dorsiflexion of the foot (Braggard's sign). Figure 9.69**B** shows goniometric measurement of SLR.

By stretching the lumbosacral nerve roots, the straight leg raising sign proves that the first sacral nerve root allows the greatest movement.

In theory, the straight leg raise (SLR) should identify not only the presence of increased root tension but also, possibly, the site of such irritation. The production of pain on passive dorsiflexion of the ankle near the limit of the pain-free range of straight leg raising confirms that the root is mechanically compromised. Pain on pressure in the popliteal fossa after flexion of the knee at the limit of straight leg raising has a similar significance, and when the well leg raising test is positive, this pain is a strong confirmation of root involvement.

The angulatory stress exerted on the lumbar nerve roots during straight leg raising was measured on cadavers within 4 hours of death (56). A short length of rubber tube was inserted between the disc and nerve root and the tension was monitored by use of semiconductor pressure transducers. Results of this testing were:

1. With the straight leg raising sign, the pressure between the nerve root and the disc does not change until the leg is raised to about 30°, with a progressive rise occurring as the angle of the leg increases.

The pressure increase is highest at the L5-S1 disc level and half as high at the L4-L5 level. The pressure increase on SLR at L3-L4 was $^{1}/_{10}$ of that at L5-S1.

It can be concluded that: (*a*) SLR that is positive under 30° reveals a large disc protrusion. The nerve root is stretched here long before it normally would be. (*b*) SLR is most useful for identifying L5-S1 disc lesions, since the pressures are highest at this level. On SLR, L4-L5 is not as apt to give as much pain as is L5-S1, since the pressure between the disc and the nerve root is half that at L5-S1. Therefore, the L5-S1 disc lesion gives more pain in the low back and leg than does the L4-L5 disc lesion. (*c*) No movement on the nerve root occurs until SLR reaches 30°. (*d*) No movement of the L4 nerve root occurs during SLR (57).

2. Adduction of the hip on SLR increases the pressure on the nerve roots.

3. O'Connell (58) reported that the second, third, and fourth lumbar nerve roots did not show an increase in tension during SLR but did show an increase during the femoral stretch test.

Straight Leg Raising and Lindner's Signs (Fig. 9.71). Whenever the straight leg raising test produces a questionable result for pain, combine it with flexion of the cervical spine (Lindner's sign). This combination places the greatest pull and stretch on the nerve roots behind the intervertebral disc and often elicits pain. Along with this combination, dorsiflex the foot, have the patient cough, or perform the Valsalva maneuver. These maneuvers further accentuate intradiscal pressure and elicit pain that otherwise might be missed.

Swan and Zervas (59) found that simultaneous flexion of the neck and elevation of the contralateral leg produced pain in the ipsilateral (presenting) sciatic notch in five patients with either free fragments or herniated disc found at operation. Raising the contralateral leg alone elicited no pain in either leg.

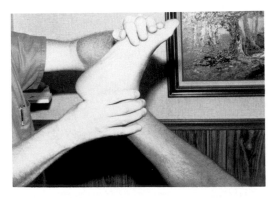

Figure 9.70.   Braggard's maneuver performed.

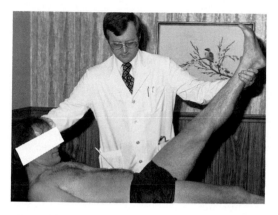

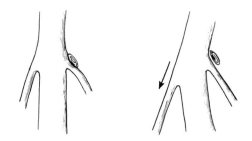

Figure 9.72. Interpretation of the well leg raising sign in lateral disc bulge.

Figure 9.71. Tests for straight leg raising and Lindner's signs, performed together.

Adduction and internal rotation of the leg while SLR is performed brings out the pain response more readily; this is called Bonet's phenomenon. Also performing dorsiflexion of the foot during SLR is called Braggard's sign; and extension of he great toe during SLR to accentuate the nerve root stretch is called Sicard's sign.

Well Leg Raising (Fajersztajn) Sign (Figs. 9.72 and 9.73). The well leg raising sign (Fajersztajn sign) is exacerbation of pain down the involved or painful lower extremity when the opposite or noninvolved extremity is placed in straight leg raise. Hudgins (60) states that increased sciatica on raising the opposite or well leg, the cross straight leg raising sign, is associated with a herniated lumbar disc in 97% of patients. Myelography is unnecessary for the diagnosis of disc hernia in patients with this sign. Although it is possible for patients with this sign to have a normal myelogram, nevertheless, 90% prove to have a herniated disc.

When the disc protrusion is displaced lateral to the nerve root (Fig. 9.72), raising the uninvolved leg actually pulls the nerve root away from the disc and can relieve back or leg pain.

When the disc protrusion is displaced medial to the nerve root (Fig. 9.73), raising the uninvolved leg pulls the nerve root into the disc bulge and causes radiculopathy down the involved leg.

Interpretation of the Straight Leg Raising Sign. In a study of 50 patients in a 2-year period, Edgar and Park (61) found that the pattern of pain on straight leg raising was closely related to the central or lateral position of the disc protrusion. In addition to its use in the diagnosis and assessment of progress, the straight leg raising sign may be helpful in localizing the protrusion by analysis of the distribution of the pain so induced. Clinically, myelographic and operative observations were carried out prospectively on 50 such patients to investigate the relation between

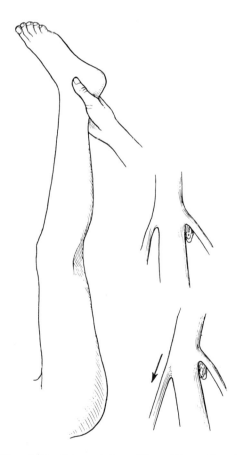

Figure 9.73. Interpretation of the well leg raising sign in medial disc bulge.

the pattern of pain in straight leg raising and the site of the protrusion. In 80% of the patients, the following correlation was found:

Location of Protrusion	Back Pain	Leg Pain
Lateral protrusion		+
Medial protrusion	+	
Intermediate protrusion (subrhizal)	+	+

Therefore, a lateral protrusion causes a patient to experience leg pain; a medial protrusion, back pain; and a subrhizal protrusion, both back and leg pain.

The straight leg raising sign can provide a wealth of information: the level of pain can indicate the disc at fault, the presence of back pain, leg pain, or both can indicate the type of protrusion, and various combinations of Valsalva, cervical flexion, dorsiflexion of the foot, and medial hip rotation can aid significantly in diagnosis.

Macnab (62) demonstrates the bowstring sign as being the most reliable test of root tension in sciatica due to intervertebral disc lesion (Fig. 9.74).

Shiqing et al. (63) reported in 1987 from a study of 113 patients that the distribution of pain on SLR allowed an accurate prediction of the location of the lesion in 100 (88.5%) of the cases. Central protrusions caused back pain, lateral pro-

trusions caused lower extremity pain, and intermediate protrusions caused both.

Validity and Importance of SLR in Objective Evaluation. Lastly, concerning the SLR, remember its importance in the diagnosis and evaluation of progress of the patient under treatment for sciatica due to disc lesion. High degrees of reproducibility of interexaminer objective assessment were found for SLR (52). SLR has been found to be the most reliable and strongly recommended objective test in evaluating spinal manipulative response for low back pain (64).

Miller et al. (65) evaluated tests including gait, toe and heel walk, plantar flexion, cervical flexion, patellar and Achilles reflexes, SLR, and sensibility to pinprick and light touch, and found that the SLR had the best intra- and interexaminer reliability. Figure 9.69**B** shows measurement of SLR with the digital goniometer for accuracy of recording.

Patrick's Sign (Fig. 9.75). Patrick's sign refers to pain in the groin and hip area, which is common with disc lesion because of the irritation of nerve supply to these structures. Evaluation of the hip by x-ray will rule out any hip disease.

Gaenslen's Sign (Fig. 9.76). The test for Gaenslen's sign is performed by flexion of one knee upon the chest, while the other is placed in extension over the side of the table. This is a differential sign between sacroiliac and lumbar spine pain. When the test is performed, the pain will appear at the location of the lesion, whether it be in the sacroiliac or lumbar spine.

Cox's Sign (Fig. 9.77). Cox's sign occurs when, during SLR, the pelvis rises from the table rather than the hip flexing. The author has noticed this

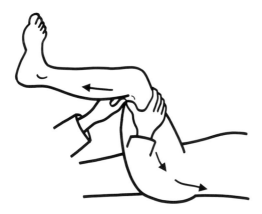

Figure 9.74. When eliciting the bowstring sign, the patient's foot should be allowed to rest on the examiner's shoulder with the knee very slightly flexed at the limit of straight leg raising. Sudden firm pressure is then applied by the examiner's thumbs in the popliteal fossa. Radiation of pain down the leg or the production of pain in the back is pathognomonic of root tension. (Reprinted with permission from Macnab I: *Backache.* Baltimore, Williams & Wilkins, 1977.)

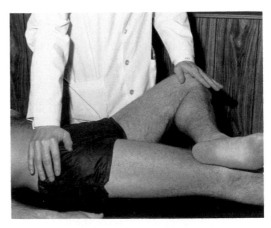

Figure 9.75. Patrick's sign.

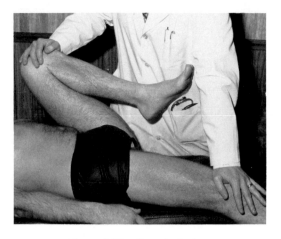

Figure 9.76. Gaenslen's sign.

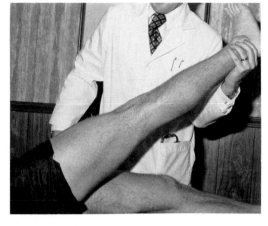

Figure 9.77. Cox's sign.

occurrence in patients with prolapse into the intervertebral foramen—a grave condition.

Amoss' Sign (Fig. 9.78). Amoss' sign is manifested by difficulty in rising from the supine position. The patient must use his arms to lift himself and prevent flexion or motion of the lumbar spine.

Dorsiflexion of the Foot (Ankle Extension) (Fig. 9.79). The sciatic nerve is made up of tibial and common peroneal nerves. The common peroneal nerve divides into the superficial and the deep peroneal branch. Dorsiflexion as shown in Figure 9.79 depends upon nerve supply via the deep branch of the peroneal nerve to the anterior tibialis muscle, the extensor hallucis longus muscle to the great toe, and the extensor digitorum longus muscle to the toes. The superficial peroneal nerve supplies the peroneal muscles that allow the foot to flex laterally at the ankle as well as flex upward (dorsiflexion). Weakness of dorsiflexion

of the foot at the ankle is indicative of fifth lumbar nerve root compression by an L4-L5 disc level lesion.

The inability of the patient to walk on his heels is also indictive of the same finding, but testing the patient's strengths as shown in Figure 9.79 is a much more intricate evaluation. The patient may be able to walk on his heels, yet demonstrate weakness of the muscle on dorsiflexion.

Dorsiflexion of the Great Toe (Fig. 9.80). Dorsiflexion strength of the great toe is determined by testing the strength of the extensor hallucis longus muscle. Weakness of dorsiflexion of the great toe is indicative of L5 nerve root irritation by an L4-L5 disc lesion.

Goodall and Hammes (66) have developed a prototype toe-strength meter to establish differ-

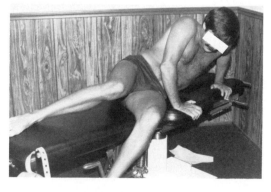

Figure 9.78. Amoss' sign.

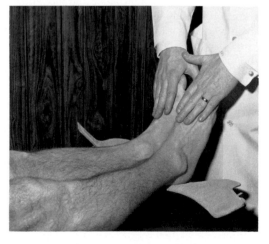

Figure 9.79. Dorsiflexion of the ankle.

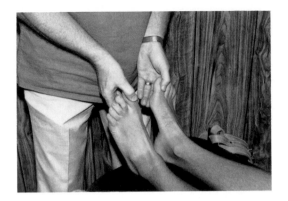

Figure 9.80. Dorsiflexion of the great toe.

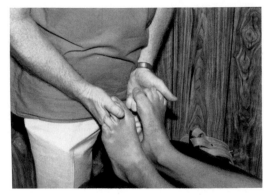

Figure 9.81. Plantar flexion of the ankle.

ences in dorsiflexion strength of the great toes so as to detect early L5 nerve root lesions. The tester is accurate within 2%.

Plantar Flexion or Ankle Flexion of the Foot (Fig. 9.81). The tibial branch of the sciatic nerve supplies the posterior tibialis, gastrocsoleus, flexor digitorum longus, and hallucis longus muscles. Weakness of plantar flexion of the foot is indicative of compression of the first sacral nerve root by an L5-S1 disc lesion.

A variation of this test is to ask the patient to walk on his toes. The inability to do so indicates the same finding as that of the plantar flexion sign. As in testing in dorsiflexion, testing the strength of one foot against the other is a much more reliable sign, since a patient may be able to walk on his toes and still have a weakness of calf muscles on one side.

Peroneal Muscle Testing. The peroneal muscles are the evertors of the ankle and foot and receive supply from the first sacral nerve root. Test them by asking the patient to walk on the medial borders of his feet; or have him sit on the edge of the table and, as the patient attempts to pull his foot into eversion and dorsiflexion, oppose this by pushing against the head and shaft of the fifth metatarsal bone with the palm of your hand.

Plantar Flexion of the Great Toe (Fig. 9.82). The flexor hallucis longus tendon is tested for strength in plantar flexion of the great toe. Weakness here is indicative of a first sacral nerve root compression by an L5-S1 disc lesion.

Thigh Measurements (Fig. 9.83). Both thighs are measured at the same distance above the superior patellar pole. Differing sizes indicate atrophy.

Calf Measurement (Fig. 9.84). Both calves are

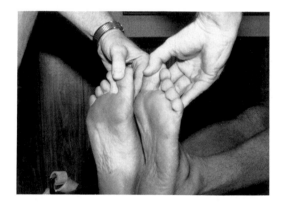

Figure 9.82. Plantar flexion of the great toe.

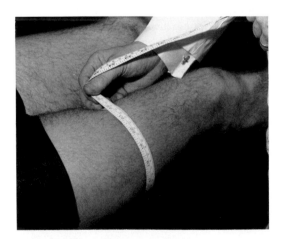

Figure 9.83. Thigh measurement for atrophy.

measured at the same distance below the inferior patellar pole. Differing sizes indicate atrophy.

Milgram's Sign (Fig. 9.85). The inability to hold the feet 6 inches off the floor while in the supine position indicates extreme nerve root irritation and is believed to be a sign of arachnoiditis due to Pantopaque dye as well as disc lesion.

Ankle Jerk Reflex (Fig. 9.86). The deep reflex of the ankle known as the Achilles reflex is diminished or absent in the presence of an L5-S1 disc irritation of the first sacral nerve root and, therefore, is of extreme importance for evaluating lower disc involvement. Note that the patient's foot is held in dorsiflexion while the ankle jerk reflex is elicited. Thus, not only the reflex but also the strength of the muscular contraction of the calf muscles is observed. This test can be performed with the patient prone or supine.

Patellar Reflex (Knee Jerk) (Fig. 9.87). The patellar reflex sign indicates involvement of the L3 disc, which would effect the fourth lumbar dermatomes. Since discs other than the L4 or L5 discs are seldom involved, this is relatively useless in evaluating disc lesions in the lower extremity.

Pinwheel Examination (Figs. 9.88 to 9.91). Pinwheel examination of the lower extremities is shown in Figures 9.88 to 9.91. The weight of the pinwheel is the only downward force applied so as to equalize the pressure of each leg. The same dermatome of each leg is stimulated, and the patient is asked which feels less sharp. Figure 9.88 shows testing of the fifth lumbar dermatome above the knee. Figure 9.89 shows testing of the L5 dermatome below the knee. Figure 9.90 shows testing of the dermatomes at the first sacral level of the thigh. Figure 9.91 shows testing of the dermatomes at the first sacral level below the knee. The first sacral dermatome is tested with the patient prone.

Vibratory Sense. Vibratory sense can be tested, but realize that older persons, as over age 50, have a naturally decreased vibratory and temperature perception.

Tensor Fascia Femoris Response. Macnab (62) discusses the reflex contraction of the tensor fascia femoris to plantar reflex and the loss of this response in S1 nerve root lesions.

Hamstring Muscle Reflex (Figs. 9.92 and 9.93). Loss of the hamstring reflex occurs in compression of the L5 nerve root by an L4-L5 disc protrusion.

Measurement of Lower Limb Circulation

Femoral Artery (Fig. 9.94). Draw a line between the anterior superior iliac spine (ASIS) and

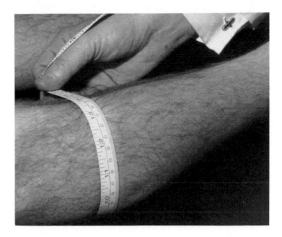

Figure 9.84. Calf measurement for atrophy.

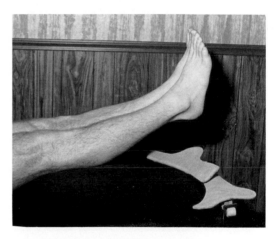

Figure 9.85. Milgram's sign.

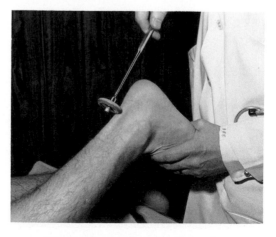

Figure 9.86. Ankle jerk reflex testing.

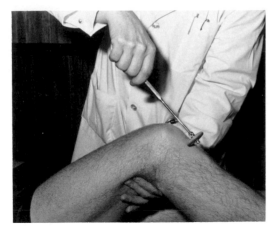

Figure 9.87. Patellar reflex (knee jerk) testing.

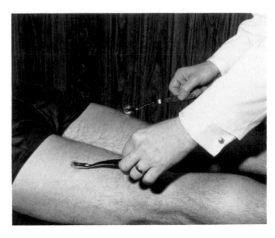

Figure 9.90. S1 dermatome.

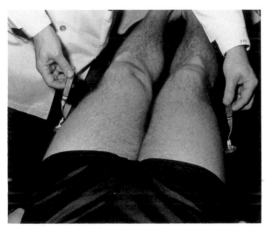

Figure 9.88. L5 dermatome.

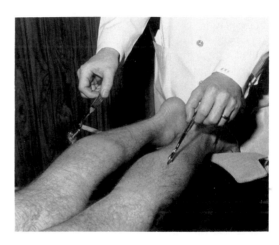

Figure 9.91. S1 dermatome.

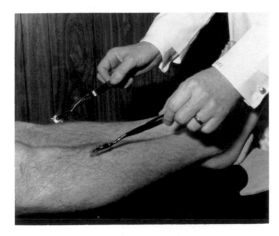

Figure 9.89. L5 dermatome.

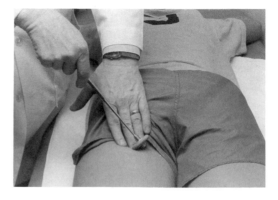

Figure 9.92. Tapping the origin of the inner hamstring muscles (semitendinosus and semimembranosus) at the ischial tuberosity to elicit the hamstring reflex.

the symphysis pubes and midway between these points, drop down 1 inch and that will be the femoral artery. Palpate the pulse and compare right to left for strength of pulse.

Popliteal Artery (Fig. 9.95). By Doppler or palpation determine the patency of the popliteal artery.

Posterior Tibialis Artery (Fig. 9.96). By Doppler or palpation compare the two pulses of the posterior tibialis arteries.

Dorsalis Pedis Artery (Fig. 9.97). By Doppler or palpation compare the pulse of the dorsalis pedis artery and its strength in the two extremities. This artery is located between the first and second metatarsal bones on the dorsum of the foot.

These pulses are important in differentiating intermittent claudication of ischemic etiology from that of neurogenic etiology. When these pulses are present and the patient has the cramplike pains of claudication, the origin of pain is not vascular but neural. Look for discal lesions, ligamentous hypertrophy, stenosis, or peripheral neuropathy.

Moses' Sign (Fig. 9.98). The test for Moses' sign is performed by grasping the calf of the patient's leg, which creates pain if phlebitis or vascular occlusion is present.

EXAMINATION WITH THE PATIENT IN THE PRONE POSITION

Nachlas' Knee Flexion Sign (Fig. 9.99). On passive flexion of the knee, the patient lying in the prone position will experience pain in the low back or lower extremity. This sign is positive for sacroiliac, lumbosacral, and disc lesions.

Yeoman's Sign (Fig. 9.100). The test for Yeoman's sign is performed by applying pressure over the suspected sacroiliac joint to fix the pelvis to the table. The patient's leg, flexed at the knee, is hyperextended by lifting the thigh from the table. Increased pain in the sacroiliac is indicative of a lesion at that level.

Ely's Heel-to-Buttock Sign (Fig. 9.101). The test for Ely's sign is performed by bringing the patient's heel to the opposite buttock by flexing the knee. Ely's sign identifies any irritation of the psoas muscle or a lumbosacral lesion.

Ely's sign also demonstrates contracture or shortening of the rectus femoris muscle. If contracture is present, the hip will flex and the buttock will rise from the table.

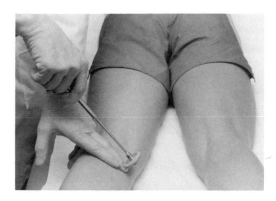

Figure 9.93. Tapping the insertion of the inner hamstring muscles of the semimembranosus and semitendinosus tendons at the medial condyle and proximal portions of the tibia to elicit the hamstring reflex.

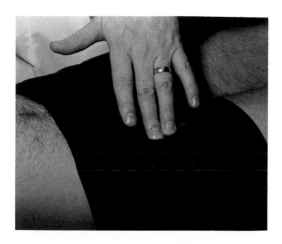

Figure 9.94. Femoral artery.

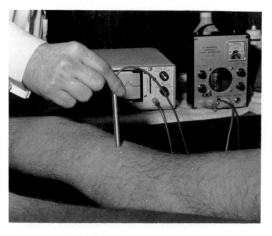

Figure 9.95. Popliteal artery.

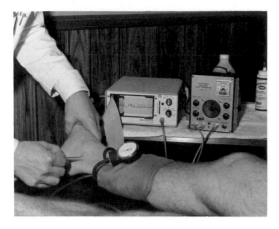

Figure 9.96. Posterior tibialis artery.

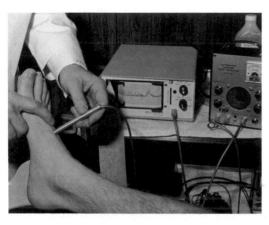

Figure 9.97. Dorsalis pedis artery.

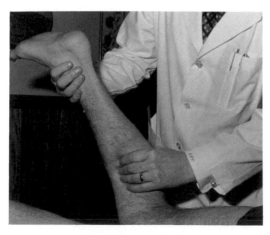

Figure 9.98. Moses' sign.

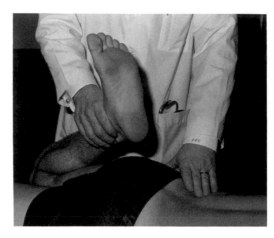

Figure 9.99. Nachlas' sign.

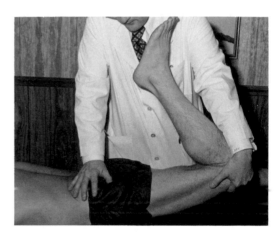

Figure 9.100. Yeoman's sign.

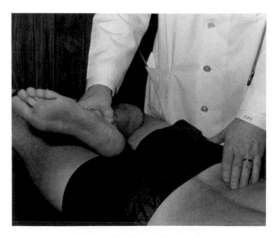

Figure 9.101. Ely's sign.

Prone Knee Flexion Test (Fig. 9.102). Prone knee flexion provides provocative testing for lumbar disc protrusion (67). The pathophysiology of this test depends upon compression of spinal nerves during hyperextension of the lumbar spine, which intensifies intervertebral disc protrusion into the spinal canal. Also, the lumbar intervertebral foramina are narrowed and the spinal canal cross-sectional area is decreased by lumbar extension. Compression of a spinal nerve by lumbar disc protrusion may be intensified; therefore, a protruded disc that has not produced sufficient neurocompression to cause weakness or reflex changes on testing with the spine normally aligned may be provoked by this test to produce changes which the examiner may elicit by testing in the prone knee flexion position.

The patient lies prone and the knees are hyperflexed, producing lumbar extension. The patient remains in the posture for approximately 45 to 60 seconds, and then the deep reflexes and muscle strength of the lower extremity are again evaluated. Weaknesses not observed prior to this maneuver may well be evident following it.

Popliteal Fossa Pressure (Fig. 9.103). In sciatica, the tibial branch of the sciatic nerve will be very tender in the popliteal space on deep pressure; this is known as the bowstring sign and, according to Macnab (62), is probably the single most important sign in the diagnosis of a ruptured intervertebral disc. The test for this sign can be performed with the patient in either the prone position, as shown in Figure 9.103, or the supine position. With the patient in the supine position, the straight leg raise is performed until the patient experiences some discomfort. At this level, the knee is allowed to flex and the examiner allows the patient's foot to rest on his shoulder. The test demands sudden firm pressure applied to the popliteal nerve. This action may startle the patient enough to make him jump. Reproduction of pain in the leg or in the back is irrefutable evidence of nerve root compression.

NONORGANIC PHYSICAL SIGNS (MALINGERING)

A patient with three or more of the following signs should be suspected of malingering. For more information on psychological screening of patients, see the article by Waddell et al (68).

Libman's Sign (Fig. 9.104). Deep palpation of the mastoid processes indicates the patient's pain

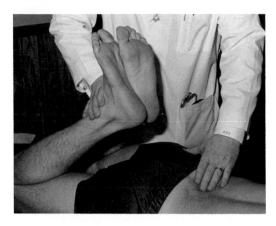

Figure 9.102. Prone knee flexion test.

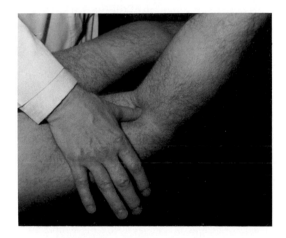

Figure 9.103. Popliteal fossa pressure.

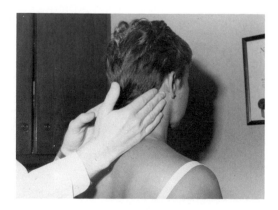

Figure 9.104. Libman's sign.

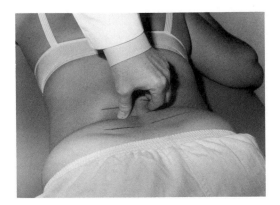

Figure 9.105. Tenderness to skin pinch.

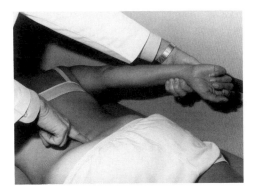

Figure 9.106. Mannkopf's sign.

threshold. Compare the patient's pain response to palpation of the mastoid processes to his pain response to examination of the low back. The two of these pain sensitivities should be the same.

Tenderness to Skin Pinch (Fig. 9.105). With a pen lay out specific spinal segments on the patient's back. Then pinch the skin segment by segment, which should elicit pain in the pathway of the appropriate segment. If the patient complains of a generalized pain over many segments of the spinal nerve, he is probably exaggerating his symptoms.

Mannkopf's Sign (Fig. 9.106). Take the patient's pulse prior to deep palpation of a painful area. Such deep palpation should increase the pulse approximately 10 bpm if it is a true marked pain. If palpation does not accentuate the pulse, the patient may be exaggerating his symptoms.

Burns' Bench Sign (Fig. 9.107). Have the patient sit on a low stool and bend forward and touch the floor with the palms of his hands. If he

says he cannot do this because of low back pain, suspect malingering, since flexion in this particular posture will not effect the low back specifically. Primary motion occurs at the hip joints and not the lumbosacral spine.

Flip Test (Fig. 9.108). Have the patient sit on the examination table with his back straight and his legs extended. If he truly suffers from a disc lesion compressing the sciatic nerve, he cannot perform this test and will have to flex the knee or raise the hip from the table in order to relieve the sciatic stretch. If he can perform this test, he probably has no true sciatica or disc lesion and is malingering.

Plantar Flexion Test (Fig. 9.109). Ask the patient to raise his legs one at a time until he feels low back or leg pain. Note the angle at which the pain is elicited, and ask the patient to lower the leg. Then place one hand under the patient's knee and one under the patient's foot and raise the lower extremity, keeping the knee slightly flexed. Raise the leg to one half of the height at

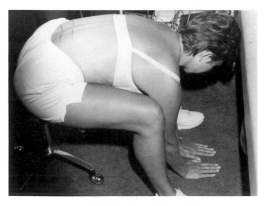

Figure 9.107. Burns' bench sign.

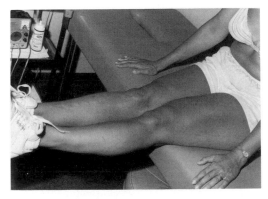

Figure 9.108. Flip test.

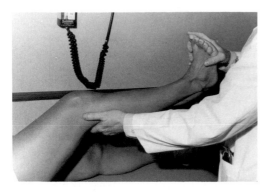

Figure 9.109. Plantar flexion test.

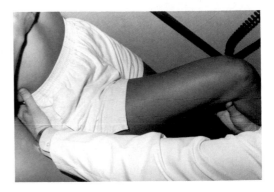

Figure 9.110. Flexed hip test.

which pain was originally elicited and plantar flex the foot. If the patient says that this causes pain, suspect malingering.

Flexed Hip Test (Fig. 9.110). Place one hand under the patient's lumbar spine and the other under the patient's knee. Lift the knee, and if the patient says he feels pain in his low back before the lumbar spine moves, suspect malingering.

Axial Loading Test (Fig. 9.111). Press the patient's cranium in a downward position. The axial loading may elicit pain in the neck but should not elicit pain in the low back. Suspect malingering if the patient says he feels pain in the low back.

Rotation Test of the Shoulders and Pelvis (Fig. 9.112). Have the patient turn his shoulders to rotate his entire spine. If he complains of low back pain, suspect malingering, since he is not truly moving his lumbar spine but rather is moving his spine from the thighs upward.

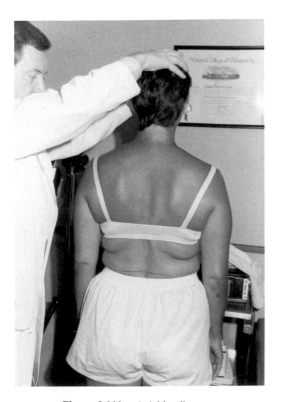

Figure 9.111. Axial loading test.

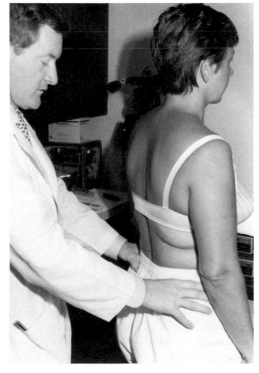

Figure 9.112. Rotational test of the shoulders and pelvis.

Correlative Diagnosis of Low Back Pain

With the history and physical examination of the patient completed, including the x-ray examination, we can now correlate our findings.

COX CLINICAL CLASSIFICATION OF LOW BACK PAIN PROGRESSION

The Cox system classifies back pain into 15 categories. Low back pain, in both its etiology and progression, is well suited to placement in one of or a combination of these categories. Description of each of these categories follows.

Category I—Annulus Fibrosus Injury

The patient with annulus fibrosus injury presents with the typical low back pain syndrome; i.e., the patient is young and usually on the first visit complains of low back pain following some flexion, twisting, or combined movement. No leg pain is usually noted, and relief is usually obtained within a few days. This type of pain may recur with progressive worsening of symptoms.

Clinically, the patient may present with muscle spasm, a loss of lordosis, and a positive Kemp's sign, but with no findings on the straight leg raising test and no altered motor or sensory changes of the lower extremity. Any leg pain is transient and not subjectively severe.

X-ray may reveal no change of discal space and no signs of discogenic spondylosis.

This patient responds well to distraction manipulation and is usually satisfied with the clinical results.

The patient in category I has undergone tearing, cracking, or severe sprain of the annular fibers, causing irritation of the sinuvertebral nerve and resultant back pain. This patient is similar to the type I or type II patient of Charnley, White and Panjabi's classification (20, 21).

Category II—Nuclear Bulge

The patient with nuclear bulge presents with a worsening of low back pain and minimal leg pain.

Clinically, the patient may have paresthesias of the lower extremities but has no frank altered deep reflexes. There is minimal irritation of the root of the nerve into the lower extremity, and a more positive straight leg raising sign, Kemp's sign, and other orthopedic tests for early disc protrusion are demonstrated. Déjérine's triad may increase the pain.

X-rays may show some early thinning of the disc space and discogenic, spondylotic change, which may be minimal.

With prolonged exacerbation of low back and leg symptoms, the patient in category II requires a longer treatment period than does the patient in category I. At this stage, it is important that the patient wear a lumbosacral support in order to stabilize the low back for healing. Sitting must be strictly avoided in order to reduce the intradiscal pressure and allow the annulus to heal. The use of the Cox exercises to open the dorsal intervertebral disc space are most helpful at this time, and nutrition with Discat may be incorporated into the treatment regimen.

The patient in category II shows progression of the tears and cracks of the annulus found in the category I patient, with the nucleus pulposus bulging into these annular fibers and causing further irritation of the sinuvertebral nerve and early and minimal irritation of the nerve roots that exit from the cauda equina within the vertebral canal.

The articular facets also become pain-producing entities because of disruption of the articular cartilage and fibrous capsule and because of the subluxation resulting from the loss of normal mobility of the motion segment. With increased intradiscal pressure or annular disruption, this patient is analogous to the type II or type III patient of Charnley's classification (21).

Category III—Nuclear Protrusion

The patient with frank nuclear protrusion has severe antalgia, marked lower extremity pain, and altered deep motor and sensory abnormalities.

Clinically, the patient demonstrates difficulty in straightening from a flexed position and marked loss of lumbar lordosis.

X-rays show antalgia and possible discal change.

Depending upon medial or lateral relationship of the disc bulge to the nerve root, the range of motion in the low back is markedly limited, and Kemp's sign is definitely positive.

The patient in category III requires prolonged treatment, and ambulation will be limited because of pain on weight bearing. It is mandatory that the patient wear a lumbosacral support and remain recumbent. At the outset of treatment, two or three visits per day may be necessary for maximum relief from pain. This patient is similar to the type IV patient of Charnley's (21).

Category IV—Nuclear Prolapse

The patient with nuclear prolapse has primarily lower extremity pain with minimal or absent low back pain. Nuclear material has completely torn through the annulus and lies within the canal as a free fragment severely irritating the nerve root and perhaps the cauda equina. The patient may have bowel and bladder problems. The decision to use surgery is based on the clinical differential diagnosis. If the patient does not show a 50% improvement within 3 weeks, surgery becomes imminent. This patient is analogous to the type V or type VI patient of Charnley's (21).

Category V—Discogenic Spondyloarthrosis

The patient with discogenic spondyloarthrosis (chronic advanced degenerative disc disease) has a history of intermittent low back pain, i.e., the patient is relatively free of pain except for acute exacerbations. The straight leg raising test is negative except for low back pain. Repeated motion of the spine, especially rotatory movements, causes low back pain. The patient must exercise care when bending and lifting and is analogous to the type VII patient of Charnley's (21).

Category VI—Facet Syndrome

The patient with facet syndrome presents with hyperextension of the lumbar spine, which usually produces pain. X-rays may well reveal a degenerative change of the facets, which follows degenerative disc disease. Macnab's line is positive, and the work of Van Akkerveeken is important here to determine the stability of the facet syndrome. See Chapter 11, "Facet Syndrome," for details on this diagnosis.

Category VII—Spondylolisthesis

X-ray is diagnostic in the patient with spondylolisthesis. See Chapter 13, "Spondylolisthesis," for details on this diagnosis.

Category VIII—Lumbar Spine Stenosis

The patient with lumbar spine stenosis may present with symptoms of neurogenic intermittent claudication. For a full explanation of lumbar spine stenosis, see Chapter 7.

Category IX—Iatrogenic Back Pain

The patient with iatrogenic back pain, due to either myelograms or surgery, suffers from irritation to the neural contents of the vertebral canal, which is perhaps severe enough to cause cauda equina symptoms. These patients are the most challenging to treat due to the difficulty in pinpointing the diagnosis and the consequent difficulty in arranging proper treatment. Many of these patients are failed back surgery syndrome (FBSS) patients whose biomechanics are so altered as to make relief from pain difficult, if not impossible, to attain.

Category X—Functional Low Back Pain

The patient with functional low back pain often has personality aberrations and does not understand or will not understand the cause and treatment of low back pain. Sometimes emotional upset manifests itself through low back pain symptoms. This type of patient represents a challenge to both the surgeon and the nonsurgeon in management.

Category XI—Sprain and Strain

The patient with sprain or strain presents with an innocuous injury of nonrecurring frequency that seems to involve muscle and ligament damage rather than discal or facetal damage. No nerve damage can be found. The pain may be present for several weeks following an athletic injury or automobile accident, but it is not chronic unless facet or disc damage has occurred.

Treatment consists of maintaining normal range of facet motion, restriction of motion in the early stages of injury, and rehabilitative exercises later.

Category XII—Subluxation

When a patient with subluxation presents with back pain, note the level and type of subluxation, e.g., a right lateral flexion subluxation of L5 on S1.

Category XIII—Tropism

In the patient with tropism, the level of asymmetry of the facet facings is marked. For a full explanation, see the discussion of tropism in Chapter 2.

Category XIV—Transitional Segment

When a patient with transitional segment presents with back pain, decide whether there are 23 or 25 spinal segments, so as to determine whether the patient has lumbarization or sacralization. See Chapter 6, "Transitional Segment," for details on this diagnosis.

Category XV—Pathologies

Category XV is allowed for patients with any other pathlology.

Establishing the Correlative Diagnosis

When the first three pages of the low back examination form (Table 9.5) are completed, the fourth page is used to arrive at the diagnosis of the 15 categories of low back pain etiologies just outlined. By following the *"Flow Chart for Correlative Diagnosis,"* we will combine our findings into a meaningful diagnosis of the patient's problem.

First, if the patient has sciatica, we use the algorithm at the top of the page entitled "Low Back and/or Leg Pain (Below Knee Diagnosis)." The dermatome involved, sciatic scoliosis, Déjérine triad, and leg pain intensity compared to back pain are used to arrive at the side, type, and location of the disc protrusion to the nerve root compressed. The diagnosis will be either category III or IV disc lesion. Each of these findings has been covered in this chapter, so their meaning can be used to arrive at this clinical impression.

Second, under "Low Back Pain (No Leg Pain Below Knee) Diagnosis," the findings will flow into the other 13 categories of low back pain problems, as explained in this chapter or explained in other chapters in this textbook.

At the bottom of the last page is the "Correlative Diagnosis of Low Back Pain and Leg Pain." Here will be given the final diagnosis of disc and nondisc causes of back problems. In the treatment chapters, the use of these correlative diagnoses to establish the treatment regimen for the patient will be shown.

An example of a diagnosis, following the examination and completing the flow chart, might be: L5-S1 right medial disc protrusion with an unstable facet syndrome of L5 on the sacrum, a right lateral flexion subluxation of L5, and tropism of the L5-S1 facet joints.

REEVALUATION OF PATIENT RESPONSE TO CARE

The reliability of tests for reevaluation of patient response to care is not good. Straight leg raising and range of motion tests are the most reliable, as the following facts substantiate.

The epineurium of the spinal nerve root is supplied with direct fibers from the spinal ganglion cells, whereas the epineurium in the anterior spinal roots is supplied by the sinuvertebral nerve. Numerous free nerve endings associated with pain sensation are found in the spinal nerve roots.

The venous plexus of the vertebral column is enmeshed by an adventitial plexus of unmyelinated nerve fibers and is a vast source of pain sensation.

In SLR, tension and movement develop first in the sciatic notch, then in the ala of the sacrum as the nerve passes over the pedicle, and finally at the intervertebral foramen itself. Movement of the nerve root through the intervertebral foramen has been given by Falconer (9) as 2 to 6-mm, by Charnley (69) as 4 to 8-mm, and by Inman and Saunders (70) as 2 to 5-mm.

It is important to remember that compressing or stretching a normal nerve is not painful. The SLR pain is a reflex or sensory input mechanism to protect us from injury. The reason for SLR pain is explained as sensitivity of the dorsal roots due to mechanical pressure. Perl (71) believes, however, that SLR pain is caused by a chemical noxious irritation by substances liberated by mechanical pressure.

Charnley (69) found SLR to be the best clinical or radiological sign for diagnosing disc protrusion. Hakelius and Hindmarsh (72) state that they found an inverse proportion to the degree of limitation of SLR and the percentage of positive disc herniation at surgery. Sprangfort (73) states that in young people the sign has no specific value for diagnosing disc herniation and that a negative SLR excludes a disc herniation. After age 30, however, possible SLR is seen less often but its diagnostic value increases, and a negative SLR no longer excludes the diagnosis of disc herniation (73).

Objective assessment of spinal motion and straight leg raising and a global objective index show a high degree of intraobserver reproducibility. Million et al. (52) conclude that the emphasis in assessing the progress of the back pain patient must be on the subjective parameters, and the technique for this assessment developed.

Nineteen low back pain patients and eight patients not suffering from low back pain were given several tests of flexibility and asymmetry by two different examiners. Three criteria of reliability and validity were used: (a) significant agreement between independent observers, (b) significantly different scores in the groups with and without low back pain, and (c) significant improvement following a successful spinal manipulation.

Tests of anterior flexion and asymmetry of foot eversion met only the first and second criteria, whereas tests of hamstring tightness and asymmetry of voluntary straight leg raising met only the first and third criteria. Passive and voluntary straight leg raising met only the first three criteria. Therefore, of the objective tests investigated here, only passive or voluntary straight leg raising can be strongly recommended for use in the evaluation of spinal manipulative therapy for low back pain (64).

We utilize four tests in determining patient response to manipulative care—Kemp's, Déjérine's triad, range of motion, and the straight leg raise. Only the latter two have proven clinically reliable.

SPECIAL DIAGNOSTIC CONSIDERATIONS

Disc Pain Distribution

The annulus fibrosus has nociceptive nerve endings in it (74), and annular tears can therefore cause pain referral of purely discogenic origin into the low back, buttock, sacroiliac region, and lower extremity even in the absence of neural compression (6, 13).

Facet Joint Pain Distribution

The zygapophyseal joints are well innervated, and facet arthropathy can cause low back pain and referred pain into the buttocks and lower extremities. Classic facet syndrome pain is in the hip and buttock, with cramping leg pain primarily above the knee, low back stiffness (especially in the morning or with inactivity), and the absence of paresthesia. Classic signs are local paravertebral tenderness, hyperextension back pain, and no neurological or root tension signs with hip, buttock, or back pain on straight leg raising.

Differentiating Disc from Facet Pain Distribution

Differential diagnosis of lower extremity pain of disc versus facet includes the fact that facet pain rarely extends beyond the calf, usually only into the thigh, and not into the foot. Radicular pain of a disc is potentially worse pain than the back pain. In facet pain, the back pain is worse than the leg pain. Radicular pain is usually accompanied by neurological signs in disc lesions but not in facet etiology (75, 76).

Differentiating Recurrent Disc Herniation from Scar Formation

Gradually increasing symptoms beginning a year or more after discectomy are considered more likely due to scar formation, while a more abrupt onset at any interval after surgery is more likely due to recurrent herniated disc (77).

Extraforaminal Disc Fragmentation Diagnosis

Persistent radiculopathy, undiagnosed by conventional CT, MRI, or myelography, could be an extraforaminal disc herniation that has escaped detection. Discography is an imaging modality of excellent selectivity to uncover this difficult entity (78). CT scanning following lumbar discography (discographically enhanced CT scan) is an excellent modality for finding previously undiagnosed or negative evaluations (79).

Pathological Change in Sciatic Foramen as Cause of Sciatica

Longstanding sciatic symptoms and signs should include pathological changes in the sacral foramen by benign and malignant neoplasms as well as infection. CT scanning should include the sciatic foramen in long-standing, undiagnosed sciatica (80).

Dorsal Root Ganglion Compression Symptoms

Dorsal root ganglion compression can result in myalgia and tendonitis symptoms into the lower extremities (81) as well as causing intermittent claudication, sciatica and groin pain (82).

Hereditary Tendency to Disc Lesions

Hanrats (83) states that the occurrence of herniated nucleus pulposus in male members of the same family seems to point to a possible hereditary or congenital association, but he has not found a tendency for disc protrusions to occur in the presence of congenital vertebral anomalies.

Clinical Instability Defined

White and Panjabi (20) state that a narrowed disc space without spondylosis is a sign of instability. Clinical instability is defined as the loss of ability of the spine, under physiological loads, to maintain normal relationships between vertebrae so that there is no damage and no subsequent limitation to the spinal cord or nerve roots and no development of incapacitating deformity or pain due to structural change.

Differentiating Contained from Noncontained Discs

When a disc lesion is present, a differential diagnosis between protrusion and prolapse is necessary. Remember that sudden onset of leg pain and absence of low back pain indicates prolapse (category IV), whereas low back pain followed later by leg pain indicates protrusion (category III).

Sciatic Scoliosis Defines Disc Lesion Type

Relief of pain on lateral flexion may indicate whether the disc protrusion is lateral or medial to the nerve root (10) (Fig. 9.113).

Cervical Disc as Cause of Myofascitis and Leg Pain

Cervical disc herniations have been reported to cause myofascial pain and altered deep reflexes in the lower extremities; once the mechanical cervical disc rubbing of the cord was surgically relieved, the myofascial pain caused by its irritation ceased (84).

Leg Length Effect on Low Back Pain

Leg length inequality alters gait efficiency and predisposes to low back pain and hip arthrosis (85).

Incidence of Disc Lesions in Children

The incidence of surgically proven lumbar disc prolapse in children varies from 0.8% to 3.2%. Trauma is not a significant etiological factor, but high familial incidence of back pain in affected children is found. Neurological signs are not as prevalent as in adults. About 40% respond to conservative care, and the best surgical results are found in those with short histories of sciatica (86).

Thoracic Disc Herniations as Cause of Leg Symptoms

Thoracic disc herniations occur in less than 4% of all disc herniations and should be included in the differential diagnosis of patients with paresthesias and weakness of the lower extremities. Some state that up to 70% of thoracic disc herniations calcify compared with 4% of normal studies (87).

Brennan (88) reported that thoracic disc herniation is uncommon in adults, comprising only 0.25% to 0.75% of herniations. Although it is extremely rare in children, he did present a paraparesis in an 11-year-old boy following minor trauma, found on MRI to be due to a T4-T5 small herniation. Myelography and CT had appeared normal. Laminectomy revealed disc material adherent to the dura with postsurgical need of left knee-ankle-foot orthosis at discharge.

Piriformis Syndrome

Sciatica could be due to a piriformis syndrome. In 10% of people, the sciatic nerve passes between the two parts of the tendinous origin of the piriformis muscle and internal rotation of the thigh compresses the sciatic nerve (89).

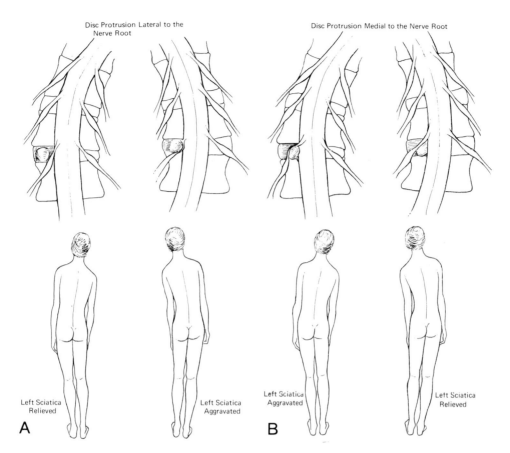

Figure 9.113. Sciatic scoliosis in a disc lesion. (Reproduced with permission from Finneson BE: *Low Back Pain*, ed 2. Philadelphia, JB Lippincott, 1980, p 302.)

Disc Protrusion Lateral to the Nerve Root

Disc Protrusion Medial to the Nerve Root

Left Sciatica Relieved

Left Sciatica Aggravated

Left Sciatica Aggravated

Left Sciatica Relieved

A

B

CASE PRESENTATIONS OF TYPICAL DIAGNOSES MADE USING AUTHOR'S EXAMINATION PROTOCOL

L5-S1 Disc Prolapse Requiring Surgical Removal

CASE 4

A 28-year-old, well-developed white male was seen who had suffered from low back pain off and on over the last 2 years. He had been treated by a chiropractor, who did give him relief, but the pain was now at the point that treatment resulted in no relief. The patient was examined by his family doctor, who prescribed pain pills. He consulted another chiropractor, who, upon seeing his low back, left S1 dermatome sciatica, and severe antalgic lean with an accompanying limp, referred the patient to us.

Examination revealed a positive Cox sign on the left at approximately 30°. The patient walked with an obvious left limp, and the ankle jerk on the left was absent. Sensory examination revealed hypesthesia over the left S1

dermatome into the small-toe side of the foot. An outstanding finding in this patient was the gluteal skyline sign, as the left buttock hung well over 2 inches inferior to the right, with a marked flaccidity of the muscle on strength examination. Both the gluteus maximus and hamstring muscles were grade 4 of 5 strengths.

Due to the marked motor loss, the severe pain to the patient, the absent left ankle jerk, and the fact that prolonged chiropractic treatment had rendered no relief, the decision was made to send this patient for a CT scan. CT scan (Fig. 9.114) revealed a large L5-S1 disc protrusion on the left. There was also an exostosis of bone on the left inferior L5 vertebral body plate as shown in Fig. 9.115.

Figure 9.116 shows the myelogram in posteroanterior projection, and Figure 9.117 shows the oblique myelogram demonstrating the massive L5-S1 disc prolapse that is compressing the cauda equina and S1 and S2 nerve roots.

At surgery, this free fragment of disc material measured 3 cm by 1½ cm. The patient had a good relief of sciatic pain and the total return of motor power following this surgery.

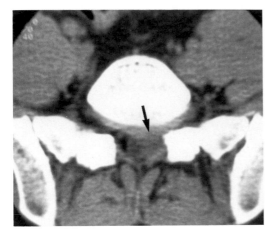

Figure 9.114. CT shows left disc protrusion of the L5-S1 disc (*arrow*) in a 28-year-old male with left S1 dermatome sciatica, an absent ankle reflex, and a marked right antalgic sciatic scoliosis.

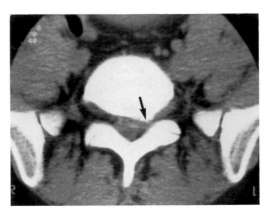

Figure 9.115. Another CT cut at L5-S1 shows L5 inferior body plate hyperostotic bone exostosis (*arrow*) narrowing the left lateral recess and intervertebral canal sagittal diameter.

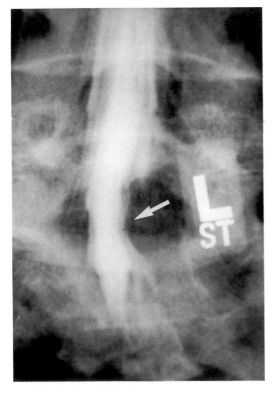

Figure 9.116. Posteroanterior myelographic study of the CT-scanned patient in Figure 9.114 and 9.115 shows the large left filling defect into the dye-filled subarachnoid space by the large disc protrusion at L5-S1 (*arrow*).

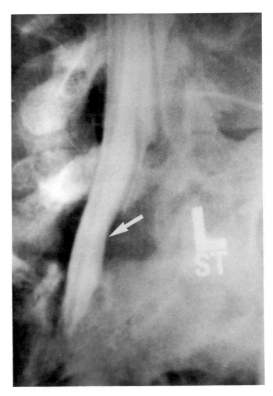

Figure 9.117. Oblique myelogram shows the defect into the myelographic dye column (*arrow*) by the disc protrusion at L5-S1.

L4-L5 Disc Protrusion with Foot Drop Treated with Manipulation

CASE 5

A 44-year-old white married female was seen complaining of 4 days of deep low back and right hip pain, which started following a sneeze. She stated that she felt better the following day, but the day before we saw her in examination, she became markedly worse, and the pain radiated into the foot and into the sulcus of the toes.

Examination revealed pain at the L4-S1 levels. The right buttock, thigh, and anterolateral leg were painful to palpation. The straight leg raising sign was positive at 50° on the right, and the right ankle jerk was absent. However, the history revealed that 15 years previously this patient had had right sciatic pain and a rupture of the L5-S1 disc that had caused loss of the ankle jerk.

The following day, the patient stated that she felt some relief in the right hip but that now the top of the foot had started to hurt. Three days later, the patient's condition had worsened until the straight leg raise became positive on the right at 30°, with Braggard's maneuver positive. The left straight leg raise was negative. There was now dorsiflexion weakness of the right great toe and foot at the ankle. The hamstring reflexes were +2 bilaterally. The ankle jerk on the right was still absent. The Déjérine triad was negative. The patient now had no low back pain, only leg pain.

Our impression 3 days following the first visit was that this patient had an L4-L5 disc prolapse and perhaps an L5-S1 extreme lateral disc lesion. Due to this dilemma, a CT scan was ordered that day. Figures 9.118 and 9.119 show the CT scan. We see a large osteophytic spur from the posterior central vertebral body plate into the vertebral canal at L5-S1 in Figure 9.118. The radiologist felt that this was a very probable cause of the patient's symptoms. The CT scan at the L4-L5 level did show a small disc asymmetrical bulge on the right side (Fig. 9.119).

Figures 9.120 and 9.121 reveal small myelographic filling defects at the L4-L5 level.

My impression was that the patient was suffering from an L4-L5 nuclear disc protrusion compressing the L5 nerve root causing radiculopathy into the right leg. The large osteophytic spur, in my evaluation, had been there probably for many years and was a result of an old annular irritation from the previous L5-S1 disc protrusion that had been treated years previously. We feel that the large osteophyte at the L5 level was really of no consequence at this time.

Treatment was given consisting of flexion distraction at the L4-L5 disc level. Positive galvanism was applied over the L5-S1 disc, as well as over the course of the sciatic nerve and the buttock and popliteal space. Alternating hot and cold packs were applied to the spine.

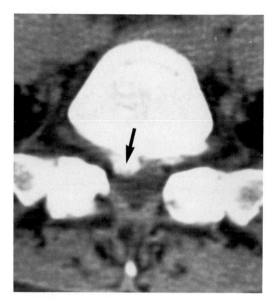

Figure 9.118. Axial CT slice at the L5-S1 level shows a right posterolateral hypertrophic spur into the lateral recess and vertebral canal (*arrow*).

This treatment resulted in gradual relief of the pain and the return of dorsiflexion strength in the right leg. At 6 weeks, the patient was able to walk on the heels and dorsiflex the great toe on the right.

This represented an excellent example of a case in which one could be misled at the L5 level by the large osteophyte that really was of no pathological signifi-

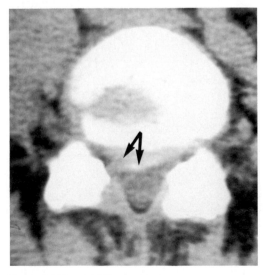

Figure 9.119. L4-L5 axial CT slice shows a right central disc protrusion into the lateral recess (*arrow*).

cance to the patient's symptoms at this time. That osteophyte had been there for many years before the present complaints. It may also be that the degeneration of the L5-S1 disc had shifted the movement to the L4-L5 disc and it was now placed under enough stress to lead to the new annular tearing and fresh disc bulge.

This case shows that careful clinical correlation of the radiographic and examination findings is absolutely necessary to arrive at the proper conclusions. Further please note that, in a patient with foot drop, one must be especially cognizant of the compression of the L5 nerve root. If this patient found the pain to continue for up to 1 or 2 weeks, with progressive weakening on dorsiflexion, a referral for a neurosurgical consultation would have been made. The doctor must be sensitive to the fact that dorsiflexion can be a permanent impairment if allowed to prevail too long before the nerve root is decompressed. Such dorsiflexion problems may well be a source of medical legal trouble to a doctor. A word on this certainly should be sufficient to make the doctor aware that a case with dorsiflexion weakness is a good case to observe very closely and to ask a second opinion on.

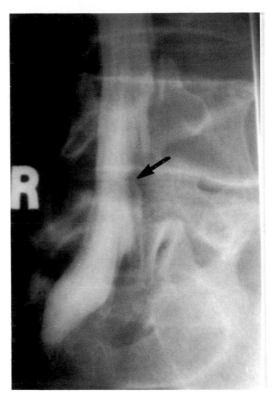

Figure 9.121. Left anterior oblique view reveals compression of the L5 nerve root by an L4-L5 disc protrusion (*arrow*).

L4-L5 Disc Prolapse Surgically Removed

CASE 6

A 42-year-old white single male, suffering from cerebral palsy, was seen complaining of low back and right leg pain with occasional pain into the left leg. This pain started 5 months previously following sleeping on a soft couch, after which he bent down to pick something up and felt immediate back pain. Two months after the injury, he developed severe right leg pain and minimal left leg pain. Approximately 1 month later, an MRI was performed with a diagnosis of an L4-L5 herniated disc and a possible L5 right herniated disc. He was treated with physical therapy for an additional 3 weeks and then sought care at our office.

Figure 9.122 is a picture of this patient standing upright, and Figure 9.123 is a posteroanterior x-ray showing the left antalgia of the thoracolumbar spine. When first seen, this patient was walking with a walker.

The results of physical, orthopedic, and neurological examination were as follows: There was inability to lie down for straight leg raising examination. The ranges of

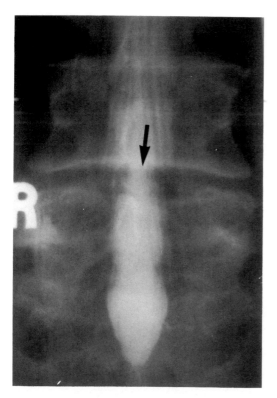

Figure 9.120. Myelogram PA view shows a minimal narrowing of the dye-filled subarachnoid space at the L4-L5 level (*arrow*).

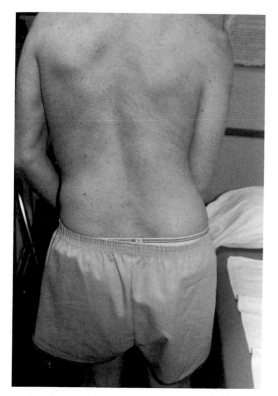

Figure 9.122. Left sciatic scoliosis of a patient with right sciatic radiculopathy.

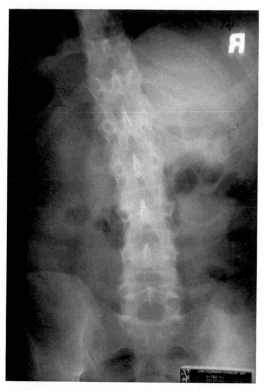

Figure 9.123. Left sciatic scoliosis of the spine of the patient in Figure 9.122.

motion were limited to 75° flexion, 0° right lateral flexion, 15° left lateral flexion, and 25° extension. The right ankle reflex was +1 and the left was +2, and the patellar reflexes were +2 bilaterally. There was hypesthesia of the right S1 dermatome. Two days later, when able to die down, the patient's straight leg raising was positive on the right at 35° and on the left at 65°.

This patient was placed on a treatment regimen that involved staying in our clinic and maintaining recumbency throughout the day to receive flexion-distraction treatment, and receiving physical therapy in the form of positive galvanism into the L4-L5 and L5-S1 disc, acupressure point treatment, and alternating hot and cold packs to the low back and the right lower extremity.

Treatment did not yield 50% relief within 3 weeks of care, and a CT scan was then ordered on this patient (Fig. 9.124). This CT was interpreted as showing a possible L4-L5 disc herniation, and a myelogram was recommended for further evaluation. Figures 9.125 and 9.126 show the myelogram, which reveals an extremely large extradural defect at the L4-L5 posterior disc space which creates a marked filling defect into the dye-filled subarachnoid space. Surgery was performed to remove a huge free fragment at the L4-L5 disc space on the right side which was underlying the L5 nerve root.

This patient had excellent relief of pain from this procedure.

Following relief of pain, a pelvic x-ray was taken to evaluate femoral head height, since the patient continued to show a marked right short leg. This x-ray (Fig. 9.127) reveals a 30-mm short right femoral head. Figure 9.128

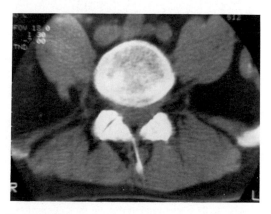

Figure 9.124. Axial CT scan fails to reveal a definitive disc prolapse.

shows a 15-mm lift placed under the patient's right short leg, which actually is an overcorrection. Ultimately a 9-mm lift was placed under the right heel and sole, which leveled the femoral heads. This combination of treatment gave this patient total relief from his low back and sciatic pain.

Extraforaminal Disc Prolapse Surgically Removed with Complications

CASE 7

This case is from the records of David Taylor, D.C., and represents a case of the "far out syndrome" in which a free fragment of disc was found to have extruded into the intervertebral foramen on the left side. Figures 9.129 and 9.130 represent the PA and oblique views at the L4-L5 level following facetectomy to remove the free fragment of disc. Note that the left L4-L5 facets have been surgically removed. It actually appears as if discitis had occurred following surgery, but certainly there is a left lateral flexion subluxation with extreme vertebral body plate sclerosis and irregular outline of the inferior L4 and superior L5 vertebral body plates.

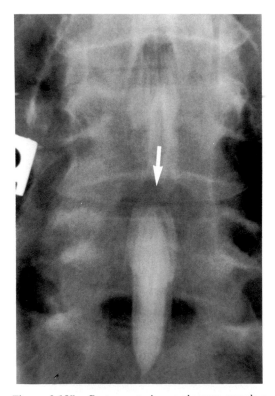

Figure 9.125. Posteroanterior myelogram reveals a large compression filling defect of the cauda equina at the L4-L5 level (*arrow*).

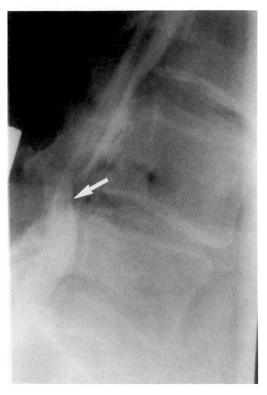

Figure 9.126. Lateral myelogram reveals flexion subluxation of L4 on L5 with an anterior defect of the dye-filled subarachnoid space (*arrow*).

Note the marked hyperostosis of the bone margins of L4 and L5. This patient still has extreme low back and leg pain following this surgery.

This is a good example of the removal of facets and the accompanying collapse of the intervertebral disc on the side of facet removal.

Discogram Reveals Nuclear Prolapse Following Two Prior Surgeries

CASE 8

A 28-year-old female, who had had spinal surgery in 1984 consisting of a laminectomy for removal of the L5-S1 disc, as well as chemonucleolysis at the L4 and L5 levels 1 year following the laminectomy, was seen for evaluation and possible treatment. Since both surgeries, her back and thigh pain had worsened.

Radiographs reveal that this patient had a transitional segment at the L5 level (Fig. 9.131). Figures 9.132 and 9.133 are discograms in the posteroanterior and lateral projections. Figure 9.133 well demonstrates the pro-

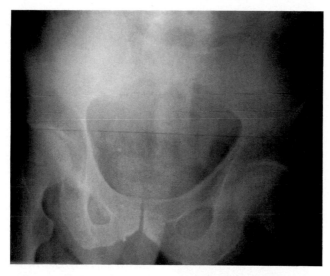

Figure 9.127. The right femoral head is 30-mm inferior to the left on this upright Chamberlain's view taken to evaluate leg length deficiency.

lapse at the L4-L5 disc with the dye extravasation into the vertebral canal and taking on the meniscoid or semilunar shape of the containing posterior longitudinal ligament.

Figure 9.132 reveals the extreme extravasation of the dye through the annulus fibrosus at the L5-S1 disc. This dye escapes both anteriorly and posteriorly, showing that the nucleus has totally ruptured throughout the circumferential annular fibers. This would represent an extreme degenerative change at both the L4-L5 and L5-S1 disc spaces.

The treatment recommended to this patient consisted of flexion distraction manipulation, a strong home exercise program, and low back wellness school. The patient, who at age 28 had grown quite tired of having this pain, and had had two back surgeries without success, was not willing to undergo the conservative treatment. She instead chose to visit a prestigious medical clinic and was told there to go home, rest, and exercise her back. Follow-up examination with the patient 3 months afterwards saw that she was still having the same type of pain.

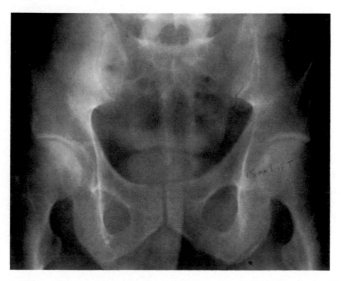

Figure 9.128. A 15-mm lift under the right heel and sole levels the femoral heads.

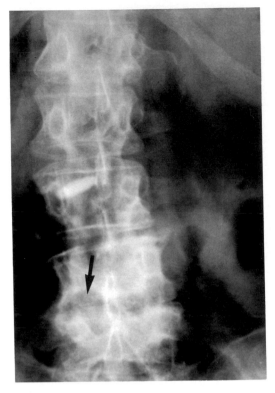

Figure 9.129. The left L4 inferior facet and L5 superior facet have been removed to surgically remove a free fragment of L4-L5 disc within the L4-L5 intervertebral canal. Note the surgical bone removal (*arrow*). L4 is in left lateral flexion subluxation. (Case courtesy of David Taylor, D.C.)

VALUE AND VALIDITY OF DIAGNOSTIC IMAGING: CT, MRI, AND MYELOGRAPHY

CT, MRI, Myelography Compared

A short discussion of modern imaging modalities and their use in chiropractic low back practice is presented. To determine the value of CT versus MRI, a 4-year study of 1500 thoracic and lumbar disc lesions using the two procedures was done (90). In classifying the benefits of each, MRI was found to be superior for spinal cord tumors, hemorrhage, and demyelinating diseases. MRI was considered a fine adjunct to CT in evaluating lumbar disc disease, stenosis, spondylolisthesis, and postsurgical bone and disc changes. CT was found to be superior for calcified disc and synovial cyst changes.

CT was found to agree with 93% of surgical

explorations in a study of 116 consecutive disc surgeries (91).

A technically adequate MRI was found to be equivalent to CT and myelography in diagnosing lumbar canal stenosis and herniated lumbar disc lesions. CT and MRI are complementary studies, and surface coil MRI is an alternative to myelography (92).

Contrast Media Selection for Myelography

When considering myelography, iopamidol seems to be slightly better tolerated than iohexol (93).

Differentiation of Recurrent Disc from Scar Tissue in Postsurgical Cases

Differentiation of recurrent disc herniation and postoperative epidural fibrosis (scar) is difficult both from clinical and imaging standpoints; however, MRI, and to a lesser degree CT enhanced with contrast myelography, will provide a more definitive diagnosis than CT alone (94).

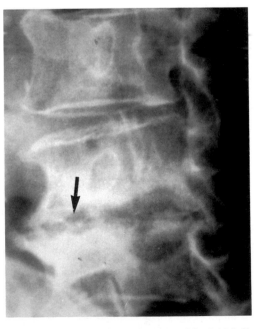

Figure 9.130. Note the marked loss of the L4-L5 disc space with irregularity of the opposing body plates, having the appearance of discitis (*arrow*).

Schmorl's Nodes—Presence and Detection

The clinical significance of Schmorl's nodes is difficult to ascertain, especially in light of the inadequacy of detecting them on plain x-ray. A study by Malmivaara et al. (95) found that 19 of 24 bone specimens were found to have Schmorl's nodes, whereas radiographs showed them in only 47% of the cases between the T10 and L1 levels when the nodes were greater than 0.5 cm in diameter, and in only 24% of the cases when they were less than 0.5 cm in diameter. From this, we can see the large percentage of Schmorl's nodes that escape detection on plain radiographic examination; furthermore, whatever their influence on the kinetics of the spine, we are unable to detect them most of the time.

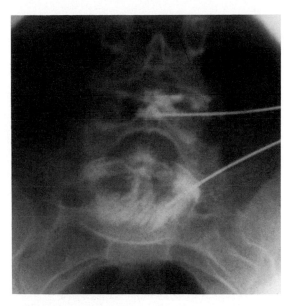

Figure 9.132. Posteroanterior discogram projection reveals the injected dye extravasating at both L4-L5 and L5-S1 laterally.

CASE STUDIES OF LOW BACK AND LEG PAIN OF ORGANIC ETIOLOGY

Appreciation of the lurking organic diseases, presenting themselves as low back and/or leg pain, forces us to look at some case presentations from our clinic of such circumstances.

To enhance the case for being aware of or-

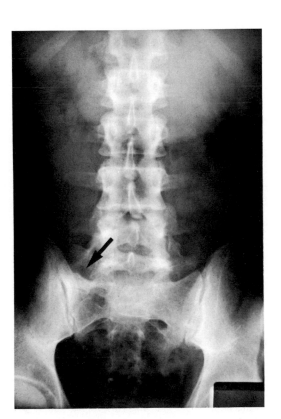

Figure 9.131. Note the transitional segment with right pseudosacralization of the transverse process of L5 with the sacrum (*arrow*).

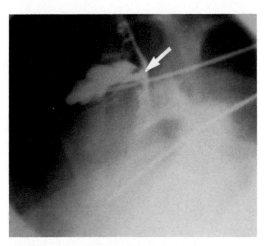

Figure 9.133. Lateral discogram shows the L4-L5 nuclear and dye material to have escaped into the vertebral canal (*arrow*) to flow cephalad and caudally along the posterior vertebral bodies, probably retained by the posterior longitudinal ligament.

ganic causes of low back symptoms, consider the fact that five patients known to be human immunodeficiency virus (HIV)-positive, that is, susceptible to AIDS, presented with symptoms that were initially thought to be indicative of lumbar disc lesions but actually were due to AIDS virus. They showed signs of nerve root or cauda equina compression in all five cases. It was suggested that all orthopedic surgeons exercise caution in diagnosing nerve root compression in patients who may be HIV-positive (96).

Let's look at some patients whose low back complaints caused them to seek chiropractic care but who needed other forms of care.

Abdominal Aneurysm

CASE 9

Case 9 is a 58-year-old man with low back pain.

X-rays reveal an abdominal aneurysm. Note the calcific expansion of the atherosclerotic abdominal aorta, measuring 4.5 cm in diameter (normal is 1.75 to 3.0 cm) (Figs. 9.134 and 9.135).

Treatment consisted of surgical care.

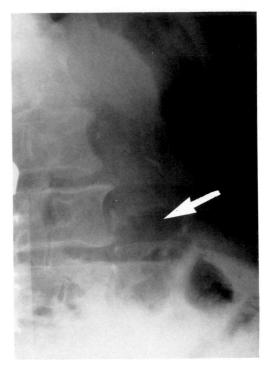

Figure 9.135. Arteriosclerotic expansion on oblique projection. (*Arrow* shows aneurysm.)

All physicians must be aware of the English study (97) showing that, in England, an abdominal aneurysm was found in 3% of those over 50 years of age and caused death in 1.5% of cases. In patients with other manifestations of arteriosclerosis, 9.5% have an abdominal aneurysm. Clinical examination may miss a third of them. Statistics on untreated aneurysms show that half of these patients were dead within 2 years and that 60 to 80% of those with symptoms lived only 1 year.

Small aneurysms rupture and grow about 4 to 5-mm a year.

Definitely the chiropractor needs to be constantly aware of the possibility of abdominal aneurysm as a cause of low back pain.

Osteomyelitis of the L3-L4 Disc

CASE 10

A 41-year-old male complained of generalized lower back pain, especially on the left side from L3 to the sacroiliac region, radiating down the anterolateral left thigh and leg. Movement aggravated the pain, and rest relieved it.

The patient presented with loss of lumbar lordosis and a mild left list of the thoracolumbar spine.

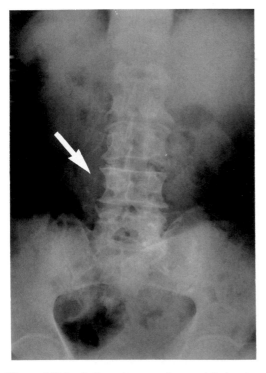

Figure 9.134. Left aortic expansion on AP view (*arrow*).

The history revealed that the back pain first occurred when the patient was getting out of his car, 18 days prior to seeking care. He had seen an osteopath, who used manipulation, with no relief. A medical doctor prescribed Motrin and muscle relaxants, with no relief.

Findings on chiropractic work-up were: left spinal tilt; loss of lumbar lordosis; positive Minor's, Bechterew's, and Valsalva signs; pain on palpation over the L3-L4 left lumbar area; Kemp's sign positive bilaterally; toe and heel walk normal; straight leg raising positive at 45° for low back pain; Patrick's sign positive for hip pain; and Gaenslen's sign positive for low back pain. Deep tendon reflexes were +2 bilaterally, motor findings were normal, and sensory examination was normal.

The impression at the time was an L3-L4 disc protrusion with L4 dermatome paresthesia. Treatment with flexion-distraction manipulation and therapy gave relief.

The patient then returned to weight lifting, and the pain worsened. A surgeon examined the patient and agreed with the diagnosis of a midline and left L3-L4 disc rupture. A myelogram was done which was indeterminate due to subdural injection of the contrast media. A CT scan was done and interpreted as normal. Plain x-rays were read as only showing minimal hypertrophic changes of the lower lumbar spine. A bone scan (Fig. 9.136) showed moderate uptake at the L3-L4 level. The patient was released from the hospital.

Two weeks later, as the pain grew worse, the patient readmitted himself to the hospital. His blood tests revealed a sedimentation rate of 116, and gram-positive cocci (*Staphylococcus aureus*) were cultured. A CT scan, shown in Figure. 9.137, now showed destruction of the L3 and L4 vertebral body plates and cancellous bone with loss of the disc space. Figures 9.138 and 9.139 are the anteroposterior and lateral views of the lumbar spine and pelvis showing the left L3-L4 disc space narrowing and the reactive periostitis of the opposing

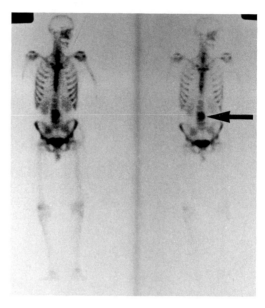

Figure 9.136.   Bone scan reveals increased uptake of the left L3-L4 vertebral level (*arrow*).

vertebral body plates indicative of infectious spondylitis.

The final diagnosis was osteomyelitis of the L3 and L4 vertebrae and intervertebral disc. The patient responded well to antibiotic therapy and, after healing, underwent chiropractic flexion distraction manipulation due to persistent stiffness and pain.

This is a great case to show how the symptoms and signs of an organic illness mimicked a disc lesion and misled several clinicians until the disease revealed itself. (Courtesy of Walter P. Kittle, D.C., Holt, Michigan.)

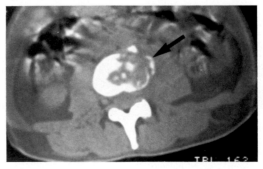

Figure 9.137.   CT scan shows destruction at the left L3 vertebral body with soft tissue swelling and bone density paravertebrally into the soft tissues (*arrow*).

Metastatic Carcinoma to the Spine

CASE 11

A 59-year-old female had had a bilateral mastectomy for malignancy performed approximately 1 year prior to seeing us, and had undergone chemotherapy following surgery. She completed chemotherapy approximately 4 months prior to seeing us for pain in the thoracolumbar spine.

X-rays in Figures 9.140 and 9.141 reveal a pathological compression fracture of the first lumbar vertebral body, which proved to be a metastatic carcinoma to the spine from the breast. This happened in the 3-month period after the original hospital films, which were normal, as shown in Figures 9.142 and 9.143.

This case is a good example of why you should never

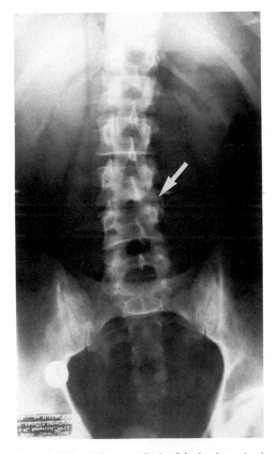

Figure 9.138. A dextroscoliosis of the lumbar spine is seen, with the apex at L3-L4. The left L3-L4 disc space is narrowed, with irregular vertebral plate outline. Soft tissue increased density is seen extending paravertebrally, representing abscess formation (*arrow*). (Case courtesy of Walter P. Kittle, D.C.)

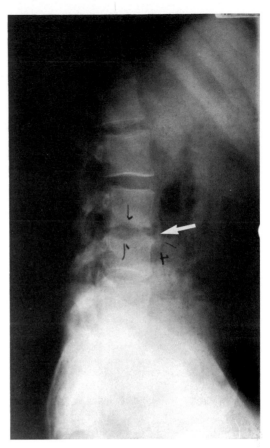

Figure 9.139. Lateral projection reveals the same finding as Figure 9.138 (*arrow*).

allow past examinations or findings to influence your present examination and diagnostic procedures. It would be quite disastrous to manipulate this lumbar spine at the level of the disease. This patient expired 4 months following discovery of the metastases on x-ray.

Congenital Hip Dislocation

CASE 12

This 11-year-old girl was seen because her gym teacher noted a strange gait pattern. Indeed, she had a "duck-waddle" gait. The pelvis appears widened, and the lumbar spine appears markedly lordotic. The abdomen protrudes somewhat. The patient denied any problem in locomotion.

Figures 9.144 and 9.145 are the anteroposterior and lateral hip projections revealing bilateral dislocation of the hips. The femoral heads rest against the lateral wall of the ilii.

The etiology of this condition is unknown, but it is

known to involve several members of the same family. Females are affected approximately 9:1 over males, and the condition is especially prevalent in the Mediterranean countries, notably Italy.

This is a most unfortunate case of bilateral hip dislocations which was allowed to go undiagnosed until seen by a chiropractor. (Courtesy of David Gafken, D.C., Auburn, Indiana.)

Spondylitis

CASE 13

A 36-year-old Hispanic female complained of weakness of the left lower extremity.

Figure 9.146 reveals a destructive bone and intervertebral disc lesion at the right T4-T5 level. Figure 9.147 is the CT scan, which reveals marked destruction of the T4 vertebral body and a large soft tissue abscess that proved to be tubercular spondylitis.

This is a good case to alert one to organic causes of leg pain and weakness. (Courtesy of Gary Guebert, D.C., D.A.C.B.R.)

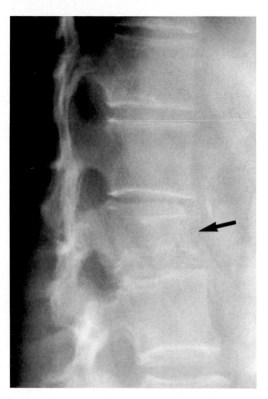

Figure 9.141. Loss of contour of the L4 vertebral body with loss of height of the body and irregular inferior body plate. There is loss of bone architecture.

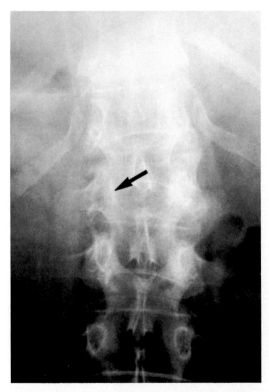

Figure 9.140. The right pedicle is not visualized ("one-eyed jack" or "winking owl" sign) (*arrow*) at L1 with loss of the right pedicle and loss of vertebral body height.

Avascular Necrosis of the Hips

CASE 14

The following case is presented from the practice of David Taylor, D.C. It is a case of avascular necrosis of both femoral heads. Figure 9.148 reveals increased radiopacity at the superolateral weight-bearing portions of both femoral heads, appearing as a wedge-shaped area. The joint space appears well maintained. Figure 9.149 is an MRI study, which, unlike the plain film, does show some loss of the sharp cortical definition of the femoral head at its articulation with the acetabulum, and there is a decreased signal intensity in the superior aspect of both femoral heads. There may be some joint space narrowing on the MRI study and an irregularity of the cortical outline superior to the area of avascular necrosis.

This condition is seen predominantly in males, usually in the 4th and 5th decade of life. Pain is the chief symptom, which begins around the hip or radiates into the thigh or knee joint. A limp may be associated with it, and a history of slight trauma or no trauma at all may be elicited.

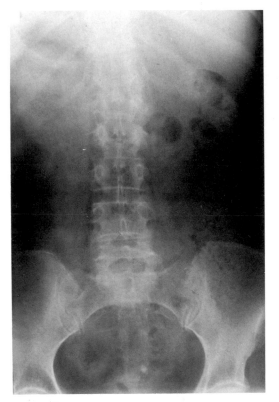

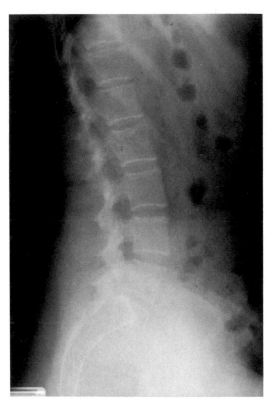

Figure 9.142. The anteroposterior x-ray taken 3 months before the x-ray in Figure 9.140 was normal.

Figure 9.143. The lateral x-ray taken 3 months before the x-ray in Figure 9.141 was normal.

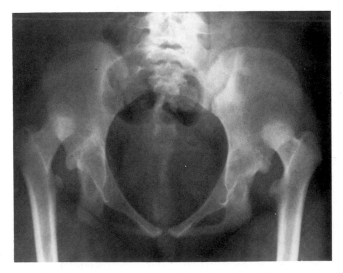

Figure 9.144. Anteroposterior pelvic x-ray shows bilateral hip dislocations. (Case courtesy of David Gafken, D.C.)

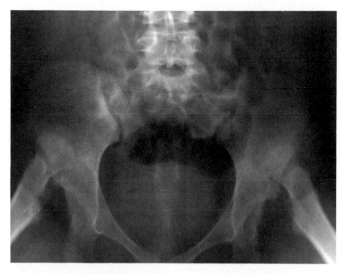

Figure 9.145. Frog-leg x-ray of the pelvis shows bilateral hip dislocations.

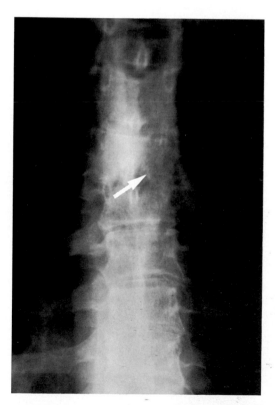

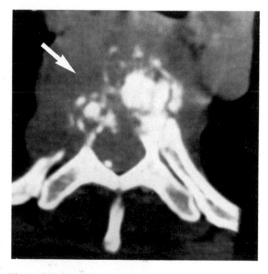

Figure 9.147. CT scan of patient seen in Figure 9.146 shows extensive vertebral body destruction and a large soft tissue abscess extending into the chest (*arrow*).

Figure 9.146. A destructive bone and intervertebral disc lesion is noted at the left (*arrow*) T4-T5 level (tubercular spondylitis). (Courtesy of Gary Guebert, D.C., D.A.C.B.R.)

Mitchell et al. found that, in 39 consecutive patients with avascular necrosis of the femoral head, representing 56 total hips, the cause included steroid administration in 31 of the patients, ethanol abuse in six, fracture dislocation of the hip in one, therapeutic radiation for lymphoma in one, and idiopathic causes in 17 (98).

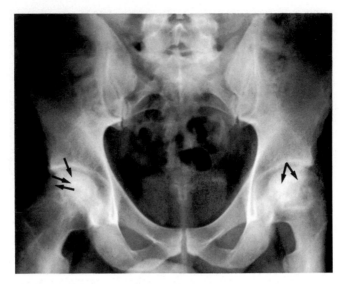

Figure 9.148. Both femoral heads show increased radiopacity and cystic changes of the superolateral weight-bearing portions as a wedge-shaped area (*arrows*). The joint space is maintained. (Courtesy of David Taylor, D.C.)

The radiographic stages of avascular necrosis are defined by Steinberg (99):

1. Normal radiographic findings;
2. Cystic and/or sclerotic changes without subcortical lucency (crescent sign);
3. Development of subchondral lucency and subchondral fracture, as evidenced by the crescent sign;
4. Subchondral collapse, depicted as flattening of the femoral heads;
5. Narrowing of the hip joint.

MRIs appear to be more sensitive than bone scans for allowing diagnosis of early avascular necrosis.

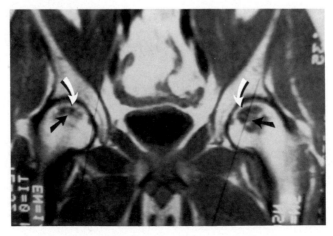

Figure 9.149. MRI shows marked signal intensity loss of both femoral heads (*straight arrows*), with irregular cortical outline at the articular surface (*curved arrows*).

Stress Fracture of Metatarsal Bone

CASE 15

Figure 9.150 reveals a stress fracture of the second metatarsal bone. You will note the osteodegenerative arthrosis of the first metacarpal phalangeal joint, which is the result of past hallux valgus bunion surgery. Following the surgery, this patient had a limp that probably resulted in stress on the second metatarsal bone, leading to the eventual stress fracture and the callus formation that we now see. This case is presented to alert us again to the possibility of a pathological cause of low back, leg, or foot pain.

Osteomyelitis

CASE 16

Figure 9.151 shows a pelvic x-ray of a 6-year-old boy who had been hospitalized for the treatment of staphylococcal pneumonia for 2 weeks prior to this x-ray being taken. We note that there is a radiolucent nidus somewhat surrounded by an area of radiopacity within the right femoral neck.

Figure 9.152 reveals osteomyelitis, this x-ray having been taken 3 weeks following that shown in Figure 9.151. This represents a hematogenous spread of the staphylococcal bacteria into the right femur and demonstrates how rapidly osteomyelitis can fulminate. (Courtesy of Gary Guebert, D.C., D.A.C.B.R.)

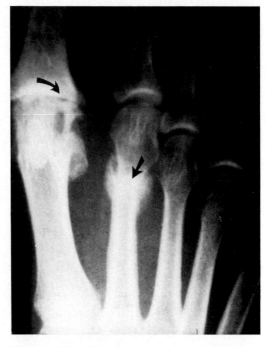

Figure 9.150. The distal second metatarsal bone reveals callous formation of a stress fracture (*straight arrow*). Note the arthrotic degeneration of the first metatarsophalangeal joint following surgery for hallux valgus (*curved arrow*).

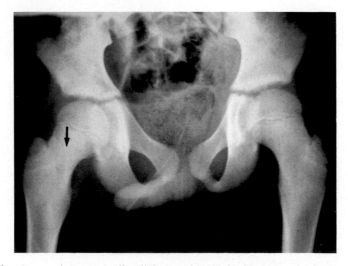

Figure 9.151. *Arrow* points to a small radiolucent nidus in the femoral neck of a 6-year-old boy.

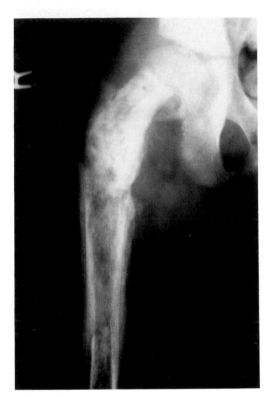

Figure 9.152. Full-blown osteomyelitis of the right femur shown in an x-ray taken 3 weeks following the x-ray in Figure 9.151. (Courtesy of Gary Guebert, D.C., D.A.C.B.R.)

Harrington Rod Fracture
CASE 17

Figures 9.153 and 9.154 reveal a fracture of the Harrington rod at the junction of the ratchet and the remaining rod.

This female patient had had this rod placed in her spine approximately 8 years prior to this fracture. The fracture was identified only upon a routine chest x-ray for an upper respiratory infection. The patient had no spinal symptoms due to the fractured Harrington rod.

Please note that these rods typically fracture at an area of pseudoarthrosis, meaning that the fusion of the scoliotic curve did not take place firmly at that level, placing more stress on the rod, with its eventual fracture. It is also again noted that this fracture usually occurs at the level of the junction of the ratchet section with the rest of the rod.

Metastatic Carcinoma
CASE 18

A 61-year-old white married female was seen complaining of low back pain. Radiographs of the lumbar spine (Figs. 9.155 and 9.156) reveal the right L1 pedicle to be absent, with loss of the vertebral body height and increase in the sagittal diameter of the vertebra. There is also some alteration in bone architecture, with areas of radiolucency mixed with areas of increased opacity of bone which probably represent compaction due to compression change. Figure 9.157 is a spot film of the first lumbar vertebra in posteroanterior position which reveals the change in the right first lumbar vertebral body and pedicle.

The history revealed that, 2 years prior to this onset of low back pain, the patient had a breast removed for carcinoma.

Figure 9.158 is a CT scan through the first lumbar vertebral body, which again reveals the alteration of bone architecture, with radiolucency throughout the vertebral body extending into the right pedicle.

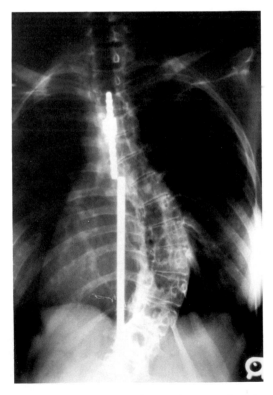

Figure 9.153. Fracture of a Harrington rod at the area of pseudoarthrosis in a scoliotic fusion.

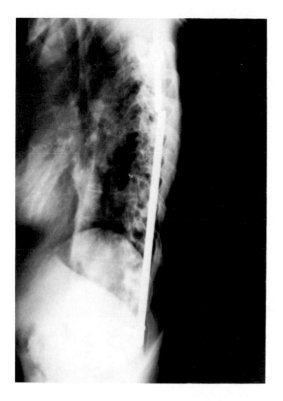

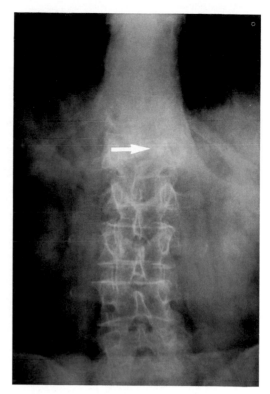

Figure 9.154. Lateral view of patient shown in Figure 9.153.

Figure 9.155. Posteroanterior lumbar spine x-ray shows absence of the right L1 pedicle ("one-eyed jack" sign) with loss of height of the lumbar vertebral body on the right (*arrow*).

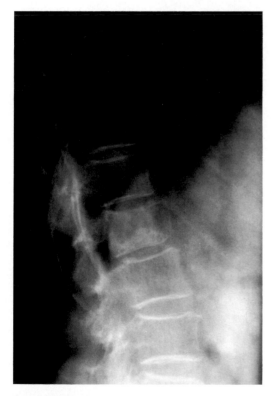

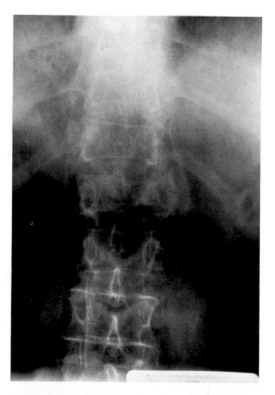

Figure 9.156. Lateral projection reveals loss of bone architecture, irregular bone outline, and radiolucency of bone of the first lumbar vertebral body.

Figure 9.157. Spot film of patient shown in Figure 9.155.

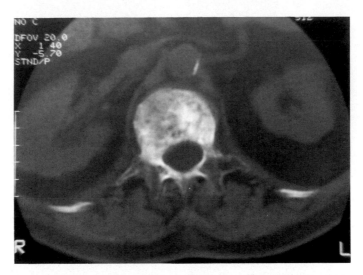

Figure 9.158. CT scan shows mixed radiolucent and radiopaque changes of the first lumbar vertebral body.

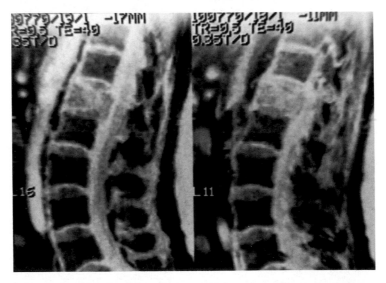

Figure 9.159. MRI reveals loss of signal intensity, loss of vertebral height, and extension of the L1 vertebral body posteriorly into the vertebral canal to create stenosis and possible compression of the conus medullaris area of the spinal cord.

Figure 9.159 is an MRI study that reveals not only the altered bone architecture but also the extension of the posterior L1 vertebral body into the vertebral canal, which is creating a stenotic change at that level.

Treatment in this case consisted of radiation treatment, and at last history of this patient, she had a remission of the malignancy.

REFLEX SYMPATHETIC DYSTROPHY

To end this diagnosis chapter, a word on this entity. It is defined as a syndrome of burning pain, vasomotor disturbances due to hypersympathetic activity, such as swelling, hyperhidrosis, hyperesthesia, and dystrophic changes of the skin and bone. *Causalgia* is an old term for the condition.

The cause of reflex sympathetic dystrophy is felt to be alteration of circuits within the spinal cord precipitated by electrical or chemical stimulation of peripheral nerves or altered spinal cord function following nerve injury (100).

Treatment by ultrasound has been found to give good clinical relief when applied to peripheral nerves (101). The physiology of help was felt to be an effect on the peripheral sympathetic nerve fibers.

References

1. Deyo RA, Tsui-Wu Y: Descriptive epidemiology of low-back pain and its related medical care in the United States. *Spine* 12(3):264, 1987.
2. McCarron RF, Laros GS: What is the cause of your patient's sciatica? *Journal of Musculoskeletal Medicine* (June):59–77, 1987.
3. Devanny JR: An orthopaedist talks about low back syndromes. *Semin Neurol* 6(4):411–412, 1986.
4. Macnab I: The mechanism of spondylogenic pain. In Hirsch C, Zotterman Y (eds): *Cervical Pain.* New York, Pergamon Press, 1972, p 89–95.
5. Vanharanta H, Sachs BL, Spivey MA, Guyer RD, Hochschuler SH, Rashbaum RF, Johnson RG, Ohnmeiss D, Mooney V: The relationship of pain provocation to lumbar disc deterioration as seen by CT/discography. *Spine* 12(3):295–298, 1987.
6. Saal JA: Electrophysiologic evaluation of lumbar pain: establishing the rationale for therapeutic management. *Spine: State of the Art Reviews* 1(1): 21–46, 1986.
7. Marshall LL, Trethewie ER: Chemical irritation of nerve root in disc prolapse. *Lancet* (August 11): 320, 1973.
8. Rothman RH, Simeone FA: *The Spine.* Philadelphia, WB Saunders, 1975, p 452.
9. Falconer MA, McGeorge M, Begg CA: Observations on the cause and mechanism of symptom production in sciatica and low back pain. *J Neurol Neurosurg Psychiatry* 11:13–26, 1948.
10. Finneson BE: *Low Back Pain,* ed 2. Philadelphia, JB Lippincott, 1980, p 428.
11. Sachs BL, Vanharanta H, Spivey MA, Guyer RD, Videman T, Rashbaum RF, Johnson RG, Hochschuler SH, Mooney V: Dallas discogram description: a new classification of CT/discography in low-back disorders. *Spine* 12(3):287, 1987.
12. Videman T, Malmivaara A, Mooney V: The value of the axial view in assessing discograms: an experimental study with cadavers. *Spine* 12(3):299, 1987.
13. Yasuma T, Makino E, Saito S, Inui M: Histological development of intervertebral disc herniation. *J Bone Joint Surg* 68A:1066–1072, 1987.
14. Bywater EGL: The pathological anatomy of idiopathic low back pain. In: *American Academy of Or-*

thopaedic Surgeons Symposium on Idiopathic Low Back Pain. St. Louis, CV Mosby, 1982, pp 152, 153.

15. Buckwalter JA: The five structures of human intervertebral disc. In: *American Academy of Orthopaedic Surgeons Symposium on Idiopathic Low Back Pain.* St. Louis, CV Mosby, 1982, pp 113–117.
16. Hirsch C: Studies on the pathology of low back pain. *J Bone Joint Surg* 41B:237–243, 1959.
17. Lindblom K: Technique and results in myelography and disc rupture. *Acta Radiol* 34:321–330, 1950.
18. Armstrong J: *Lumbar Disc Lesion.* Baltimore, Williams & Wilkins, 1965.
19. Turek S: *Orthopaedics—Principles and Their Application.* Philadelphia, JB Lippincott, 1956, p 748.
20. White AA, Panjabi MM: *Clinical Biomechanics of the Spine.* Philadelphia, JB Lippincott, 1978, pp 285–291.
21. Charnley J: Acute lumbago and sciatica. *Br Med J* 1:344, 1955.
22. Naylor A: Intervertebral disc prolapse and degeneration: the biochemical and biophysical approach. *Spine* 1:108, 1976.
23. Kazarian L: Personal communication to authors. In White AA, Panjabi MM: *Clinical Biomechanics of the Spine.* Philadelphia, JB Lippincott, 1978, p 285.
24. Hirsch C: An attempt to diagnose the level of disc lesion clinically by disc puncture. *Acta Orthop Scand* 18:132, 1948.
25. Wiesel SW, Tsourmas N, Feffer HL, Citrin CM, Patronas N: A study of computer-assisted tomography. I. The incidence of positive CAT scans in an asymptomatic group of patients. *Spine* 9(6): 549–551, 1984.
25a. Sprangfort EV: The lumbar disc herniation: a computer-aided analysis of 2,504 operations. *Acta Orthop Scand [Suppl]* 142:1972.
26. Epstein BS: *The Spine, A Radiological Text and Atlas,* ed 3. Philadelphia, Lea & Febiger, 1969, pp 35, 38, 554.
27. Nachemson A, Morris JM: In vivo measurements of intradiscal pressure, a method for the determination of pressure in the lower lumbar discs. *J Bone Joint Surg* 46A:1077, 1964.
28. Keele CA, Neil E: *Samson Wright's Applied Physiology,* ed 10. London, Oxford University Press, 1961, p 51.
29. Nachemson A: The lumbar spine, an orthopaedic challenge. *Spine* 1(1):59–69, 1976.
30. Fahrni WH: Conservative treatment of lumbar disc degeneration: our primary responsibility. *Orthop Clin North Am* 6(1):93–103, 1975.
31. Gresham JL, Miller R: Evaluation of the lumbar spine by diskography. *Orthop Clin* 67:29, 1969.
32. Arns W, Huter A: Conservative therapy of lumbar intervertebral disc lesions. *Dtsch Med Wochenschr* 101:587–589, 1976.

33. Semmes RE: *Rupture of the Lumbar Intervertebral Disc.* Springfield, IL, Charles C Thomas, 1964, pp 17–18.

34. Herlin L: *Sciatic and Pelvic Pain due to Lumbosacral Nerve Root Compression.* Springfield, IL, Charles C Thomas, 1966, pp 14, 16, 19, 31, 120, 128, 168, 169.

35. Emmett J, Love J: Vesical dysfunction caused by a protruded lumbar disc. *J Urol* 105:86–91, 1971.

36. Ross JC, Jackson RM: Vesical dysfunction due to prolapsed disc. *Br Med J* 3:752-754, 1971.

37. Amelar R, Dubin L: Impotence in the low back syndrome. *JAMA* 216:520, 1971.

38. Gray H: *Anatomy of the Human Body,* ed 28. Philadelphia, Lea & Febiger, 1967, pp 1007–1009.

39. Stoddard A: *Manual of Osteopathic Practice.* New York, Harper & Row, 1970, pp 140.

40. Katznelson A, Nerubay J, Lev-El A: Gluteal skyline. *Spine* 7(1):74–75, 1982.

41. Young A, Getty J, Jackson A, Kirwan E, Sullivan M, Parry CW: Variations in the pattern of muscle innervation by the L5 and S1 nerve root. *Spine* 8(6):616–617, 1983.

42. Kortelainen P, Puranen J, Koivisto E, Lahde S: Symptoms and signs of sciatica and their relation to the localization of the lumbar disc herniation. *Spine* 10(1):88–92, 1985.

43. Schoedinger GR: Correlation of standard diagnostic studies with surgically proven lumbar disc rupture. *South Med J* 80(1):44–46, 1987.

44. Gainer JV, Nugent GR: The herniated lumbar disc. *Am Fam Pract* (September):127–131, 1964.

45. Bell G, Rothman R, Booth R, Cuckler J, Garfin S, Herkowitz H, Simeone F, Doninskas C, Han S: A study of computer-assisted tomography. II. Comparison of metrizamide myelography and computed tomography in the diagnosis of herniated lumbar disc and spinal stenosis. *Spine* 9(6):552, 1984.

46. White SH, Leslie IJ: Pain in scrotum due to intervertebral disc protrusion. *Lancet* (March 1):504, 1986.

47. Gleis G, Johnson JR: Pro forma office examination for low back pain. *Journal of Musculoskeletal Medicine* (June):37–43, 1986.

48. Fisk JW: The straight leg raising test: its relevance to possible disc pathology. *N Z Med J* 81:557–560, 1975.

49. Raney RL: The effects of flexion, extension, Valsalva maneuver, and abdominal compression on the larger volume myelographic column. Paper presented at the International Symposium for study of the Lumbar Spine, June 1978.

50. Lindblom K: Intervertebral disc degeneration considered as a pressure atrophy. *J Bone Joint Surg* 39A:933–944, 1957.

51. Porter RW, Miller CG: Back pain and trunk list. *Spine* 11(6):596, 1986.

52. Million R, Hall W, Nilsen KH, Baker RD, Jayson MIV: Assessment of the progress of the back-pain patient. *Spine* 7(3):204–212, 1982.

53. Goddard MD, Reid JD: Movements induced by straight leg raising in the lumbo-sacral roots, nerves, and plexus, and in the intrapelvic section of the sciatic nerve. *J Neurol Neurosurg Psychiatry* 28:12–18, 1965.

54. Lasègue C: Considerations sur la sciatique. *Arch Med (Paris)* 2:558–580, 1864.

55. Breig A, Troup JDG: Biomechanical considerations in the straight leg raising test. *Spine* 4(3):242–250, 1979.

56. Suguira K: A study on tension signs in lumbar disc hernia. *Int Orthop* 3:225–228, 1979.

57. Goddard MD, Reed JD: Movements induced by straight leg raising in the lumbo sacral roots, nerve and plexus and in the intrapelvic section of the sciatic nerve. *J Neurol Neurosurg Psychiatry* 28:16–18, 1965.

58. O'Connell JEA: Sciatica and the mechanism of the production of the clinical syndrome in protrusion of the lumbar intervertebral disc. *Br J Surg* 30:315–327, 1963.

59. Swan KW, Zervas NT: Modified crossed leg raising test and sciatica. *Neurosurgery* 15(2):175–177, 1984.

60. Hudgins WR: The crossed straight leg raising test: a diagnostic sign of herniated disc. *J Occup Med* 21(6):407–408, 1979.

61. Edgar MA, Park WM: Induced pain patterns on passive straight leg raising in lower lumbar disc protrusions. *J Bone Joint Surg* 56B:4, 1974.

62. Macnab I: *Backache.* Baltimore, Williams & Williams, 1977, pp 121–126, 174–176.

63. Shiqing X, Quanzhi Z, Dehao F: Significance of the straight-leg-raising test in the diagnosis and clinical evaluation of lower lumbar intervertebral-disc protrusion. *J Bone Joint Surg* 69A:517–522, 1987.

64. Hoehler FK, Tobis JS: Low back pain and its treatment by spinal manipulations: measures of flexibility and asymmetry. *Rheumatol Rehabil* 21:21, 1982.

65. Miller B, Leo K, Clarke WR, Fairchild ML, Stultz M, Hanson L: Reliability of neurological testing in patients with low back pain. *Phys Ther* 66(5):1–11, 1986.

66. Goodall RM, Hammes MR: Electronic comparison of toe strengths for diagnosis of lumbar nerve root lesions. *Med Biol Eng Comput* 24:555–557, 1986.

67. Herron LD, Pheasant HC: Prone knee-flexion provocative testing for lumbar spine protrusion. Spine 5(1):65–67, 1980.

68. Waddell G, McCulloch JA, Kummel E, Venner RM: Nonorganic physical signs in low back pain. *Spine* 5(2):117–125, 1980.

69. Charnley J: Orthopaedic signs in the diagnosis of disc protrusion. *Lancet* 1:186–192, 1951.

70. Inman VT, Saunders JB: The clinico-anatomical aspects of the lumbosacral region. *Radiology* 38: 669–678, 1942.

71. Perl ER: Mode of action of nociceptors, cervical pain. *Wennergren Cent Int Symp Ser* 17:157–164, 1971.

72. Hakelius A, Hindmarsh J: The significance of neurological signs and myelographic findings in the diagnosis of lumbar root compression. *Acta Orthop Scand* 43:239–346, 1972.

73. Sprangfort E: Lasègue's sign in patients with lumbar disc herniation. *Acta Orthop Scand* 42:459, 1971.

74. Bogduk N, Tyran W, Wilson AS: The innervation of the human lumbar intervertebral disc. *J Anat* 132:39–56, 1981.

75. Mooney J, Robertson J: The facet syndrome. *Clin Orthop* 115:149–156, 1976.

76. Schofferman J, Zucherman J: History and physical examination. *Spine: State of the Art Reviews* 1(1): 14, 1986.

77. Teplick JG, Haskin ME: Intravenous contrast-enhanced CT of the postoperative lumbar spine: improved identification of recurrent disc herniation, scar, arachnoiditis, and diskitis. *Am J Neuroradiol* 5(4):373–385, 1984.

78. Kurobane Y, Takaahashi T, Tajima T, Yamakawa H, Sakamoto T, Sawaumi A, Kikuchi I: Extraforaminal disc herniation. *Spine* 11(3): 260–268, 1986.

79. McCutcheon ME, Thompson WC: CT scanning of lumbar discography: a useful diagnostic adjunct. *Spine* 11(3):257–259, 1986.

80. Cohen BA, Lanzieri CF, Mendelson DS, Sacher M, Hermann G, Train JS, Rabinowitz JG: CT evaluation of the greater sciatic foramen in patients with sciatica. *AJNR* 7(March/April):337–342, 1986.

81. Johannson B: Practical experience of intervertebral joint dysfunction as a possible cause of disturbed afferent nerve activity influencing muscle tone and pain. *Manuelle Medizin* 21(August):4, 1983.

82. Vanderlinden RG: Subarticular entrapment of the dorsal root ganglion as a cause of sciatic pain. *Spine* 9(1):19, 1984.

83. Hanrats: In Nashold BS, Hrubec Z: *Lumbar Disc Disease, A Twenty-Year Clinical Follow-up Study*. St. Louis, CV Mosby, 1971, p 65.

84. Margoles MS: Cervical discs as perpetuating factors in chronic moderate to severe myofascial pain syndromes (Letters to the editor). *American Back Society Newsletter* 2(3):4, 1987.

85. Moseley CF: Leg-length discrepancy. *Pediatr Clin North Am* 33:1385–1394, 1986.

86. Clark NMP, Cleak DK: Intervertebral lumbar disc prolapse in children and adolescents. *J Pediatr Orthop* 3:202–206, 1983.

87. Chin LS, Black KL, Hoff JT: Multiple thoracic disc herniations. *J Neurosurg* 66:290–292, 1987.

88. Brennan M, Perrin JCS, Canady A, Wesolowski D: Paraparesis in a child with a herniated thoracic disc. *Arch Phys Med Rehabil* 68:806–808, 1987.

89. Nakano KK: Sciatic nerve entrapment: the piriformis syndrome. *Journal of Musculoskeletal Medicine* (February):33–37, 1987.

90. Caton WL, Garner JT: Comparison of CT and MRI scanning in the evaluation of thoracic and lumbosacral spinal lesions. *Neurosurgery* 20(6): 992–993, 1987.

91. Firooznia H, Benjamin V, Kricheff I, Rafii M, Golimbu C: CT of lumbar spine disc herniation: correlation with surgical findings. *Radiology* 163: 221–226, 1987.

92. Modic MT, Masaryk T, Boumphrey F, Goormastic M, Bell G: Lumbar herniated disc disease and canal stenosis: prospective evaluation by surface coil MR, CT, and myelography. *AJNR* 7(4):709–717, 1986.

93. Hoe J, Tan L: A comparison of iohexol and iopamidol for lumbar myelography. *Clin Radiol* 37:505, 1986.

94. Sotiropoulos S, Chafetz N, Genant HK, Winkler M: Assessment of the post-operative lumbar spine: distinction between post-operative fibrosis and recurrent disc herniation—I.V. contrast enhanced CT vs MRI. *Invest Radiol* 21(9):515, 1986.

95. Malmivaara A, Videman T, Kuisma E, Troup JDG: Plain radiographic, discographic, and direct observations of Schmorl's nodes in the thoracolumbar junctional region of the cadaveric spine. *Spine* 12(5):453–457, 1987.

96. Crawford EP, Baird PE, Clark AL: Cauda equina and lumbar nerve root compression in patients with AIDS. *J Bone Joint Surg* 69B:36–37, 1987.

97. Hopkins NF: Abdominal aortic aneurysms. *Br Med J* 294(March 28):790, 1987.

98. Mitchell DG, Rao VM, Dalinka MK, Spritzer CE, Alavi A, Steinberg ME, Fallon M, Kressel HY: Femoral head avascular necrosis: correlation of MR imaging: radiographic staging, radionuclide imaging, and clinical findings. *Radiology* 162: 709–715, 1987.

99. Steinberg ME, Brighton CT, Hayken GD, Tooze SE, Steinberg DR: Early results in the treatment of avascular necrosis of the femoral head and electrical stimulation. *Orthop Clin North Am* 15: 163–175, 1984.

100. Schwartzman RJ, McLellan TL: Reflex sympathetic dystrophy. *Arch Neurol* 44(May):555, 1987.

101. Portwood MM, Lieberman JS, Taylor RG: Ultrasound treatment of reflex sympathetic dystrophy. *Arch Phys Med Rehabil* 68(February):116, 1987.

10

Laboratory Evaluation

David Wickes, D.C.

A man is not hurt so much by what happens, only his opinion of what happens

—Montaigne

A thorough diagnostic evaluation lays the foundation for a logical treatment plan. However, the phrase *laboratory diagnosis* is a misnomer. In actuality, the evaluation of blood, urine, and other specimens is but one of the five major means of evaluating patients with low back pain, the others being the history, physical examination, routine radiographs, and special studies (electromyography, computed tomography, magnetic resonance imaging, etc.). Laboratory tests, in and of themselves, should never be considered as the primary or only investigatory means, but rather as tools to assist the physician in analyzing and correlating other clinical findings.

Although there are many different etiologies of low back pain, the clinical laboratory is most useful in evaluating infectious, inflammatory, metabolic, and neoplastic disorders. Most simple traumatic, mechanical, and degenerative conditions are not associated with significant laboratory abnormalities. Indeed, those conditions seen most frequently in the office, such as strain/sprain syndromes, disc disorders, degenerative joint disease, and primary fibromyositis, are characterized by normal laboratory test results.

Because the prevalence of these common conditions is so much greater than that of other disorders, few laboratory tests are sufficiently cost-effective to be utilized as routine procedures. As the prevalence of a condition diminishes, the chance of encountering a false-positive test result becomes greater, and may even exceed the chance of a true-positive test. Because of the differences in sensitivity, specificity, and predictive value of laboratory tests, it is most reasonable to utilize laboratory tests in pursuing a statistically reasonable diagnosis rather than in haphazard screening. In other words, the selection of laboratory tests should be guided by the working diagnoses generated by the history and physical examination, rather than simply done as indiscriminate screening. As will be seen, the "rheumatic" or "arthritic" profile, which commonly consists of tests for the rheumatoid factor, antinuclear antibodies (ANA), uric acid, and antistreptolysin O (ASO), is almost never indicated in the patient with isolated low back pain because the conditions that are associated with abnormalities of those tests almost never produce symptoms in the low back without considerable concomitant peripheral involvement.

If the initial history and physical examination raise the possibility of a nonmechanical, nondegenerative disorder resulting in low back discomfort, then appropriate follow-up procedures are selected. The most common laboratory tests utilized to evaluate patients with low back pain are discussed in the following section.

Tests can be broadly considered as "nonspecific" and "specific" tests. In the former category, which includes such tests as the erythrocyte sedimentation rate and the C-reactive protein assay, the tests frequently yield abnormal results in many different disorders without identifying any one particular disease. "Specific" tests seldom meet the ideal goal of being 100% specific (i.e., abnormal only in patients with the disease in question) but do help narrow down the possibilities when used appropriately.

NONSPECIFIC LABORATORY INDICATORS OF DISEASE

Erythrocyte Sedimentation Rate

The erythrocyte sedimentation rate (ESR) is a widely utilized nonspecific test. The basis of the test is that red blood cells will settle with gravity in a vertical tube of blood at a rate dependent on such variables as the number of cells, the size and shape of the cells, and the type and amount of plasma proteins. Abnormalities result in an elevation (increase) in the rate of sedimentation. Not only may anemias result in an increased ESR but also many diseases resulting in an antibody response will do so. With low back patients, the ESR is of most use in suspected cases of vertebral osteomyelitis and lumbar disc infections. The ESR is elevated in the vast majority of cases of vertebral osteomyelitis, with sensitivity ranging from 88 to 98% (1, 2, 3). Tuberculosis of the spine does not produce as dramatic a change in the ESR as do suppurative forms of osteomyelitis, with the ESR being significantly elevated in 70% of cases and seldom elevated more than 50 mm/hr (3).

Infection of the intervertebral disc following lumbar discectomy can be a difficult diagnosis to make. In the typical scenario, the patient has undergone a lumbar discectomy and is seen in the office 1 or 2 weeks after discharge complaining of progressively increasing discomfort in the lumbar spine. The ESR can be used to determine if the symptoms are probably the result of a postoperative discitis. Elevation of the sedimentation rate above 50 mm/hr at 2 or more weeks postoperatively appears to be a reliable indication of a secondary discitis, and this precedes diagnostic radiographic changes (4).

Malignancies, including plasma cell dyscrasias, primary bone tumors, and metastatic disease to the lumbar spine, can also cause elevations of the ESR; however, the sensitivity is not sufficiently great to comfortably rule out a tumor on the basis of a normal result or to support the use of the ESR as a screening procedure for cancer.

The ESR has been shown to be of considerable value in the diagnosis of polymyalgia rheumatica and temporal arteritis, with the vast majority of cases having rates in excess of 50 mm/hr.

Table 10.1 summarizes the results of the ESR in orthopedic conditions affecting the low back and pelvis.

C-Reactive Protein

C-reactive protein (CRP) is a protein synthesized in the liver in response to tissue damage. It is considered, along with haptoglobin, fibrinogen, ceruloplasmin, complement, and several other proteins, as an "acute phase reactant" because its levels rise rapidly in response to inflammatory states and tissue destruction. Measurement of CRP by sensitive quantitative methodologies, such as nephelometry and immunoassays, has made slide agglutination techniques obsolete and has increased the usefulness of the test. Because the ESR is affected by changes in acute phase proteins, especially fibrinogen, it is understandable that many of the conditions that cause elevated sedimentation rates also cause increased serum levels of CRP. Measurement of CRP is of particular use in monitoring disease activity in patients with low back pain caused by ankylosing spondylitis and Reiter's disease, being more sensitive than the ESR (5).

Urinalysis

Urinalysis is a low-cost procedure that is an important part of the evaluation of patients with low back and lower extremity radicular pain. It should be performed whenever there is no obvi-

Table 10.1.
Erythrocyte Sedimentation Rate (ESR) in Low Back and Pelvic Orthopedic Disorders

ESR Usually Normal	ESR Often Elevated[a]
Degenerative joint disease	Suppurative osteomyelitis
Sacroiliac syndromes	Tuberculous osteomyelitis
Spondylolisthesis	Intervertebral discitis
Fibromyomalgia	Multiple myeloma
Intervertebral disc syndromes	Ankylosing spondylitis
	Reiter's syndrome
Osteoporosis	Metastatic disease
Facet syndromes	Psoriatic arthritis
Common compression fractures	Polymyalgia rheumatica
	Polymyositis
	Primary malignancy

[a]Frequency of elevation varies considerably in these disorders.

ous direct etiology for the patient's discomfort. A complete discussion of urinalysis is beyond the scope of this chapter; instead, the focus will be upon those components directly relating to low back pain. These consist of the chemical evaluation for protein, blood, and glucose, and determination of the presence of bacteria and white blood cells. In most cases, a simple dipstick assessment will suffice.

Routine determination of protein in urine actually elevates only for the presence of albumin. Dipsticks are not sensitive to globulins or to immunoglobulin free light chains (Bence Jones protein) Albuminuria in trace amounts is often seen in normal persons; however, greater amounts should be evaluated by means of a 24-hour urine protein quantification. Albuminuria indicates a disorder of the renal glomerulus or tubules. This might be due to an organic disorder, such as glomerulonephritis or secondary damage to the nephrons in multiple myeloma, or may occur as a physiological variant. Relating to the latter, heavy exercise may induce transient proteinuria, and some persons spill protein into the urine in the erect posture (orthostatic proteinuria).

Hematuria should always be taken seriously. Blood can get into the urine from any part of the urinary tract, so the range of conditions producing hematuria is quite large. Hematuria may be the only finding early in the course of a renal cell carcinoma, a condition to be considered in patients over the age of 20. Other conditions associated with hematuria and which may produce back pain include renal and ureteral stones, pyelonephritis, glomerulonephritis, cystitis, and prostatic diseases.

Glucosuria, even in trace amounts, should be evaluated further by means of a fasting plasma glucose level. Glucosuria is most often seen in diabetes mellitus, and these patients will have either a fasting plasma glucose level in excess of 140 mg/dl or an abnormal glucose tolerance test.

Infections of the kidney, prostate, and bladder usually are associated with bacteriuria and pyuria. Current dipstick technology allows for screening for bacteria through the detection of nitrites that are converted by bacteria from normal urinary nitrates. Leukocyte esterase determination is useful in the chemical (dipstick) detection of white blood cells. If both the nitrite and leukocyte esterase tests are negative, then urinary tract infection as a cause of low back symptoms can be ruled out. If either is positive, then microscopic evaluation and possibly culture should follow.

Common Serum Chemical Analyses

ALKALINE PHOSPHATASE

Alkaline phosphatase actually represents several isoenzymes sharing similar activity, but with slight differences in physical structure. The isoenzymes are produced in a variety of tissues, the most clinically significant of which are bone, liver, placenta, and small intestine. Elevations of the serum enzyme level result from increased metabolic activity or cellular damage. Alkaline phosphatase levels are normally increased in children and in the healing stage of fractures because of the increased activity of osteoblasts. When evaluating the alkaline phosphatase levels of a pediatric patient, one must be sure to use the age-adjusted reference values. In all age groups, fractures of long bones are more likely than vertebral or small bone fractures to be associated with increased alkaline phosphatase activity. An elevated alkaline phosphatase level in an older patient with an apparent osteoporotic compression fracture should prompt the physician to consider other possible causes of the enzyme elevation. Alkaline phosphatase levels gradually rise in pregnancy, peaking at 32 to 34 weeks of gestation and then remaining constant until a few days after delivery (6). As with all tests, there is the possibility of pharmacological and physiological causes of abnormal results. In addition to those elevations seen with pregnancy and healing fractures, serum alkaline phosphatase may rise with drugs that may induce cholestasis, in some adults after a fatty meal, and in the elderly patient (7).

Because of the multiorgan origin of the enzyme, it is understandable that many different diseases can result in elevation of the serum level. Table 10.2 lists the more common disorders associated with elevated alkaline phosphatase levels.

The further evaluation of an elevated alkaline phosphatase can be done in two ways. As shown in Figure 10.1, determination of the tissue of origin of alkaline phosphatase can be done by searching for elevations in other serum enzymes which parallel those of alkaline phosphatase in certain diseases, or by separation and quantification of the various isoenzymes. G-glutamyl transpeptidase (G-GTP) is elevated in many hepatic disorders but is not affected by osseous diseases. Many routine chemistry profiles include both alkaline phosphatase and G-GTP. Serum 5'-nucleotidase and leucine aminopeptidase can also be measured, and changes tend to parallel those in

Table 10.2.
Pathologies Associated with Elevated Serum Alkaline Phosphatase Levels

Musculoskeletal
  Primary and metastatic osteoblastic tumors
  Paget's disease
  Fractures
  Rickets
  Osteomalacia
  Hyperparathyroidism
Hepatobiliary
  Drug-induced cholestasis
  Primary and metastatic liver tumors
  Biliary cirrhosis
  Choledocholithiasis
  Carcinoma of head of pancreas
  Carcinoma of ampulla of Vater
  Acute hepatitis (mild elevation)
  Hepatic cirrhosis (mild elevation)
Gastrointestinal
  Extensive gastric or bowel ulceration
  Intestinal infarction
Miscellaneous
  Hyper- and hypothyroidism
  Renal infarction
  Severe diabetes mellitus

G-GTP, although neither is quite as sensitive. Measurement of alkaline phosphatase isoenzymes can be performed; however, the accuracy of the analysis varies with the method utilized and the experience of the laboratory. Isoelectric focusing and immunoassay will likely evolve as the techniques of choice in the future.

Of particular concern to the practitioner is the patient with a history of cancer who presents with low back pain. Osseous primary and secondary osteoblastic malignancies have been associated with elevations of serum alkaline phosphatase, and the finding of such in a patient with a history of cancer should prompt further evaluation, such as radionuclide bone scanning. In breast cancer patients, serial measurement of alkaline phosphatase isoenzymes and G-GTP has been shown to be useful in detecting the occurrence of liver and bone metastases, with abnormal levels found in slightly more than 40% of all patients with these metastases, and in 75% of those patients who are symptomatic because of the metastases (8).

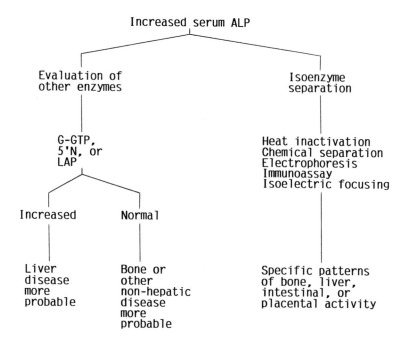

[ALP = alkaline phosphatase, 5'N = 5-nucleotidase,
LAP = leucine aminopeptidase]

Figure 10.1. Methods to determine origin of increased serum alkaline phosphatase.

ACID PHOSPHATASE

Measurement of serum acid phosphatase, an enzyme produced predominantly by prostatic epithelial cells, but also by platelets, red blood cells, bone, and other tissues, has only limited diagnostic usefulness. Elevation of the serum acid phosphatase level is found in many cases of advanced prostatic cancer. Although it was hoped that techniques such as radioimmunoassay and monoclonal antibody-based immunoassays would improve the detection of prostatic cancer while the disease was still confined to the prostate, such has not been the case, and serum prostatic acid phosphatase testing cannot be considered a reliable screening procedure for prostatic cancer (9). Even the new assays for the recently discovered prostate-specific antigen, a glycoprotein produced solely by prostatic epithelial cells, have not been found to be effective screening procedures for prostatic cancer (10). Digital examination of the prostate remains the cornerstone of the diagnosis of prostatic cancer, and no combination of laboratory tests has been demonstrated to be as sensitive. The finding of a suspicious nodule warrants urological consultation, regardless of the results of blood tests.

URIC ACID

Serum uric acid is a common part of the laboratory rheumatic profile but has little use in the evaluation of the patient with low back pain. Gout is the primary disease associated with hyperuricemia, and is characterized by an acute inflammatory response triggered by uric acid crystal precipitation in synovial fluid. Gout preferentially affects distal joints, most notably those of the foot, ankle, knee, and wrist. Seldom are joints of the spine affected, most likely because the higher temperature in those joints helps to keep the uric acid crystals in solution. It would be extremely unusual for gout to affect the lumbar spine or sacroiliac joints without there being preceding involvement of peripheral joints. A more likely situation would be the incidental finding of hyperuricemia in a patient being evaluated for other reasons. An elevation of the serum uric acid level can result from several mechanisms, including decreased renal excretion, increased formation, and metabolic changes (11). Table 10.3 lists the more common causes of hyperuricemia.

Table 10.3.
Common Causes of Hyperuricemia

Increased production of uric acid
  High-purine diet
  Increased turnover of nucleis acids
    psoriasis
    Multiple myeloma
    Megaloblastic anemias
    Polycythemia vera
    Leukemia
  Primary gout (some)
Decreased excretion of uric acid
  Renal failure
  Alcohol use
  Aspirin
  Primary gout (most cases)
  Diuretics
Miscellaneous (multifactorial) causes
  Obesity
  Primary hypertension
  Hypertriglyceridemia
  Idiopathic hypercuricemia

CALCIUM

The blood calcium level is normally closely regulated by the complex interactions of parathyroid hormone, vitamin D, bone, plasma proteins, and calcitonin. Disturbances of those factors may result in alterations in the calcium balance, as reflected by increased or decreased serum calcium levels. The routine serum calcium assay is actually a measurement of the combined levels of calcium bound onto plasma proteins and ionized, or "free," calcium. Calcium is transported in the blood by binding to albumin and some globulins. As calcium is needed for metabolic functions, it is freed from the plasma proteins and becomes physiologically active in this ionized form. A wide variety of diseases may result in abnormal serum calcium levels. Table 10.4 lists the most common causes of hypocalcemia and hypercalcemia. It should be noted that the serum calcium level is typically normal in osteoporosis and in degenerative joint disease. Primary hyperparathyroidism and metastatic carcinoma account for the majority of cases of hypercalcemia.

PHOSPHORUS

Serum phosphorus (phosphate) levels are affected by many of the conditions that alter serum calcium levels. In hyperparathyroidism, serum phosphorus levels are usually decreased, an inverse relationship to calcium. Vitamin D-resistant

Table 10.4.
Causes of Serum Calcium Abnormalities

Hypercalcemia

Increased release of calcium from bone
    Metastatic carcinoma to bone
    Primary hyperparathyroidism
    Multiple myeloma
    Sarcoidosis
    Tumorous release of PTH-like substance
    Hyperthyroidism
    Prolonged immobilization
Decreased urinary excretion of calcium
    Renal failure (secondary hyperparathyroidism)
    Thiazide diuretics
Increased GI absorption
    Excess vitamin D intake
    Sarcoidosis
    Hyperparathyroidism

Hypocalcemia

Nutritional syndromes
    Osteomalacia
    Rickets
    Malabsorption
Hypoalbuminemia
Hypoparathyroidisms

rickets may also have a low serum phosphorus level. Hyperphosphatemia may result from chronic renal failure, vitamin D excess, hypoparathyroidism, and some healing fractures. Children tend to have higher phosphorus levels than adults.

Immunological Studies

RHEUMATOID FACTORS

The rheumatoid factors (RF) are a family of immunoglobulins reactive with autologous immunoglobulin G (IgG). Although most of these anti-IgG autoantibodies are of the immunoglobulin M (IgM) class, RF belonging to most of the other classes have also been discovered. Traditional tests for RF search for IgM RF and are based upon agglutination of either sensitized sheep erythrocytes or antibody-coated latex particles. The sheep erythrocyte procedure appears to be a more specific test for rheumatoid arthritis than the latex method but is less sensitive. It has been shown that the combination of positive results for RF by both methods is highly specific for rheuma-

toid arthritis (12). More precise quantification of RF is possible through radioimmunoassay or enzyme-linked immunosorbent assay (ELISA); however, these sensitive methods are not yet widely available.

Because the RF in a patient can be of one or more antibody types, and because it is polyclonal in origin, it is not surprising that standard RF tests often fail to detect the presence of the antibody in patients with rheumatoid arthritis. Rheumatoid arthritis patients who have negative RF tests are said to be "seronegative." Some seronegative patients will convert to positive; however, this usually occurs during the 1st year of the disease. As more sensitive tests for rheumatoid factors are developed, the number of seronegative cases of rheumatoid arthritis will diminish. Another source of confusion is that RF is not specific for rheumatoid arthritis. Table 10.5 summarizes the more common disorders associated with the presence of RF. It should be noted that titers of RF tend to be higher in the rheumatic diseases than in the nonrheumatic disorders.

Rheumatoid arthritis seldom causes low back pain and almost never produces low back pain without concurrent symptomatic involvement of the peripheral joints and cervical spine. There is, therefore, no justification for ordering a rheumatoid factor test in a patient with isolated low back pain. It must also be realized that a positive rheumatoid factor test is neither the only, nor a mandatory, criterion for the diagnosis of rheumatoid arthritis (13).

Table 10.5.
Frequency of Rheumatoid Factor (RF)[a]
in Various Disorders

Condition	Percentage with +RF
Rheumatoid arthritis	75–80%
Systemic lupus erythematosus	30–50%
Progressive systemic sclerosis (scleroderma)	20–30%
Mixed connective tissue disease	20–30%
Hepatic cirrhosis	20–30%
Polymyositis/dermatomyostils	15–20%
Juvenile rheumatoid arthritis	10–15%
Normal subjects	3–15%[b]

[a]Measured by latex method; numbers are lower with sheep red blood cell method.

[b]The higher values are seen in the elderly and are usually associated with low titers of RF.

ANTINUCLEAR ANTIBODIES

Antinuclear antibodies (ANA) are autoantibodies directed against antigenic components of cell nuclei. These antibodies occur in many connective tissue diseases as well as a variety of other disorders. The standard ANA test, typically done by an immunofluorescent technique (IF-ANA, F-ANA), screens for the presence of many of the different ANA types, which can be further identified by specific testing. As shown in Figure 10.2, dozens of specific ANAs reactive with isolated cellular antigenic components have been described. Many of these autoantibodies are of research interest only at this time, while less than a dozen are of practical value for the physician.

Although the connective tissue disorders seldom cause isolated low back pain, the vague arthralgias accompanying many of the conditions often prompt the ordering of an arthritic laboratory profile, which usually includes an ANA test. Low back pain, by itself, is not an indication for ANA testing. The approximate incidence of ANA in various disorders is shown in Table 10.6.

Laboratories typically report the results of the ANA as both an antibody titer and the pattern of fluorescence. The latter is determined by the specific ANA interaction with the cell antigens and can be helpful, along with the clinical picture, in deciding which specific ANA assays should be ordered (Fig. 10.3).

HUMAN LEUKOCYTE ANTIGEN (HLA) SYSTEM

The HLA system, also referred to as the major histocompatibility complex (MHC), consists of a

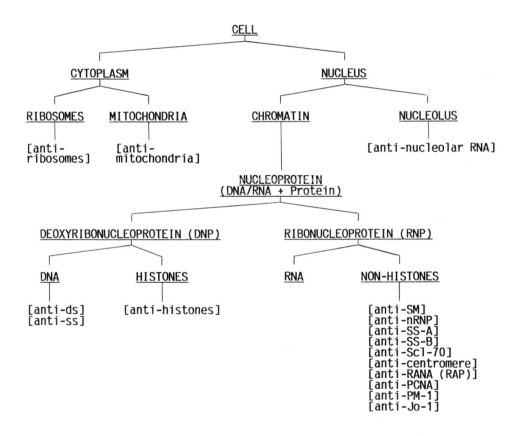

Abbreviations: PCNA = proliferating cell nuclear antigen; RANA = rheumatoid arthritis nuclear antigen; nRNP = nuclear ribonucleoprotein; RAP = rheumatoid arthritis precipitin; ds = double stranded; ss = single stranded

Figure 10.2. Autoantibodies in rheumatic diseases.

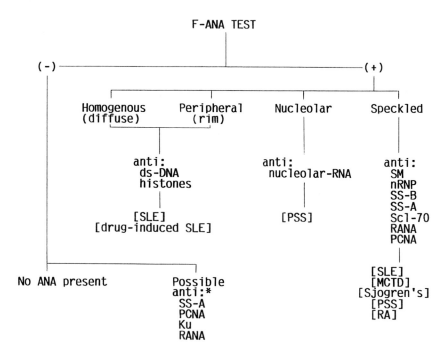

Figure 10.3. Patterns of ANA immunofluorescence.

series of genes on chromosome 6 which regulates the production of proteins, serving as antigenic markers on cell membranes and participating in important immune reactions. As can be seen in Figure 10.4, the MHC has several major categories, each of which has a series of numbered subcategories. Each parent contributes a haplotype, which means that the offspring will have up to two HLA antigens from each major category. Testing of peripheral blood lymphocytes establishes the HLA typing of an individual.

HLA-A, -B, and -C antigens are located on most nucleated cells in the body. HLA-D and -DR antigens are found primarily on lymphocytes and macrophages. The HLA system functions to regulate the immune response of the body, including the killing of viral-infected target cells by cytotoxic T lymphocytes, the recognition of foreign antigens, and the control of synthesis of comple-

Table 10.6.
Frequency of Antinuclear Antibodies (ANA)
in Various Disorders

Condition	Percentage with +ANA
Systemic lupus erythematosus	85–96%[a]
Mixed connective tissue disease	>95%
Progressive systemic sclerosis (scleroderma)	40–90%[a]
Rheumatoid arthritis	30–60%
Polymyositis/dermatomyositis	20–40%
Sjögren's syndrome	40–75%
Hepatic cirrhosis	15–20%
Elderly patients	10–20%[b]

[a]The higher values are obtained with HEp-2 substrate.
[b]Usually low titers.

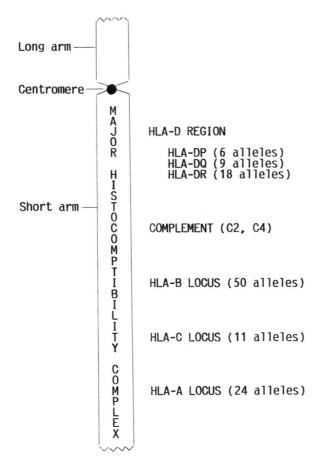

Long arm

Centromere

Short arm

MAJOR HISTOCOMPTIBILITY COMPLEX

HLA-D REGION

    HLA-DP (6 alleles)
    HLA-DQ (9 alleles)
    HLA-DR (18 alleles)

COMPLEMENT (C2, C4)

HLA-B LOCUS (50 alleles)

HLA-C LOCUS (11 alleles)

HLA-A LOCUS (24 alleles)

[note: because of re-classification, numbering of alleles is no longer consecutive]

Figure 10.4. The major histocompatibility complex (HLA system).

ment factors (14). In addition to the use of HLA typing in organ transplantation, it has become increasingly recognized that certain HLA types are associated with an increased frequency of disease states. Table 10.7 lists the rheumatic diseases that show a greater frequency of specific HLA types than is found in the normal population.

The association of HLA-B27 with ankylosing spondylitis initially led to its use as a screening test in patients with low back pain. More recently, however, it has been recognized that several factors prevent B27 testing from being an effective diagnostic test except in certain unusual circumstances. These factors include the occurrence of the B27 antigen in up to 10% of the normal population, variation in the distribution of the B27 type among various ethnic groups, the association of B27 with other seronegative types of sacroiliitis and spondylitis, and the increased frequency of B27 in asymptomatic relatives of patients with ankylosing spondylitis. HLA-B27 testing is of no value as a screening test in low back pain patients. Similarly, typing would contribute little information in the presence of obvious radiographic and clinical evidence of ankylosing spondylitis. At best, the test may prove helpful in cases where there are equivocal radiographic findings; a negative result in these cases would argue strongly against ankylosing spondylitis (15).

Table 10.7.
HLA Associations with Selected Rheumatic Diseases in Caucasians[a]

Disease	Associated Antigen	Antigen Frequency (%)	
		Disease Group	Controls
Ankylosing spondylitis	B27	96	4
Reiter's syndrome	B27	76	6
Reactive arthritis			
—Yersinia	B27	94	14[c]
—Salmonella	B27	94	14
—Shigella	B27	85	14
Rheumatoid arthritis	Dw4[b]	59	16
	DR4	70	28
Sjögren's disease	B8	58	21
	Dw3	69	10
Psoriatric arthropathy (peripheral arthropathy alone)	B27	24	7

[a]Adapted with permission from Dewar P: HLA antigens. *Clin Rheum Dis* 9:96–116, 1983.

[b]"w" denotes workshop designation.

[c]Variation in control frequency of identical antigen types due to different investigators.

LABORATORY EVALUATION OF SPECIFIC DISORDERS

Lumbar Spine and Sacroiliac Infections

Infections of the lumbar spine may involve either the intervertebral disc or the vertebral body. Discitis is primarily a concern in children because the vascular supply to the disc diminishes in the adult. Discitis in adults is usually a complication of surgical intervention or is secondary to vertebral body osteomyelitis.

Discitis in children is characterized by low back pain, difficulty in walking, local tenderness, and loss of spinal motion (16). Many, but not all, cases have constitutional symptoms, such as nausea, irritability, and fever. X-rays may not show diagnostic changes until several weeks into the disease process, so the more sensitive procedure of radionuclide bone scanning should be considered early. The white blood cell total and differential counts are often normal; however, the ESR is almost always elevated. Adult cases of discitis are often more difficult to diagnose because the condition typically follows lumbar disc surgery, and therefore there is often already some local discomfort. The most reliable indicator of a postoperative discitis is the ESR. The ESR is elevated in most postoperative patients during the 1st

week; however, its elevation 2 or more weeks after surgery should prompt further investigation (4, 17). Bone scans in this type of patient are not reliable because the procedure is not adequately sensitive in the early case and because discectomy itself may cause an abnormal scan. Magnetic resonance imaging appears to be sensitive to the vertebral end-plate abnormalities in these patients.

Vertebral osteomyelitis is most common in the thoracic and lumbar regions and is most often seen in patients with preexisting infections, especially involving the urinary tract. The onset of the disease is often subtle, and the diagnosis may not be made for several months. The patient typically complains of back pain, often with sciatica, and psoas muscle irritability is frequently found (1). With acute infections, the patient may be febrile and may have localized tenderness, redness, and warmth, whereas with chronic infections, fever and local findings other than tenderness are uncommon (18). Chronic vertebral osteomyelitis may occur as a sequela to an inadequately treated acute osteomyelitis or may occur as the result of an insidious infection with an organism of lower virulence. As with discitis, the white cell count is not a reliable indicator of infection, but the ESR is elevated in the majority of cases. Further evaluation of suspected cases of osteomyelitis consists of plain film radiography and radionuclide bone scanning. In acute osteomyelitis, there may be a lag of a week or more between the onset of symptoms and the development of plain film findings of vertebral destruction. During this radiographic latent period, technetium-99 bone imaging has high sensitivity, and if the scan is negative in the face of a strong clinical impression of osteomyelitis, a gallium-67 scan should be obtained (19, 20). In chronic osteomyelitis, the plain films frequently show abnormalities. Gallium and indium-111 scans are more sensitive in chronic osteomyelitis than the standard technetium bone scan.

Sacroiliac joint infections can mimic mechanical lesions of the low back, pelvis, and hip. As with vertebral osteomyelitis, sacroiliac infections may be the result of pyogenic organisms or a more insidious process, such as tuberculosis. Infection should be ruled out in all cases of unilateral sacroiliitis. Pain may be present in the low back, pelvis, and hip, and radicular symptoms are common, along with difficulty in weight bearing and pain upon joint compression (21). Children with sacroiliac joint infection complain of hip, thigh, and buttock pain, and often have a positive Patrick's test as well as a painful limp (22). Almost all cases of sacroiliac infection, whether in adults or children, have an elevated ESR. As with vertebral infections, the white blood cell count is unreliable. CT scanning is of particular value in the diagnosis of sacroiliac joint infection.

Multiple Myeloma

Multiple myeloma is a hematologic malignancy characterized by the monoclonal proliferation of plasma cells and the resultant hypersecretion of immunoglobulins and their subunits. The disease occurs after age 30, with most cases found in the 6th and later decades. The replacement of normal bone marrow with neoplastic cells, the alteration of normal ratios of immunoglobulin synthesis by plasma cells, the secretion of an osteoclast activation factor, and the damaging effects of immunoglobulin fragments on renal cells result in anemia, abnormal serum and urine protein levels, increased susceptibility to infections, osteolytic lesions, and impairment of renal function (23).

The most common presenting symptom of myeloma is bone pain. Any bone containing marrow is susceptible, with vertebral involvement being quite common, especially in the thoracic and lumbar areas. Plain film radiographs of the area may reveal classic multiple osteolytic lesions, but they are also likely to simply show osteopenia and are frequently entirely normal in early cases.

Clinical laboratory abnormalities occur before the osseous lesions become radiographically evident. Thus, unexplained bone pain in the middle-aged and older patient should prompt the ordering of appropriate blood and urine studies. The increased synthesis of immunoglobulins by the proliferating plasma cells produces quantitative and qualitative abnormalities in the plasma proteins. As shown in Figure 10.5, these changes may be detected by several methods.

A routine chemistry panel might show elevations in the total protein and globulin levels; however, hypergammaglobulinemia is nonspecific. It is best to pursue any case of hypergammaglobulinemia with serum protein electrophoresis, which allows for a determination of which type of globulin is responsible for the elevation. The pattern of electrophoresis is extremely helpful in evaluating globulin elevations. Conditions that cause stimulation of multiple clones of plasma cells produce a "polyclonal gammopathy" in which there is a diffuse elevation of several antibody types. Such elevations are seen in chronic infections, connective tissue diseases, sarcoidosis, chronic liver disease, and some lymphomas (Fig. 10.6).

Multiple myeloma, in contrast, produces a monoclonal gammopathy that is revealed on protein electrophoresis as a narrow, homogeneous peak in the γ or β region. This finding would then be followed by serum immunoelectrophoresis, which will identify the specific type of immunoglobulin present and verify the monoclonal nature of the gammopathy. Light chains can also be assessed at this time. Most cases of multiple myeloma are IgG, with a lesser number being IgA.

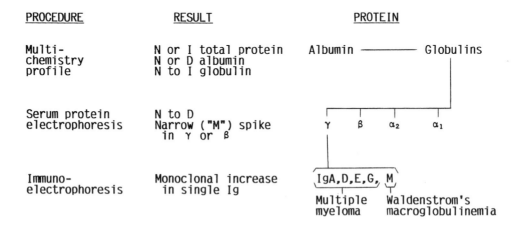

[N = normal; D = decreased; I = increased]

Figure 10.5.   Serum protein evaluation in plasma cell dyscrasias.

HYPERGAMMAGLOBULINEMIA

SERUM PROTEIN ELECTROPHORESIS

POLYCLONAL GAMMOPATHIES

Connective tissue diseases
Chronic infections
Sarcoidosis
Chronic liver disease
Lymphomas

MONOCLONAL GAMMOPATHIES

Multiple myeloma
Waldenstrom's macroglobulinemia
Heavy chain disease
Some carcinomas
Plasma cell dyscrasia
 of unknown signficance
 ("benign monoclonal
  gammopathy")

Figure 10.6. Serum gamma-globulin electrophoretic patterns.

Less than 5% are IgD, and only a few cases of IgE myeloma have been reported. An IgM monoclonal gammopathy is characteristic of Waldenström's macroglobulinemia.

Excess production of free light chain portions of the immunoglobulins is common in multiple myeloma. These light chains (Bence Jones protein) are rapidly cleared by the kidney and can be demonstrated by immunoelectrophoresis to be present in the urine (Fig. 10.7). Heat testing for Bence Jones protein is insensitive and obsolete. Some types of Bence Jones protein can cause renal tubular damage. Because 15 to 20% of the cases of multiple myeloma produce only light chains rather than complete immunoglobulins, if the clinical suspicion of myeloma is raised, urine immunoelectrophoresis should be ordered along with the serum protein electrophoresis to ensure detection of almost all cases of myeloma.

The secretion of osteoclast activation factor by the malignant plasma cells results in the lytic changes in bone and is accompanied by hypercalcemia in many cases. Alkaline phosphatase levels usually remain normal because of the lack of osteoblast activity. Bone scans are often normal for this same reason.

Suppression of erythropoiesis results in a normocytic anemia in most patients. The production

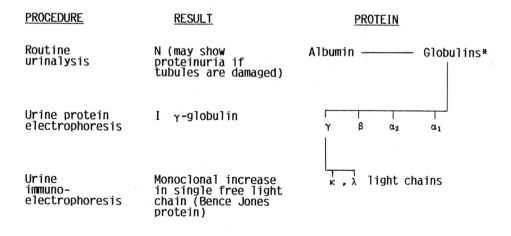

PROCEDURE	RESULT	PROTEIN
Routine urinalysis	N (may show proteinuria if tubules are damaged)	Albumin ———— Globulins*
Urine protein electrophoresis	I γ-globulin	γ β α₂ α₁
Urine immuno-electrophoresis	Monoclonal increase in single free light chain (Bence Jones protein)	κ , λ light chains

[N = normal; I = increased]
*dipstick method not sensitive to globulins

Figure 10.7. Urine protein evaluation in multiple myeloma.

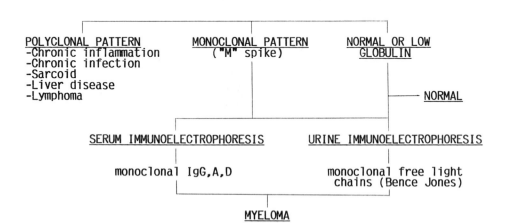

Figure 10.8. Sequence of evaluation in multiple myeloma.

of abnormal immunoglobulins causes the red blood cells to tend to clump together (rouleau), and this causes the ESR to increase (Table 10.8).

Figure 10.8 summarizes the diagnostic evaluation of multiple myeloma. Although the diagnosis of multiple myeloma is fairly straightforward in the middle-aged or older patient with bone pain, bony lesions on x-ray, anemia, or increased ESR, and a monoclonal gammopathy, there is still a need for confirmation by means of bone marrow evaluation. As shown in Figure 10.6, there are other causes of a monoclonal gammopathy, and consultation with a hematologist is recommended.

Metastatic Carcinoma

Because of the extensive vascular network of the spine, metastatic disease of the vertebra is a relatively common occurrence. Besides bone pain, clinical findings may include pathological compression deformity and osteoblastic and osteolytic lesions. The alkaline phosphatase level may be elevated in osteolytic as well as osteoblastic lesions, although it is more consistently and markedly elevated in the latter. Lytic lesions may also cause the serum calcium level to rise. The ESR may be increased, but it is not sensitive enough to be relied upon in the decision process. Radionuclide bone scanning is sensitive to malignant change and is an important means of differentiating the bony involvement from that due to osteomalacia, osteoporosis, multiple myeloma, and other osseous disorders.

Table 10.8.
Common Hematologic Findings in Multiple Myeloma

Normocytic, normochromic anemia
Norma or decreased recitulocyte count
Rouleaux
Elevated erythrocyte sedimentation rate
Normal or low total white blood cell count
Normal differential count or relative lymphocytosis

Metabolic Disorders

A number of metabolic disorders may produce orthopedic complaints. *Osteomalacia* is the adult version of rickets, in which there is defective bone mineralization due to disturbances in the vitamin D pathway (e.g., vitamin D deficiency or malabsorption), hypophosphatemia (e.g., malnutrition or malabsorption), or calcium deficiency. Symptoms of osteomalacia include bone pain and pelvic girdle muscle weakness. X-rays may show diffuse osteopenia, which must be clinically differentiated from other causes of such (Table 10.9). Compression deformities of the vertebrae may occur. The presence of pseudofractures in the ribs, pelvis, or femurs would indicate osteomalacia rather than osteoporosis. Serum studies may show the calcium and phosphorus levels to be low-normal, and the alkaline phosphatase is usually elevated. Specific assays of the various forms of vitamin D are available.

Primary *osteoporosis*, in contrast, is characterized by normal levels of the serum calcium, phosphorus, and alkaline phosphatase. The ESR will also be normal in simple primary osteoporosis. *Hyperparathyroidism* is an unusual cause of back pain because most cases are detected before compression deformities can occur. In hyperparathyroidism due to a parathyroid tumor or hyperplasia (primary hyperparathyroidism), the serum calcium level becomes elevated, while the phosphorus level drops. Measurement of the serum parathyroid hormone (PTH) level is important. *Cushing's syndrome* is hypercortisolism resulting from iatrogenic steroid excess, a pituitary lesion causing excessive ACTH secretion (Cushing's disease), or an adrenal adenoma. The primary orthopedic complication is the development of osteoporosis and vertebral compression fractures. Most of these patients will also be obese and hypertensive. If hypercortisolism is suspected, the initial test of choice is a 24-hour measurement of urine free cortisol, which will show elevated levels in most Cushing's patients.

Inflammatory Lumbar and Sacroiliac Disorders

Several inflammatory diseases, collectively referred to as spondyloarthropathies, affect the spine and pelvis. These conditions include ankylosing spondylitis, reactive arthritis (Reiter's syndrome), enteropathic arthritis, and psoriatic arthritis. Many of these patients will be HLA-B27-positive, and it has been suggested that the HLA-B27 antigen somehow makes an individual susceptible to infection with an arthritogenic organism (24). It is apparent that the process is multifactorial because, as previously pointed out, ankylosing spondylitis and the other spondyloarthropathies may occur in the absence of the HLA-B27 antigen. Clinical indicators of an inflammatory disease process include chronic low back pain of insidious onset in a young patient, morning stiffness, and relief of symptoms with exercise. In the absence of symptoms of inflammatory bowel disease (enteropathic arthritis), a personal or family history of psoriasis (psoriatic arthritis), or a recent episode of urethritis, cervicitis, conjunctivitis, or oral mucosal lesions (Reiter's syndrome), ankylosing spondylitis is the most likely diagnosis. Diagnostic emphasis is placed upon the plain film radiographs and, to a lesser extent, on bone scanning. As mentioned previously, HLA-B27 testing is of little value in the diagnostic evaluation of sacroiliitis and low back pain.

Polymyalgia Rheumatica

Polymyalgia rheumatica is a clinical syndrome of unknown etiology which is characterized by muscle pain in the shoulder and pelvic girdles, constitutional symptoms, an elevated erythrocyte sedimentation rate, and a high incidence of temporal arteritis. It is primarily a disease of the elderly, with occurrence in patients less than 50 years of age being quite rare. Most patients have aching, tenderness, and stiffness in the neck and shoulders. Other patients may have hip and thigh symptoms, as well as low back pain. Although the onset is often sudden, in other cases it is gradual and the patient may initially be treated for a diagnosis of fibromyalgia for weeks to months. Patients may complain of vague constitutional

Table 10.9.
Causes of Osteopenia

Osteomalacia
Osteoporosis
  Primary
  Endocrine related (e.g., Cushing's syndrome,
    hyperparathyroidism, hyperthyroidism)
Multiple myeloma
Metastatic lytic carcinoma

symptoms such as fatigue, low-grade fever, and anorexia (25). Although the symptoms of polymyalgia rheumatica may cause disability, of greater concern is the temporal arteritis (giant cell arteritis) that so often accompanies the disease. The arteritis, in addition to causing headache and local tenderness, may result in loss of vision, cerebral ischemia, and jaw claudication. In almost all cases of polymyalgia rheumatica, the sedimentation rate is elevated. If the clinical suspicion of the condition is slight, then a normal ESR rules out the diagnosis; however, if the suspicion is strong, a normal ESR should not preclude further investigation (26).

Polymyositis

Polymyositis is an inflammatory muscle disease producing weakness in the shoulder and pelvic girdles. Clinical features include progressive proximal muscle weakness, difficulty in ambulation, and minimal pain or tenderness (unlike polymyalgia rheumatica). A skin rash may occur on the face and hands (dermatomyositis). Although low back pain is not present, the condition is considered in the differential diagnosis of lower extremity weakness. The diagnosis is based on the symmetrical involvement of the proximal muscles, abnormal serum levels of the muscle enzymes (creatine kinase, aspartate aminotransferase (SGOT), and lactic dehydrogenase), and a characteristic electromyogram (27). Specific antinuclear antibodies (ANAs) have been found, including PM-1 and Jo-1, but the sensitivity of these has varied, and they have not been widely adopted for clinical use.

Acquired Immunodeficiency Syndrome (AIDS)

AIDS is a disease of the immune system caused by the human immunodeficiency virus (HIV). Infected persons are susceptible to opportunistic infection from several organisms and may manifest symptoms from both the primary HIV infection and the secondary infection. Of particular importance to the chiropractic physician is the high frequency of musculoskeletal complaints in HIV-infected persons, with some type of rheumatic manifestation in 75% of these patients. A frank arthritis affecting one or more joints occurs in about 10% of HIV-infected patients, and intermittent or acute arthralgias occur in almost 45%

(28). Involvement of the knees is most common, followed in order of frequency by the shoulders, elbows, ankles, neck, wrists, sacroiliac joints, hips, hands, feet, and lumbar spine. An increased incidence of Reiter's syndrome has been noted to occur and may be the result of the immunosuppression allowing for infection with arthritogenic organisms. Testing for HIV infection should be considered in male homosexuals, hemophilics, intravenous drug users, or other high-risk individuals who complain of joint pain.

Lyme Disease

Lyme disease is a newly recognized arthritic disorder, being named after an outbreak of recurrent joint pain in many residents of Old Lyme, Connecticut, in 1975. Since that time, the disease has been reported across the United States, particularly in the upper midwest and northeast. The disease is attributed to infection by a spirochete (*Borrelia burgdorferi*) transmitted through the bite of a tick. In most patients, the disease is heralded by a slowly enlarging annular skin lesion (erythema chronicum migrans) developing at the site of innoculation, accompanied by malaise, headache, arthralgias, and fever. Back pain occurs in about one-fourth of the patients (29). The rash and constitutional symptoms last about a month if untreated, but may recur. Over the next several months (perhaps years), the patient may experience recurrent arthralgias, heart block, and neurological abnormalities. In about 10% of the patients, there is the development of a chronic knee arthritis.

Early in the course of Lyme disease, at a point when backache occurs, there may be elevation of the ESR. The diagnosis is based upon an elevated antibody titer to the Lyme agent. Treatment with tetracyclines or penicillin markedly reduces the duration of the rash and usually prevents development of the subsequent arthritis and cardiac involvement.

Paget's Disease

Paget's disease (osteiitis deformans) is characterized by abnormal structural arrangement of bone in which there is disorganized activity of the osteoblasts and osteoclasts. This condition is of unknown etiology and primarily affects elderly patients. The disease progresses through stages of excessive bone resorption and excessive bone formation. The majority of patients are asymptomatic, with their disease discovered incidentally in the evaluation of another complaint. Although low back pain is classically described as a common feature of Paget's disease, it appears that the pain is most often due to an accompanying osteoarthritis rather than to the pagetic process itself (30). Laboratory evaluation shows the serum alkaline phosphatase level to be markedly elevated. If a patient with known Paget's disease develops increased pain and a sudden rise in the already elevated alkaline phosphatase level, the development of a sacroma should be suspected.

Infective Endocarditis

Subacute infective endocarditis is an infection, usually bacterial, of the endocardium in patients with an existing cardiac defect. The development of symptoms is often quite insidious, and the diagnosis may not be made for weeks or months. The classic features of subacute endocarditis, consisting of low-grade fever, anorexia, murmur, and embolic phenomena, are well known by physicians, but often unappreciated is the frequent occurrence of musculoskeletal complaints. As many as one-fourth of patients with subacute endocarditis have low back pain, and in many this is the presenting complaint (31, 32). X-rays of the area usually are negative. The ESR is almost always elevated, whereas the white blood cell count is often normal. The diagnosis is usually confirmed by blood cultures.

References

1. Ross PM, Fleming JL: Vertebral body osteomyelitis. *Clin Orthop* 118:190–198, 1976.
2. Frederickson B, Yuan H, Olans R: Management and outcome of pyogenic vertebral osteomyelitis. *Clin Orthop* 131:160–167, 1978.
3. Paus B: Tumour, tuberculosis and osteomyelitis of the spine. *Acta Orthop Scand* 44:372–382, 1973.
4. Bircher MD, Tasker T, Crawshaw C, Mulholland RC: Discitis following lumbar surgery. *Spine* 13:98–102, 1988.
5. Nashel DJ, Petrone DL, Ulmer CC, Sliwinski AJ: C-reactive protein: a marker for disease activity in ankylosing spondylitis and Reiter's syndrome. *J Rheumatol* 13:364–367, 1986.
6. Griffiths J, Black J: Separation and identification of alkaline phosphatase isoenzymes and isoforms in serum of healthy persons by isoelectric focusing. *Clin Chem* 33:2171–2177, 1987.
7. Wolf PL: Clinical significance of an increased or decreased serum alkaline phosphatase level. *Arch Pathol Lab Med* 102:497–501, 1978.
8. Mayne PD, Thakrar S, Rosalki SB, Foo AY, Sparbhoo S: Identification of bone and liver metastases from breast cancer by measurement of plasma alkaline phosphatase isoenzyme activity. *J Clin Pathol* 40:398–403, 1987.
9. Kaplan LA, Chen I, Sperling M, Bracken B, Stein EA: Clinical utility of serum prostatic acid phosphatase measurements for detection (screening), diagnosis, and therapeutic monitoring of prostatic carcinoma; assessment of monoclonal and polyclonal enzymes and radioimmunoassays. *Am J Clin Pathol* 84:334–339, 1985.
10. Wells DJ, Bennett BD, Gardner WA: Uses and limitations of prostate-specific antigen in the laboratory diagnosis of prostate cancer. *South Med J* 81:218–220, 1988.
11. Scott JT: Uric acid and the interpretation of hyperuricaemia. *Clin Rheum Dis* 9:241–255, 1983.
12. Goodman LA, Pisko EJ, Foster SL, Turner RA, Panetti M, Semble EL: Analysis of combined rheumatoid factor determinations by the rheumatoid arthritis latex and sheep cell agglutination tests and the American Rheumatism Association criteria for rheumatoid arthritis. *J Rheumatol* 14:234–239, 1987.
13. Rheumatoid Arthritis Criteria Subcommittee of the Diagnostic and Therapeutic Criteria Committee of the ARA: The American Rheumatism Association 1987 revised criteria for the classification of rheumatoid arthritis. *Arthritis Rheum* 31:315–324, 1988.
14. Schiffenbauer J, Schwartz B: The HLA complex and its relationship to rheumatic diseases. *Rheum Dis Clin North Am* 13:463–485, 1987.
15. Hollingsworth PN, Owen ET, Dawkins RL: Correlation of HLA B27 with radiographic abnormalities of the sacroiliac joints and with other stigmata of ankylosing spondylitis. *Clin Rheum Dis* 9:307–322, 1983.
16. Moskal MJ, Villar LA: Childhood diskitis: report of 2 cases and review of the literature. *J Am Osteopath Assoc* 86:170–174, 1986.
17. Kornberg M: Erythrocyte sedimentation rate following lumbar discectomy. *Spine* 11:766–767, 1986.
18. Wheat J: Diagnostic strategies in osteomyelitis. *Am J Med* 78(Suppl 6B):218–224, 1985.
19. David R, Barrow BJ, Madewell JE: Osteomyelitis, acute and chronic. *Radiol Clin North Am* 25:1171–1201, 1987.
20. Merkel KD, Fitzgerald RH Jr, Brown ML: Scintigraphic evaluation in musculoskeletal sepsis. *Orthop Clin North Am* 15:401–416, 1984.
21. Pouchot J, Vinceneux P, Barge J, et al.: Tuberculosis of the sacroiliac joint, outcome, and evaluation of closed needle biopsy in 11 consecutive cases. *Am J Med* 84:622–628, 1988.

22. Reilly JP, Gross RH, Emans JB, Yngve DA: Disorders of the sacro-iliac joint in children. *J Bone Joint Surg* 70A:31–40, 1988.

23. Osserman EF, Merlini G, Butler VP: Multiple myeloma and related plasma cell dyscrasias. *JAMA* 258:2930–2937, 1987.

24. McGuigan LE, Geczy AF, Edmonds JP: The immunopathology of ankylosing spondylitis—a review. *Semin Arthritis Rheum* 15:81–105, 1985.

25. Allen NB, Studenski SA: Polymyalgia rheumatica and temporal arteritis. *Med Clin North Am* 70:369–384, 1986.

26. Sox HC, Liang MH: The erythrocyte sedimentation rate: guidelines for rational use. *Ann Intern Med* 104:515–523, 1986.

27. Hochberg MC, Feldman D, Stevens MB: Adult onset polymyositis/dermatomyositis: an analysis of clinical and laboratory features and survival in 76 patients with a review of the literature. *Semin Arthritis Rheum* 15:168–178, 1986.

28. Berman A, Espinoza LR, Diaz JD, et al.: Rheumatic manifestations of human immunodeficiency virus infection. *Am J Med* 85:59–64, 1988.

29. Goldings EA, Jericho J: Lyme disease. *Clin Rheum Dis* 12:342–367, 1986.

30. Altman RD, Brown M, Gargano F: Low back pain in Paget's disease of bone. *Clin Orthop* 217:152–161, 1987.

31. Churchill MA, Geraci JE, Hunder GG: Musculoskeletal manifestations of bacterial endocarditis. *Ann Intern Med* 87:754–759, 1977.

32. Harkonen MI, Olin PE, Wennstrom J: Severe backache as a presenting sign of bacterial endocarditis. *Acta Med Scand* 210:329–331, 1981.

11

Facet Syndrome

James M. Cox, D.C., D.A.C.B.R.

Through education I learn to do by choice what other men do by constraints of fear.

—Aristotle

To start this chapter, which deals with probably the single most common factor seen in chiropractic practice with low back pain patients, a discussion of the biomechanics of the posterior elements of the lumbar spine is offered.

Superimposed loads on the lumbar spine are borne by the body-disc-body anteriorly and by the two articular facets posteriorly; ligaments provide stability for the posterior elements and the intervertebral disc. It is obvious that weight distribution on these elements changes with degenerative disc disease, in which narrowing of the disc places disproportionately more weight on the articular facets.

COMPRESSIVE FORCES ACTING ON THE ARTICULAR JOINTS

The compressive force passing through the posterior column (articular facet joints) has been obtained by taking the area of the inferior articular facets. The vertebral body surface area gradually increases from T5 to L4, indicating increased weight bearing by the anterior column from above downward. The L5 vertebral body is significantly smaller than that of L4, indicating that compressive force is diverted before reaching the L5 inferior surface (1).

The mean articular facet area increases suddenly at L4 and L5 as compared to the upper lumbar levels, indicating that there is more compressive force at the articular facets in the lower than in the upper lumbar spine (Table 11.1). Transfer of part of the compressive force from the anterior to the posterior column is suggested. The increased transfer of weight through the pedicles at L5, which is an area of forward and downward inclination of forces as L5 sits on the sacrum at an inclined plane, has been offered as an explanation for the stress leading to fracture of the pars interarticularis (spondylolysis) and resultant spondylolisthesis.

Disc versus Facet Compressive Weight Bearing

It is important to know, under compressive loading, how much weight is born by the articular facets versus the intervertebral disc. The percentage of weight-bearing compressive load transmitted through the articular facets, in persons with normal intervertebral discs, no evidence of degeneration, and a slightly flattened lumbar lordosis (Fig. 11.1), has been measured at 16% in two studies (1, 2) and between 3 and 25% in another (3). Morris (4) states that 70% of the superimposed body weight is carried on the vertebral bodies and 30% on the articular facets. Fiorini (5) concluded that 12% of the weight bearing was on the facets.

In degenerative disc disease, the articular weight bearing is as high as 47% (3) or up to 70% (2). Much of this abnormally high resistance is due to extraarticular impingement of the facet tips on the adjacent lamina or pedicle, and the apophyseal joints show gross osteoarthritic changes. It is possible that the joint capsule is nipped by such high stress placed on the tips of the articular facets. This may explain why standing for long periods can produce

Table 11.1.
Percentage Area of Body and Articular Facets at Various Vertebral Levels

Vertebral Levels	Total Area (Body + Facets)		Body Area		Area of Two Articular Facets	
	cm²	%	cm²	%	cm²	%
T₅	7.00	100	5.34	76.28	1.66	23.71
T₈	9.32	100	7.30	78.32	2.02	21.68
T₉	10.11	100	7.91	78.23	2.20	21.76
T₁₁	10.92	100	8.82	80.76	2.10	19.23
T₁₂	12.04	100	10.24	85.04	1.80	14.95
L₁	13.66	100	11.46	83.89	2.20	16.10
L₃	16.84	100	13.82	82.06	3.02	17.93
L₄	17.55	100	14.17	80.74	3.38	19.25
L₅	17.93	100	14.07	78.47	3.86	21.52

Percentage Area of Body and Cross-Sectional Area of Lamina at Various Vertebral Levels

Vertebral Levels	Total Area (Body + Lamina)		Body Area		Area of Lamina	
	cm²	%	cm²	%	cm²	%
T₅	6.59	100	5.34	81.03	1.25	18.96
T₈	8.73	100	7.30	83.61	1.43	16.38
T₉	9.51	100	7.91	83.17	1.50	15.77
T₁₁	10.10	100	8.82	87.32	1.28	12.67
T₁₂	11.49	100	1.24	89.12	1.25	10.87
L₁	12.88	100	11.46	88.97	1.42	11.02
L₃	15.61	100	13.82	88.53	1.79	11.46
L₄	16.43	100	14.17	86.24	2.26	13.75
L₅	17.08	100	14.07	82.37	3.01	17.62

ᵃFrom Pal GP, Routal RV: Transmission of weight through the lower thoracic and lumbar regions of the vertebral column in man. *J Anat* 152:98, 1987. Reproduced with the permission of Cambridge University Press.

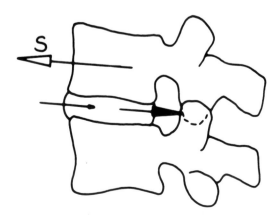

Figure 11.1. Schematic drawing of a lumbar spine having normal disc spaces and normal compressive weight bearing on the anterior and posterior columns of the spine. (Reproduced with permission from Adams MA, Hutton WC: The mechanical function of the lumbar apophyseal joints. *Spine* 8(3):328, 1983.)

a dull ache in the low back which is relieved by sitting or by using some device, such as a bar rail, to rest one foot upon, to induce slight flexion of the lumbar spine (2). This contact between facet tip and lamina is labeled in chiropractic as a facet-lamina syndrome.

It is shown that if the lumbar spine is slightly flattened (as occurs in erect sitting or heavy lifting), all the intervertebral compressive force is resisted by the disc. However, when lordotic postures, such as erect standing, are held for long periods, the facet tips do make contact with the laminae of the subjacent vertebra and bear about one-sixth of the compressive force (Fig. 11.2) (2).

Simulation of Triple Joint Complex in Laboratory

A two-dimensional biomechanical model was assembled using two rigid bodies as the vertebrae

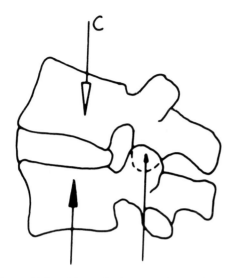

Figure 11.2. Schematic drawing of a lumbar spine with intervertebral disc space thinning and increased articular joint weight bearing. (Reproduced with permission from Adams MA, Hutton WC: The mechanical function of the lumbar apophyseal joints. *Spine* 8(3): 328, 1983.)

and six elastic springs to represent the tissues of the disc and posterior elements. Compression loads were inflicted, and the following facts were determined (6):

1. The apophyseal joints are not loaded heavily by compression or flexion-extension loads but can be heavily loaded by anteroposterior shear loads.

2. Resistances developed by the apophyseal joints are not very effective in relieving loads on the intervertebral disc when the motion segment is compressed, but they can be effective in relieving the disc when the segment is flexed, extended, or anteroposteriorly sheared.

3. In response to anteroposterior shear loads, the location of the facet joints relative to that of the intervertebral disc in the superior-inferior direction is a major determinant of what loads each structure will bear.

Under compressive load, the highest compressive strains were recorded near the bases of pedicles and on the superficial and deep surfaces of the partes interarticulares; the loads were increased by extension (7). It is possible that extension movement is limited by the bony contact of the facet joints (2).

Rotational Stresses on the Disc and Facet

In shear stress applied to the intervertebral joint, two-thirds of the stress is born by the disc and one-third by the facets.

Normal intervertebral discs fail completely at 22.6° of rotation when studied in cadaveric studies, while in real life they can tolerate only 5° of rotation without damage (8). The lumbar apophyseal joints function to allow limited movement between vertebrae and to protect the discs from shear forces, excessive flexion, and axial rotation. They are not well designed to resist compression, and this is normally born by the disc (2).

Unequal Facet Loading Leads to Unequal Degeneration

Panjabi (9) presents the following algorithm of the stages of injury to the functional spinal unit (FSU):

1. Asymmetric disc injury at one FSU level;
2. Disturbed kinematics of FSUs above and below this level;
3. Asymmetric movements at facet joints;
4. Unequal sharing of facet loads;
5. High load on one facet joint resulting in intraarticular cartilage degeneration, joint space narrowing, and facet atrophy (arthrosis).

Figures 11.3 and 11.4 are common radiographic findings in a daily chiropractic practice. The slight rotational, lateral flexion subluxation of a lumbar vertebra with unilateral disc degeneration results in greater facet loading on the concave side of the subluxation, and the resultant degenerative changes are seen in the triple joint complex at the facet.

Facet Subluxation in Unequal Weight Distribution

Hadley's "S" line allows visualization of facet disrelationships and is especially beneficial in evaluating oblique views of the lumbar spine and, to a lesser extent, anteroposterior views. Figures 11.5 through 11.8 schematically and radiographically show how these lines are established. The Hadley "S" curve is formed by tracing a line along the undersurface of the transverse process at the superior process and bringing this down the infe-

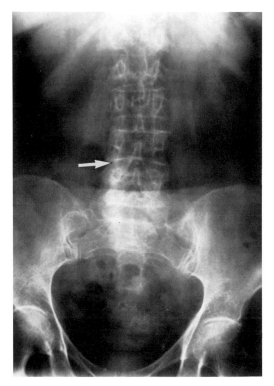

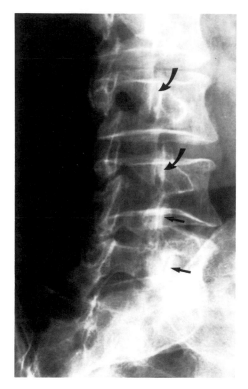

Figure 11.3. An anteroposterior projection of a lumbar spine with a slight dextrorotation and lateral flexion subluxation of the L4 vertebral body on L5 and L3 on L4, resulting in increased weight bearing on the left articular facet joints (*arrow*) compared to the right.

Figure 11.4. An oblique projection shows the narrowed intraarticular joint space, subchondral sclerosis, and facet imbrication at the L4 and L5 levels where increased weight bearing has taken place for a period of time (*straight arrows*). Compare these changes with the more normal joints above at L3 and L2 (*curved arrows*).

rior articular process to the top of the superior articular surface; this is joined by a line traced upward from the base of the superior articular process of the inferior vertebra to the lower edge of its articular surface. These lines should join to form a smooth S. If the S is broken, subluxation is present (10).

PAIN SENSITIVITY OF THE FACET SYNOVIAL LINED JOINT

Pressure-sensitive recording paper was placed between the facet facings, and the pressure between the facets was measured. This was done on 12 pairs of facet joints, and it was found that narrowing the

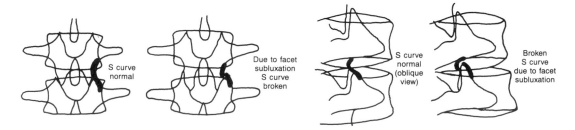

Figure 11.5. The "S" lines of Hadley are shown for determining the facet subluxation that occurs when increased weight bearing is placed on a facet joint. (Adapted from Yochum TR, Rowe L: *Essentials of Skeletal Radiology*. Baltimore, Williams & Wilkins, 1987, p 192.)

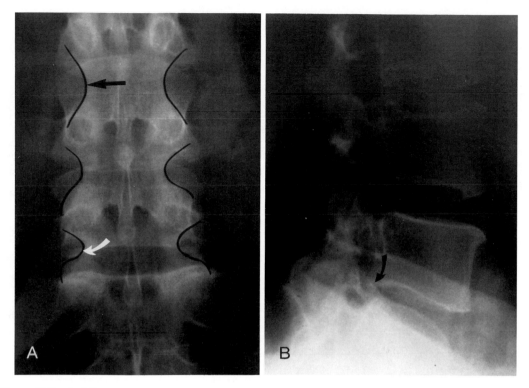

Figure 11.6. **A**, "S" lines are shown on an anteroposterior radiograph of the lumbar spine which reveals normal (*straight arrow*) and broken "S" lines (*curved arrow*). **B**, Lateral view of **A** shows the retrolisthesis (*arrow*) of L5 accompanying the Hadley "S" line changes.

disc space and increasing the angles of extension caused an increase in pressure or impingement on the facet joint surfaces (11). Stretching of the joint capsule (or transmission of load across it) may be a source of pain due to the presence of a nociceptive type IV receptor system (12).

Histological study of sectioned zygapophyseal joints indicates the presence of an extensive vascular supply to the articular cartilage in a joint that shows minor osteoarthrosis. The anatomy of a vascular synovial inclusion of the type seen in most lumbosacral zygapophyseal joints is clearly demonstrated. Since vascular structures may be related to pain, this may explain spinal pain of zygapophyseal origin (13).

The capsule of the articular facets is richly innervated with sensory fibers, according to von Luschka (14). The posterior primary division of the spinal nerve and the recurrent nerve of the anterior primary division innervate the capsule. This sensory nerve supply is sufficiently developed to support the hypothesis that irritation of the capsule of the lumbar articular facets could well produce pain stimuli which could return to the central nervous system through the posterior primary division and produce referred pain through the dermatomes of the involved nerves, which correspond exactly with the pathway of sciatic radiation, namely, the fourth and fifth nerves.

The synovial folds of the lumbar zygapophyseal joints are innervated by nerves ranging from 1.6 to 12 μm in diameter, with the number of fibers ranging from 1 to 5. They run a course separate from blood vessels, indicating that they are afferent nerves that probably have a nociceptive function (15).

Ghormley (16), in his classic paper, stated that there was ample evidence to regard facets as a cause of sciatic pain. He used the term *facet syndrome* to describe the sudden onset of low back pain brought on by some activity usually involving a twisting or rotatory strain of the lumbosacral region.

Facet joints are subject to abnormal stresses following disc degeneration. The normal pedicle-facet complex with a normal intervertebral disc carries 20% of the vertical pressure applied at the inter-

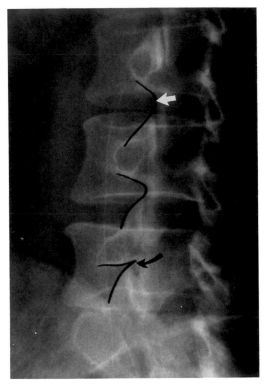

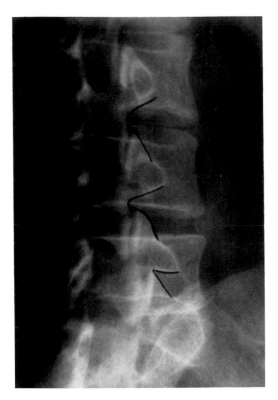

Figure 11.7. Right anterior oblique view of the lumbar spine shows normal (*straight arrow*) and abnormal (*curved arrow*) "S" lines.

Figure 11.8. Left anterior oblique view of the lumbar spine shows normal and abnormal "S" lines.

space, and this constitutes 10 times the weight per square inch applied to the knee joints (17).

Uneven apophyseal joint spaces, from right compared to left or vertically adjacent, indicate disc damage, instability, or possible bulge. Facet override is a finding in disc lesion (18).

FLEXION AND EXTENSION EFFECTS ON FACET LOADING

Under axial compression force, the location of the segmental mechanical balance point shifts posteriorly as the facets come into contact.

In coupled flexion rotation, under axial compression, each facet carries a negligible percentage of compression which remains nearly constant as applied force increases.

The contact forces developed at the facet articulation increase considerably with extension rotation. For example, the addition of up to 5.6° of extension rotation increases the load on each facet from 10 to 30% of the compression preload.

Large flexion loadings similar to those ex-

pected during heavy lifting, as well as large extension loadings, are likely to be related to facet injury and degeneration.

The transfer of forces from one facet to the adjacent one occurs through different areas in flexion and in extension postures. That is, on the articular surface, the contact area shifts from the upper and central regions in flexion to the inferior tip in extension (19).

The anteromedial region of the zygapophyseal joints has been shown to be the primary site of degenerative change (20).

RADIOGRAPHIC CONCEPTS OF FACET SYNDROME

Two studies done by Cox et al. (21, 22) reveal that 26% of patients with low back pain have facet syndrome either alone or in conjunction with other findings. The exact amount of low back pain caused by the facet syndrome is still unknown. A close look at the stresses imposed on the lumbosacral articulation by facet syndrome should, therefore, be of great importance to the chiropractic physician treating this condition.

Figure 11.9 is a radiograph of a patient suspected to have facet syndrome. There is posterior narrowing of the L5-S1 intervertebral disc space compared with the anterior disc space, and imbrication of the first sacral facet into the upper third of the intervertebral foramen at L5-S1, resulting in apparent vertical stenosis of the L5-S1 foramen as compared to the adjacent levels.

Figure 11.10 shows the lines of Macnab (23) identifying the hyperextension subluxation of L5 on the sacrum, with the tip of the superior facet of the sacrum imbricating above the line drawn along the inferior plate of L5. The telescoping of the superior sacral facet into the intervertebral foramen at L5-S1 creates vertical stenosis of the foramen. Also note that the lines drawn along the inferior

plate of L5 and the superior plate of the sacrum intersect at a point that is near the articular facets. The closer to the facets these lines cross, or if they are actually anterior to the articular joints, the greater will be the severity of the facet syndrome, meaning a greater posterior disc space narrowing, vertical narrowing of the foramen, and hyperextension subluxation of the facet joints.

Hellems and Keats (24) found the normal sacral base angle to be 41° (Fig. 11.11). At this degree of angulation of the sacrum, 80% of the superimposed body weight is carried upon the vertebral bodies and the sacral promontory. Although only 20% of the weight is carried upon the articular facets, the resulting pressure per square inch on the facets is 10 times greater than the pressure carried upon the knee with the person standing in the upright posture. This gives a good idea of the strain produced on the articular facets in normal kinematics.

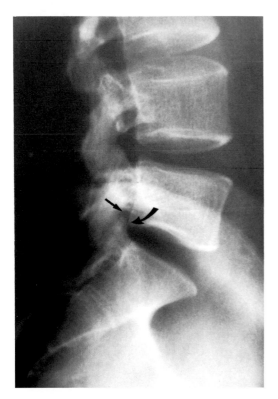

Figure 11.9. Radiograph showing a facet syndrome at L5-S1. There is posterior narrowing of the L5-S1 intervertebral disc space, with the first sacral facet stenosing the L5-S1 foramen by its vertical telescoping subluxation (*straight arrow*). Note also the nuclear disc invagination of the L5-S1 disc into the inferior vertebral body plate of L5. L5 shows a retrolisthesis subluxation on the sacrum (*curved arrow*).

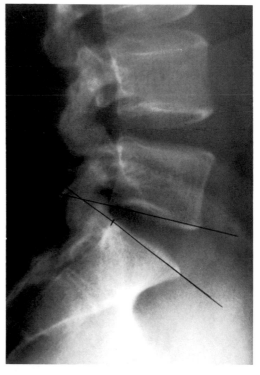

Figure 11.10. Macnab lines are drawn along the superior S1 vertical plate and inferior L5 vertebral plate and intersect near the zygapophyseal joints instead of more posteriorly. Also, the S1 superior facet lies well above the line drawn along the inferior L5 body plate, indicating probable vertical stenosis at the L5-S1 intervertebral foramen. This is termed facet imbrication.

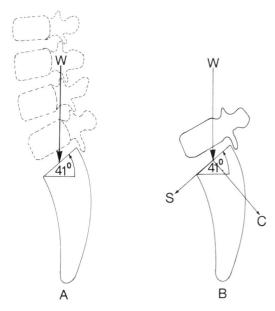

Figure 11.11. Position of the normal sacrum during erect standing. **A**, the superincumbent weight (*W*) passing through the posterior edge of the lumbosacral joint. **B**, the compression (*C*) and shearing (*S*) components of the superincumbent weight. (Reproduced with permission from LeVeau B: *Biomechanics of Human Motion.* Philadelphia, WB Saunders, 1977, p 94.)

An increase of the sacral angle shifts weight bearing posteriorly onto the posterior elements and

facets (Fig. 11.12). The articular facets were never created to stand this shearing stress. As the sacral base inclines farther, a hyperextension subluxation of the upper motion segment and/or hyperflexion subluxation of the lower motion segment must take place. Look at Figure 11.13; in this figure you see a 65° sacral base angle with facet syndrome. Figure 11.14 demonstrates marked structural faults with a degenerative spondylolisthesis at the L4 level and a facet syndrome and increased sacral angle at the L5-S1 level. Treatment of this last case would involve addressing both conditions by placing a flexion pillow under L4 while contacting the spinous process of L3 in applying the distraction manipulation.

Figures 11.15 and 11.16 show two basic conditions to be dealt with in manipulation. There is a facet syndrome present at L5-S1 as shown in Figure 11.15 but also a transitional segment with a unilateral pseudosacralization of the left transverse process to the sacrum (Fig. 11.16). As presented in this text in Chapter 6, this condition proved to be the most time-consuming and treatment-demanding condition to yield to manipulative care in a study of 576 cases (22). Couple this with a facet syndrome, and we see a very difficult case to treat. This author treated this case by contacting the spinous process at the L5 level and *very gently* applying flexion distraction at the L5-S1 joint. This was followed with complete range of motion manipulation of the articular facets.

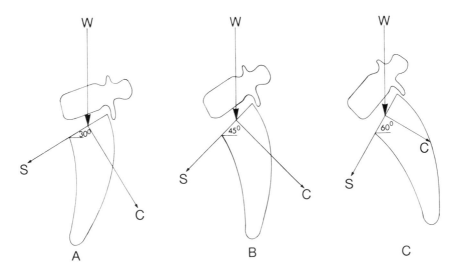

Figure 11.12. Change in the compression (*C*) and shearing (*S*) force components with change in the sacral angle. *W*, weight. (Reproduced with permission from LeVeau B: *Biomechanics of Human Motion.* Philadelphia, WB Saunders, 1977, p 95.)

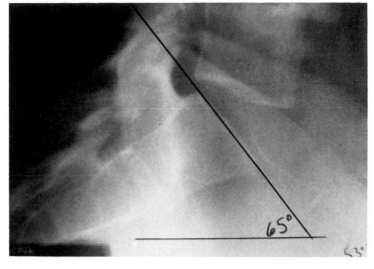

Figure 11.13. Increased sacral angle and hyperextension subluxation of L5 on the sacrum.

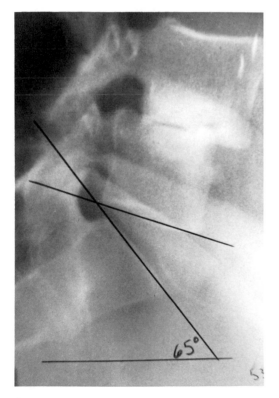

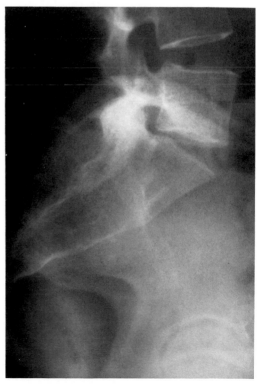

Figure 11.14. Radiograph showing a facet syndrome subluxation complex at L5-S1 and a degenerative spondylolisthesis at L4 on L5. Treatment for this combination problem is discussed in the text.

Figure 11.15. Radiograph showing facet syndrome of L5 on S1. There is marked disc thinning, imbrication of the first sacral facet into the L5-S1 foramen, and probably some arthrosis of the L5-S1 facet joints.

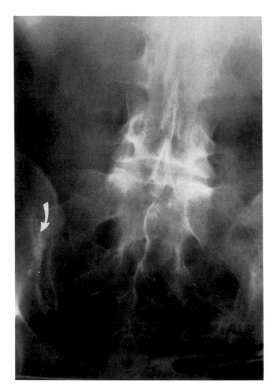

Figure 11.16. In addition to the findings on the lateral view in Figure 11.15, we also have a unilateral pseudosacralization transitional segment of the L5 transverse process with sacrum (*arrow*).

We used a belt support, as shown later in this chapter, to stabilize this joint while healing.

Figure 11.17 reveals a stable, normal disc space with no evidence of facet imbrication. You will note that the lines drawn along the inferior L5 and superior sacral plates intersect far posterior to the lumbosacral junction. We feel that in this type of finding we have a stable articulation and that the weight bearing primarily is found on the body-disc-body, with minimal weight bearing on the articular facets at L5-S1.

STABILITY IN THE FACET SYNDROME AND AN INDICATION OF RESPONSE TO MANIPULATION

Although the articular facets are well supplied with nerve fibers from the dorsal ramus of the spinal nerve, discussion continues as to the role that the articular facet plays in the etiology of low back and lower extremity pain. Van Akkerveeken determined a measurement for stability or insta-

bility of the lumbar spine from use of lateral lumbar films in order to determine damage to the posterior longitudinal ligament and the annulus fibrosus. This measurement is illustrated in Figure 11.18.

According to Van Akkerveeken (25), in a normal lumbar spine in full extension, with the annulus fibers and longitudinal ligaments intact, a line drawn along the posterior longitudinal ligament shows a fairly smooth arch. If the annulus fibers are cut, there is a definite posterior sliding of each vertebra posteriorly upon the vertebra below. If lines are drawn along the inferior plate of the vertebra above and along the superior plate of the vertebra below, and the intersection of these lines is called point *a*, there should be less than a 3-mm difference in length between the line drawn from point *a* to the posterior margin of the superior vertebra and the line drawn from point *a* to the posterior margin of the inferior vertebra. If the difference is 3 mm or more, instability is

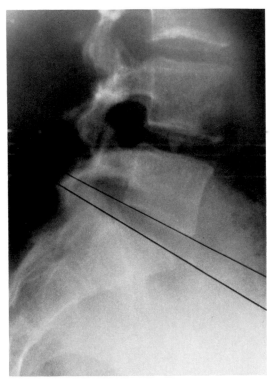

Figure 11.17. Stability is suggested in the radiograph by the parallel Macnab's lines and their intersection far posterior to the L5-S1 facet joints. Note the symmetric L5-S1 disc space indicating probable maximum weight bearing on the disc and minimal weight bearing on the articular facet joints.

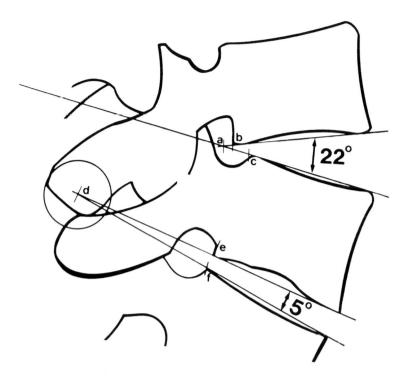

Figure 11.18. Line drawing of the lateral aspect of lumbar segment in full extension, illustrating radiologic instability and methods of measuring it (degrees of tilt and length of parallel displacement). The lower segment is stable; *de* = *df* in length. At the upper segment, radiological instability is demonstrated; in this case, line *ab* is 3 mm shorter than line *ac* (see text for explanation). (Reproduced with permission from Van Akkerveeken PF, O'Brien JP, Park WM: Experimentally induced hypermobility in the lumbar spine. *Spine* 4(3):238, 1979.)

present, meaning that there is damage to the annular fibers and/or the posterior longitudinal ligament. We utilize this measurement as a prognostic aid to determine the response of a patient to treatment as well as to predict future difficulty in the lumbosacral spine.

It has also been shown that the greater the discal angle, the more severe the facet syndrome. The discal angle (*edf*) shown in Figure 11.18 is 5°, a sign of stability and no facet syndrome. The other angle (*bac*) is 22°, a sign of severe facet syndrome. This author believes that any discal angle over 15° is a sign of severe facet syndrome (Fig. 11.19).

Figure 11.20 demonstrates the use of Van Akkerveeken's line measurement to determine stability. The spines shown in Figure 11.20**A** and **B** are stable. Figure 11.21 demonstrates the use of this measurement in a patient with an unstable spine. A line is drawn from the point of intersection (*a*) to the posterior border of the 5th lumbar body above (*b*) and to the posterior border of the sacrum below (*c*). The distance from *a* to *b* measures 11 mm; the distance from *a* to *c* measures 16 mm. By Van Akkerveeken's measurement, therefore, the lumbosacral articulation is unstable, showing that the annulus and posterior longitudinal ligament are damaged.

The facet syndrome has been accused of causing much low back pain; a review of our present knowledge about the sensitivity of the articular bed of the facet, therefore, is in order.

Increasingly in the literature, articles are appearing concerning the innervation of the articular facets. There are important anatomical relationships in the lumbosacral region of the adult which are traceable to embryonic development. In their discussion of the pain relationships evolving from biomechanical faults of the lumbosacral complex, Carmichael and Burkhart (26) state that the paraxial mesoderm that condenses alongside the notochord becomes segmented into somites. Each somite then differentiates into a scleratome (which contributes to vertebrae formation), a myotome (which forms axial and appendicular muscle), and a dermatome (which forms the dermis). The developing neural tube innervates each somite and its derivatives so that the nerve pattern becomes segmental.

Each scleratome divides transversely, and each hemiscleratome reaggregates with a hemiscleratome adjacent to it, becoming the centrum that forms most of the vertebral body. These divisions and reaggregations determine important anatomical relationships in the adult: (a) the spinal nerve, which originally would have run through the scleratome, now runs between the vertebrae, and (b) the myotome forms muscle that spans adjacent vertebral segments, thus establishing the patterns for back muscles.

The notochord, surrounded by the centrum, undergoes mucoid degeneration and usually disappears completely except for the nucleus pulposus of the intervertebral disc.

The centrum eventually forms part of the membranous vertebral column. Each vertebra undergoes chondrification and ossification, a process completed several years after birth. The costal elements form a substantial part of the transverse process of the adult lumbar vertebra and the major portion of the lateral part of the sacrum.

Thus, by the process reviewed above, the individual vertebrae are formed and the overall shape of the vertebral column is established. The five lumbar vertebrae typically are massive and show some differentiation. Generally, the vertebral foramen (which determines the shape of the spinal canal) becomes more triangular at L5 as the pedicles shorten, but the distance between the foramina shows little change.

STRUCTURAL FACTORS OF THE LUMBOSACRAL REGION

The joint between L5 and S1 is the single most common site of problems in the vertebral column because of, but not limited to, the following anatomical reasons: (a) this joint bears more weight than any other vertebral joint; (b) the center of gravity passes directly through these vertebrae; (c) a transition occurs here between the mobile presacral vertebrae and the relatively stable pelvic girdle; and (d) there is a change in the angle that exists between these two vertebrae.

In 1976, Mooney and Robertson (27) pointed out that Ghormley had coined the phrase *facet syndrome* in 1933 and that lesions of the intervertebral disc could not explain all low back and leg

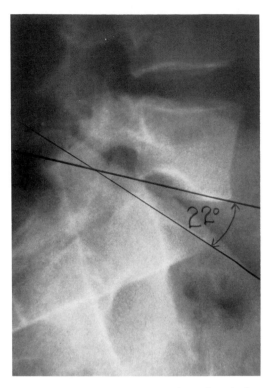

Figure 11.19. Lines are drawn to determine whether there is facet syndrome. Note that the angle is 22°. The greater this angle becomes, the greater the severity of the facet syndrome due to hyperextension of L5 and/or due to hyperflexion of the sacrum. The closer this angle is to 5°, the more stable the articulation.

pain complaints. From his review of surgical literature, Sprangfort (28) found that only 42.6% of surgical patients obtained complete relief of back and leg pain following surgery.

Mooney and Robertson (27) also discovered that the injection of an irritant fluid into the facet joint caused referred pain patterns indistinguishable from pain complaints frequently associated with the disc syndrome. Even straight leg raising and diminished reflex signs were obliterated by precise local anesthetic injection into the facet joint. Injection of steroids and local anesthetic into the facet joint in a group of 100 consecutive patients suggested that this treatment alone achieved long-term relief in one-fifth of the patients with lumbago and sciatica and partial relief in another one-third of these patients. This author (J.M.C.) would point out, however, that far less than half of the patients received long-term relief from pain from use of this technique. The point to be emphasized here is that the physician

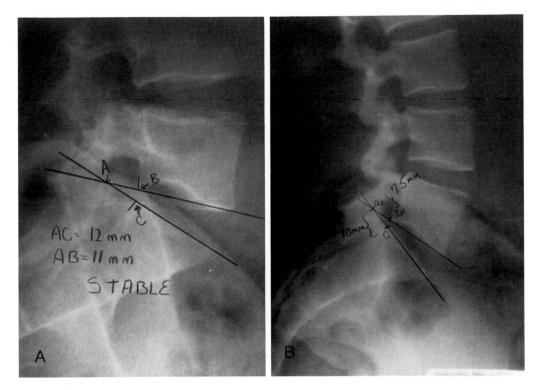

Figure 11.20. Van Akkerveeken's lines are drawn and show stability of the annulus fibrosus and posterior longitudinal ligament in **A**, where there is only 1 mm difference between *AB* and *AC*. **B** also shows a stable facet syndrome, as it shows 2.5 mm difference between lines *ab* and *ac*.

must be clinically careful to realize that a combination of therapies may be necessary to bring maximum relief of the patient's complaints.

FACET PAIN PATTERNS

In June of 1976, Lora and Long (29) wrote that the results of stimulation in and around the facets yielded interesting pain patterns. Typical radicular radiation is not generated by stimulation of the nerves in and around the facet, but widespread referral of sensation even into the leg is possible. This referral of sensation, however, characteristically has a diffuse nonradicular character, is difficult for the patient to localize, and has not gone below the knee in any patient.

Stimulation of the L5-S1 facet characteristically produces sensation or reproduces pain in the coccyx, which is usually unilateral, or in the hip. The latter is usually described by the patient as being in the hip joint, and diffusely down the posterior thigh. Stimulation may occasionally travel circumferentially around the body along the course of the inguinal ligament into the groin.

Stimulation at the L4-L5 facets characteristically produces a local sensation at the level of the electrode, which radiates diffusely into the posterior hip and thigh. Coccygeal radiation of sensation is less commonly observed with L4-L5 stimulation than with L5-S1 stimulation, but it does occur. Stimulation at L3-L4 characteristically produces radiation upward into the thoracic area. Pain or sensation radiates around the flank and into the groin and anterior thigh much more diffusely with L3-L4 stimulation than with L5-S1 stimulation. Coccygeal sensations in the perineum are produced more commonly with L3-L4 stimulation than with L4-L5 stimulation but less commonly with L3-L4 stimulation than with L5-S1 stimulation. It appears that radiation of pain, at least as judged by stimulation of the posterior ramus by use of this technique, may be much more diffuse than is generally supposed. Although hip, thigh, and groin radiations are well known from studies of patients with disc protrusion, the observation that stimulation characteristically reproduces pain in the coccygeal area or produces sensation in this region is not as well

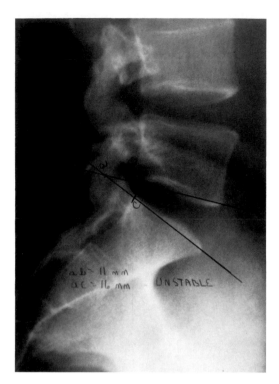

Figure 11.21. Unstable facet syndrome, as there is 5 mm difference in lines *ab* and *ac*.

known. *It certainly seems possible that coccydynia is, in fact, another manifestation of lumbar degenerative disc disease* (Table 11.2).

Stimulation at the T12, L1, L2, and L3 levels does not produce leg or coccygeal sensations. Radiation of sensations is limited to the upper back,

Table 11.2.
Facet Joint Pain Patterns Described by Lora and Long[a]

L5-S1 facet pain distribution	L4-L5 facet pain distribution
Coccyx	Posterior hip and thigh
Hip	Coccyx
Posterior thigh	
Groin	
Flank	
L3-L4 facet pain distribution	T12, L1, L2, L3 facet pain distribution
Upward to thoracic spine	No leg or coccygeal pain
Diffuse flank and groin pain	Radiating pain to thoracic and cervical spines
Coccyx	

[a]Based on Lora J, Long D: So-called facet denervation in the management of intractable back pain. *Spine* 1(2):121–126, 1976.

to thoracic and cervical regions, and around the course of the T12, L1, and L2 nerve roots in a diffuse fashion on the anterior abdominal wall.

This author would note that these are scleratogenous pains that do not cause any sensory or motor deficits in the lower extremity. These pains never radiate below the knee and are usually isolated to the buttock and upper thigh. When motor and sensory changes are noted down the lower extremity, a disc lesion should be suspected. Figure 11.22 shows the distribution of sensations from L4-L5 and L5-S1 facet irritation.

McCall et al. (30) studied the referral of induced pain from the posterior lumbar elements in order to (*a*) trace the exact area of pain referral from the

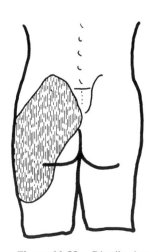
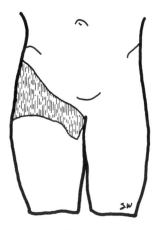

Figure 11.22. Distribution of sensations from L4-L5 and L5-S1 facet irritation.

L1-L2 and the L4-L5 levels and (*b*) compare the distribution and intensity of the pain produced by intraarticular versus pericapsular provocation. In their study, normal subjects were given injections of 0.4 ml of 6% saline. Pain started within 25 seconds of each injection, with the episode usually lasting 5 minutes. At both the L1-L2 and the L4-L5 levels, injection into the joint interior (intraarticular provocation) produced less intense pain than did pericapsular injection.

The upper lumbar level was more sensitive than was the lower lumbar level. The distribution of referred pain from either intraarticular or pericapsular injection was the same, but the intensity was worse with the pericapsular injection than with the intraarticular injection.

In general, injection into the upper lumbar level referred pain to the flank region, whereas injection at the L4-L5 level referred pain to the buttocks. Thigh pain never extended beyond the knee. No contralateral pain was noted. *No demonstration of significant leg pain was produced in these normal subjects.*

There is an absence of nerve endings in the articular cartilage and synovium. The fibrous capsule of the synovial joint, however, is innervated.

McCall et al. (30) question the existence of scleratomes because of the considerable overlap of pain patterns between upper and lower lumbar spine facets.

Schofferman and Zucherman (31) feel that leg pain may prove more useful diagnostically. The distribution and quality of the pain are used to separate referred pain from radicular pain. Pain in the absence of neurological deficit is referred pain, while pain in the presence of neurological change is radicular. It must be born in mind, however, that there may be an absence of neurological signs in the early stages of radicular problems. *Referred pain shares the same distribution as the innervation of the affected zygapophyseal articulations. Pain arising from the L4-L5 and L5-S1 articulations will be felt in the posterior thigh, and occasionally in the medial or lateral calf, and back pain is usually greater than leg pain. Numbness or tingling may accompany this pain. Posterior joint complex pain (facet, ligament, annulus) rarely, but occasionally, extends beyond the calf and into the foot.* Contrast this pain distribution with that of radicular pain caused by nerve root compression—for example, by a disc protrusion in which the predominant and more severe pain is usually felt in the thigh and in the posterior lateral calf, extending to the toes. While dermatomal pain may

Table 11.3.
Facet Joint Pain Patterns Described by Schofferman and Zucherman[a]

L4-L5, L5-S1 pain distribution:
Posterior thigh, calf, rarely to foot
Back pain greater than leg pain

[a]Based on Schofferman J, Zucherman J: History and physical examination. *Spine: State of the Art Reviews* 1(1):14, 1986.

not be exact, certain patterns are characteristic. L3 pain involves the groin and anterior medial thigh; L4 pain involves the anterior thigh and medial calf and gluteal area; L5 pain involves the lateral thigh, lateral and possibly medial calf, and great toe; and S1 nerve pain involves the posterior thigh, posterior calf, and lateral aspect of the foot and heel (Table 11-3).

From the results of the above study, one can see that irritation of the articular facets at L4-L5 and L5-S1 can result in pain in the coccyx, perineum, groin, buttock, and flank and into the posterior thigh, radiating as far as the knee. Our therapeutic interest in the facet is the maintenance of its ability to maintain its normal ranges of motion and thereby render it as free of subluxation as possible.

BACKGROUND OF FACET SYNDROME TREATMENT

The major benefits of flexion manipulation are: improvement of transport of metabolites into the intervertebral discs, reduction of stress on the apophyseal joints and on the posterior half of the annulus fibrosus, and giving the spine a high compressive strength (2).

Facet joint injection in 245 patients who presented with chronic symptoms of low back pain, with or without nondermatomal lower limb pain referral, was performed (32). No previous back surgery had been performed, and each patient underwent both facet studies and provocative lumbar discography at the lower three lumbar levels. To localize accurately any level of symptom relief, only one level per day was studied in each patient. Lumbar discography was performed, and the presence or absence of symptom reproduction on injection of contrast medium was recorded at each level.

In this group of 245 patients, the intervertebral discs were a more frequent source of symptoms than the facet joints. In 45 patients, complete symptom relief followed injection of local anesthetic into the facet joints. Following facet injection, no significant difference was apparent in the incidence of complete symptom relief between the three groups of patients: the incidence was 19% for those with symptomatic disc disease, 25% for those with nonsymptomatic disc disease, and 17% for those with total disc resorption. By contrast, of 45 patients with normal three-level lumbar discography, only two (5%) had complete symptom relief following facet injection. *The study indicates that the facet joint and capsule are infrequent pain sources in patients with severe chronic low back pain, particularly when the discs are normal, but also in the presence of significant disc degeneration* (32).

This highlights a controversy with respect to the relief possible through facet injection. This author (J.M.C.) has been negatively influenced by facet and epidural injection attempts to relieve low back pain.

Manipulative Care of the Facet Syndrome

The manipulation used in treating facet syndrome is Cox® flexion distraction procedures as performed on the Zenith®-Cox® instrument.

Patients are divided into two types for purposes of manipulative care: *patients having low back pain only, and those with low back pain and sciatica.* The flow chart shown in Figure 11.23 describes our treatment outline. Please observe that we do not place zygapophyseal joints through their physiological ranges of motion when the patient has sciatic radiculopathy until the leg pain shows at least 50% relief as noted by subjective patient evaluation and objective signs of straight leg raising, range of thoracolumbar motion, Déjérine's triad, and Kemp's sign. Any patient who has only low back pain, with leg pain not extending below the knee, is treated with full physiological range of motion applied to the facet articulations. Flexion distraction is the first manipulative movement administered, followed by the remaining four normal ranges of motion, which will be discussed next.

Normal Joint Movements

The lumbar articular joints are capable of five movements—flexion, extension, lateral flexion, rotation, and circumduction. Pearcy (33) measured the ranges of active flexion and extension, axial rotation, and lateral bending in the lumbar

spines of normal volunteers in vivo, to assess the relation between the primary and accompanying movements in the other planes. He stated that L5-S1 revealed larger movements of flexion and extension than did other levels of the lumbar spine, although L5-S1 did not demonstrate consistent patterns of equal movement of flexion and extension as seen at other levels of the lumbar spine. Lateral bending at L4-L5 and L5-S1 showed significantly less mobility than in the upper three levels.

In voluntary flexion and extension, Pearcy (33) found little accompanying axial rotation or lateral bending. During both axial rotation and lateral bending, there were large accompanying rotations in the other planes. Axial rotation saw a consistent pattern of accompanying lateral bending.

Pearcy (33) found lateral bending of approximately 10° occurring at the upper three lumbar levels, while there was significantly less lateral bending, 6° and 3°, at L4-L5 and L5-S1, respectively. In flexion and extension, accompanying axial rotation of 2° or more, and lateral bending of 3° or more, occurred rarely, and larger accompanying rotation at an intervertebral joint should be considered abnormal. During twisting and side bending, axial rotation to the right is accompanied by lateral bending to the left and vice versa at the upper three levels. At L5-S1, axial rotation and lateral bending generally accompany each other in the same direction, while L4-L5 is a transitional level. During lateral bending, there is generally extension at the upper levels and flexion at L5-S1.

Range of Motion Variation in Painful versus Nonpainful Spines

Mayer (34) studied the range of motion in the lumbar spine in painful versus nonpainful low back patients. He concluded that low back pain subjects exhibit lower gross motion than normal subjects (54%), with the ratio of lumbar flexion to gross flexion decreased (63% to 43%). Range-of-motion exercising can significantly increase functional pain-free range both in lumbar (71%) and pelvic motion (39%) over a 3-week period.

Yang and King (3) state that normal, nonarthritic facet joints carry 3 to 25% of the superimposed body weight. If the facet joint was arthritic, the load could be as high as 47%. The transmission of the compressive facet load occurs through contact of the tip of the inferior facet with the pars interarticularis of the vertebra below. Fur-

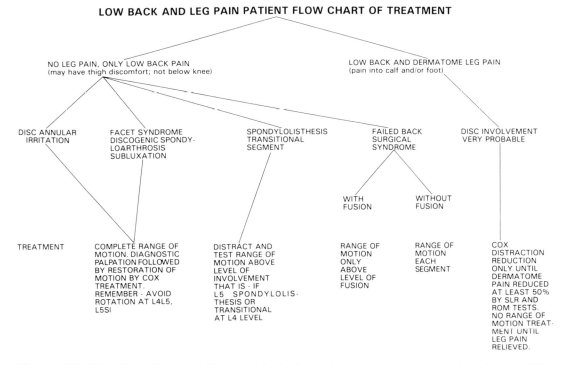

Figure 11.23. Flow chart of treatment for patients having low back pain alone or low back pain and sciatica. This chart outlines the treatment approach followed for our manipulative care depending upon patient findings.

ther, facet overload caused rearward rotation of the inferior facet, which stretched the facet capsule.

Nociceptor Origin of Low Back Pain

Wyke (35) states that the cause of low back pain is irritation of nociceptors. The term *nociceptive* means "sensitive to tissue abnormality." Two abnormalities causing pain are mechanical and chemical. There are three morphological types of nociceptors:

1. Unmyelinated fibers in interstitial tissues;
2. Free naked nerve endings;
3. Paravascular nociceptive system in the adventitial layers of blood vessels. These are unmyelinated also.

Wyke points out that the apophyseal capsule contains unmyelinated nerve fibers. They are sensitive to both chemical and mechanical irritation, and high tensions develop in the facets following disc degeneration and the carrying of more weight.

SUMMARY OF MANIPULATIVE PRINCIPLES

Based upon the references cited above, one can conclude that manipulation may be beneficial by increasing spinal range of motion; relieving nociceptor irritation; perhaps equalizing the weight bearing between the anterior weight bearing column of the lumbar spine (made up of the vertebral body-disc-vertebral body) and the posterior column of the spine (namely the articular facet); and finally relieving the compressive forces against the nerve root within the vertebral canal and intervertebral foramen.

Rules on Submission of a Patient to Flexion Distraction

Prior to discussing any form of spinal manipulation in this chapter, we note that it is extremely important to test the patient's tolerance to distraction manipulation so as to determine the necessary limitations prior to its application.

This is done by the rules of Kramer (36) as follows:

1. If a decrease of pain can be demonstrated under distraction, traction treatment should be instituted. As a rule, the pain first changes its character. For instance, a lateral pain will be transferred centrally, and a sharp lancinating root pain can turn into dull low back pain.

2. Traction is contraindicated when it causes an increase of pain (*a*) when shearing forces will influence a displaced fragment and dislocate it completely (pain will always be increased when the prolapse is medial and near the nerve root); (*b*) when a prolapse is still within the boundaries of the vertebral margins but during traction may become dislocated into the spinal cord; (*c*) when there are adhesions around the nerve root; (*d*) adhesions in the spinal canal following surgery; (*e*) Traction is also contraindicated in patients who have had an increase of symptoms during a long period of relaxation, e.g., when sleeping at night, when there is "increase of disc volume." Moreover, traction should not be used in patients with hypermobile segments and muscle insufficiency. Young people with disc degeneration experience very good results with traction treatment.

Testing Procedure Prior to Manipulative Care

In our clinic, we use the following procedure to test the patient's ability to withstand flexion distraction. With the patient lying prone on the treatment table, a thenar contact of the doctor's hand is made upon the spinous process from the first to the fifth lumbar vertebra, while the caudal section of the table is gently pressed downward no more than 1 to 2 inches. No cuffs are placed on the patient for tractive force, but rather, the patient's pelvic and lower extremity weight is the only distractive force utilized as the caudal section is distracted downward (Fig. 11.24). If this amount of traction causes pain to the patient, do not place the cuffs on him or use this distraction technique. If it is an acute low back pain case, it may be hours or days before the patient will tolerate any tractive treatment. Perhaps occasionally a patient will not be able to tolerate the tractive force at all. It is necessary to test the patient's ability to withstand flexion distraction repeatedly until he or she has no adverse reaction. If no pain is felt using the patient's weight as a tractive force, proceed to test lateral distraction by grasping the patient's ankle as shown in Figures 11.25 and 11.26 and testing each side of the lumbar spine for symptoms of pain. We feel that this places stress upon the unilateral facet articulations and will reveal any latent pain probability.

What to Do If Pain Is Caused on Testing for Flexion Distraction

The most common incidence of pain on testing is seen in the acute intervertebral disc protrusion patient in whom an antalgic lean and dermatomal leg pain are present. Pain is seen, however, on occasion in facet syndrome subluxation patients. When it appears, do not use the flexion distraction instrument but instead use positive galvanic current over the involved segment (disc or facet

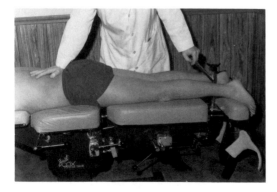

Figure 11.24. Testing patient tolerance to distraction without the ankle cuffs applied. Contact on the spinous process of the lumbar vertebrae is made while applying cephalad pressure to stabilize the vertebral segment. The caudal section is distracted downward 1 to 2 inches while patient evidence of pain or muscle spasm is documented.

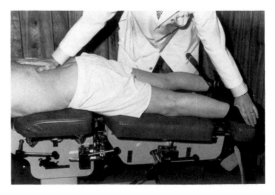

Figure 11.25. Unilateral facet stress is placed on the lumbar spine by grasping the left ankle and applying unilateral distraction with the caudal section being pressed downward as patient reaction is gauged.

joint) with application of hot and cold alternating packs to the low back. This should be 10 to 15 minutes of heat, followed by 10 minutes of cold or ice pack, and repetition of the heat again. This may be done with three or four sessions of hot packs with cold packs placed between each hot application. This stimulates circulation, relieves muscle tension, and drives out inflammatory changes while sedating nerves. Acupressure points, as described in the chapter on the treatment of intervertebral disc lesion, should be used. These are bladder meridian points 22 to 49. Following such treatment, again test the patient's tolerance to the flexion distraction manipulation. It may be that the patient can now tolerate the maneuver, or it may take two or three such therapy sessions, or 2 or 3 days, before the patient is able to withstand this manipulative technique.

LIMITATION OF DISTRACTIVE FORCE

Never distract downward more than 2 inches with the caudal section at any time in treating the lower lumbar spine. As you progress into the thoracic or cervical spine, you will go down more than 2 inches with the caudal section of the table as you dissipate the distractive force over a longer area of the spinal column.

Description of the Manipulative Instrument

Prior to application of the technique, please note the movements available with the flexion-distraction table, as shown in Figures 11.27 through 11.30. This is the Zenith®-Cox® flexion instrument as manufactured by the Williams Manufactur-

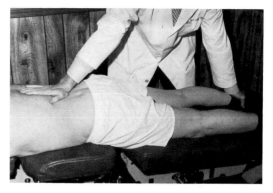

Figure 11.26. The same procedure as in Figure 11.25 is used on the right side.

ing Company for the manipulation procedures shown in this textbook.

Figure 11.27 demonstrates the flexion application, Figure 11.28 extension, and Figure 11.29 lateral flexion; Figure 11.30 demonstrates rotational motions of both the thoracic and lumbar sections.

TREATMENT OF FACET SYNDROME

Facet syndrome is a subluxation complex of the articular processes in which increased weight bearing occurs due to intervertebral disc narrowing and degeneration or hyperextension subluxation of the superior vertebra on the inferior segment. Facet capsule irritation, stenosis of the intervertebral foramen, and arthrosis may be the result. Figure 11.9 shows the posterior narrowing of the L5-S1 intervertebral disc space with imbrication of the first sacral facet into the upper third of the intervertebral foramen at L5-S1.

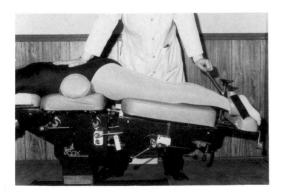

Figure 11.27. Application of the flexion maneuver with the manipulation instrument.

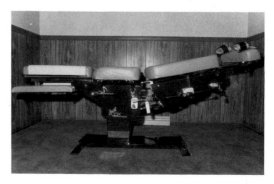

Figure 11.28. Application of extension with the manipulation instrument.

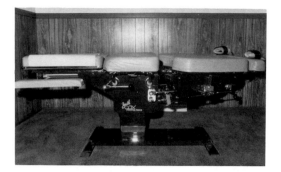

Figure 11.29. Application of lateral flexion with the manipulation instrument.

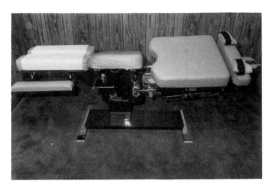

Figure 11.30. Application of thoracic and lumbar capabilities of rotation alone or individually with the manipulation instrument.

The radiograph in Figure 11.10 shows the lines of Macnab (23) identifying the hyperextension subluxation of L5 on the sacrum with the tip of the superior facet of sacrum imbricating above the line drawn along the inferior plate of L5. The telescoping of the superior facet of the sacrum upward into the intervertebral foramen at L5-S1 creates vertical stenosis of the foramen.

Whether the facet syndrome as seen in Figures 11.9 and 11.10 is stable or unstable, the treatment by manipulation is the same. After the patient's tolerance of manipulation is tested, he or she is allowed to lie prone on the table; if the patient has a pendulous abdomen that creates a flattening and slight kyphosis of the lumbar lordotic spine, treatment is given with no flexion pillow under the abdomen. If the patient is thin and lies on the table with a lordotic lumbar curve, a flexion Dutchman roll is placed under the abdomen as shown in Figure 11.31 so that a flattening

and slight kyphosis is artificially created prior to manipulation. This serves to start reduction of the facet syndrome by bringing the superior facet of the vertebra below into a caudal direction so as to increase the vertical height of the intervertebral foramen.

Figure 11.32 shows goading pressure applied to the paravertebral muscles and bladder acupressure meridian points from L2 to the coccyx. These acupressure points are fully described in Chapter 12, "Care of the Intervertebral Disc."

Figures 11.33, 11.34, and 11.35 show the setup for the treatment of facet syndrome. A flexion pillow is under the abdomen (Fig. 11.33). Figure 11.34 shows the patient lying without the flexion pillow under the abdomen. Remember that with the flexion pillow, less force is needed to achieve flexion, since the patient already is in a degree of traction due to the pillow. Remember

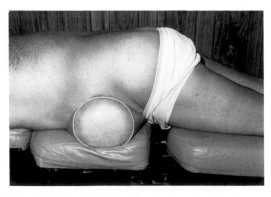

Figure 11.31. A flexion pillow is placed under the patient's abdomen at the level of facet syndrome to create a flattening of the lumbar lordosis and reduction of the hyperextension of L5 on S1.

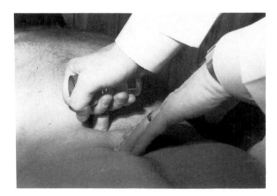

Figure 11.32. Treatment by goading pressure on the paravertebral muscles and acupressure bladder meridians is given.

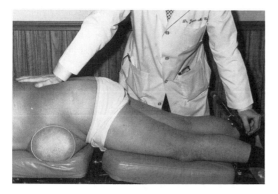

Figure 11.33. Here a flexion pillow is placed under the abdomen to produce a reduced lordosis of the lumbar spine and relief of facet syndrome.

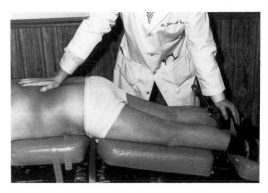

Figure 11.34. Here the patient lies on the table without the benefit of the flexion pillow.

to use gentle distraction always, but even less force with the pillow in place.

The first movement used in treating facet syndrome subluxation is flexion distraction, applied by contacting the spinous process of the vertebra above the facet syndrome and applying flexion as seen in Figures 11.33 and 11.34. We limit the downward flexion movement of the caudal section of the table to 2 inches or less, and we apply this limitation to downward force when treating the lower three lumbar segments. When treating above the L3 level, we will use more downward force, since we are dissipating the tractive force over several segments instead of applying it to one or two levels. Always remember to test the patient's tolerance prior to any manipulative maneuver. Figure 11.35 shows a side-lying maneuver to treat facet subluxation syndrome when the patient is in too much pain to lie prone.

When applying flexion distraction to facet syndrome, we utilize a push-pull pumping effect on the spinous process in order to induce an increased interspinous spacing. This is accomplished by maintaining the contact on the spinous process with the thenar contact of the hand while placing the caudal section into repetitive flexion position. First, after placing the contact hand on the spinous process, we take the table into flexion until tautness of the tissue occurs under our contact hand. This means that all tissue and joint slack is removed from the body from the ankle cuffs to our contact hand on the spine. From this point of tautness, we will press the table downward 1 to 2 inches to create a push-pull pumping effect on the intervertebral space under our spinal contact. We repeat this pumping until we feel

the gap between the spinous processes open and the usual spreading of the spinal units take place under our treating hand. When normal flexion opening is elicited, we will do one of two steps: either move to the segment above and repeat the process, or put the just-treated segment through its other normal ranges of motion, which will be described in the next section.

We feel that this push-pull pumping action allows us to open the intervertebral foramen and disc and to bring the zygapophyseal joints into an open, nonhyperextended position. With this position, we feel that we can apply lateral flexion, circumduction, and limited rotation without causing subarticular entrapment neuropathy by bringing a superior facet of the vertebra below into the lateral recess and subarticular gutter

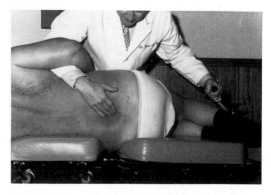

Figure 11.35. If the patient feels too much pain to lie on the abdomen for treatment, we can have the patient lie on the side and laterally flex the caudal table section so as to create flexion at L5-S1. The hand contact at the spinous process of L5 localizes and directs the tractive force.

where the nerve root could be compressed. In the vertical stenosis induced by facet syndrome, the nerve root can be vulnerable to more compression if we do not first flex open the facets and disc spaces prior to applying other facet movements.

The duration for which flexion distraction should be applied to a specific level depends on the fixation or normal range of mobility elicited by the doctor as he or she performs the manipulation. A fixated joint may require repetitive mobility before the joints distract and freedom of motion is felt under the treating hand. It is only following the feeling of free flexion motion that the other ranges of motion are applied to a specific level as described next.

Motion Palpation and Range of Motion Manipulation Following Flexion Distraction

Following flexion distraction in facet syndrome, we will place each facet pair through their physiological ranges of motion. One author mentioned earlier in this chapter (33) stated that rotation is a very limited motion at the lower lumbar spine. We know that flexion and extension are strong movements in the lower lumbar spine. The zygapophyseal joints are capable of five normal ranges of motion, with combinations of these motions possible. These five motions are flexion, extension, lateral flexion, circumduction, and rotation. A description of the application of each of these motions with the manipulation instrument is shown in Figures 11.36 through 11.40.

Factors in Patient Care Ancillary to Manipulation

Figure 11.41 illustrates steps taken to get the patient on the table. We ask the patient to tighten the abdominal muscles and buttock muscles as much as possible while he or she leans over the table. While grasping the table sides, the patient lowers him- or herself as the doctor stands beside the patient to assist. This maintains the lumbar spine rigid and prevents motion that aggravates the pain.

Before the patient arises, we will have placed a lumbar support on him or her. The patient arises by again tightening the abdominal and buttock muscles so as to stabilize the pelvis while pushing himself or herself up with the hands grasping the sides of the table (Fig. 11.42). The doctor assists

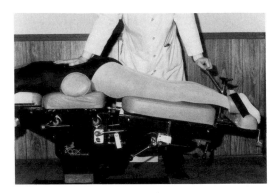

Figure 11.36. Flexion distraction is applied to the lumbar segment by contacting the spinous process above the segment to be manipulated with the thenar process of the treatment hand. The caudal section of the table is flexed until tautness of the interspinous space occurs and motion is felt between the adjacent vertebrae. This necessitates 1 to 2 inches of downward distractive force with the table section. This maneuver is repeated until freedom of motion is felt.

as needed. The belt used is one developed by the author (J.M.C.); it utilizes a compact memory foam insert that molds to any configuration of the lumbar spine, whether it be kyphotic or lordotic.

Figure 11.43 shows the application of either positive galvanism or tetanizing current. The benefits of these modalities are explained in Chapter 12. For muscle spasm, we like to use tetanizing current to the paravertebral muscles to create re-

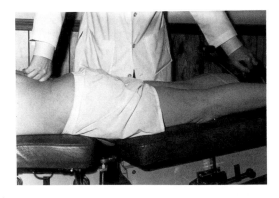

Figure 11.37. Extension is applied by contacting the spinous process of the segment to be manipulated and gently applying a downward force as the caudal table section is brought into slowly increasing extension. This maneuver is done repeatedly until freedom of motion is felt in extension. It may be done once or several times, depending upon the resistance encountered.

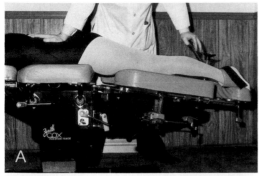

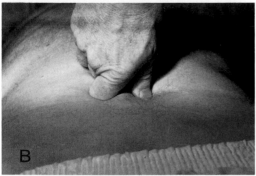

Figure 11.38. Lateral flexion is shown. The spinous process is held as shown, either **A**, with the palm of the hand, or **B**, between the index finger and thumb, as shown during lateral flexion motion of the caudal section of the table. Resistance is applied to the right spinous process as the table is right flexed and the left spinous process as left lateral flexion is applied. Either the palm or thumb-finger contact can be used to direct the motion. Remember that if the spinous process at the L4 level is stabilized, the L4-L5 facet joints will be tested for their ability to go through physiological motion and return to full mobility. The joints below the spinous process contacted are being tested and treated. This motion may be sufficient to regain normal motion if hypomobility of a facet articulation is found.

laxation and positive galvanism to relieve pain and release myofascial inflammation.

Some patients are in too much pain to lie on their abdomen during treatment or therapy application. We lay these patients on their sides and apply the therapy as shown in Figure 11.44. The tetanizing current is applied and the hydrocollator or cryotherapy applied over it, with straps holding the therapy in place. In clinical practice, we use alternating hot and cold therapies consisting of 10 to 15 minutes of heat followed by 5 to

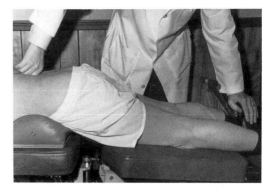

Figure 11.39. Circumduction is a combined coupled motion of flexion and lateral flexion applied at a motion segment. The spinous process is held as flexion is first applied followed by lateral flexion. This is performed in clockwise and counterclockwise directions. We feel this to be the best means of regaining motion when fixation or hypomobility is present.

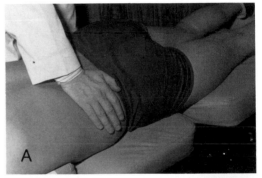

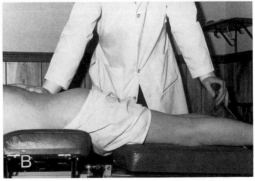

Figure 11.40. **A**, Rotation is applied by placing the palm of the hand on the paravertebral area of the segment to be manipulated while the thoracic section of the table is rotated under the patient. This allows the vertebra to be rotated right or left as the needed force is applied with the treating hand. **B**, Traction can be applied to the motion segment as rotation is applied to the lumbar spine. This allows coupling of two movements to a single vertebral segment or to multiple vertebral segments.

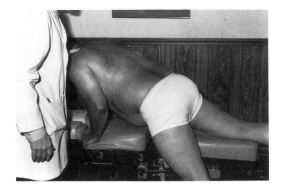

Figure 11.41. Getting the patient on the manipulation instrument.

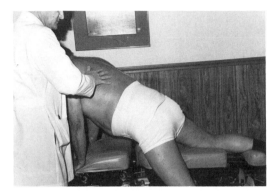

Figure 11.42. Placing the lumbar brace on and getting the patient up following care.

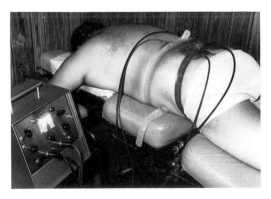

Figure 11.43. Application of electrical stimulation following manipulation.

10 minutes of ice, using three or four heat sessions with two or three ice sessions between. Always begin and end with the heat, as we find it to leave the patient more relaxed.

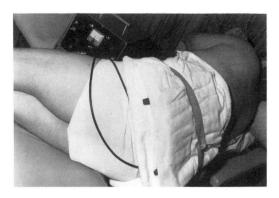

Figure 11.44. When in too much pain to lie on the abdomen, the patient may lie on the side and have therapy applied.

Analgesic liniment is massaged into the lumbar spine paravertebral muscles, with emphasis on the acupressure bladder meridian points from the second lumbar paravertebral area, between the transverse and spinous processes, to the coccyx, which is bladder point B35 (Fig. 11.45).

The adductores muscle group is treated, as shown in Figures 11.46 and 11.47, by deep goading of the origin and insertion with a firm rotatory pressure applied for 20 to 30 seconds. We find the adductores muscles to be weak and painful. Such soft tissue massage goading dissipates pain and strengthens the muscle. Further information on these muscles and their treatment is offered in Chapter 15 on specific low back conditions.

Those patients with hyperlordosis, facet syndrome, or anterior weight-bearing stress on the lumbar spine who have ankle pronation or pes planus arch defects are treated with foot manipulation and arch orthotics. Figures 11.48, 11.49,

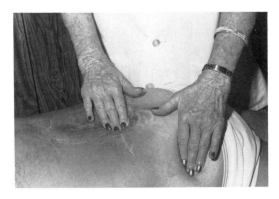

Figure 11.45. Massage of acupressure points.

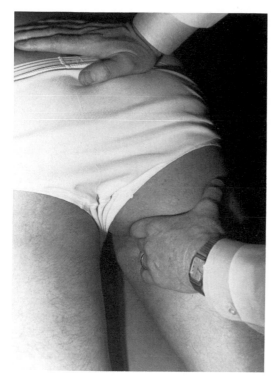

Figure 11.46. Adductores muscle pressure goading at the origin.

and 11.50 reveal this condition and the orthotic used for correction.

All facet syndrome patients attend low back wellness school, especially those patients with unstable or severe pain type. This class is held every third Thursday and becomes a routine part of management of the patient.

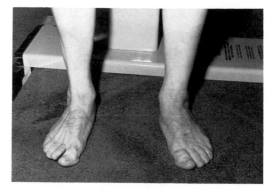

Figure 11.48. Pes planus of both feet.

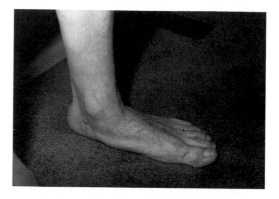

Figure 11.49. Medial view of marked arch planus in a patient with facet syndrome of the lumbar spine.

Cox® exercises 1, 2, 3, 3, 6, 8, 9, and 10, shown in Chapter 12, "Care of the Intervertebral Disc," are recommended.

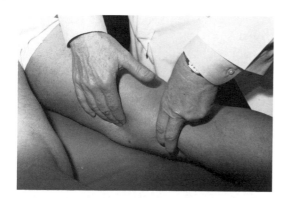

Figure 11.47. Adductores and gracilis muscle pressure goading at the insertion.

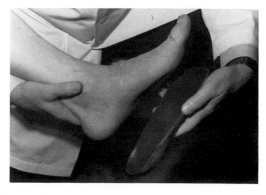

Figure 11.50. Orthotics used for the correction of the pes planus and additional care of the patient with facet syndrome.

RETROLISTHESIS SUBLUXATION

We have chosen to discuss the treatment of retrolisthesis subluxation at this time due to its seemingly increased incidence with facet syndrome; it will often be a dual subluxation with the facet subluxation.

Figure 11.51 shows an unstable facet syndrome of L5 on S1, with L5 being 5 mm posterior on the sacrum. This creates an apparent facet imbrication of the L5-S1 intervertebral foramen by the superior facet of S1 entering the upper third of the foramen. This subluxation is far from being totally accepted or explained. Let's consider some opinions on this subluxation prior to studying its manipulative care under our type of manipulation.

I feel that retrolisthesis can be caused by three primary factors:

1. Congenital underdevelopment of the pedicles of the lumbar vertebra, so-called *pedicogenic*

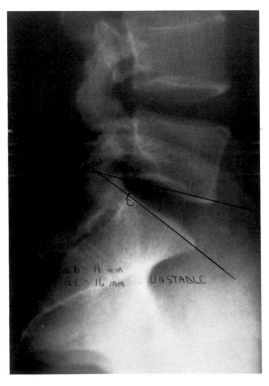

Figure 11.51. Radiograph showing an unstable facet syndrome of L5 on the sacrum with L5 being 5 mm posterior on the sacrum, a retrolisthesis subluxation of L5. Note the apparent stenosis of the intervertebral foramen due to the facet imbrication of the first sacral facet and the posteriority of L5 on the sacrum.

stenosis. This underdevelopment certainly creates alteration of motion capacity and can be relieved only by the best of treatment.
2. Multifidus and rotatores muscle spasm.
3. Subluxation of a primary traumatic etiology, such as hyperflexion.

Willis (37) found the depth of the last lumbar vertebra greater than the first sacral segment, which he felt gave rise to an optical illusion on x-ray of backward displacement of the fifth lumbar vertebra on the sacrum. He stated that, in measuring 50 skeletons, the depth of the L5 and S1 bodies were found to be equal in 34% of the cases; in the other 66%, lumbar depth exceeded sacral depth, or in a few cases was less.

This author (J.M.C.) feels that in facet syndrome in which there is discal degeneration, the increased facetal weight bearing will force the inferior fifth articular facet to impact the first sacral facet and will cause a posterior displacement of the fifth body as the two segments approximate one another. In turn, the only means of returning some degree of alignment is to open the disc space and relieve the impaction hyperextension subluxation of L5 on the sacrum. In the end, the clinical result and relief of patient symptoms will depend upon effective clinical application of manipulative principles based on anatomical abnormality.

Examination should reveal the following in retrolisthesis:

1. Underdevelopment of the pedicles resulting in probable sagittal stenosis as measured by Eisenstein's procedure, described in Chapter 7. With this shortened pedicle and the resultant posterior placement of L5 on the sacrum, George's line will show a posteriority of L5 on the sacrum. George's line is shown in Figure 11.51 as the line behind the L5 body. In the figure, it is not a smooth line continuing behind the sacrum; rather, it breaks as it shifts anterior to the posterior sacral position. George's line can be continued behind all the lumbar bodies. It normally is a smooth, uninterrupted line behind the normal lumbar lordosis.
2. Flattening of the lumbar lordosis on physical examination.
3. In some cases, spasm over the paravertebral musculature, which is very tender to touch; gluteus maximus spasm and tenderness; and/or an adductor muscle that is spastic and tender to touch.

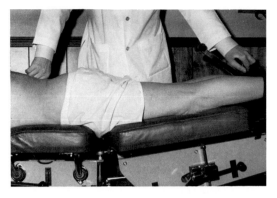

Figure 11.52. Shown is extension manipulation being applied to a retrolisthesis subluxation of L5. The table is gently brought into extension as a downward pressure is applied to the spinous process of L5.

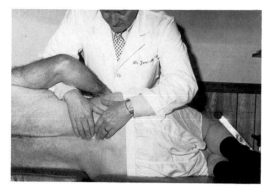

Figure 11.54. Placing the patient on his or her side for the application of extension manipulation is an excellent method. It allows complete control of the depth of extension while affording the contact hand to detect and control the extension forces being applied.

4. Radiation of pain into the groin, buttock, posterior thigh, and flank, as described previously in this chapter.

Treatment

Treatment is shown in Figures 11.52 through 11.55. Figure 11.52 shows extension manipulation being applied gently on the manipulative in-

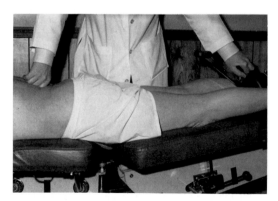

Figure 11.53. Following extension tolerance by the patient, the facets may be placed through lateral flexion and circumduction. We use this motion only on patients who have regained full range of mobility without pain in the flexion posture with the table. The doctor must be sensitive to the infliction of stenosis by such extension motion at L5-S1 and must test the patient's ability to take this type of manipulation prior to its application. We use it only on those patients who feel marked relief from extension position manipulation. This negates its use in elderly persons with intermittent neurogenic claudication due to stenosis.

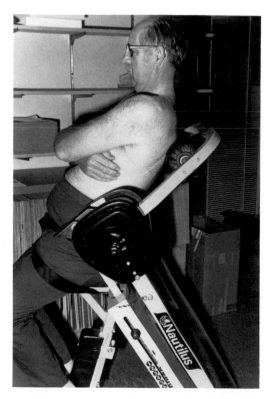

Figure 11.55. In facet syndrome and retrolisthesis, following relief of pain, we use extension Nautilus conditioning for the paravertebral muscles. We like to use a maximum of 130 pounds of extension force. We start the patients, even elderly little ladies, on 20 to 30 pounds of resistance and build them up.

strument. We avoid thrusting into this segment, as it can be very painful to the patient. By using extension manipulation we can also use lateral flexion with extension, as shown in Figure 11.53, to place the articular facets through their physiological ranges of motion.

Figure 11.54 shows treatment being applied with the patient on his side. Two purposes are found for this technique. First, it is excellent for the patient who has too much pain to lie on his abdomen for care. Also, it is an excellent modality for placing the patient into extension while controlling the motion of the vertebrae with the contact hand on the spine.

In addition to manipulation, we use the other modalities used in facet syndrome: goading of acupressure points B22 to B49, alternating hot and cold packs, massage, electrical stimulation, belt support in severe pain, exercises, low back wellness school, and Nautilus exercise, as shown in Figure 11.55.

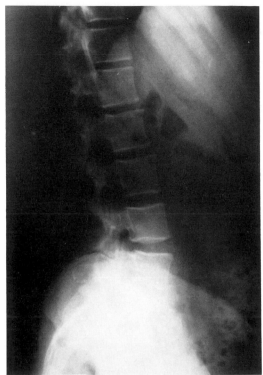

Figure 11.57. Lateral projection of patient shown in Figure 11.56.

CONCLUSION

This concludes our discussion of the mechanics and treatment of probably the most common condition encountered in low back pain patients—facet subluxation syndromes. To end this chapter, a case presentation of facet syndrome is given.

CASE PRESENTATION

A 51-year-old white female was seen for the chief complaint of low back pain and no leg pain. It had worsened this time following yard work, but she had had low back pain off and on for most of her life.

Examination revealed +2 deep reflexes bilaterally, no motor weakness, and no sensory abnormalities. The ranges of motion of the thoracolumbar spine were normal, and straight leg raises were negative.

Figures 11.56 and 11.57 are anteroposterior and lateral views of the lumbar spine and pelvis. Figure 11.58 reveals a stable facet syndrome at the L5-S1 level. You will note that the discal angle is 22°. The greater the discal angle, the greater the severity of the facet syn-

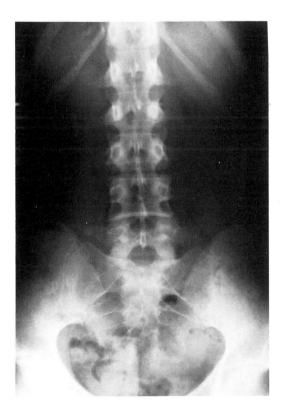

Figure 11.56. Anteroposterior view of a 51-year-old female with low back pain.

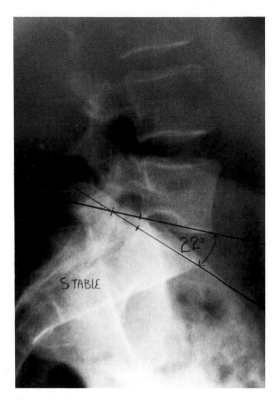

Figure 11.58. Spot lateral view shows the 22° discal angle and a stable facet syndrome. The superior S1 facet is telescoped into the L5-S1 foramen, and nuclear invagination of the L5-S1 disc into the inferior end plate of L5 is seen.

drome, as indicated by the thinning of the posterior L5-S1 disc space. In this case, we do have nuclear invagination of the inferior vertebral plate of L5 by the intervertebral disc. The posterior disc space is markedly thin compared to the anterior.

Treatment consisted of flexion distraction with a small flexion pillow under the L5 vertebral body. Deep goading of the paravertebral muscles over the acupressure points B22 through B49 was utilized in preparation for flexion distraction manipulation. This patient was given knee-chest exercises, abdominal strengthening exercises, and hamstring stretching. Three visits resulted in almost total relief of the low back pain.

References

1. Pal GP, Routal RV: Transmission of weight through the lower thoracic and lumbar regions of the vertebral column in man. *J Anat* 152:93–105, 1987.
2. Adams MA, Hutton WC: The effect of posture on the role of the apophyseal joints resisting intervertebral compressive force. *J Bone Joint Surg* 62B: 358–362, 1980.
3. Yang KH, King AI: Mechanism of facet load transmission as a hypothesis for low-back pain. *Spine* 9: 557–565, 1984.
4. Morris JM, Lucas DB, Bresler B: Role of the trunk in stability of the spine. *J Bone Joint Surg* 43A:327, 1961.
5. Fiorini GT, McCammond D: Forces on lumbo-vertebral facets. *Ann Biomed Eng* 4:354–363, 1976.
6. Miller JAA, Haderspeck KA, Schultz AB: Posterior element loads in lumbar motion segments. *Spine* 8(3):331–337, 1983.
7. Jayson MIV: Compression stresses in the posterior elements and pathologic consequences. *Spine* 8(3): 338–339, 1983.
8. Farfan HF, Cossette JW, Robertson GH, Wells RV, Kraus H: The effects of torsion on the lumbar intervertebral joints: the role of torsion in the production of disc degeneration. *J Bone Joint Surg* 52A: 468–497, 1970.
9. Panjabi MM, Krag MH, Chung TQ: Effects of disc injury on mechanical behavior of the human spine. *Spine* 9(7):707–713, 1984.
10. Hadley LA: Intervertebral joint subluxation: bony impairment and foramen encroachment with nerve root change. *Am J Roentgenol* 65:337–402, 1951.
11. Dunlop RB, Adam MA, Hutton WC: Disc space narrowing and the lumbar facet joints. *J Bone Joint Surg* 66B:707–710, 1984.
12. Nade S, Bell E, Wyke BD: The innervation of the lumbar spinal joint and its significance. *J Bone Joint Surg* 62B:255, 1980.
13. Giles LGF, Taylor JR: Osteoarthrosis in human cadaveric lumbo-sacral zygapophyseal joints. *J Manipulative Physiol Ther* 8:239–243, 1985.
14. von Luschka H: Die Nerven des menschlichen Wirbelkanals. Tubingen, H Laupp, 1850.
15. Giles LGF, Taylor JR: Innervation of lumbar zygapophyseal joint synovial folds. *Acta Orthop Scand* 58: 43–46, 1987.
16. Ghormley RK: Low back pain with special reference to the articular facets, with presentation of an operative procedure. *JAMA* 101:1773–1777, 1933.
17. Weinstein PR, Ehni G, Wilson CB: *Lumbar Spondylosis.* Chicago, Year Book, 1977, p 68.
18. Abel MS: *Occult Traumatic Lesions of the Cervical and Thoraco-Lumbar Vertebrae with an Evaluation of the Role of C.T.,* ed 2. St. Louis, MO, Warren H. Green.
19. Shirazi-Adl A, Drouin G: Load-bearing role of facets in a lumbar segment under sagittal plane loadings. *J Biomech* 20(6):601–613, 1987.
20. Giles LGF: Pressure related changes in human lumbosacral zygapophyseal joint articular cartilage. *J Rheumatol* 13:1093–1095, 1986.
21. Cox JM, Fromelt KA, Shreiner S: Chiropractic statistical survey of 100 consecutive low back pain pa-

tients. *J Manipulative Physiol Ther* 6(3):117–128, 1982.

22. Cox JM, Shreiner S: Chiropractic manipulation in low back pain and sciatica: statistical data on the diagnosis, treatment and response of 576 consecutive cases. *J Manipulative Physiol Ther* 7(1):1–11, 1984.

23. Macnab I: *Backache*. Baltimore, Williams & Wilkins, 1977, p 200.

24. Hellems HK, Keats TE: Measurement of the normal lumbosacral angle. *AJR* 113:642–645, 1971.

25. Van Akkerveeken PF, O'Brien JP, Park WM: Experimentally induced hypermobility in the lumbar spine. *Spine* 4(3):236–241, 1979.

26. Carmichael S, Burkhart S: Clinical anatomy of the lumbosacral complex. *J Phys Ther* 59:966, 1979.

27. Mooney V, Robertson J: The facet syndrome. *Clin Orthop* 115:149–156, 1976.

28. Sprangfort EV: Lumbar disc herniation. *Acta Orthop Scand* 142(Suppl), 1972.

29. Lora J, Long D: So-called facet denervation in the management of intractable back pain. *Spine* 1(2): 121–126, 1976.

30. McCall I, Park W, O'Brien J: Induced pain referral from posterior lumbar elements in normal subjects. *Spine* 4(5):441–446, 1979.

31. Schofferman J, Zucherman J: History and physical examination. *Spine: State of the Art Reviews* 1(1):14, 1986.

32. Colhoun EN, McCall IW: Lower lumbar facet joint injection: a review of 245 cases. *Br J Radiol* 60:604, 1987.

33. Pearcy MJ: Stereo radiography of lumbar spine motion. *Acta Orthop Scand* 212 (Suppl 56), 1985.

34. Mayer TG, Tencer AF, Kirstoferson S, Mooney V: Use of noninvasive techniques for quantification of spinal range-of-motion in normal subjects and chronic low-back dysfunction patients. *Spine* 9(6): 588–595, 1984.

35. Wyke B: Paper presented at Challenge of the Lumbar Spine, New Orleans, December 1984.

36. Kramer J: *Intervertebral Disc Diseases*. Chicago, Year Book, 1981.

37. Willis TA: Lumbosacral anomalies. *J Bone Joint Surg* 41A:935–938, 1959.

12

Care of the Intervertebral Disc

James M. Cox, D.C., D.A.C.B.R.

If a man empties his purse into his head, no man can take it away from him.

An investment in knowledge always pays the best interest.

—Benjamin Franklin

Let's begin this chapter with a discussion of clinical findings concerning the effectiveness of spinal manipulation in the treatment of low back pain, especially the disc lesion. Pal (1) reports that patients receiving continuous lumbar traction for the treatment of back pain and sciatica showed similar improvement to patients receiving simulated traction; he therefore questioned the justification of admitting patients with back pain into hospitals for the purpose of traction alone. Glover et al. (2) reported in 1974 that a controlled trial showed that those who were manipulated had significantly better relief 15 minutes later, but after 3 days the advantage over those not manipulated was lost. Grayson (3) felt that relief was better for 2 weeks following manipulation, but after that there was no longer a benefit. Hoehler, Tobis, and Buerger (4) stated that manipulation gave better relief than soft tissue massage up to 3 weeks after treatment, and then no difference in relief was found. Sims-Williams et al. (5) felt that for 2 months there was better relief in those patients manipulated than in those not so treated. Doran and Newell (6) compared manipulation (the technique used was at the discretion of the manipulator, including soft tissue technique and mobilization, given a minimum of two treatments weekly and an average of six treatments per patient), definitive physiotherapy (including any technique except manipulation used in the practice of the department, with an average of 7.3 treatments per patient), corset, and analgesics in a multicenter trial of 456 patients with low back pain randomly assigned to one of the above-listed four forms of care. No important differences were noted among the four groups, except that a few patients responded well and quickly to manipulation, but there was no way of identifying those who would respond positively to manipulation. Paterson (7) reported good results in the care of 1037 patients who presented with symptoms of pain arising in the spine and compared his results with Robertson (8), who reported a 75% success rate within three manipulative treatments. Fisk (9) reported statistically significant alteration in the straight leg raising tension measurements after manipulation of the painful side as compared to the change after manipulation of control subjects. In another study, Fisk (10) reviewed 369 cases of patients experiencing low back pain who were treated with spinal manipulative therapy. He concluded that 90% were completely relieved, 5% at least benefited, and only 5% failed to attain any relief.

MANIPULATION SEEMS MOST BENEFICIAL IN EARLY STAGES OF TREATMENT

In general, manipulation seems to have been found to have its benefit early in the acute phases of low back pain conditions. Acute low back pain studies show that manipulation tends to shorten the episode of pain (11, 12). Similar results are found in chronic back pain (13, 14). Kirkaldy-Willis and Cassidy (15) reported on 283 patients

467

with chronic low back and leg pain who underwent manipulation; 202 became symptom-free or maintained mild intermittent pain, returning to work without restriction. Eighty-one were helped but had restriction of activities due to pain or were unaffected by manipulation. Nwuga (16), using oscillatory rotatory manipulation, was able to document an increase in spinal motion and significant straight leg raising following manipulation. Jayson et al. (17) felt that manipulation may hasten improvement in low back pain but did not influence the long-term outcome. Glover (2) found that patients undergoing manipulation gained significantly greater relief than a control group receiving short-wave diathermy 15 minutes after treatment, but no difference was found between the groups 3 to 7 days later. Moritz (18) reported that manipulation of the lumbar spine might have an immediate, short-term effect on low back pain in a limited number of patients. However, no superior long-term effects were found, as compared to other forms of care. Zylbergold and Piper (19) claim that no universally recognized treatment exists for low back pain problems, and patients, therefore, frequently seek assistance from more than one medical specialist and often receive conflicting advice as to the appropriate care.

Kane (20) reported a Utah study showing workman's compensation records from patients treated by chiropractic physicians and patients treated by allopathic physicians for work injuries to the spine and found chiropractic manipulation to be as effective as conventional medical approaches. Fonti and Lynch (21) claim an 85% success rate for reduction of pain from intervertebral disc displacement by manipulation of the spine.

Is Manipulation More Beneficial Initially or Later in Care?

There is controversy over the contention that manipulation is of benefit in the 1st week, or after the first treatment, and then of no benefit afterward. Evans, in contrast to this finding, reported on 32 patients with chronic low back pain who were treated three times weekly with rotational manipulation; he found that the 1st week of manipulative treatment was more painful than the corresponding week in a control group, but in the 2nd and 3rd weeks there was less pain in the manipulated group (13). *Thus, strong disagreement is found between research projects that are supposedly controlled and blinded studies on whether or not manipulation is beneficial when first applied or later following a few treatments.*

The Capabilities of the Manipulating Physician Are Important

This author would add that there are various capabilities of manipulating physicians. Deyo and Tsui-Wu (22) stated that one-third of low back pain sufferers seek chiropractic are as the portal of entry into the health care delivery system. Furthermore, white, better-educated persons were the majority of those persons going to the chiropractor first. This author (J.M.C.) interprets this as possibly meaning that those who study the benefits of types of health care delivery might select the chiropractor over other types of healers.

There is a call for some to specialize in areas of the spine, be that the pelvic articulations or lumbar, cervical, or other regions. The reason is the multiple specific anatomical differences, clinical presentations, and necessary therapeutic implications of handling each diagnosis. To expect that manipulation be related to a general practitioner or other type doctor whose primary interest and training is in some other specialty is to place a low priority on manipulative treatment of disease and to also be prepared for less than good clinical expectation. Furthermore, studies such as that of Doran and Newell (6) have been rightfully criticized for the specification of manipulation delivered (23, 24). Their study only stated that the manipulative technique was at the discretion of the manipulator, using ancillary osteopathic procedures such as mobilizing and soft tissue techniques. In addition, the procedures were carried out at multicenter locations, thus decreasing any standardization of care. This is felt to render inconsistent manipulative techniques. Kirkaldy-Willis and Cassidy (15) state that manipulation requires much practice to acquire the necessary skill and competence, with few medical practitioners having the time or inclination to master it. They feel that most medical practitioners, whether family physicians or surgeons, wish to refer their patients to a practitioner of manipulative therapy with whom they can cooperate, whose work they know, and whom they can trust. The physician who does this will have many contented patients and will save himself many headaches. Donnelly et al. (25) state that patients with asthma and nonasthmatic lung conditions who seek alternative medical care (most commonly chiropractic care, followed by homeopathy, naturopathy, acupuncture, herbal medicine, osteopathy, hypnosis, iridology, faith healing, and megavitamin therapy) were not disgruntled with orthodox medicine. They merely sought an alternative form of care. This author feels that this addresses a problem often felt by practitioners, namely, feeling rejected or angered if a patient wants to substitute or supplement the care of one doctor with the advice or care of another. Perhaps, the Donnelly paper points out, this feeling exists only in the minds of the doctors, not the patients.

Cost Factors in Low Back Pain Care

Another point of importance in the care of low back pain patients is cost. Swezey et al. (26) in a study of 39 patients treated successfully at home for low back pain, with outpatient ambulatory care designed for treatment of back pain and arthritis, found that the average total cost per patient, including physician's fees, x-rays, laboratory, and therapy, was approximately equivalent to the day rate for 1½ days in the hospital. This author notes that insurance or third-party payers are quite aware of such statistics. Snook (27) claims that a few high-cost cases account for most of the expense of back care—specifically, that 25% of the cases account for 90% of the costs. He says that cheap care is primarily short sighted and looks for a quick and simple medical solution to the back problem, while cost-effective care is synonymous with early intervention, conservative treatment (unless otherwise indicated), patient follow-up, education (for both the patient and employer), and timely decisions regarding case management. Cost-effective care recognizes the value of early return to work as part of the therapy, and utilizes such techniques as modified work and modified hours. The goal is not only to get the patient back to work but also to keep him or her there. Deyo et al. (28) stated that patients without neuromotor deficits found that 2 days of bed rest were just as effective and cost-saving as longer periods, say 7 days.

MANIPULATIVE EXPECTATIONS IN THE CLINICAL SETTING

Today the clinical expectations for manipulative approaches are good compared to the results reported in the early studies in the 1950s to 1980s.

Splendid research in the biomechanics of the low back is presently being performed, and varying techniques in the surgical treatment of low back conditions are being investigated and tried. Therefore, it is incumbent on chiropractic to develop manipulative care of the low back to its utmost perfection.

"The last part of surgery, namely operations, is a reflection on the healing arts. No surgeon should approach an operation without reluctance." John Hunter made this statement in 1749 (30), and it seems just as applicable today to the chiropractic physician utilizing manipulation to the low back. Manipulation can be a great tool when used properly or an iatrogenic nightmare if abused.

According to Dommisse and Grabe (31), a spinal surgeon rather than an orthopedic or a neurosurgeon is the appropriate leader of the surgical team in an operation on the spine. This reflects the idea that a surgeon whose training is primarily in spinal surgery is the appropriate physician to enter the spine. It might also be said that some chiropractic physicians should specialize in the care of the low back and make this their primary study and practice. To this end, the manipulative care of other specialists throughout the world is briefly examined.

Hadler et al. (29) reported a randomized controlled study in which 54 subjects were placed under manipulative care. The patients were divided into two subgroups: those with acute low back pain of less than 2 weeks duration, and those whose discomfort had persisted for 2 to 4 weeks. Outcome was measured with a functional impairment questionnaire, which showed that those patients who had suffered a backache were afforded more rapid improvement if they were subjected to spinal manipulation. Due to the extreme prevalence of low back pain in society today, this finding of relief in fewer days than without such care was pointed out to be a major ramification. This author (J.M.C.) finds this controlled study to provide a more realistic appraisal of manipulation than previous studies of more questionable design and purpose.

Arkuszeqski (30) allocated 100 patients with lumbago or sciatica alternately into two groups; all received standard drug treatment and physiotherapy, undergoing manual examination twice a week. Traction, mobilization, and/or manipulation was applied to all parts of the spine in the manual treatment group. In 60% of patients, there was concomitant neck pain. Blockages of the cervical segments were found in 95% of the patients, the atlanto-occipital segment being the one most frequently affected. In the manual treatment group, the treatment period was shorter, and posture, intensity of pain, and neurological signs showed greater improvement both on discharge and 6 months later. When manipulation was compared to standard conservative medical care, the manipulation group had a 30% reduction in hospitalization time, a greater number who remained well at 6 months, and greater improvement in neurological findings.

Ongley et al. (32) contrasted two patient groups: an experimental group of 40 patients receiving manipulation along with proliferant injections, and a control group of 41 patients receiving parallel treatment with less forceful manipulation and saline solution instead of proliferant. Disability scores then showed that the experimental group had greater improvement than the control group at 1, 3, and 6 months after the end of treatment. At 6 months posttreatment, an improvement of 50% or more was recorded in 35 of the experimental group versus 16 of the control group, with 15 of the experimental group free of pain versus four of the control group. The experimental group receiving manipulation showed significant advantages over the control group, which had not been manipulatively cared for.

Rupert et al. (33) carried out a chiropractic controlled clinical trial to evaluate the efficacy of chiropractic adjustments in the treatment of low back pain among 148 Egyptian workers. The patients were randomly assigned to one of three treatment regimens—chiropractic adjustments, drugs and bed rest, or placebo. Treatment results were evaluated by the visual analogue scale, active and passive straight leg raising, and the fingertips-to-floor assessment of forward flexion. Chiropractic treatment was associated with the greatest improvement.

Cox and Shreiner (34) carried out a chiropractic multicenter observational pilot study of 576 patients with low back and/or leg pain to compile statistics on examination procedures, diagnosis, types of treatments rendered, results of treatment, number of days of care, and number of treatments required to arrive at a 50% and a maximum clinical improvement. This study showed that 275 (50%) of the patients reported on showed an excellent outcome, 74 (14%) very good, 60 (11%) good, 36 (6%) fair, and 22 (4%) poor; 17 (3%) underwent surgery, 57 (10%) stopped or did not undergo treatment, and seven

(1%) were examined but not treated. Fifty percent relief of pain was seen after 14.4 days and 9.5 treatments (mean values). Maximum improvement was obtained after 42.8 days and 18.6 treatments (mean values).

Potter (35) reported chiropractic manipulation in 744 cases of neck and back pain, whether acute or chronic, with or without radicular signs, to have overall statistical results of recovery in 268 cases (36%), much improvement in 257 (34.5%), slight improvement in 54 (7.3%), no change in 161 (21.6%), or worsened condition in four (0.6%).

Nyiendo and Haldeman (36) found that 80% of low back pain patients seen at a chiropractic college teaching clinic were diagnosed as having lumbosacral strain, with 23% of 2000 patients receiving one visit, 54% receiving two to five treatments, and less than 1% receiving more than 20 visits. The range was one to 81 visits, with a mean of 5.3 visits.

Bronfort (37) stated that 298 patients with acute or chronic low back pain from 10 different chiropractic clinics were selected for study. Fifty-three percent of them had consulted a medical doctor or had received other types of treatment due to their current episode of pain. Seventy-five percent of these patients reported being free of symptoms or feeling much better following chiropractic care.

Waagen et al. (38) performed a double blind study of the efficacy of spinal adjustment therapy in a college clinic. Nineteen patients with low back pain underwent a 2-week treatment period, with nine patients receiving chiropractic adjustments and 10 in a control group receiving a comparable series of manual interventions. It was reported that the experimental nine patients improved significantly compared to the control group.

Wooley and Kane (39) stated that major areas of difference were found between allopathic and chiropractic care for low back pain with respect to the number of visits and duration of treatment given. Patients were seen an average of about 13 times by chiropractors, as opposed to approximately seven times by allopaths. However, the treatment by allopaths took over 9 weeks, as opposed to 6½ weeks for chiropractors. This averaged out at 1.2 visits per week for allopaths and 2.5 visits per week for chiropractors.

Chrisman et al. (40) found that 10 of 27 patients with positive myelograms had good to excellent results 3 years or more after manipulation. Fifty-one percent of patients with clinical evidence of lumbar disc rupture had good to excellent results from manipulation.

A full-scale multicenter trial to include 2000 patients was proposed and was found to be feasible after a feasibility study for a randomized controlled trial of chiropractic and hospital outpatient management for low back pain of mechanical origin (41). Patients who were eligible for this study were interviewed by a nurse coordinator who explained the purpose of the study and pointed out that agreement to take part involved an equal chance of being treated by chiropractic or by conventional hospital methods, the decision being made at random. The study involved the Northwick Park Hospital and a local chiropractic clinic.

Vernon et al. (42) found manipulation to be associated with a statistically significant increase in serum β-endorphin levels when blood testing was performed before and after spinal manipulation. This allows a hypothesis that pain relief induced by manipulation is due, in part, to a short-term increase in β-endorphin levels.

Response of Lumbar Disc Lesions to Manipulation

Kuo and Loh (43) reported on a total of 517 patients with protruded lumbar discs admitted for manipulative treatment from 1975 through 1983. The results were that 76.8% had satisfactory results, and the conclusion was that manipulation of the spine can be an effective treatment for lumbar disc protrusions.

Gillstrom et al. (44) reported that, of 20 patients with positive CT scans for lumbar disc lesions, 11 had good, four fair, and five poor outcomes following autotraction manipulative reduction.

Li et al. (45) studied 1455 cases of lumbar intervertebral disc protrusion treated with traction and manipulative reduction. Eight hundred ninety-one cases (61%) were deemed cured based on resolution of leg pain and Lasègue's sign over 70°, and the patients returned to work. Two hundred fifty-seven cases (18%) were deemed remarkably improved, and they either resumed normal work or shifted to lighter jobs. Two hundred forty-two (17%) cases were improved, with milder radiating pain, but they were not able to resume work or required continual treatment. Sixty-five cases (5%) had no relief. The total effec-

tive rate was 95.5%. Traction manipulation reduction of the disc protrusion was felt to be accomplished by effecting a negative intradiscal pressure in the widened disc space with stretching of the posterior longitudinal ligament. Through tension created within the outer layers of the annulus fibrosus and the posterior longitudinal ligament, and the suction effect of the negative pressure, a favorable condition was created for the reduction of the disc protrusion.

INFLAMMATORY CHANGES SURROUNDING THE NERVE ROOT BY DISC LESION

McCarron et al. (46) formulated a hypothesis to explain the inflammatory effect of the nucleus pulposus on nerve roots. He based his conclusions on clinical observations and literature interpretation. It is given as follows:

1. The annulus fibrosus forms incomplete fissures over a period of time which eventually completely tear with trauma.
2. Nuclear material leaks through the tears into the epidural space to bathe the nearby dural sac and roots.
3. A painful inflammatory reaction results.
4. Persistent symptoms occur if the fissure in the annulus fibrosus fails to heal due to persistent intradiscal hydrostatic pressure or due to inability of the annular tissue to heal.
5. This irritative nuclear material is constantly replenished by living nuclear cells.

The ability of nuclear material to irritate thecal membranes and nerve roots is supported by the work of Fernstrom (47), who reported on 35 patients who were operated on for herniated nucleus pulposus. No disc protrusion was found, but rather only a tear of the annulus fibrosus. This author (J.M.C.) has written elsewhere in this book concerning the pain sensitivity of the annulus fibrosus and the ability of such tearing to cause low back, pelvic, and thigh pain. Coupling this ability to cause such low back pain with the chemical irritation of the nerve root by nuclear material leaking into the spinal canal, we can see two possibilities for pain production in addition to the mechanical compression of the nerve root—namely, tearing of the annulus and the presence of free nuclear material within the spinal canal.

Harris and Wagnon (48) have shown circulatory blood flow increase through the fingertips following specific adjustments to the spine; they have shown that the response varies, depending on the location of the adjustment. Thus, they felt that adjustments to the spine can, via stimulation of the nervous system, affect the physiology of the tissues distant to the spine. This may be of importance in affecting the healing of nerve damage or circulatory disturbances accompanying disc lesions and nerve root compression.

MANIPULATION AND DISTRACTION TECHNIQUES AND CONCEPTS FOR LOW BACK AND LEG PAIN TREATMENT.

As we consider some of the manipulative treatments of low back and leg pain resulting from intervertebral disc lesions, we must think of two approaches that could be responsible for relief attained by manipulative efforts. These are, first, the reduction of annular and nuclear disc protrusion, with relief of the annular irritation that can cause back pain; and secondly, the possible effect of manipulation on stimulating circulation and causing resorption of the inflammatory effects of free nuclear material within the spinal canal.

Burton's Concepts of Traction Reduction

Burton (49) performs nonsurgical treatment of back-leg pain patients with acute contained disc herniations by using a chest harness to suspend the patient and using patient body weight as the distractive force. He finds the technique of benefit in the following three entities:

1. Disc "bulging" producing distention of the annulus and posterior longitudinal ligament. This entity produces pain by stimulating branches of the sinuvertebral nerve. A dorsal ramus pain syndrome, typically referred to the low back, hips, and knees, is produced. Pain is rarely referred as far as the ankles.

2. A herniated disc, in which nuclear material extends beyond the annulus but is contained by the posterior longitudinal ligament (sometimes called a "roof disc"). Compression of a spinal nerve either exiting or traversing the interspace produces sciatic pain that radiates to the toes and feet and neurological findings that are associated with this compression.

3. A herniated disc in which nuclear material extends beyond the annulus and is beginning to erode through the posterior longitudinal ligament but has not yet become a free protrusion.

Experience has shown that when herniated disc material extrudes past the posterior longitudinal ligament (free protrusion) or migrates in the spinal cord (sequestered fragment) the application of gravity traction accentuates pain and neurological deficit rather than alleviating it. This phenomenon occurs during the first few days of treatment and is most important to document, because it signals the need to discontinue the traction program and consider more aggressive treatment modalities such as chemonucleolysis or surgery.

Figure 12.1 shows Burton's schematic observation of what "before and after" CT scans show when gravity reduction is applied to contained discs. This indicates substantial change in spinal nerve root compression and suggests that the total reduction of disc protrusion is of secondary importance to nerve root decompression.

According to Hirschberg (50), herniation of a nucleus pulposus causing nerve compression can heal spontaneously, provided that low intradiscal pressure can be maintained for 3 months. He described two regimens: one of complete continuous bed rest, and an ambulatory regimen that includes the use of a canvas corset or plastic body jacket and specific exercise. The use of the ambulatory regimen alone or in combination with the bed rest regimen has produced complete disappearance of symptoms in more than 90% of patients.

Furthermore, he states that conservative management in the treatment of patients suffering from symptoms of a herniated nucleus pulposus should be tried before resorting to a surgical procedure and that this concept is commonly accepted. The danger of surgical complications, the certainty that laminectomy causes damage to the stability of the spine, and the occasional failure of surgical procedures to relieve symptoms indicate the advisability of an initial trial of conservative treatment.

According to Hirschberg, under favorable circumstances the protruded portion of the nucleus pulposus shrinks by dehydration, and the symptoms of nerve root compression are relieved. Over a period of months, the posterior wall of the annulus fibrosus heals, which may result in com-

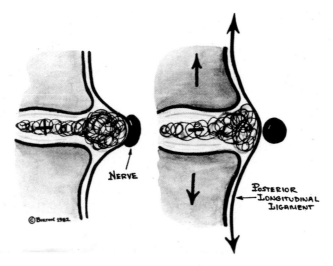

Figure 12.1. CT scanning shows that the application of axial traction on the vertebrae, annulus fibrosus, and longitudinal ligaments causes the protruding disc to diminish in volume but rarely to return to its normal state. The clinical problem relates to distention of annular and ligamentous dorsal ramus nerve fibers and spinal nerve compression. It is believed, in the basis of biomechanical calculation, that significant intradiscal negative pressures may be produced. The intermittent reduction appears to allow reparative processes to reestablish support. (Reproduced by permission of Churchill Livingstone from Burton CV: Gravity lumbar reduction. In: Kirkaldy-Willis WH: *Managing Low Back Pain.* Edinburgh, Churchill Livingstone, 1983, p 196.)

plete clinical recovery. If excessive pressure on the disc occurs before healing of the annulus fibrosus has progressed sufficiently, however, the tear will recur, additional disc material will be expelled, and symptoms will return or become aggravated. Conservative management, therefore, keeps the intradiscal pressure low enough for a period long enough to permit adequate healing of the annulus fibrosus. In our experience, it is approximately 3 months before a patient can carry out the activities of daily living without the danger of recurrence.

Neugebauer (51), who has treated more than 30,000 patients in 14 years, has proved that a disc prolapse can be converted into a disc relapse. He has achieved a 99% incidence of healing and believes that decompression treatment provides the only lasting recovery for the patient with a disc prolapse. Neugebauer has found that, as evidenced by x-ray measurement, he can increase the height of the L5 disc; he has increased the intervertebral disc distance from 3 mm dorsally and 9 mm ventrally to 6 mm dorsally and 15 mm ventrally over a course of treatment of 6 months. He is the first person to document that a disc can be reestablished by decompression treatment.

Neugebauer achieves three therapeutic effects by his decompression treatment:

1. The disc is reestablished.
2. The intervertebral foramen is enlarged, giving enough space for the nerve root to escape the prolapse.
3. Restretching of the anterior and posterior longitudinal ligaments brings the vertebra back into its normal position.

Other Concepts of Disc Treatment

Deyo et al. (28, 51a) state that, in principle, traction stretches the back so that vertebrae are pulled away from each other, and roentgenographic studies have suggested that spinal traction is capable of distracting vertebrae and diminishing disc protrusion in patients with herniated discs.

Tien-You (52), writing in the *Chinese Medical Journal*, states that manipulative reduction is the key to the treatment of patients with a protruded nucleus but asks the question: Can a protruded nucleus be reduced by simple manipulation? His answer is that a specific feature of the nucleus pulposus is its strong elasticity. This elasticity has been used during manipulative reduction to change the shape of the space between the affected vertebrae and to produce a retractile force by which the prolapsed nucleus is pulled back to its original position.

Others (53–60) using similar techniques have provided strong documentary evidence as to the effectiveness of manipulative treatment and/or the nonsurgical approach to the care of patients with myelographically proven disc protrusion who are awaiting surgery.

How much can the intervertebral disc space be opened on distraction? Gupta and Ramarao (61) write that traction by various methods was a very popular form of treatment for lumbar disc prolapse in the early years of this century. Subsequently, it fell into disrepute until the middle of the century, when more modern and sophisticated traction techniques were introduced and became popular. For example, Mathews (56) is reported to have demonstrated the efficacy of traction in the reduction of lumbar disc prolapse in three patients, with the help of epidurography. In his series, symptoms persisted and there was no change in the patterns on epidurograms in only two of 14 patients, supporting the popular belief that disc protrusion may safely be treated by traction.

According to Gupta and Ramarao (61), De Seze and Levernieux reported a distraction of 1.5 mm/disc space after lumbar traction (Fig. 12.2), and Mathews reported a vertebral distraction of 2 mm/disc after traction. Gupta and Ramarao, however, could demonstrate a vertebral distraction of only 0.5 mm/disc space.

Lind (62) documented a 20.7% increase in the intervertebral disc space during manipulative reduction of lumbar disc protrusion. Furthermore, of 20 patients awaiting surgery for lumbar disc protrusion, 14 received complete relief from pain within 1 hour of application of her autotraction technique.

In an article from China (63) on the treatment of lumbar disc protrusion by an automatic chiropractic traction instrument, it is reported that 73% of the 400 patients treated were completely cured of disc protrusion. Also, myelography showed that the defects reduced spontaneously; it was believed that the increased forward pressure of the longitudinal ligaments caused the protruded disc to return to its proper place.

Myelography has consistently shown that flexion of the lumbar spine causes disappearance of the bulge of the posterior annulus and longitudinal ligament as the anterior margins of the vertebral bodies approach each other and the posterior margins separate. The myelographic column becomes flat, and the dural sac closely approximates the back of the posterior longitudinal ligament and annulus. Even though flexion increases the force propulsing the disc posteriorly, it also tightens the posterior annulus and posterior longitudinal ligament and improves the barrier, with the net effect being reduction of the posterior protrusion. Raney (64) points out that complete prolapse is not helped by this procedure and that *abdominal compression and the Valsalva maneuver also diminish the amount of protrusion of the bulging disc.*

Discs absorb shock in two ways: (*a*) by squeezing fluid out of the nucleus, and/or (*b*) by allowing the fibers of the outer shell to stretch (65). Hukins and Hickey (66) show that the disc fibers have limited elasticity and suffer irreparable damage at 1.04 times their initial length. When a person is standing upright, the discs can withstand 10 times more compression than the vertebrae can, so a heavy load crushes the bones before it ruptures the disc. Disc fibers are less capable of coping with torsion because the stress then concentrates at points of maximum curvature. It has been reported that astronauts are 5 cm taller on their return to earth than they were when they left (65). Nachemson (67) reports that they are 10 cm taller.

Protrusion or rupture of the disc is usually preceded by degenerative changes characterized structurally by radiating cracks in the annulus that develop and weaken its resistance to nuclear herniation. As Tindall (68) points out, the sinuvertebral nerve supplies the posterior longitudinal ligament, periosteum, meninges, articular connective tissue, annulus, and vascular structures of the vertebral

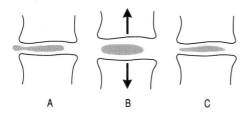

Figure 12.2. Effect of traction after discography. **A,** Disc herniation: dye protruding backwards (to the left). **B,** On traction, the protruding disc material returns to the center of the disc. **C,** On relaxing the traction, the disc material tends to remain in the center of the disc. (Reproduced from Kirkaldy-Willis WH: *Managing Low Back Pain.* Edinburgh, Churchill Livingstone, 1983, p 179. After Leverenieux J: *Les tractions vertébrales.* Paris, L'expansion, 1960.)

canal. The characteristic clinical features of back and leg pain, therefore, are related to irritation and stretching of the sinuvertebral nerve by the bulging annulus and by direct pressure on the nerve root, respectively (68).

Effects of Distraction of the Intervertebral Disc

According to Cyriax (69), there are three effects from traction and its attendant distraction on the intervertebral disc (Fig. 12.3):

1. Increase in the interval between the vertebral bodies, thus enlarging the space into which the protrusion must recede.
2. Tautening of the joint capsule, which allows the ligaments joining the vertebral bodies to exert centripetal force all around the joint, thus tending to squeeze the pulp back into place.
3. Suction.

Levernieux's experiments (69a) on spines under distractive forces were done on cadavers whose discs were injected with an opaque dye and then placed under tractive forces. Radiographs made before, during, and after traction showed that an internally disrupted disc, with the nuclear material protruding posteriorly into the vertebral canal, sees the dye pass into the center of the disc as the disc space is widened. After traction was complete, part of the contrast material was retained in the center of the disc (Fig. 12.2).

De Seze (70, 71) felt that low back pain was caused by nuclear fragments becoming lodged within the annular cracks. This created annular bulging and pressure on the sinuvertebral sensory nerve innervation of the annular fibers. His explanation of how manipulation corrected disc protrusion is shown in Figure 12.4.

IS THE DISC THE SOURCE OF LOW BACK PAIN?

Graham (72) explored the question of whether back pain emanated from disc, facet joint, adjacent musculature or the lateral recess. Two hundred consecutive patients underwent discographic examination of their discs, and during the procedure their pain responses were monitored. In 111 of the 200 patients, their original pain was precisely intensified during discography, while an additional 43 patients who had no

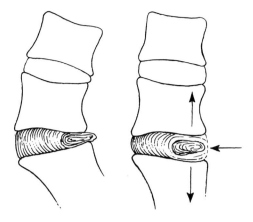

Figure 12.3. Positive effect of traction (lumbar flexion) upon protruding fragment of disc. (Reproduced with permission from Finneston BE: *Low Back Pain*, ed 2. Philadelphia, JB Lippincott, 1980, p 312.)

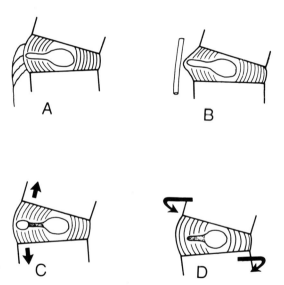

Figure 12.4. Explanation of the way in which manipulation may reduce pressure of a disc herniation on a nerve. **A,** Herniation with irritation of branches of sinuvertebral nerve. **B,** Herniation with pressure on a spinal nerve. **C,** Traction separates the vertebral bodies and allows the herniated material to return to the nucleus. **D,** Rotation encourages further return of herniated material to the nucleus. (From Kirkaldy-Willis WH: *Managing Low Back Pain*. Edinburgh, Churchill Livingstone, 1983, p 179. Originally modified from Sandoz R: Some physical mechanisms and effects of spinal adjustments. *Ann Swiss Chirop Assoc* 6:91, 1976, after de Sèze S: Les manipulations vértebral. Sem Hôp Paris 1:2313, 1955.)

pain during discography had an increased intensity of the presenting pain during the ensuing 24 hours of mobilization. Graham felt that these findings suggested that in the majority of patients, *low back pain did emanate from the disc, as suggested by Mixter and Barr in 1934.*

Acute Symptomatic Disc Protrusion

Kessler (73), in a discussion on the effects of pelvic traction, states that *"static pelvic traction must not be used in the acute stage of a disc prolapse."* The patient may feel less pain while the distractive force is applied, but as the traction is released, he often experiences a marked increase in pain. He may have some difficulty in rising from the treatment table. Such an effort is probably due to absorption of additional fluid by the nucleus while the traction is applied and the development of a high intradiscal pressure as the distractive force is relaxed. This unfortunate result is less likely to occur with intermittent traction, but few patients in the acute stage tolerate this well. We often hear of the patient with low back pain who enters the hospital and is placed in pelvic traction. How often these patients are the same or even worse following such traction! In clinical practice we often see patients who have been hospitalized, had every test done, and were discharged in the same or worse condition. Static traction actually opens the intervertebral disc space, can allow the nucleus to imbibe fluids, and can thereby increase the intradiscal pressure, which will cause a worsening of pressure against the already compressed nerve root.

According to Kessler (73), if a patient is hospitalized or can attend therapy sessions without risking worsening of the lesion from increased intradiscal pressure, treatment may include specific segmental manual distraction techniques applied by a therapist skilled in such techniques. Oscillatory techniques may relieve pain by increasing large fiber and proprioceptive input and thus by relieving some of the protective muscle spasm. Possibly, decreasing the longitudinal slack in the posterior longitudinal ligament and annular lamellae overlying the bulge in the disc effects a centripetal movement of the disc material away from the pain-sensitive structures.

Thus, Kessler (73) believes that the management of the patient with an acute disc protrusion should include

1. Bed rest with short periods of ambulation;
2. Avoidance of positions or activity that may increase intradiscal pressure, especially sitting, forward bending, and the Valsalva maneuver;
3. Relaxation of reflexed muscle splinting;
4. *Specific segmental distraction techniques.*

Please note that the *Cox technique is a specific intermittent distraction.* Distraction of the disc provides a push-pull pumping effect on the intervertebral disc space as the caudal section of the table is gently moved up and down during traction. This movement creates a milking action on the intervertebral disc space. *Remember that in the acute stage of a disc lesion, the patient may not tolerate traction until some of the swelling and inflammation has dissipated.*

ANOTHER OPINION ON TRACTION APPLICATION

McElhannon (74) gives four basic purposes for traction:

1. Enlargement of the intervertebral disc space;
2. Tautening of posterior longitudinal ligament to create a centripetal force on the annulus fibrosus;
3. Separation of apophyseal joints;
4. Enlargement of intervertebral foramina.

He listed 12 contraindications for traction: malignancy, cord compression, infectious disease, osteoporosis, hypertension or cardiovascular disease, rheumatoid arthritis, old age, pregnancy, active peptic ulcer, hiatal hernia, aortic aneurysm, or hemorrhoids.

The "rule of three" is advocated by McElhannon. It says that the patient must be seen for distraction for 3 consecutive days at the beginning of care. The patient may feel some discomfort after the first session, but it should diminish on the second or third session. The lordotic curve must be flattened in order to distract the vertebrae. He advocates static traction for the first three sessions, in order to adapt the muscles and ligaments to the force, and then the use of intermittent or kinetic traction, holding for 30 seconds and releasing for 10 seconds. Acute discs are, in McElhannon's opinion, best handled by static traction until the spasm and radiculitis begin to subside; then treatment should be changed to intermittent traction.

EFFECT OF EXTENSION MANIPULATION ON THE NUCLEUS PULPOSUS

Gill, Videman, Shimizu, and Mooney (75) studied the effect of mechanical treatment on the intervertebral disc by performing extension/compression moments on discographically injected discs of 19 cadavers. A total of 103 discs were studied in this manner. Repeated extension moments applied to lumbar motion segments forced the dye from the nucleus pulposus into the spinal epidural space, or into the peridural space in abnormal discs. Normal discs did not see the dye extravasate out of the nucleus pulposus through a defect in the annulus. Only when the disc was pathological did extension cause the leakage of dye posteriorly into the spinal canal. This finding of evidence causing dye to be forced into the spinal canal has been shown in many other studies, as described in Chapter 2, "Biomechanics of the Lumbar Spine." Extension, by this author's (J.M.C.) study and clinical judgment, can be used when disc protrusion is either not present or when healing of a disc protrusion has shown at least 50% improvement of subjective symptoms and objective findings of straight leg raise and range of motion of the thoracolumbar spine. Extension, this author feels, can be helpful in the later stages of disc healing by narrowing the posterior disc space and allowing the nucleus to be contained within the interspace while strong healing of the annular fibers takes place.

STODDARD'S OSTEOPATHIC TECHNIQUE (76)

Stoddard (75) has described his osteopathic technique as follows:

The treatment of intervertebral disc herniation should start long before it occurs. We should manipulate and mobilize osteopathic spinal lesions long before they lead to these degenerative changes and not leave them to take their course. If on examination of the spine we find areas of restricted mobility or even single lesions, our duty is to release the restricted joints and insure normality as far as is within our power.

I am of the firm opinion that a herniated disc can sometimes be replaced by manipulation, but when a true prolapse of the disc occurs, I am convinced that it is impossible to replace the nuclear material by manipulation. At that stage all that can be achieved by manipulation is the empirical attempt to shift the position of nerve root and prolapsed nuclear material so that less pressure occurs on the nerve root.

By herniation of a disc I envision a bulging of the annulus sufficient to press on and irritate the posterior longitudinal ligament and dura mater without a complete rupture of the annulus and the posterior longitudinal ligament. If there is sufficient outer annular fibers and posterior ligaments to hold the herniation from protruding right through them I think it ought to be possible to reposition the nuclear material—not that such a state of affairs is desirable, it is a highly vulnerable condition—but clinically at least such cases are rewarding in that the patient obtains a dramatic relief of symptoms. even though at a later date he may well have a relapse. After all, a track has been formed in the circular fibers of the annulus and such a tract does not repair well, if at all, because cartilage once torn is not repaired with cartilage but merely with fibrous tissue. At best we can hope for fibrous tissue repair and provide additional support either by improving the muscles surrounding the joint or by using artificial external supports.

When nuclear material has escaped into the spinal canal and has become wedged between the nerve root and the intervertebral foramen, manipulation can sometimes alter the site of pressure or shift the prolapsed material to another site where there is less irritation of the nerve roots. If the technics are designed to achieve this and they are sufficiently gentle to avoid further damage, they are well worth attempting because in roughly half of the cases the attempts succeed. If the attempts are successful, the patient has still to observe caution; the hope is that the prolapsed material will in time shrink and cause less trouble. In the meantime a laminectomy has been avoided. If the attempt is unsuccessful and the technic is designed to avoid further damage, the patient is no worse off and, if necessary, can still take advantage of surgical procedures(76) [a].

Stoddard's guide to the prognosis of the effect of manipulation on the disc lesion is based on straight leg raising tests. If the test is positive at 30° or less, the prospects of success are distinctly limited. The smaller the angle, the less likely is manipulation to be successful, and the lower the level of disc lesion, the less chance of success. A probable reason for this observation is that the lowest intervertebral foramen has the smallest hole and the largest nerve root. There is, therefore, less opportunity for maneuver and alteration of position.

Given a patient with a disc prolapse at the L4-L5 level, and a straight leg raise that is positive at 45°, the chances of success by manipulation are more than 50%, and by success I do not mean

---

[a] From Stoddard A: *A Manual of Osteopathic Technic.* New York, Harper & Row, 1969.

complete relief of pain but a substantial reduction of pain and a reduction of physical signs.

Stoddard's technique of stretching the sciatic nerve involves placing the patient on his side while stretching the lower extremity over the side of the table. The idea is to make sure that the articular facets are at least mobile and that adhesions are released on the nonpainful side. The technique is applied on both sides. Stoddard believes that this procedure alters the position of the nerve root and the prolapsed disc. According to Stoddard, during application of the flexion and extension technique with use of the McManis table, *"the lower leaf of the table ought not be pressed far down into too much flexion in case gapping of the joint causes a herniation of the disc"* (76) (italics added).

The technique is useful on both the thoracic and the lumbar spine, but here you must rely on patient cooperation and on the patient's ability to grip the top of the table firmly and yet relax the spine. Such controlled relaxation is not easy by any means but should be possible for the average cooperative patient.

A combination of movements can be obtained by using the lower leaf of the McManis table to open to two of its ranges, but such combined movements are complex, are not easy to control, and are rarely indicated anyway. The goal is to place the pivot of movement just below the level of the lesion and, while articulating all levels of the lower thoracic and lumbar joints, to pay special attention to those joints at which there is a *restricted range of movement*.

GAUGING PATIENT RESPONSE TO SURGERY AND MANIPULATION

Of the 200,000 back surgeries done in the United States annually, 30% fail to relieve any pain, and at 5-year follow-up, only 10% of the remainder have provided satisfactory relief (77). Malec et al. (78) define success from back surgery thusly: The patient is free from the use of pain medication and is more active than he was before treatment, i.e., working, training, running a house, or capable of continued exercise 50% to 100% of the time with no increase in pain. Trief (77), however, defines success as improvement in the straight leg raise of 20°, and the ability to bring the knee 10 cm closer to the chest.

Recent interest in manipulation as an adjunct to the conservative treatment of low back and sci-atic pain led us to study the effects of this procedure on a group of patients who had this typical syndrome and have received little relief from ordinary conservative care (40).

In an analysis of 205 patients with clinically diagnosed ruptured intervertebral disc who were treated conservatively, which included rotatory manipulation, Mensor (79) reports prompt and satisfactory relief of symptoms in 64% of his private patients and 45% of his patients injured in industrial accidents. These results are considerably better than those reported by Colonna and Friedenberg (80), who found that only 29% of 28 patients whose myelograms were positive for disc rupture were pain-free after conservative treatment without manipulation. It should be noted that these two series are not necessarily comparable because Mensor did not use myelograms as an aid in establishing diagnosis. It is possible that patients with the best manipulative results did not have myelographically demonstrable protrusions.

In an attempt to determine how manipulative treatment alleviates symptoms, Wilson and Ilfeld (81) studied 18 patients with a ruptured intervertebral disc, the diagnosis of which was clinically firmly established; myelography was performed both before and after rotatory manipulation. Only two of the 18 patients received anesthesia for the manipulation. Thirteen showed myelographic defects before manipulation; five did not. Myelographic changes after manipulation were seen in only one patient whose myelogram was positive and in whom the size of the defect increased slightly. Three of the patients had brief improvement, and 12 of the 18 subsequently underwent operation.

The following conclusions can be drawn from these last studies.

1. Twenty of 39 patients (51%) who were unequivocally diagnosed as having a ruptured intervertebral disc unrelieved by conservative care had good or excellent results after rotatory manipulation of the spine under anesthesia, thus confirming Mensor's results (51.2%) with this method.

2. The appearance of the myelograms of these patients before and after manipulation, whether positive or negative, were unchanged.

3. Ten of the 27 patients whose myelograms were positive had good to excellent results 3 years or more after manipulation.

4. Patients whose myelograms were negative consistently did better after manipulation than those whose myelograms showed a defect.

Singer et al. (82) evaluated various predictors of therapeutic outcome in acute low back pain patients and found that pain intensity at entry proved to be the best universal predictor of outcome.

SURGICAL OUTCOMES

Cauda equina syndrome secondary to a central disc lesion, in a study of 31 cases, showed all to have urinary retention preoperatively; this proved to be the most seriously affected function and remained so postoperatively. The prognosis for return of motor power was good; since 27 of 30 patients who were operated on regained normal motor function. Even though early surgery is recommended, this study showed that decompression does not have to be performed in less than 6 hours if recovery is to occur, as has been suggested in the past (83).

Hellstrom et al. (84) measured urinary bladder function urodynamically in 17 patients operated on 2 to 3 years previously for cauda equina syndrome caused by a prolapsed lumbar intervertebral disc. Ten reported normal urination, and seven had symptoms of urinary obstruction or incontinence. Regeneration of the autonomous nerves supplying the bladder and genitals may require an interval of several months to years.

Myrseth (85) reported that sciatica lasting not more than 6 months from onset to operation was correlated with a better surgical result. After removal of a prolapsed disc fragment in 97 patients, 62% were completely fit, and 35% were improved by the operation.

Children with lumbar disc protrusion that was surgically treated were reported by Fisher and Saunders (86) as being similar to adults with respect to symptoms, signs, myelograms, and surgical findings.

RESULT OF EPIDURAL STEROID INJECTION

Andersen and Mosdal (87) seem to adequately evaluate epidural injection results when they report on 16 patients following treatment. Ten (62%) had relief of half their pain and sciatica the following day. One month later, only seven patients reported one-third relief of their symptoms, and only one patient was found to have benefited at retesting at 6 months. The remaining six patients had no relief at all. The results are not

encouraging, and for long-lasting relief the procedure was useless.

INTERVERTEBRAL DISC PAIN SENSITIVITY AND PRODUCTION

The sinuvertebral nerve supplies the posterior longitudinal ligament, annulus fibrosus, and neurovascular contents of the epidural space (88, 89). The outer annulus and the nerve root are the most pain-sensitive and can reproduce the patient's presurgical symptoms when stimulated 3 to 4 weeks postsurgically (67).

The existence of unmyelinated nerve endings, usually associated with pain reception in the posterior annulus and even penetrating the nucleus, are increasingly evident. The posterior longitudinal ligament is well innervated (90).

When a radial tear penetrates the outer annulus, there is an attempt at healing by ingrowth of granulation tissue. Naked endings of the sinuvertebral nerve have been identified in this granulation tissue. These endings may be pain receptors, which would explain discogenic pain in the absence of herniation (91).

Tsukada (92) believes that there are nerve fibers not only in the posterior longitudinal ligament but also in the nucleus and notochord. Malinsky (93) and Hirsch et al. (94) suggest that nerve fibers accompany granulation tissue in free nerve endings within the inner layers of the annulus and in the nucleus of some degenerated discs. In this same article, Yoshizawa et al. (95) are reported to have found profuse free nerve terminals in the outer half of the annulus but no such terminals in the nucleus. According to Sunderland (96), the recurrent meningeal nerve supplies the dura, the intervertebral disc, and associated structures.

The sinuvertebral nerve divides into ascending, descending, and transverse branches adjacent to the posterior longitudinal ligament (97). According to Lazorthes (98), this nerve supplies the neural laminae, the intervertebral disc at adjacent levels, the posterior longitudinal ligaments, the internal vertebral plexus, the epidural tissue, and the dura mater. It should be noted, however, that although there is still disagreement concerning what tissue is supplied by this nerve, some investigators believe that there is such a wide distribution. Tsukada (92) and Shinohara (99) have found that in a normal disc the outer annulus is innervated but that in a degenerated disc, fine nerve fibers accompany granulation tissue present in degenerating nuclear material.

According to Macnab (100), the pain of osteoporosis can be ascribed to trabecular buckling or fracture. Pain is also due to the venous spaces in the vertebral body spongiosa. The intraosseous venous pressure of a normal vertebra is 20 mm and that of an osteoporotic vertebra is about 40 mm.

Farfan (101) points out that the disc contains A, B, and G nerve fibers and that the G nerve fibers are found in high-velocity communicating networks. If the disc is not sensory, why then are they present?

One series (102) reports that in at least some circumstances low back pain is provoked by direct mechanical stimuli. This effect was demonstrated in experiments made during spine surgery when the patient was under local anesthesia. According to Spurling and Grantham (103), patients often complained of back pain when the annulus fibrosus was manipulated. Falconer et al. (104) report that during spine surgery, pressing on a disc prolapse produced low back pain, whereas pressing on a nerve root produced sciatica. Longitudinal nerve root stretching did not produce pain. Hirsch (105) found that lumbar pain was sometimes elicited by pressing on an intervertebral disc. According to Wiberg (106) however, pressing on the nerve root caused acute "root pain," whereas pressing on the intervertebral disc caused back pain. Disc palpation caused pain whether or not the area was anesthesized. At surgery, Smyth and Wright (107) tied threads into various structures of the low back. After the surgery, the effects of pulling on these threads was recorded. *"Pulling on the dura mater, the ligamentum flavum, or the interspinous ligaments provoked no pain. Pressing on the nerve root caused pain, and the nerve root involved in the herniation was much more sensitive than the uninvolved nerve root. Pressure on the annulus fibrosus caused sciatic pain and sometimes caused backache"* (107).

A second series concerns studies of pain accompanying fluid injection into an intervertebral disc during discography. Although not all authors are in agreement, there is a significant amount of literature on the subject.

For example, Hirsch (105) found that pain typical of back pain was produced in 16 patients by injection of normal saline into the lumbar disc, especially if considerable pressure was needed for the injection. This pain disappeared after a few minutes. Lindblom (108) found that on discography in 150 patients, back pain occurred when the needle passed through the posterior surface of the disc but not when the needle entered the center of the disc. Injection of contrast medium and an anesthetic produced pain similar to low back pain. If the disc did not hold the fluid, no pain was produced. According to Hirsch (105), when normal saline was injected, pain was elicited only in the presence of raised pressure. When the pressure dropped, the pain disappeared. These reports imply that the pain was due to the pressure increase rather than to the chemical irritation.

Cloward and Buzaid (109) found that injection of contrast medium into a disc was often painful and frequently elicited back pain similar to that elicited by bending or lifting. *Collis and Gardner (110) injected contrast medium into the lumbar discs of 400 patients with surgically verified herniated discs. Of these injections, 68% produced both back and leg pain, 26% produced only back pain, and only 6% produced no pain at all.* On injection of contrast medium into 148 cervical discs in 50 volunteer subjects who were free of any cervical pathology, Holt (111) found that needle insertion produced only slight discomfort but that injection produced severe pain in every subject at every disc space injected! This pain lasted about 5 minutes, then disappeared completely. Again, this seems to point to mechanical rather than chemical pain receptors.

In a later report on lumbar discography, however, Holt found that little discomfort resulted from injection of a normal lumbar disc. Discomfort resulted only when the contrast medium came into contact with any tissue having sensory innervation, implying that the irritation was chemical rather than mechanical. Hudgins (112) also found that the pain response elicited by lumbar discography was inconstant and unreliable. Occasionally, injection reproduced back pain.

A third series concerns studies of pain referred from the low back regions. The objectives of these studies were to determine when pain was referred and from what structures. Injections of hypertonic saline solution into structures superficial to the disc were the stimuli. The original work was done by Kellgren (113) and several investigators (114) did follow-up studies. Considerable controversy has arisen over some of the issues. Aside from the controversy, all authors seem to agree that the injections caused pain much of the time. Sometimes it was local pain, and sometimes it was referred pain. Whether the pain resulted from the mechanical pressure of the injected fluid or from chemical irritation is not clear.

Perhaps more work on injection responses and pain-sensing mechanisms would be of value, if it could be done without excessive risk. Attempts should be made to distinguish chemical stimuli from mechanical stimuli. Only Hirsch's results seem to allow this distinction to be made, if one assumes that normal saline would not produce any chemical irritation (105).

According to LaMotte (115), the word *nociceptors* is defined broadly as those endings of certain peripheral nerve fibers in humans, and by inference in animals, which when active are associated with sensations of pain. There are numerous peripheral sources of low back pain. Distortion of the annulus and facet joints could stretch the posterior longitudinal ligament and activate nociceptors in the ligament. There is evidence that the outer border of the annulus fibrosus is supplied with nerve endings and that pain can arise from intradiscal injection of a contrast material. Also, intradiscal injection of chymopapain in the treatment of lumbar disc herniations can, in certain cases, relieve pain in minutes.

The observations and illustrative cases surgically explored by Torkildsen (116) give support to the idea that cervical spondylosis giving rise to brachialgia may simultaneously be the cause of pains in the leg that resemble sciatica. This may be the case even if spondyloarthritic changes are limited to the cervical intervertebral canal. This type of sciatica—brachialgic sciatica—differs in nature from true sciatica as seen in cases of lumbar disc lesion. The differential diagnostic points are pyramidal tract signs; i.e., deep reflexes of the painful leg are increased, the plantar reflex is extensor in response, and the tone of the painful leg extends beyond the limits of one or two dermatomes, with the Achilles reflexes being bilaterally equal. These signs occur in addition to the peripheral nerve lesions of the arm.

The sources of pain in various structures associated with ruptured discs have been identified by Murphy (117). *The sequence of events as involves pain in the lumbar region is as follows: When an incomplete tear in the annulus occurs, and if the tear is in the midline posteriorly, a fragment of nucleus will protrude into this tear, stretching the annulus and posterior longitudinal ligament, causing midline back pain. If the tear in the annulus is lateral, then the pain will be over the sacroiliac joint and in the buttock and hip, with nerve root compression, and depending on the level, it will cause radiation of pain down the leg.* For example, if a patient claims that his back pain stopped when his leg pain began, it is almost a certainty that the disc fragment has extruded through the posterior longitudinal ligament into the canal and will have to be removed.

COX CLOSED REDUCTION OF DISC PROTRUSION

The Zenith®-Cox® Table

In the early 1970s, this author developed the Zenith®-Cox® table, which was a blending of osteopathic and chiropractic principles into one instrument. This table has application in the treatment of lumbar disc protrusion, spondylolisthesis, facet syndrome, subluxation, and scoliotic curves of a nonsurgical nature and can be used to place the articulations of the spine through the normal ranges of motion. These normal ranges of motion are *flexion, extension, lateral bending, rotation, and circumduction* (Figs. 12.5 to 12.9).

Closed Reduction: Its Definition and Use in the Patient with an Acute Disc Lesion

Cox flexion distraction manipulation is a form of chiropractic spinal manipulative therapy allowing the following benefits:

1. It increases the intervertebral disc height to remove annular distortion in the pain-sensitive peripheral annular fibers.
2. It allows the nucleus pulposus to assume its central position within the annulus and relieve irritation of the pain-sensitive annular fibers.
3. It restores vertebral joints to their physiological relationships of motion.
4. It improves posture and locomotion while relieving pain, improving body functions, and creating a state of well-being.

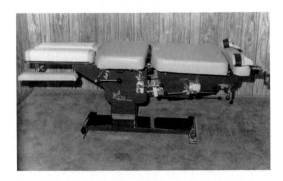

Figure 12.5. Zenith®-Cox® table in its closed position.

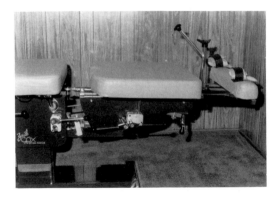

Figure 12.6. Zenith®-Cox® table in distraction position.

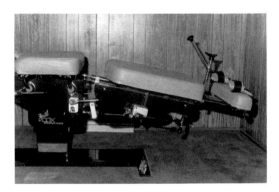

Figure 12.7. Zenith®-Cox® table in flexion distraction position.

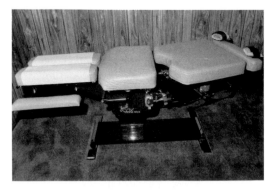

Figure 12.8. Zenith®-Cox® table in lateral flexion position.

Note that we use the term *closed reduction*. This term has been used in much of the literature as well as by this author. Frankly, it has met with some misunderstanding, in that it has been mis-

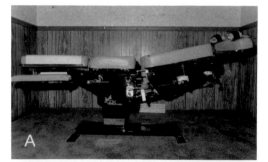

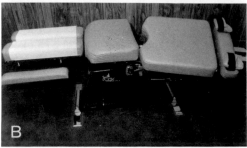

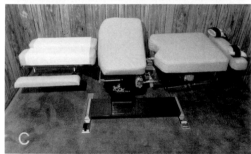

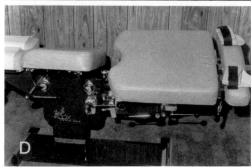

Figure 12.9. **A**, Zenith®-Cox® table in position for application of extension to the spine. **B**, Table with caudal section in rotation position for lumbar spine rotation. **C**, Table with thoracic rotation section for motion palpation of the thoracic spine. **D**, Table with combined lumbar and thoracic rotation section for manipulation of "S" scoliotic thoracolumbar curves.

taken for a surgical procedure, such as setting a broken bone. Closed reduction should be understood to be in opposition to a surgical open reduction or surgical removal of a disc protrusion or prolapse.

Treatment of the patient with acute disc protrusion or prolapse demands specific care. The steps preparatory to distraction are explained next.

Acupressure Point Therapy (Fig. 12.10)

A deep goading pressure is applied as shown in Figures 12.11 and 12.12, in preparation for distraction. The goading pressure is applied over the paravertebral areas of the upper lumbar spine through the coccyx. These areas coincide with bladder meridian points B24 through B35 at the coccyx.

The goading is then applied into the belly of the gluteus maximus muscle (Fig. 12.13). Further information on the treatment of this muscle is given in a later chapter; suffice it here to state that the gluteus maximus is supplied by the inferior gluteal nerve having a common spinal origin with the sciatic nerve. The pain and spasm of the gluteus maximus muscle will recede as the disc lesion heals and the sciatic nerve is relieved. Therefore, a deep goading pressure is placed into the belly of this muscle for 15 to 20 seconds both before and after treatment. The relaxation and loss of pain in this muscle is an indicator of patient response.

Next, the gluteus medius and minimus muscles are goaded (Fig. 12.14), at their origin and insertion prior to distraction. These are abductor muscles of the lower extremity, are quite painful to palpation, and are usually weak to muscle testing.

Bladder meridian point B54 in the popliteal space is goaded vigorously for 15 to 20 seconds (Fig. 12.15). This point is used in acupuncture to relieve sciatic pain.

The goading of the adductores and gracilis

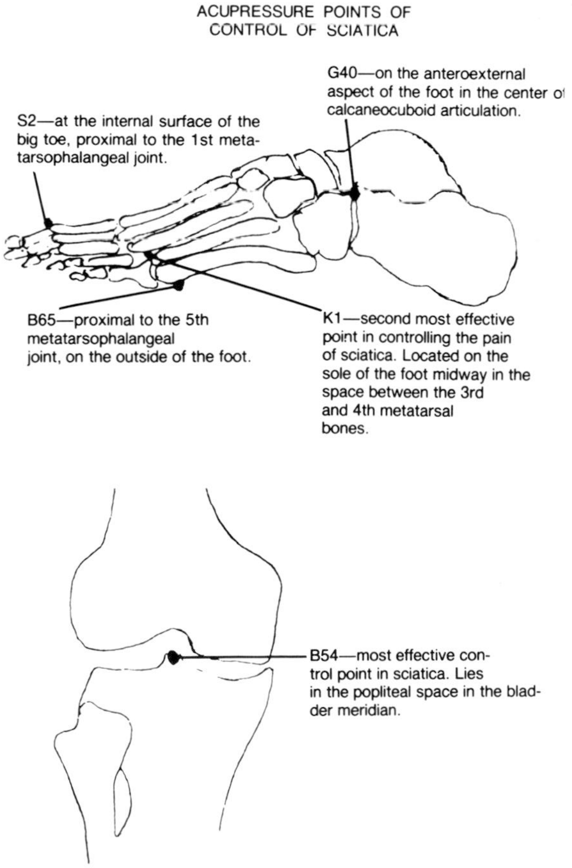

ACUPRESSURE POINTS OF
CONTROL OF SCIATICA

G40—on the anteroexternal aspect of the foot in the center of calcaneocuboid articulation.

S2—at the internal surface of the big toe, proximal to the 1st metatarsophalangeal joint.

B65—proximal to the 5th metatarsophalangeal joint, on the outside of the foot.

K1—second most effective point in controlling the pain of sciatica. Located on the sole of the foot midway in the space between the 3rd and 4th metatarsal bones.

B54—most effective control point in sciatica. Lies in the popliteal space in the bladder meridian.

Figure 12.10. Acupressure point therapy for sciatica.

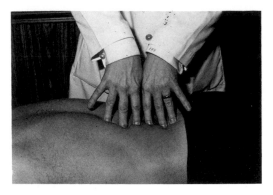

Figure 12.11. Paravertebral bladder meridian acupressure points being goaded.

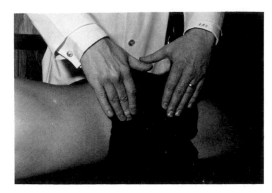

Figure 12.14. Abductor muscle origin and insertion pressure applied.

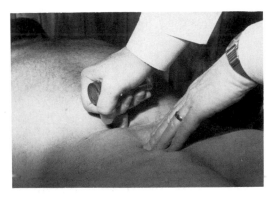

Figure 12.12. Deep pressure is applied with an instrument for ease of application.

muscles at their origins and insertions is shown in Figures 12.16 and 12.17. These muscles are supplied by the obturator nerve from the second, third, and fourth lumbar nerve roots. They are extremely tight and painful in the patient with a disc lesion. These muscles are also discussed in a later chapter on muscle treatment.

Testing Patient Tolerance to Flexion Distraction Manipulation

Prior to application of Cox flexion distraction manipulation, the doctor must determine if the technique will cause any iatrogenic changes. This is avoided by testing as follows: Place the patient on the instrument, lying prone, with the anterior superior iliac spines 2 to 3 inches cephalad of the bottom of the thoracic section, as shown in Figure 12.18.

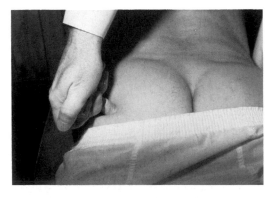

Figure 12.13. Gluteus maximus B49 acupressure point being goaded.

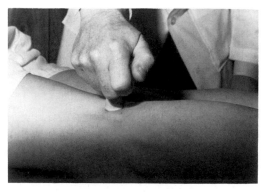

Figure 12.15. Bladder meridian point B54 being goaded.

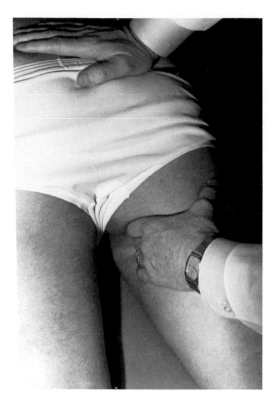

Figure 12.16. Pressure goading of the adductores muscle origins.

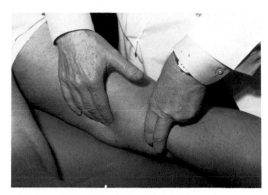

Figure 12.17. Pressure goading of the adductor and gracilis insertions.

The cuffs are not placed on the patient. A downward tractive force with the caudal section of the instrument is applied as shown in Figure 12.18, using only the patient's lower extremity and pelvic weight as the force used to traction the spine. The contact hand thenar eminence is on the spinous process of the lumbar vertebrae while the tractive force is applied. Each of the lumbar segments is tested from T12-L1 to the L5-S1 level. If no pain is felt on central spinous process distractive force, the contact with the thenar eminence is moved laterally over the facet joints. Unilateral traction is tested by grasping the ankle on the side of facet contact and applying a gentle downward pressure with the table caudal section while asking the patient if this causes any pain in the low back or lower extremities. This lateral facet irritation testing is shown in Figure 12.19.

If the patient feels no low back or lower extremity pain, the cuffs can be placed on the ankles for the application of normal flexion distraction. If there is pain felt on testing, either central or lateral, *the cuffs are not placed on the patient.* Instead, a flexion pillow is placed under the abdo-

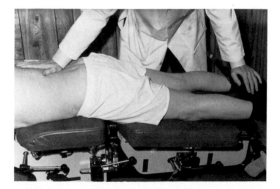

Figure 12.18. Testing patient tolerance to flexion distraction. The cuffs are not applied to the ankles, and only the patient's lower extremity weight is used as a tractive force.

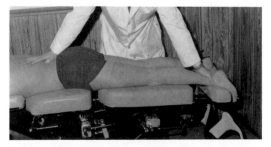

Figure 12.19. Lateral facet tolerance to flexion distraction is tested by unilateral distraction. The ankle on the side of traction is held during traction while the facet joints are held in place.

men to allow minimal flexion to the lumbar spine (Fig. 12.20).

Caring for the Patient If Testing Elicits Pain

The most common condition in which pain is elicited on testing for tolerance to flexion distraction is the acute disc lesion in which the patient has sciatica. Second most common, in this author's experience, is pain in acute lumbago conditions in which severe muscle spasm and forward flexion of the lumbar spine are seen. When this negative reaction to the use of flexion distraction is found, the following treatment program is recommended: Apply positive galvanic current through the involved disc and paravertebral muscles for 15 minutes, as shown in Figure 12.21. If the patient is in too much pain to lie on the stomach, he or she may lie on the side, as shown in Figure 12.22, while the therapy is applied. During this 15-minute period, moist heat is applied to the low back and pelvis into the thigh over the course of the painful sciatic nerve (Fig. 12.23). Following the heat application, we remove the heat and place cold packs over the same area, as shown in Figure 12.24. Often, if severe spasm of the paravertebral muscles is found, we will apply tetanizing current to the muscles while the ice is applied for relief of spasm and swelling.

Treatment If Testing Does Not Elicit Pain

If the patient felt no pain on testing, we will place the cuffs on the ankles and proceed as described below.

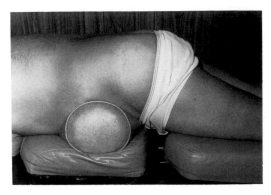

Figure 12.20. A flexion roll is placed under the patient who feels pain when tested for his tolerance to flexion distraction manipulation. This allows slight flexion of the lumbar spine, which often allows relief of pain when disc protrusion or facet syndrome exists.

If pain was felt on testing, the cuffs are not used until traction is found to be nonpainful when applied by grasping the ankle and applying unilateral distraction while holding the spinous process with the treating hand. Therefore, if pain is felt without the cuffs in place, no cuffs are used until such time as there is no pain upon controlled distraction by holding the ankle and applying traction to one leg at a time.

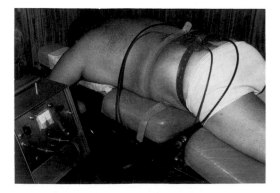

Figure 12.21. Positive galvanism is applied to the disc as the patient lies prone.

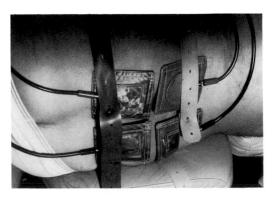

Figure 12.22. Positive galvanism is applied to the disc as the patient lies on the side.

Treating the Patient with Sciatica Due to a Disc Lesion

GETTING THE PATIENT ON AND OFF THE TABLE

To lie down on the table, the patient is told to tighten the abdominal and gluteal muscles and to lower him- or herself onto the table by supporting his or her weight on the arms until the prone posture is reached (Fig. 12.25). In arising from the table, a belt support is placed on the patient, and he or she stands upright by pushing up with the arms while sliding the lower extremities from the table (Fig. 12.26). The doctor or assistant supports the patient if need be. The belt used by this author is the Dee Cee Laboratories support, which has a memory foam insert that is effectively held against the lumbar spine with uniform pressure by the elastic belt.

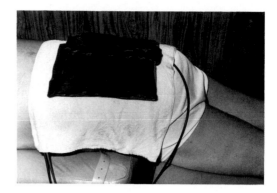

Figure 12.24. Cryotherapy is applied to the low back as galvanic or tetanizing currents are applied.

Mechanics of Applying Cox Distraction Manipulation to the Disc Patient

Figure 12.27 shows the patient lying on the instrument with the cuffs on and a small flexion roll under the abdomen. If the patient has a built-in flexion roll, that is, a large abdomen, no flexion lift is added. The flexion assists the patient in lying on the table. Often patients cannot lie prone on the table due to the lordosis afforded to the lumbar spine in this position; sometimes we must even treat the patient lying on the side, as shown in Figure 12.28. Once the patient is comfortably placed on the instrument, he or she is tested for the ability to undergo flexion distraction manipulation as described earlier. If the patient is able to undergo manipulation, application is as follows.

Medial and lateral discs are treated with the same basic approach. Always be sure to contact

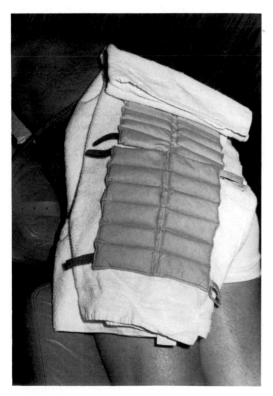

Figure 12.23. Moist heat is applied to the low back and extremity.

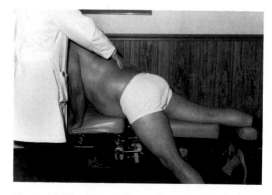

Figure 12.25. Doctor directs the patient to hold the abdominal and buttock muscles taut while lowering himself onto the instrument.

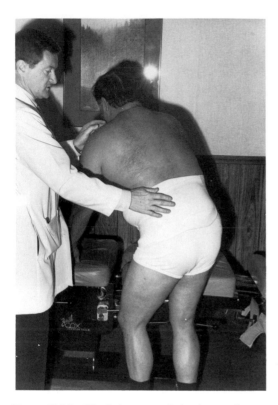

Figure 12.26. The belt support is in place as the patient arises from the prone posture.

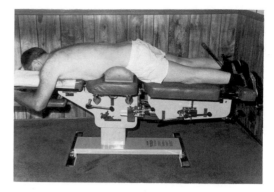

Figure 12.27. The patient lies on the table with a flexion roll under the abdomen.

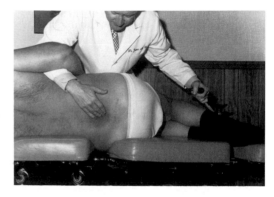

Figure 12.28. The patient can lie on the side for flexion distraction manipulation if pain prohibits him from lying prone.

the spinous process above the disc to be distracted, because contact of the spinous process below the level of protruding disc could force the disc cephalad and into the nerve root if the disc had a medial type of protrusion.

Please note that the patient's anterior superior iliac spines (ASISs) are placed 2 to 3 inches cephalad of the opening of the thoracic and caudal sections of the table (Fig. 12.27). This places the disc to be tractioned on the middle section of the instrument for easy control of movement and tractive force. Also note that the ankle cuff section has been drawn taut so that all slack is taken out of the table sections. The patient's arms lie comfortably on the arm rests.

THREE 20-SECOND FLEXION SESSIONS ARE UTILIZED

The actual manipulative application consists of three 20-second distractive sessions. Between sessions, the doctor will reposition his or her treating hand for proper spinous process placement. With the patient properly placed on the table, the

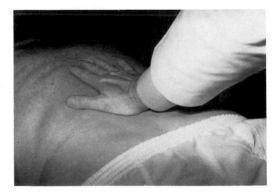

Figure 12.29. The thenar contact of the doctor's hand is under the spinous process directly above the disc space to be distracted.

doctor makes a contact on the spinous process as shown in Figure 12.29. The caudal section of the instrument is flexed downward until tautness is felt under the spinous process contact on the spine by the doctor's thenar contact. From this point of tautness, meaning that all tissue and joint play has been removed and the joint under the contact hand is afforded all the tractive force, *no more than 1 to 2 inches of tractive force is applied* with the downward caudal section motion (Fig. 12.30).

During each 20-second session of traction application, the interspinous and intradiscal space is subjected to a push-pull pumping action or a milking action by applying the tractive force and then letting the table return to the point of tautness between tractive applications. That is, five or six such pumping actions are performed during the 20-second tractive force by first attaining the tautness point, then allowing the table to be taken downward 1 to 2 inches and to be brought back to neutral tautness position. Patient tolerance to the procedure is carefully monitored.

This traction is applied three times for approximately 20 seconds each time, for a total of 1 minute of distraction. (A fine differential point should be noted: The patient with a protruding disc usually states that he or she feels mild pain from traction, whereas the patient with a prolapsed disc does not.) *Remember to not use a strong traction.* Most doctors tend to use too much force in applying the traction technique. Start gently and increase the traction as patient relaxation and confidence takes place. Understand that following the traction the patient may have a feeling of weakness or perhaps discomfort in the low back. This is because swollen, irritated tissues are being tractioned during the reduction of the disc.

LATERAL FLEXION IN TREATING LATERAL DISCS

Medial and lateral disc protrusions are treated in the same ways. After initial plane traction at the specified disc level, the lateral disc may be flexed, via the caudal section of the table, away from the side of pain so as to increase the lateral flexion of the vertebra above the site of disc protrusion, as is shown in Figure 12.31. This flexion increases the distraction effect and hastens reduction of the lateral disc.

For treatment of a left lateral L4 or L5 disc protrusion, the caudal end of the table is bent to the right so as to accentuate the right lateral flexion of L4 on L5 (Fig. 12.31).

DUAL DERMATOME SCIATICA TREATMENT

According to most authorities, 90% of all disc lesions occur at one level and involve one nerve root. For that other 10%, the following discussion is presented (Figs. 12.32 to 12.34).

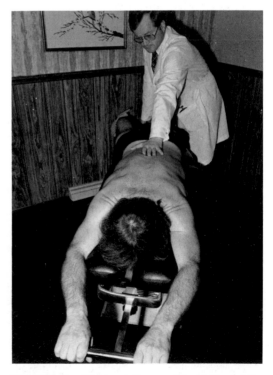

Figure 12.31. The arm is kept straight while applying traction to the spine and the table is right laterally flexed for a left lateral disc protrusion.

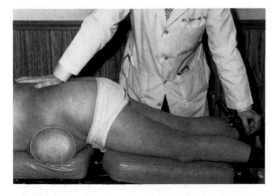

Figure 12.30. One to two inches of downward motion of the caudal section of the table is used in applying the tractive force to a specific joint area. This distractive force is applied following attaining tautness of the spine.

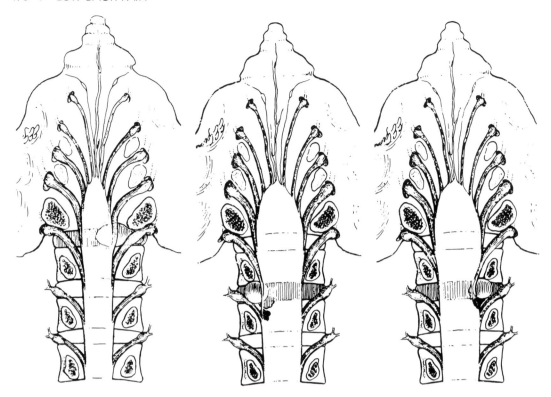

Figure 12.32. *Above left*, Usual relationship of fourth lumbar disc compression of L5 nerve root. The schematic illustration of the disc hernia pushing the L5 nerve root aside medially was predicted analytically and verified at operation. This patient had suffered from an intermittent, extremely painful left-sided L5 syndrome for 18 years. During periods of serious pain, the patient walked with a definite lean toward the right. Although the pain had been of long standing, the only nerve root involved in this overall picture of the disease was the left L5 nerve root. A year earlier, the extensor paresis had become severely involved. Before that time, the extensor paresis had been rather variable and involved to a moderate degree. This patient had had a surgery done previously and the fourth lumbar disc exposed, but no hernia was found.

In this patient, the unnatural lean to the right indicated that the L5 nerve root was pushed medially. The patient recovered rapidly and became free of pain as he gradually regained satisfactory extensor muscle function. (Reproduced with permission from Herlin L: *Sciatic and Pelvic Pain due to Lumbosacral Nerve Root Compression.* Springfield, IL, Charles C Thomas, 1966, p 42.)

Figure 12.33. *Above middle*, Unusual lateral position of the disc prolapse extending into the intervertebral foramen to compress the L4 nerve root. This 32-year-old nurse's aide developed an acute attack of right-sided L5 syndrome 3 years prior to seeing the author. Six months prior to admission, she had experienced an acute recurrence of the right-sided L5 syndrome with severe pain and extensor paresis.

During examination, the L5 syndrome was confirmed, but slight symptoms and signs from L4 were also noticed as minor radiating pain on the anterior side of the thigh. In addition, pain occurred during palpation over the muscular attachments of the adductor muscles. The Lasègue sign was positive, at a low angle, for L5. The knee jerk was normal. No sciatic scoliosis was apparent. When the patient bent to the right, distinct pain in the L5 distribution area was elicited; less pain was provoked by bending to the left. *Myelography was negative.* The diagnosis indicated a nerve root compression by a lateral disc protrusion on the right side in the fourth lumbar disc. This condition exerted a slight compression on L4 and severe compression together with a slight medial displacement on L5.

At surgery, the fourth disc level was explored, and the L5 nerve root was displaced a little medially by the disc lesion. The intervertebral joint was resected in order to explore the L4 nerve root exiting the cauda equina through the intervertebral foramen. A major portion of the disc protrusion had been hidden by the intervertebral joint. Also found was the cranially displaced fragment of the nucleus pulposus that had pushed its way from the cavity and become lodged under the posterior longitudinal ligament of the spinal canal. It produced a sharp-angled cone that pinched the L5 nerve root at its angle of departure from the cauda equina.

The patient was immediately free of pain, and the extensor power returned quickly. (Reproduced with permission from Herlin L: *Sciatic and Pelvic Pain due to Lumbosacral Nerve Root Compression.* Springfield, IL, Charles C Thomas, 1966, pp 100–101.)

Figure 12.34. *Opposite page, right.* L5-S1 disc protrusion prolapse compressing both the L5 nerve root at the intervertebral foramen and the S1 nerve root at its origin at the cauda equina.

This schematic is of a 32-year-old housewife who had had two children and who had a history of intermittent low back pain and lumbago for several years. She had suffered two spontaneous miscarriages, the latest 4 months prior to admission, which had been immediately followed by the onset of left-sided sciatica.

The examination indicated mixed nerve root syndromes of a painless lateral L5 syndrome, an ordinary dominant S1 syndrome, and a left-sided S2 syndrome. The left S3 was also involved. Left S2 pain could be provoked at palpation over the inguinal region, the tuber ischii, the medial part of the fossa poplitea, and medially over the soleus muscle of the calf. S3 pain was provoked over the symphysis and the most median part of the gluteal musculature. There was no obvious scoliosis.

Diagnosis was of a large hernia in the 5th lumbar disc extending from the left lateral to the median line with its maximum bulk where the S1 nerve root runs over the disc.

Surgery confirmed the presence of a large disc hernia. The disc was evacuated and recovery was excellent.

Comment: The two miscarriages appear to have been due to a lower sacral nerve root compression that caused the onset of the lumbago, with the sciatica developing later.

Herlin (118) documents other urogenital diseases due to lumbosacral nerve root compression. On page 79 (118), he discusses a situation he had encountered in which severe pelvic pain and urogenital infection might be due to a cause similar to that of sciatica—nerve root compressions from the outside due to different types of disc degeneration. He believes that there is the possibility that whole pelvic diseased states depend upon multiple nerve root compressions of the S2 and the lower sacral nerve roots. Surgical relief of lumbosacral nerve roots resulted in normalization of such diseases as salpingitis, painful irregular menstruations, vaginal discharge, sluggish frequent urination, cystitis, prostatis, urethritis, infertility, impotency, and vertigo. (Reproduced with permission from Herlin L: *Sciatic and Pelvic Pain due to Lumbosacral Nerve Root Compression.* Springfield, 1L, Charles C Thomas, 1966, pp 14, 16, 19, 31, 120, 128, 166, and 169.)

Figure 12.32 is an illustration showing fourth lumbar disc compression of the fifth nerve root.

Figure 12.33 is an illustration showing the fourth lumbar disc compressing the fourth lumbar nerve root. This is unusual and has occurred in two patients who required surgery for repair, as documented by this author. A differential diagnosis we have encountered in practice is that, at about 15° straight leg raise in a patient with disc protrusion into the intervertebral foramen, the entire pelvis lifts off the table instead of flexion occurring at the hip as in normal patients (Cox sign).

It is possible for a large disc protrusion to compress two nerve roots: both the one exiting at its intervertebral level as well as the nerve root originating at its level to exit at the foramen one level below (Fig. 12.34). The indication for the disc protrusion demonstrated in Figure 12.34 would be a patient who has nerve root dysesthesias in two dermatomes of the same extremity. This would indicate either two disc protrusions or a prolapse, such as is demonstrated here, impinging on two nerve roots at one level. If the former were the case, treatment of both disc protrusions would result in a closed reduction of both discs. This would afford relief even if it were not known

whether one or two disc protrusions were involved. Keep in mind that if the patient failed to show 50% relief in 3 weeks of conservative care, a neurosurgical evaluation would be sought. This would then allow discovery of such an unusual situation. As the attending physician, your duty is to be aware of this clinical possibility.

A difficult diagnostic situation is encountered when, during treatment of a third lumbar disc protrusion, an L4 nerve root dermatome pattern is found. If no response is found in treating the third lumbar disc, keep in mind the possibility of an L4 disc impingement on the intervertebral foramen. It is the author's opinion that intervertebral foramen encroachment by disc prolapse is probably a surgical case.

A thought to be entertained about the diagnosis and treatment of lumbar disc protrusion is the possibility that diseases of the female pelvis, such as urogenital infection and severe pelvic pain, might be due to nerve root compressions resulting from different types of disc degeneration (118). Herlin (118) describes a patient who had two miscarriages which, he believes, were due to a lower sacral nerve root compression that caused the lumbago and sciatica that developed afterward. He claims that there is a connection between low back pain and urogenital disorders and believes that if such a connection exists, the rationale of resecting uterine tubes and ovaries must be questioned, especially as pain is not improved when oophorosalpingitis is caused by sacral nerve root compression.

POSTREDUCTION CARE

Following distraction manipulation, the muscles and acupressure points shown in Figures 12.11 through 12.17 are treated again.

Physical therapy in the form of positive galvanic current and hot and cold therapy is applied to the involved disc and acupressure points, as shown in Figures 12.21 through 12.24. One positive pad is placed directly over the disc protrusion with the negative pad next to it, and the other positive pad may be placed on the gluteal region so as to sedate the sciatic nerve there, or may be placed over B54 in the popliteal space with the negative pad opposite to it (Fig. 12.35). The benefits of galvanic current are given as follows:

Application of Galvanism

Galvanism is a continuous, waveless, undirectional current of low voltage commercial spoken of as a *direct current*. Galvanic current is decidedly chemical in action and, as it passes through the body, breaks up some of the molecules that it encounters into their component atoms or *ions* as they are more properly called. All ions have either a *positive* or *negative* electric charge and attract or repel each other, with *like* charges repelling and *unlike* charges attracting. When two dissimilar ions unite, a neutral molecule is formed, but when the galvanic current breaks this union, the original positive and negative ions are liberated.

Table 12.1 outlines the action produced at the respective poles.

The active pole, either positive or negative, is the one that produces the effects desired. The other is the inactive or indifferent pole. The active should be the smaller in order to concentrate the current locally and thus intensify the action.

The number of milliamperes to be used depends on the smoothness of the current and the susceptibility of the patient, with from 5 to 20 ma being the average. The length of the treatment is determined by the milliamperes used, with from 5

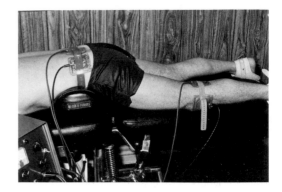

Figure 12.35.   Positive galvanism being applied.

Table 12.1.
Actions Produced by Galvanic Current

Positive	Negative
Attractis acids	Attracts alkali
Repels alkali	Repels acid
Hardens tissue	Softens tissue
Contracts tissue	Dilates tissue
Stops hemorrhage	Increases hemorrhage
Diminishes congestion	Increases congestion
Sedative	Stimulating
Relieves pain in acute conditions due to reduction of congestion. If scar is formed, it is hard and firm	Reduces pain in chronic conditions due to softening of tissues and increase of circulation. If scar is formed, it is soft and pliable.

to 15 minutes usually being sufficient time for application of the current.

RULES FOR THE APPLICATION OF GALVANIC CURRENT

1. Caution should be used to prevent galvanic burns.
2. Never dispute the patient. If he complains, investigate.
3. Be careful with paralyzed patients.
4. Avoid shocks.
5. See that the pads are properly placed, i.e., active and indifferent.
6. See that the intensity control is completely turned off before placing the pads.
7. Do not place or remove the pads while the instrument is running.

8. Be sure to have pads thoroughly moist but not dripping wet.
9. Turn current on and off slowly.
10. Have the patient remove enough clothing and protect the remainder from getting damp.
11. Never change poles while the current is flowing, except when testing.
12. Protect scars or wounds.

Remember: Positive ions are driven in under the positive pole. *Negative* ions are driven in under the negative pole.

POLARITY

The most important feature of the galvanic current is its *polarity*, with each pole having distinctive attributes and, consequently, being productive of certain specifically definite therapeutic effects. The action of one pole is opposed to that of the other pole. This matter of polarity must be well understood. The direct current (DC) decomposes liquid as it passes through it. This decomposing of a liquid by an electric current is termed *electrophoresis*. The liquid decomposed is the *electrolyte*; and the parts of the separated electrolyte are the *ions*. The current enters the electrode by the *anode (positive pole)* and leaves by the *cathode (negative pole)*.

There are *positive ions* and *negative ions*. Those ions possessing an excess *negative* charge are termed *electronegative*, and those possessing an excess *positive* charge are termed *electropositive*. *It is a universal law of electrical physics that like poles repel and unlike poles attract; therefore negative ions will travel toward the positive pole and positive ions will travel toward the negative pole.* Oxygen, being electronegative, is repelled from the negative pole and forms at the positive pole; hydrogen, being electropositive, is repelled from the positive pole and collects at the negative. Consequently, when we treat a pain, we use the *positive* pole over the seat of pain because the positive pole is a sedative and is acid in reaction. We desire this reaction because where there is pain, there is always an alkaline reaction, and by using the positive pole the alkalinity is driven toward the negative pole.

The slogan for pain is *positive pole*; however, there are exceptions. For instance, if inflammation has been prolonged sufficiently to cause distinct organic tissue changes (fibrosus, adhesions) that, in turn, cause pain on motion of the parts

involved, the *negative* pole is used because of its liquefying and vasodilative properties.

APPLICATION OF ELECTRODES

The active electrode is always the smaller of the two electrodes; the opposite electrode is known as the indifferent electrode and should be placed as nearly opposite to the active electrode as possible. The indifferent electrode is usually a well-moistened pad.

Electrodes must be secured or must be held in contact with the patient before the instrument is turned on and current is allowed to flow. Also, contact between the patient and the electrode must not be broken while the current is flowing. Lastly, the current must not be turned off until it has been reduced to zero; otherwise the patient will receive a shock.

SUMMARY OF CLOSED REDUCTION OF DISC PROTRUSION

The closed reduction technique for the disc protrusion is summarized below. Careful study will allow you to apply this technique with the use of the Zenith®-Cox® table; seeing a presentation, however, will greatly enhance utilization of the technique and the table.

1. Have the patient lie prone on the table, as described earlier, and test for tolerance to traction.

2. Traction is applied until you feel traction or a slight tautening of the muscles around the spinous processes.

3. Maintain contact on the spinous process of the vertebra directly above the disc protrusion. For example, if you are treating a fourth lumbar disc protrusion, maintain contact on the spinous process at L4 and press down on the spinous process while exerting pressure cephalad against the inferior portion of the fourth lumbar spinous process.

4. Apply gentle traction by pressing down on the table, and ask the patient if he or she feels pain. The patient may feel discomfort; if so, stop and maintain contact for a slow count of 8 or 10 or for approximately 20 seconds. The push-pull pumping action of the caudal section of the table while the patient is under traction creates a milking action on the disc and assists in speeding recovery.

5. Repeat the above procedure to the patient's

tolerance. You may feel a clicking release as you traction. This usually represents an instant relief from pain for the patient. If it is not felt, however, continue with treatment.

6. Repeat the above procedure one more time to the patient's tolerance or until you feel that a good traction has been applied to the involved segment. Three traction sessions of 20 seconds each are the rule.

7. After closed reduction, slowly return the caudal section of the table to its closed position, then release the ankle straps until this section of the table is closed, as this can cause a sharp pain in the patient's low back.

8. Treat the adductors, gluteals, and acupressure points, if necessary. The acupressure points for control of sciatic pain are illustrated in Figure 12.10. Use of these points has been beneficial; treatment can be administered by pressure, galvanism, or needle acupuncture as state law allows.

9. Apply physical therapy.

10. Apply the belt to the patient before he or she rises from the table.

11. Give the patient instructions for home care and review them with him or her.

Frequency of Treatment

Patients with an acute disc lesion are best kept in the office throughout the day so that treatment can be given two or three times. The patient should avoid sitting, which increases the intradiscal pressure and slows healing. By lying recumbent, the patient enhances healing. It is far superior to have the patient lie recumbent than to have the patient leave the office, get in a car, and drive home; the driving posture can destroy what you have accomplished through manipulation.

Following treatment of the disc, the patient is fitted with a lumbosacral support, which he or she must wear for 24 hours a day until the leg pain eases. The patient is weaned from wearing of the support and is allowed to remove the support permanently when the back pain has ceased.

All patients with an acute disc lesion are treated for 3 months. At the outset, these patients are told to be prepared to come into the office every day for treatment. As they begin to respond, the length of time between treatments is then extended.

As a rule, all patients are told that when they have low back and leg pain due to a disc protrusion, they must show at least a 50% relief from pain within 3 *weeks or a neurosurgical consultation will be requested.* This statement relieves the patient of the worry as to what to do if treatment is not effective. Secondly, it lessens the chance that the patient will come for three or four visits and then stop coming for treatment. Lastly, it allows you to have the patient's complete confidence because he knows that, regardless of what it takes to fix this condition, you will see to it that is done, which makes for an excellent doctor-patient relationship.

Next Step in Care of the Disc following Flexion Distraction

Treatment progresses from strict flexion distraction manipulation to range of motion manipulation of the facet joints when the patient attains at least 50% relief of the disc lesion as measured by subjective relief, and 50% return of straight leg raising capability and range of motion of the thoracolumbar spine. At this point, the disc case will begin treatment in a similar manner to facet syndrome (this care is described in Chapter 11). Full range of motion of the facets is applied following careful determination of patient tolerance to each movement when applied with the distraction instrument.

National College Protocol in Teaching Flexion Distraction Treatment

The National College of Chiropractic teaches flexion-distraction adjustment techniques under the direction of James Jedlicka, D.C. To expand upon the application of the technique as taught at National College, I would like to present the entire protocol, from patient placement on the table to the application of the actual adjustment. This technique is very exacting in its application because it is taught to undergraduate students who are in the process of learning biomechanics and therapeutic manipulative procedures. Following is the procedure as taught by James Jedlicka, D.C.:

PATIENT POSITIONING SEQUENCE

1. Place the patient in a prone position on the table.
2. Identify and mark the involved motor unit at the interspinous space.

3. Position the pelvis so that the ASISs are resting on the caudal inch of the thoracic section of the table.
4. Adjust the footpiece so that the tibiotalar joint of the ankle is slightly caudal to the caudal edge of the footpiece cushion.
5. Attach the assist bar to the table.
6. Release the flexion-extension lock and determine the pelvic spring tension. Adjust if necessary.

FLEXION TOLERANCE TESTING SEQUENCE

1. Contact assist bar. Release flexion-extension lock. Apply specific palmar contact over the thoracolumbar region. Stabilize the patient. Flex the pelvic section of the table to patient tolerance and/or a maximum of 2 inches. Hold for 3 seconds. Slowly return the pelvic section of the table to the horizontal (neutral) position and then slowly remove the specific contact.
2. Contact assist bar. Release flexion-extension lock. Apply specific palmar contact on the spinous process of the superior vertebra of the involved motor unit. Stabilize the patient. Flex the pelvic section of the table to patient tolerance and/or a maximum of 2 inches. Hold for 3 seconds. Slowly return the pelvic section of the table to the horizontal (neutral) position and then slowly remove the specific contact.
3. Grasp the uninvolved lower extremity. Release flexion-extension lock. Apply specific palmar contact on the spinous process of the superior vertebra of the involved motor unit. Stabilize the patient. Flex the pelvic section of the table to patient tolerance and/or the point where patient stabilization is overcome (caudal movement of patient's upper body). Hold for 3 seconds. Slowly return the pelvic section of the table to the horizontal (neutral) position and then slowly remove the specific contact.
4. Grasp the involved lower extremity. Release flexion-extension lock. Apply palmar contact on the spinous process of the superior vertebra of the involved motor unit. Stabilize the patient. Flex the pelvic section of the table to patient tolerance and/or the point where patient stabilization is overcome (caudal movement of patient's upper body). Hold for 3 seconds. Slowly return the pelvic section of

the table to the horizontal (neutral) position and then slowly remove the specific contact.

Note: If the specific contact remains firm and has not slipped during step 2, it may be left in place during steps 3 and 5.

PALPATORY CONTACT FOR INCREASING LOCAL SOFT TISSUE TENSION

1. Utilize the cephalad hand to palpate the interspinous space of the motor unit to be treated.
2. Place the tip of the third digit in the interspinous space.
3. Place the tips of the second and fourth digits over the middle region of the paravertebral muscles at the level of the motor unit to be treated.

PROCEDURE FOR INCREASING LOCAL SOFT TISSUE TENSION: AXIAL TRACTION METHOD

1. Apply ankle cuffs securely.
2. Instruct the patient to grasp the table and pull his or her body cephalad against the ankle cuffs. Then have the patient release his or her grip and relax.
3. Apply palpating contact.
4. Utilize the caudal hand to grasp the rear caudal crank of the table and begin to slowly separate the pelvic section from the thoracic section of the table.
5. Continue separating the table sections until separation of the spinous processes and/or an increase in muscle tension is sensed with the palpatory contact.

PROCEDURE FOR INCREASING LOCAL SOFT TISSUE TENSION: FLEXION TRACTION METHOD

1. Apply ankle cuffs securely.
2. Instruct the patient to grasp the table and pull his or her body cephalad against the ankle cuffs. Then have the patient release his or her grip and relax.
3. Release the flexion-extension lock.
4. Apply palpating contact.
5. Utilize the caudal hand to grasp the assist bar, and slowly induce flexion of the pelvic section

of the table until separation of the spinous processes and/or an increase in muscle tension is sensed with the palpatory contact. This new table position of pelvic flexion now becomes the neutral starting position for all further table movement.

PROTOCOL I: FLEXION/ DISTRACTION—INTERMITTENT TRACTION (AXIAL TRACTION METHOD)

Orders:

Flexion/distraction: L4-L5 intermittent traction by the axial traction method. Three sets of one repetition: flexion—20-second hold time per repetition; 20-second rest period between sets.

1. Patient positioning sequence.
2. Flexion tolerance testing sequence.
3. Apply ankle cuffs securely.
4. Instruct the patient to grasp the table and pull his or her body cephalad against the ankle cuffs. Then have the patient release his or her grasp and relax.
5. Apply palpatory contact at the L4-L5 spinal motor unit.
6. Utilize the axial traction method for increasing soft tissue tension at the involved motor unit.
7. Disengage the flexion-extension lock.
8. Apply specific palmar contact on the L4 spinous process. Stabilize the patient. Induce flexion movement of the pelvic section and maintain this position for 20 seconds.
9. Return the pelvic section of the table to a neutral (horizontal) position, remove the stabilization force, and engage the flexion-extension lock.
10. Allow the patient a 20-second rest period.

Note: Steps 5 through 10 constitute one set. In order to fulfill the orders cited (three sets of one repetition), steps 5 through 10 would be repeated two more times.

11. Utilize the rear caudal crank of the table to slowly return the pelvic section to the fully closed position.
12. Remove the assist bar from the table.
13. Remove the ankle cuffs.

PROTOCOL II: FLEXION/ DISTRACTION—INTERMITTENT TRACTION (FLEXION TRACTION METHOD)

Orders:

Flexion/distraction: L4-L5 intermittent traction by the flexion traction method. Three sets of one repetition: flexion—20-second hold time per repetition; 20-second rest period between sets.

1. Patient positioning sequence.
2. Flexion tolerance testing sequence.
3. Apply ankle cuffs securely.
4. Instruct the patient to grasp the table and pull his or her body cephalad against the ankle cuffs. Then have the patient release his or her grasp and relax.
5. Disengage the flexion-extension lock.
6. Apply palpatory contact at the L4-L5 spinal motor unit.
7. Utilize the flexion traction method for increasing soft tissue tension at the involved motor unit.
8. Apply specific palmar contact on the L4 spinous process. Stabilize the patient. Induce flexion movement of the pelvic section and maintain this position for 20 seconds.
9. Return the pelvic section of the table to the neutral starting position, remove the stabilization force, and engage the flexion-extension lock.
10. Allow the patient a 20-second rest period.

Note: Steps 5 through 10 constitute one repetition. In order to fulfill the orders cited (three sets of one repetition), steps 5 through 10 would be repeated two more times.

11. Return the pelvic section of the table to the horizontal position.
12. Remove the assist bar from the table.
13. Remove the ankle cuffs.

PROTOCOL III: FLEXION/ DISTRACTION—INTERMITTENT TRACTION (AXIAL TRACTION METHOD)

Orders:

Flexion/distraction: L4-L5 intermittent traction by the axial traction method. Three sets of five repetitions: flexion—4-second hold time per repetition; 10-second rest period between sets.

1. Patient positioning sequence.
2. Flexion tolerance testing sequence.
3. Apply ankle cuffs securely.
4. Instruct the patient to grasp the table and pull his or her body cephalad against the ankle cuffs. Then have the patient release his or her grasp and relax.
5. Apply palpatory contact at the L4-L5 spinal motor unit.
6. Utilize the axial traction method for increasing soft tissue tension at the involved motor unit.
7. Disengage the flexion-extension lock.
8. Apply specific palmar contact on the L4 spinous process. Stabilize the patient. Induce five flexion movements of the pelvic section of 4 seconds duration, producing a total hold time of 20 seconds.
9. Return the pelvic section of the table to a neutral (horizontal) position, remove the stabilization force, and engage the flexion-extension lock.
10. Allow the patient a 10-second rest period.

Note: Steps 5 through 10 would constitute one set. In order to fulfill the orders cited (three sets of five repetitions), steps 5 through 10 would be repeated two more times.

11. Utilize the rear caudal crank of the table to slowly return the pelvic section to the fully closed position.
12. Remove the assist bar from the table.
13. Remove the ankle cuffs.

PROTOCOL IV: FLEXION/ DISTRACTION—INTERMITTENT TRACTION (FLEXION TRACTION METHOD)

Orders:

Flexion/distraction: L4-L5 intermittent traction by the flexion traction method. Three sets of five repetitions: flexion—4-second hold time per repetition; 10-second rest period between sets.

1. Patient positioning sequence.
2. Flexion tolerance testing sequence.
3. Apply ankle cuffs securely.
4. Instruct the patient to grasp the table and pull his or her body cephalad against the ankle cuffs. Then have the patient release his or her grasp and relax.
5. Disengage the flexion-extension lock.

6. Apply palpatory contact at the L4-L5 spinal motor unit.
7. Utilize the flexion traction method for increasing soft tissue tension at the involved motor unit.
8. Apply specific palmar contact on the L4 spinous process. Stabilize the patient. Induce five flexion movements of the pelvic section of 4 seconds duration, producing a total hold time of 20 seconds.
9. Return the pelvic section of the table to the neutral starting position, remove the stabilization force, and engage the flexion-extension lock.
10. Allow the patient a 10-second rest period.

Note: Steps 5 through 10 constitute one set. In order to fulfill the orders cited (three sets of one repetition), steps 5 through 10 would be repeated two more times.

11. Return the pelvic section of the table to the horizontal position.
12. Remove the assist bar from the table.
13. Remove the ankle cuffs.

PROTOCOL V: FLEXION/ DISTRACTION—MOBILIZATION (AXIAL TRACTION METHOD)

Orders:

Flexion/distraction: L4-L5 mobilization by the axial traction method. Three sets of five repetitions: flexion, right-left lateral flexion, and right-left circumduction.

1. Patient positioning sequence.
2. Stand on the left side of the table.
3. Flexion tolerance testing sequence.
4. Apply ankle cuffs securely.
5. Instruct the patient to grasp the table and pull his or her body cephalad against the ankle cuffs. Then have the patient release his or her grasp and relax.
6. Apply palpatory contact at the L4-L5 spinal motor unit.
7. Utilize the axial traction method for increasing soft tissue tension at the involved motor unit.
8. Disengage the flexion-extension lock.
9. Apply specific palmar contact on the L4 spinous process. Stabilize the patient. Induce flexion movement of the pelvic section of the table in a rhythmical and oscillatory type of

motion for a total of five repetitions. The velocity is approximately one repetition per second.

10. Return the pelvic section of the table to a neutral (horizontal) position, remove the stabilization force, and engage the flexion-extension lock.
11. Disengage the lateral flexion lock.
12. Apply thumb point contact on the right side of the L4 spinous process. Induce right lateral flexion of the pelvic section of the table in a rhythmical and oscillatory type of motion for a total of five repetitions. The velocity is approximately one repetition per second.
13. Return the pelvic section of the table to a neutral (midline) position.
14. Disengage the flexion-extension lock.
15. Apply specific palmar contact on the L4 spinous process. Stabilize the patient. Induce right circumduction (right lateral flexion, flexion, return to midline, and then return to horizontal position) movement of the pelvic section of the table in a rhythmical and oscillatory type of motion for a total of five repetitions. The velocity is approximately one repetition per 2 seconds.
16. Engage flexion-extension and lateral flexion locks.
17. Move to the opposite side of the table.
18. Repeat steps 11 through 16.

Note: All of the above procedures constitute one set of five repetitions. In order to fulfill the requirements of the orders cited (three sets of five repetitions), steps 6 through 18 would be repeated two more times.

19. Utilize the rear caudal crank of the table to slowly return the pelvic section to the fully closed position.
20. Remove the assist bar from the table.
21. Remove the ankle cuffs.

PROTOCOL VI: FLEXION/ DISTRACTION—MOBILIZATION (FLEXION TRACTION METHOD)

Orders:

Flexion/distraction: L4-L5 mobilization by the flexion traction method. Three sets of five repetitions: flexion, right-left lateral flexion, and right-left circumduction.

1. Patient positioning sequence.

2. Stand on the left side of the table.
3. Flexion tolerance testing sequence.
4. Apply ankle cuffs securely.
5. Instruct the patient to grasp the table and pull his or her body cephalad against the ankle cuffs. Then have the patient release his or her grasp and relax.
6. Disengage the flexion-extension lock.
7. Apply palpatory contact at the L4-L5 spinal motor unit.
8. Utilize the flexion traction method for increasing soft tissue tension at the involved motor unit.
9. Apply specific palmar contact on the L4 spinous process. Stabilize the patient. Induce flexion movement of the pelvic section of the table in a rhythmical and oscillatory type of motion for a total of five repetitions. The velocity is approximately 1 repetition per second.
10. Return the pelvic section of the table to the neutral starting position, remove the stabilization force, and engage the flexion-extension lock.
11. Disengage the lateral flexion lock.
12. Apply thumb point contact on the right side of the L4 spinous process. Induce right lateral flexion of the pelvic section of the table in a rhythmical and oscillatory type of motion for a total of five repetitions. The velocity is approximately one repetition per second.
13. Return the pelvic section of the table to a neutral (midline) position.
14. Disengage the flexion-extension lock.
15. Apply specific palmar contact on the L4 spinous process. Stabilize the patient. Induce right circumduction (right lateral flexion, flexion, return to midline, and then return to the neutral starting position) movement of the pelvic section of the table in a rhythmical and oscillatory type of motion for a total of five repetitions. The velocity is approximately one repetition per 2 seconds.
16. Engage flexion-extension and lateral flexion locks.
17. Move to the opposite side of the table.
18. Repeat steps 11 through 16.

Note: All of the above procedures constitute one set of five repetitions. In order to fulfill the requirements of the orders cited (three sets of five repetitions), steps 6 through 18 would be repeated two more times.

19. Return the pelvic section of the table to the horizontal position.
20. Remove the assist bar from the table.
21. Remove the ankle cuffs.

EXERCISE PROGRAM FOR THE DISC LESION PATIENT

The patient is started on the first three of the Cox exercises (Figure 12.36) at the outset of treatment, regardless of the severity of his pain. Following the relief of Déjérine's triad, i.e., relief of pain in the low back on coughing, sneezing, and straining at the stool, he is given the remainder of the exercises to do. These exercises must be chosen carefully by the doctor with regard to the patient's condition.

HOME CARE FOR THE DISC PATIENT

Following examination and diagnosis of the patient's condition, the x-rays are shown to the patient and an explanation of the condition made. We feel it very important that the patient understand his or her problem as fully as possible so that he or she can help in his or her care and recovery. A copy of the book *Low Back Pain: What It Is and How It Is Treated* is given to the patient; it is shown in Figure 12.37. Figure 12.38 shows the index of the book. The patient's diagnosis and treatment procedures, along with his or her instructions at home, are written down for the patient to study and follow. This forces the patient to become involved with his or her care. Figure 12.39 shows the instructions for the patient to follow at home; the appropriate instructions are checked for each patient.

COX LOW BACK WELLNESS SCHOOL

Every patient is invited to attend low back wellness school, which is a 2-hour class intended to teach the patient how to control a low back problem so that it does not control him or her. The school consists of three segments: first is a 25-minute segment to teach the patient the causes of low back pain based on knowledge of the disc and facet joint as sources of pain. Next, ergonomic training is given, teaching the patient the proper low back motions to avoid disc damage; emphasis is placed on lifting, bending, and twisting as the causes of back pain, and on the combined stresses they create on the lumbar spine. Finally, the Cox exercise program is presented with participation of the class attendees so that they learn how to do them properly. Questions and answers are shared in a mutually beneficial atmosphere. Once the patient has attended this 2-hour class, he or she understands two important facts: first, that the patient is equally responsible with the doctor for his or her own care and relief, and second, that there is not always a cure but rather control for low back pain. Patients learn that degenerative disc disease, spondylolisthesis, transitional vertebrae, scoliosis, and disc protrusions are not curable conditions but can be controlled by proper understanding and use of the low back in daily living.

NUTRITIONAL HOME CARE OF THE INTERVERTEBRAL DISC PATIENT

Cole, Ghosh, and Taylor (119) reported that Arteparon, a polysulphated polysaccharide, was administered systemically to mature beagle dogs over a 26-week period. At necropsy, disc proteoglycans were isolated, purified, and analyzed. Their findings were the first report that a systemically administered drug could influence the disc proteoglycans and suggested that Arteparon might be of value in the management of degenerative disc disease.

Lowther (120) reported 50% loss of proteoglycan from the cartilage of the rabbit articular cartilage when arthritis of the joint was present. This caused the cartilage matrix to be less capable of restoring the proteoglycan content of the cartilage and resulted in loss of joint stiffness and resistance to compression.

Wilhelmi and Maier (121) found, in rabbits with osteoarthrosis of the knee, that injection of sulphated glycosaminoglycans (GAG) inhibited enzymes that destroy cartilage and promoted repair of the defects. GAG has been found to increase proliferation of hyaline cartilage of the hip joint in mice and the femoral condyles, femur, and tibia of rabbits. Puhl and Dustmann (121) induced regeneration of damaged cartilage in rabbits with glycosamine sulphate.

Discat Supplement in Treatment of Disc Degeneration

Discat is a nutritional formula used by this author (J.M.C.); it is given to all disc degeneration or disc

THE COX EXERCISES

TO ACCOMPANY CHIROPRACTIC MANAGEMENT OF LOW BACK PAIN

Exercises for the acute severe low back pain patient.

Exercise 1.

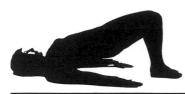

Lie on your back with your knees flexed and your feet flat on the floor as close to the buttocks as possible. Keep the knees together. Tighten the muscles of the lower abdoman and buttocks so as to flatten your low back against the floor. Slowly raise your hips up from the floor and hold for slow count of 8. Repeat this exercise 4 times. If you cannot raise your hips from the floor, merely tighten the belly, the abdominal and buttock muscles and wait until you can raise the hips.

General Instruction

Do Not Sit when you have low back pain. This increases the pressure within the disc and the joint of your spine. If your doctor prescribes a belt to wear, remove it to do these exercises. If your doctor agrees, it is good to alternate hot and cold on your low back before doing these exercises. This is done by applying moist heat in the form of a hot towel for 10 minutes followed by 5 minutes of ice therapy in which a moist cool towel is placed on the skin with an ice bag on top of it. Place the heat on the back 4 times and ice on the back 3 times beginning and ending with heat.

Exercise 2.

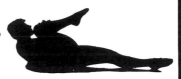

Lie on back and draw the right knee up to the chest and pull the knee down upon chest while attempting to touch the chin to the knee. Do this for a slow count of 8 and repeat 4 times. Repeat the same exercise with left knee brought to the chest. Relax between each session. Repeat with both knees brought up to the chest.

Exercise 3.

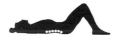

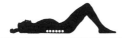

While standing or lying tighten the abdominal and buttock muscles so as to flatten your back. Repeat this several times throughout the day. Contract the muscles and relax the approximately 8 times at each session.

If your doctor suggests nutritional supplementation, be sure to follow it closely.

Do these exercise on a firm surface such as the floor or a mat. Do not be alarmed if discomfort is noted during exercise. If this pain is great, stop it and consult your doctor before continuing.

Exercises after the acute pain has diminished. Do the following exercises if you feel no pain in your low back upon coughing, sneezing, or straining to move the bowel.

Exercise 4.

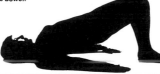

Repeat #1 exercise above but be sure to hold the knees firmly together.

The Cox exercises are to be used in conjunction with your chiropractic care and should be discussed with the chiropractic physician before use.

Exercise 5.

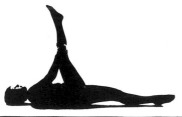

Do the exercises marked (x) in numerical order _____times a day.

Lie flat on your back and raise the right leg straight upward without bending the knee. Place your hands behind the knee while keeping the knee straight, pull the leg straight up so as to stretch the muscles behind your thigh. Repeat this 8 times on the right leg and then do it on the left. Relax your low back muscles following this exercise.

Exercise 6.

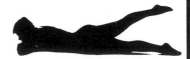

Lie on stomach and raise the right leg off of floor while keeping the knee straight. Hold the leg up in this position for a count of 4 and slowly let it down. Repeat this 4 times. Repeat the same exercise with the opposite leg. Relax following this exercise.

Figure 12.36. Cox exercise program.

Exercise 7.

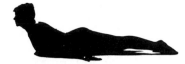

Lie flat on stomach with arms along side, palms down. Slowly raise chest from floor. Feel the muscles of the low back tighten. Hold the chest up from the floor for a slow count of 6 and slowly let it down. Rest between each session. Repeat this 6 times.

Exercise 8.

Sit on floor on your knees. Extend your right leg as far to the side as possible, keeping the knee straight and the arch of the foot on the floor. Slide your foot along the floor until you feel the stretch of the muscles inside your thigh. Do it slowly and hold for a count of 5. Repeat it 3 times on the right leg and then repeat with the left side. These muscles, which are tight at the beginning, will loosen and stretch with subsequent exercise sessions.

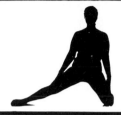

Exercise 9.

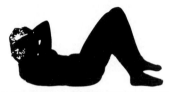

Abdominal Strengthening Exercises. Lie on Back with Knees bent and feet on floor. Bring chin to chest as shown. Now tighten the abdominal muscles so as to lift and curl the shoulders up to about 1 foot off the floor. Remember - curl up the spine from the neck downward to between the shoulder blade. Feel the abdominals tighten. Do this 10 to 30 times depending on your stamina.

Exercise 10.

Lie on side. Turn the toes inward on the right foot and lift leg upward. Repeat this 6 times on right and then 6 times on the left. You will feel pulling in the outer thigh and pelvis.

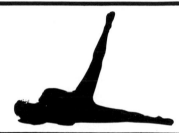

Exercise 11.

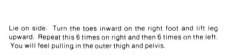

Lie on back and draw knees to chest, arms extended level with shoulders, roll hips to side in attempt to touch the knees to floor. Turn your head, in the opposite direction to which your knees are bending. Repeat this 4 times going first to the right and then to the left. This exercise brings all spinal movements together in a smooth forceful manipulation of the spinal articulations. Since the exercise involves rotation, it should only be done under physician instruction.

Exercise 12.

Lie on back. Bend knees and bring feet up to the buttocks. Now lift and straighten the legs so that the legs are at a right angle to the body. Raise the buttocks from the floor and place the hand beside the buttocks and support your pelvis as you raise the pelvis from the floor. Allow the legs to go over the head with feet over the head and the legs parallel to the floor. Hold this position for 10 seconds and repeat 2 - 3 times. Slowly lower your pelvis and legs to the original starting position. This exercise should only be used by those who have been working with the exercises for some time and have their low back pain under control.

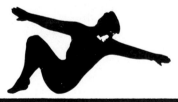
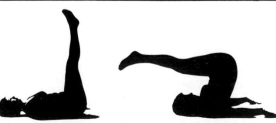

Figure 12.36. *(continued)* Cox exercise program.

LOW BACK & LEG PAIN

WHAT IT IS AND HOW IT IS TREATED

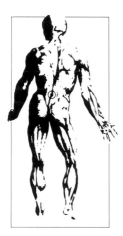

by James M. Cox D.C., D.A.C.B.R.

Figure 12.37. This book contains a simple explanation of various problems occurring in the low back, such as disc degeneration, disc protrusion, spondylolisthesis, transitional segment, subluxation, facet syndrome, short leg, stenosis, and scoliosis. This teaches the patient to understand his or her problem.

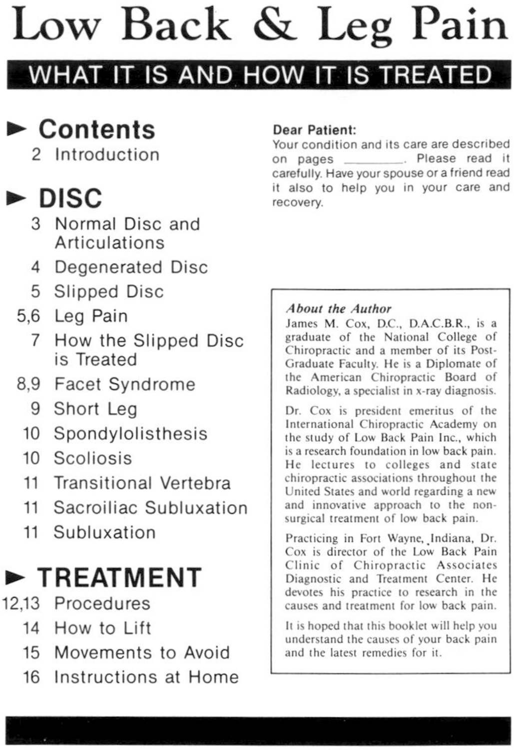

Low Back & Leg Pain

WHAT IT IS AND HOW IT IS TREATED

Contents

2 Introduction

DISC

3 Normal Disc and Articulations
4 Degenerated Disc
5 Slipped Disc
5,6 Leg Pain
7 How the Slipped Disc is Treated
8,9 Facet Syndrome
9 Short Leg
10 Spondylolisthesis
10 Scoliosis
11 Transitional Vertebra
11 Sacroiliac Subluxation
11 Subluxation

TREATMENT

12,13 Procedures
14 How to Lift
15 Movements to Avoid
16 Instructions at Home

Dear Patient:
Your condition and its care are described on pages ________. Please read it carefully. Have your spouse or a friend read it also to help you in your care and recovery.

About the Author
James M. Cox, D.C., D.A.C.B.R., is a graduate of the National College of Chiropractic and a member of its Post-Graduate Faculty. He is a Diplomate of the American Chiropractic Board of Radiology, a specialist in x-ray diagnosis.

Dr. Cox is president emeritus of the International Chiropractic Academy on the study of Low Back Pain Inc., which is a research foundation in low back pain. He lectures to colleges and state chiropractic associations throughout the United States and world regarding a new and innovative approach to the non-surgical treatment of low back pain.

Practicing in Fort Wayne, Indiana, Dr. Cox is director of the Low Back Pain Clinic of Chiropractic Associates Diagnostic and Treatment Center. He devotes his practice to research in the causes and treatment for low back pain.

It is hoped that this booklet will help you understand the causes of your back pain and the latest remedies for it.

Figure 12.38. Index of the book.

protrusion patients. Discat contains 150 mg of manganese sulphate, 150 mg of calcium, 50 mg of potassium, 75 mg of magnesium, 4 mg of iron, 10 mg of zinc, and 50 mg of perna canaliculus. The latter ingredient is glucosaminoglycan. the mucopolysaccharide found in the disc; the others are the minerals found in the disc along with the chemical glucosaminoglycan. For the first 3 months of care, the patient is told to take six to eight tablets daily, and then a maintenance dose of two tablets a day is prescribed.

Disc Imbibition of Nutrients

Direct vascular contacts, vascular buds, exist between the marrow spaces of the vertebral body and the hyaline cartilage of the end plates of the vertebra and are important for the nutritition of the disc (67). Until a person reaches the early 20s, the intervertebral disc receives nutrients via the epiphyseal end plates. Following their closure, however, a thinning of the hyaline cartilage between the nucleus and the vertebral body and an ingrowth of granulation tissue, which becomes important in the nutrition of the disc, occur. There is a diffusion of solutes both from the cancellous bone of the vertebral body into the nucleus through the end plate as well as from the anterior and posterior annulus fibrosus. Oxygen and glucose enter primarily through the former route, whereas the sulfate radical enters primarily through the anterior and posterior annulus fibrosus.

According to Naylor et al. (122), studies of the components of the disc by use of chemical analysis, x-ray crystallography, and electron microscopy have shown that in disc degeneration a fall in the total sulfate (both chondroitin sulfate and keratin sulfate) occurs with age. Happey, Wiseman, and Naylor (123) have shown that there is a gradual diminution of the sulfate content of the disc with aging and degeneration and that the prolapsed nucleus pulposus usually contains values of sulfate less than half those of the normal disc. Keep in mind that the posterior annular fi-

═══════════════════════════════════════ To My Patients

INSTRUCTIONS AT HOME

Authorities state that it takes at least 3 months for a torn disc to heal sufficiently to allow such daily movements as prolonged sitting, bending, lifting, or other usual everyday activities. The first 3 weeks of daily treatment allow maximum ability for the disc to heal quickly. Wearing a belt also assures a quick heal. Those things you must do at home are checked as follows:

☐ 1. Do not sit! Sitting increases the pressure of the spinal fluid four times more than when you lie down. The pressure within the disc itself is up to 11 times higher than when you lie down. Therefore, in order to allow the disc to heal strongly and quickly, **you must not sit.**

☐ 2. You are advised to place alternating hot and cold packs on your low back every 3-4 hours as follows. Place heat for 10 minutes followed by an ice bag for 5 minutes. Alternate the hot and cold, beginning and ending with heat, placing the heat on 4 times and the cold 3 times. Therefore, you will place the heat on for 10 minutes, cold for 5, heat for 10, cold for 5, heat for 10, cold for 5, heat for 10.

☐ 3. Analgesic liniment may be prescribed to be massaged into the low back following this hot and cold therapy.

☐ 4. Constipation. You are urged to avoid constipation, since straining at the stool can aggravate low back and sciatic problems. If you are constipated, your doctor will prescribe something to help your problem.

☐ 5. Take the supplement, Discat, as prescribed, to help heal the disc or other low back condition. This contains manganese sulfate and the trace minerals that are found within the disc and that

are felt to be of importance in its healing. Most sciatic patients are also given high vitamin B, C, and A. In addition, you are urged to eat a diet high in lean meat, vegetables, gelatin, fruits, fruit juices especially grape, apple and cranberry and to avoid sweets, fried fatty foods, pork, carbonated and alcoholic drinks, and foods that normally constipate you. Eat those foods that you know have a mild cathartic effect on your bowels and increase your intake of fluids.

☐ 6. It is important to realize the seriousness of sciatic pain. It is often discouraging when one gets along fine and then feels that old pain start back again. You will be told to expect this as it is common to have slight recurrences during healing. Consult page 14 regarding the movements that lead to or aggravate low back and sciatic pain. Study them well and avoid them.

☐ 7. Mattress. Sleep on a firm mattress. If it is soft, place a piece of plywood under it.

☐ 8. Chairs. Following successful relief of your problem, a good chair is indicated. For suggestion of proper chair contour, consult your doctor.

☐ 9. Occupation. If your low back and leg pain is not so severe that the job irritates it, possibly you will be allowed to work. If your job entails sitting and bending of the spine which aggravates your condition, you cannot work. If your work irritates the condition, there is no choice except to avoid working until relief is secured. You must discuss this with your doctor.

☐ 10. Exercises. Exercises will be prescribed for you to do at home for the correction of your condition. Follow them as prescribed by your doctor.

Figure 12.39. This page describes the patient's home instructions for care of the low back problem. The rules to be followed by the patient are indicated by placing a checkmark in the box in front of the number.

bers have the poorest nutrition, although they are subjected to the greatest strain by a bulging turgor-filled nucleus pulposus.

Robles (124), in an extensive study of the nutrition of the disc, used electron microscopy and atomic spectrometry to measure the mineral salts and water content of the annulus fibrosus and nucleus pulposus. He found that the disc, which is deprived of vessels, receives nutrients by the diffusion of plasma filtrates from the surrounding structures. The intervertebral disc is supplied by the vertebral epiphysis until a person reaches the age of approximately 25. After fusion of the epiphysis, the vessels join those of the vertebral bodies. Certain vascular loops reach the cartilaginous structures of the vertebral plates and that area above where the disc tissue is formed. It has been suggested that, by the process of diffusion, these loops form nutrient channels from the cancellous bone of the vertebral body into the adjacent disc.

The nucleus pulposus demonstrates a *hydrophilia*, which is an osmotic force that brings about a diffusion of fluid from the vertebral body into the nucleus. The nucleus pulposus demonstrates twice the hydrophilic capacity of the remaining disc. Nutrient channels are formed from the vertebral bone into the disc, and a high rate of mineral salt flow is noted within these channels.

It has been demonstrated by the use of atomic spectrometry that there are five mineral constituents, namely potassium, calcium, magnesium, iron, and sodium, that flow into the disc. Only one of these elements, sodium, is found in increased concentration within the nucleus.

It is interesting how Robles determines the flow of nutrients from the vertebral body into the disc. He injected dye into the nucleus and observed it to flow through the nutrient channels.

Urban et al. (125) found diffusion to be the main mechanism of transport of small solutes into the intervertebral disc. About 40% of the end-plate area was found to be permeable to small solutes in experiments on dogs. The amount of solute entering via the end plate was shown to be less for negatively charged solutes, such as the sulfate ion, than for the neutral solutes, such as glucose, because of charge exclusion in the region of the nucleus.

This route of nutrition is important, as many authors believe that there is a correlation between the impermeability of the central region of the end plate and disc degeneration. The only solute whose metabolism has been studied at all is the sulfate ion. In the dog, it has been shown that there is a turnover of sulfate in the nucleus pulposus in about 500 days. Consequently, Nachemson (67) believes ruptured discs take a long time, if ever, to heal.

The in vivo procedure used to study sulfate metabolism was performed on dogs. They were anesthetized and given injections of radioactive sulfate tracers. Blood samples were collected at regular intervals until the dogs were killed at regular intervals of 1 hour to 6 hours after the initial injection. The spines were dissected as quickly as possible, usually within 5 to 10 minutes after death, and plunged into liquid nitrogen. Liquid nitrogen was poured onto the discs to stop diffusion from occurring during the measuring and cutting operations that followed. Urban et al. (125) reports that the cell density in the peripheral regions of the annulus and near the end plate is about three to four times higher than that in the rest of the disc. From the values determined in their study, it appears that the cells in the periphery of the disc are taking up sulfate and, hence, producing proteoglycan less actively than those in the center of the disc. The cells in the surface layers of the articular cartilage likewise are less active in producing proteoglycans than are those in the deeper zones.

We can see that there is a loss of sulfate from discs as they undergo degenerative change. It has been postulated that nutritional deficiencies could lead to disc degeneration. If the end plate were blocked, there could be a buildup of waste products or a nutritional deficiency that could predispose the disc to degenerative change (126). Consequently, we use Discat, which incorporates manganese sulfate along with five other trace minerals, in the treatment of low back pain. No studies have been done on the benefits of such treatment, however, although nutritional prevention of low back pain via such nutrients should be considered and may provide another avenue of treatment for low back pain.

According to Nachemson (as reported in Ref. 127), exercise improves the delivery of nutrients to the spinal discs, perhaps delaying the deterioration that eventually afflicts all backs.

Exercise Influence on Nutrient Imbibition

Lowther (120) found that synovial lined joints, under exercise, stimulated penetration of nutrients into the cartilage. Kramer (128) states that a continuous well-balanced metabolism is necessary in the disc for the maintenance of the synthesis and depolymerization of the extracellular components. Cells lacking satisfactory nutrition produce macromolecules inferior in quality and quantity.

Holm and Nachemson (129) reported that the free sulphate concentration for exercised canines was higher than among those not exercising. Brody (127) quoted Nachemson that improved delivery of nutrients by exercise might delay the deterioration that eventually affects all backs. Ogota and Whiteside (126) state that nutritional deficiency can lead to disc degeneration because there is a block of the end plate creating a buildup of waste products or a nutritional deficiency that may predispose the disc to degenerative change.

Finally, Eismont (130) showed that there is circulation into the disc when he found that rabbit models showed over 50% of the serum level following 8 hours of antibiotic intramuscular injection, in the nucleus pulposus.

It would seem that we are only beginning to understand possible nutritional etiologies of discal degeneration.

OSTEOPOROSIS

Osteoporosis is a problem commonly seen in chiropractic practice, particularly in elderly females. They are seen with compression fractures, kyphotic sagittal curves, and spine pain of sometimes indeterminate origin.

Osteoporosis is defined as an absolute decrease in the amount of bone (*osteopenia*) that makes one vulnerable to fracture with minimal trauma (131). Two types of osteoporosis are currently recognized (132). Type 1 is postmenopausal osteoporosis, which occurs in women within 15 to 20 years of menopause and is related to accelerated bone loss. Fractures of vertebrae are common due to loss of trabecular bone. Type 2 is slow bone loss that starts around age 30 and is continuous throughout life. Trabecular and cortical bone are lost, and hip fractures are common.

Primary osteoporosis (involutional osteoporosis) is loss of bone mass of age-related etiology, as opposed to secondary osteoporosis due to disease states such as hyperparathyroidism or hyperthyroidism.

For more than 80 years, it has been known that if calcium intake is reduced below need, osteoporosis will develop, and that this osteoporosis, in turn, can be largely reversed by replacing the missing nutrient (133). This disorder occurs less frequently in some populations at outward nutritional disadvantages such as poor rural blacks, who are accustomed to low calcium intake yet have excellent teeth, satisfactory cortical indices, and a low frequency of hip fracture (134).

Factors Determining Osteoporosis Occurrence

A woman will typically lose 50% of her bone during life. Five factors determine the risk of developing osteoporosis: age, initial bone density, menopause, bioavailability of calcium, and sporadic factors such as low weight, smoking, alcohol intake, and physical activity (135). One of three women will have a vertebral facture after age 65 and a hip fracture in extreme old age.

The Food and Drug Administration and the National Institute of Health Consensus Conference on Osteoporosis have published a recommended daily allowance for calcium which is 1000 mg for estrogen-normal women and 1500 mg for estrogen-deprived women. Middle-aged and elderly women have an average intake of only 550 mg per day, and women with osteoporosis often consume less. The calcium requirement of premenopausal women is 1000 mg, whereas for postmenopausal women it is 1500 mg (133, 135).

The reasons women need this amount of calcium are:

1. Middle-aged women cannot achieve calcium balance at intakes of less than 1000 mg per day (136).
2. Calcium absorption efficiency declines with age (137).
3. Estrogen hormone deficiency leads to decreased calcium absorption and decreased retention of absorbed calcium (138).

Men also develop osteoporosis, although less commonly than women. Nevertheless, it can cause significant morbidity when present. It occurs in men due to lowered testosterone hormone (139).

Calcium Supplementation

This author agrees with Heaney (133), who feels that a calcium intake of 2.5 g/day is quite safe and reasonable. He also stated that this level would not cause kidney stones because the stones are caused not so much by calcium in the diet as by failure of the kidneys to produce a product that keeps its components in solution. Calcium absorption aggravates kidney stone formation but does not cause it. Mueleman (140) feels that most adult American women should take a calcium supplement, since low calcium intake probably contributes to reduced bone mass in older adults. He does state that the relationship of calcium intake to osteoporotic fractures is inconclusive.

To assure adequate intake of calcium, this author (J.M.C.) places premenopausal women on 500 mg and postmenopausal women on 1000 mg of nonphosphorous calcium carbonate daily.

Estrogen, Calcitonin, and Exercise for Osteoporosis

Lindsay (141) feels that estrogen stimulates production of calcitonin, a hormone that inhibits osteoclastic bone resorption. Synthetic salmon calcitonin has been used in treating Paget's disease since 1975, and in 1985 it was approved in treating osteoporosis. Fatourechi and Heath (142) find no data to indicate that calcitonin therapy reduces the number of fractures or increases bone strength. Lindsay (142) felt that, in addition to estrogen, calcium supplementation and exercise may have roles to play in the prevention and management of osteoporosis. Exercise was found to give conflicting results as to whether it influenced bone mass. The majority of studies failed to show that it can significantly enhance radial compact bone mass, although nonexercising persons showed significant losses over the study period (143). It was felt to be unwise to give confident recommendations for the prophylactic use of exercise, and it was suggested that indiscriminate counseling of individuals to undertake programs of exercise with hope of preventing osteoporosis should be discouraged (143).

Osteoporosis Screening

Digital imaging screening for osteoporosis is being vigorously pursued. Quantitative computed tomography provides a reliable means of evaluating and monitoring the many forms of osteoporosis and the various interventions aimed at ameliorating the condition (144). Wahner (145) finds single- and dual-photon absorptiometry to allow bone mineral measurements to define the osteoporotic syndrome in terms of bone mass. It can assess the risk of fracture and the severity of bone loss.

Mass screening for osteoporosis is discouraged because of its high cost and lack of cost effectiveness. Treatment for a woman with osteoporosis is preventative and will proceed without knowing how much osteoporosis she might have. The money spent on the dosimetry has been called a retailing enterprise, and it has been asserted that the cost is better spent on almost anything else (146).

TWO FINAL FACTORS IN TREATING LUMBAR DISC DISEASE

Anterior innominate subluxations are particular problems when they occur on the same side of

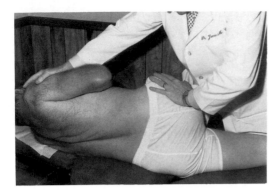

Figure 12.40. Shown is the correction of an anterior innominate subluxation. The patient's knee is flexed, and the doctor directs cephalad pressure against the popliteal space as an anterior thrust of the ischial spine of the ischium is given.

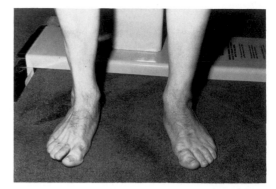

Figure 12.41. Patient with pes planus accompanying low back pain.

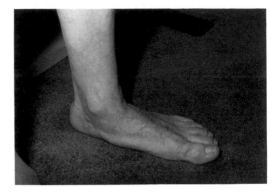

Figure 12.42. Medial view of patient in Figure 12.41.

disc lesion. This author feels that the anterior ilium causes the sacrospinous ligament to traction the sciatic nerve over itself and to aggravate the leg pain. Therefore, when the patient shows a long leg on the side of sciatica, we adjust the innominate as shown in Figure 12.40. Note that rotation of the lumbar spine is avoided by flexing the hip joint, contacting the ischium, and delivering the corrective manipulation without inflicting any rotation to the lumbar spine which might tear the disc annular fibers.

Whenever dropped arches create pes planus deformity of the foot, as shown in Figures 12.41 and 12.42, we place orthotics made from foot casts into the shoes to correct this fault (Fig. 12.43).

PRESENTATIONS OF DISC CASES TREATED BY AUTHOR

CASE 1

A 40-year-old male, who had been under treatment for low back and left S1 dermatome pain for approximately 4 months, was seen in our clinic for these symptoms. Figures 12.44 and 12.45 show the posteroanterior and lateral lumbar spine and pelvic views, which reveal right lateral flexion subluxation of L3 on L4.

Figures 12.46 through 12.49 show the posteroanterior, lateral, and oblique views of the myelogram of this patient's spine, which do not reveal any evidence of nuclear disc impression into the dye-filled subarachnoid space.

Figures 12.50 through 12.52 are the CT scans of this patient's spine. Please note that in Figure 12.50, the

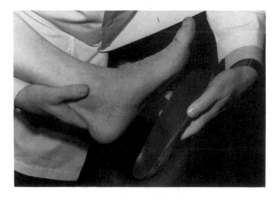

Figure 12.43. The foot orthotic used to correct pes planus.

L5-S1 level allows good visualization of both first sacral nerve roots. Figure 12.51 reveals the left first sacral nerve root to not be well visualized, while Figure 12.52 reveals a large nuclear disc protrusion completely obliterating the left S1 nerve root.

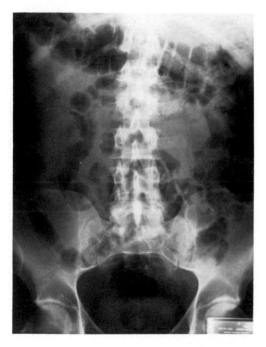

Figure 12.44. Right lateral flexion of L3 on L4 is seen. Dye from prior myelographic study is visible.

These CTs had been originally interpreted as being normal. In cooperation with the patient's family medical doctor, we gained authorization to treat the patient, and he was able to return to his job as a truck driver 2 months following the treatment in our clinic of this L5-S1 left nuclear disc protrusion. Treatment consisted of the use of flexion distraction and therapy as described under "Cox Closed Reduction of Disc Protrusion" earlier in this chapter.

Figure 12.53 shows a bone scan of this patient, which was normal.

CASE 2

A 49-year-old white female was seen for the complaint of left leg pain in the distribution of the L5 dermatome. It had started 10 months prior to our seeing the patient, following riding a long distance in the car. She had taken nonsteroidal antiinflammatory drugs and consulted a neurosurgeon, who suggested surgery if the pain continued. Figure 12.54 shows a magnetic resonance image (MRI) that was performed; an L4-L5 disc protrusion is seen, with loss of signal intensity from the L4-L5 disc due to its degenerative state.

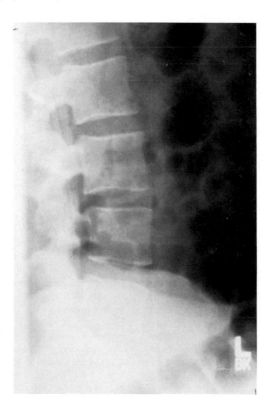

Figure 12.45. The L5-S1 disc space is narrowed, with early degenerative changes.

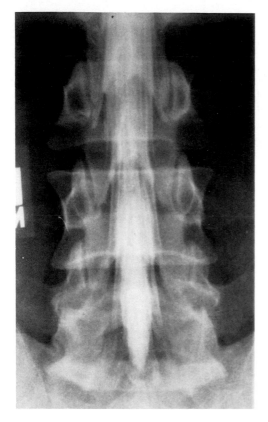

Figure 12.46. Posteroanterior view of the myelographic procedure reveals no sign of filling defect.

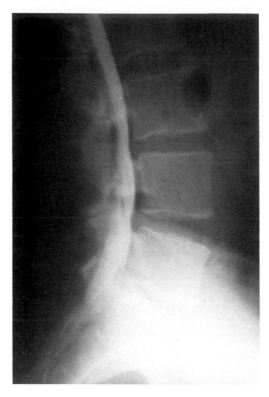

Figure 12.47. No extradural lesion is noted on lateral myelogram study.

The patient's past treatment consisted of physical therapy and an epidural steroid injection 1 month prior to our seeing her. These treatments did not alleviate her leg pain. Examination revealed hypesthesia of the left L5 dermatome. The deep reflexes at the knee and ankle were +2 bilaterally. No muscle weakness was noted, the ranges of motion of the lumbar spine were normal, and the straight leg raises were negative.

It was our impression that this patient, in the absence of a Déjérine's triad and having only leg pain with no back pain, was suffering from a free fragment of disc material at the L4-L5 level. X-rays taken in neutral upright position and right and left lateral flexion, shown in Figures 12.55 through 12.57, revealed good right lateral flexion with L4 going into lateral flexion with normal rotation of the spinous process into the right concavity (Fig. 12.56). Left lateral flexion (Fig. 12.57) found that L4 did not left laterally flex, with the only flexion occurring above the L4 level. From this, our impression was that the patient was suffering from an L4-L5 left non-contained disc prolapse. We feel that leg pain, without low back pain, is the most difficult sciatic case that we

see due to the strong probability of a free fragment within the vertebral canal compressing the nerve root but no longer aggravating the annulus fibrosis of the disc or the posterior longitudinal ligament to cause low back pain.

With this in mind, we told the patient that we would attempt 3 weeks of conservative care and that, if 50% relief was not obtained, subjectively and objectively, a surgical intervention would probably be needed.

Flexion distraction manipulation was given at the L4-L5 disc level with positive galvanism into the L4-L5 disc, goading of acupressure points B22 through B54, and the use of alternating hot and cold packs to the spine. Under treatment, the patient started to state that her left foot felt as though there were water running over the skin. She progressively felt less pain in her leg until approximately 10 days after the beginning of treatment, at which time she began to feel the pain to worsen in the leg again. She began to have problems sleeping at night. Following a long car trip, she had marked leg pain even at night. She took off work for 1 week, but the leg pain continued. At the end of 3 weeks, she was not 50% improved. At that time, the clinical decision was made to begin to stretch her very short ham-

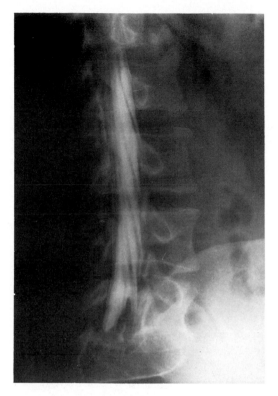

Figure 12.48. Left anterior oblique projection reveals normal nerve root filling with no extradural lesion.

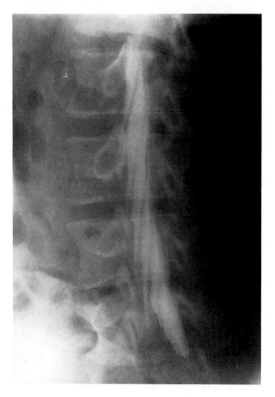

Figure 12.49. Right anterior oblique projection reveals normal nerve root filling with no extradural lesion.

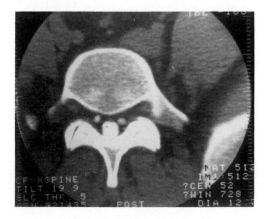

Figure 12.50. CT scan shows the first sacral nerve root to be well visualized, although the left root is slightly posteriorly displaced.

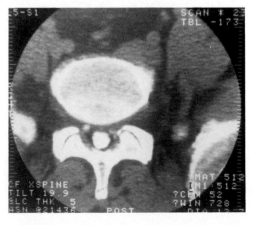

Figure 12.51. The left S1 nerve root is not seen clearly due to discal protrusion into the left lateral recess, causing peridural fat and root displacement.

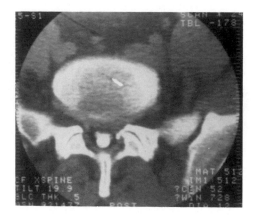

Figure 12.52. The findings of Figure 12.51 are more demonstrable now. Note the large left lateral discal protrusion.

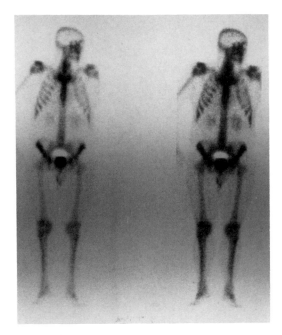

Figure 12.53. Bone scan of case 1.

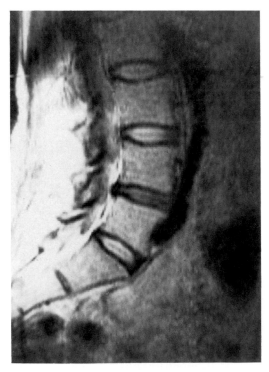

Figure 12.54. MRI shows degenerative L4-L5 disc disease with protrusion of the disc posteriorly into the vertebral canal.

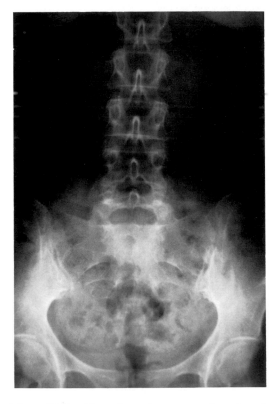

Figure 12.55. Neutral upright x-ray reveals no lateral scoliotic list.

string muscles, even though she was still having much leg pain. To the surprise of the clinicians, the following day, after strong stretching of the hamstring muscles with proprioceptive neuromuscular facilitation used, the patient stated that she felt much improved. Therefore, it was the final stretching of the hamstring muscles that actually gave us the best relief in this case.

Figure 12.58 is shown as a reminder of the sciatic scoliosis that patients develop in order to relieve their low back and sciatic pain.

CASE 3

A 29-year-old white married male was seen for low back and right leg pain. He had been treated previously by a chiropractor for the same symptoms, with possibly 90% relief. The pain had returned, and even under chiropractic treatment had gotten progressively worse. A CT and myelogram were performed, and the patient had been informed that he had a ruptured L4-L5 disc; surgery was recommended. He saw us for a second opinion.

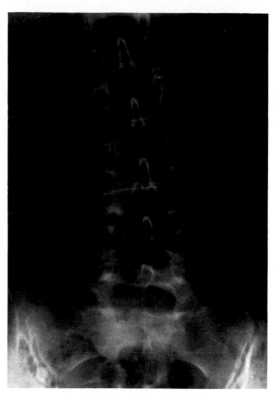

Figure 12.57. Left lateral flexion is Lovett reverse as the spinous processes of L2, L3 and L4 fail to rotate to the left concavity on left lateral flexion.

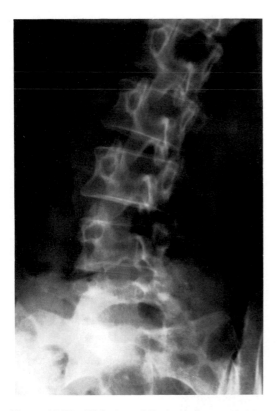

Figure 12.56. Right lateral flexion is Lovett positive rotation with lateral flexion as the spinous processes rotate into the right concavity of the curve.

Examination revealed that the patient leaned to the left from the waist and complained of pain down the right L5 dermatome into the big toe. On flexion, however, the patient's lean was markedly to the right side. His motions were restricted to 60° of flexion, and the straight leg raises were positive bilaterally with a positive well leg raise sign being present, meaning that the pain shot down the right leg as we raised the left leg. The deep reflexes were +2 bilaterally, and no sensory changes were noted on pinwheel examination. The muscle strength of the lower extremities were grade 5 of 5 and equal. The patient's Déjérine triad was negative, and closer questioning revealed that this patient actually had very little back pain but primarily leg pain. Figures 12.59 and 12.60 reveal a complete block of the subarachnoid dye-filled space posterior to the L4-L5 disc space, and the CT scan shows a marked posterior protrusion of the L5-S1 disc into the vertebral canal.

The diagnosis was an L4-L5 nuclear disc prolapse. This patient was referred back to his treating chiropractor with the following recommendation: In light of the fact that there were no absent deep reflexes, no motor weakness, and a normal sensory examination, 3 weeks of daily flexion distraction manipulation were to be ap-

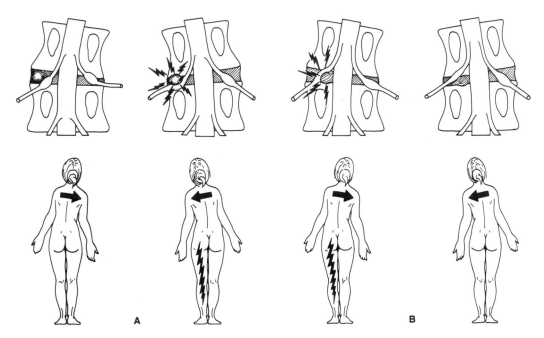

Figure 12.58. Patients with herniated disc disease may sometimes list to one side. This is a voluntary or involuntary mechanism to alleviate nerve root irritation. The list in some patients is toward the side of the sciatica; in others, it is toward the opposite side. A reasonable hypothesis suggests that when herniation is lateral to the nerve root (**A**), the list is to the side opposite the sciatica because a list to the same side would elicit pain. Conversely, when the herniation is medial to the nerve root (**B**), the list is toward the side of the sciatica because tilting away would irritate the root and cause pain. If this hypothesis could be documented in clinical practice, it would be helpful at the time of surgical exploration. (Reproduced with permission from White AA, Panjabi MM: *Clinical Biomechanics of the Spine.* Philadelphia, JB Lippincott, 1978, p 299.)

plied. If this did not show at least 50% improvement within 3 weeks of care, surgical intervention should then be undertaken. The final outcome of this case was unknown to this author.

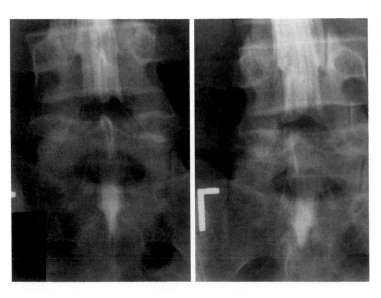

Figure 12.59. The L4- and L5-level myelogram shows a large extradural filling defect of the dye-filled subarachnoid space.

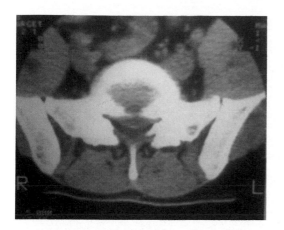

Figure 12.60. CT scan at the L5-S1 level shows a large, relatively symmetrical disc protrusion. No S1 dermatome radiation was seen in this patient.

CASE 4

The following case is presented from the practice of Charles C. Neault, D.C., of Simi Valley, California. It is a case report in which a diagnosed case of an L4 lumbar nuclear prolapse, verified by magnetic resonance imaging and treated with Cox flexion distraction manipulation, was managed successfully and the reduction verified with a posttreatment MRI scan.

A 58-year-old white female presented complaining of low back and left leg pain of 1½ weeks duration following moving a couch in her home. She indicated that she had had some minor back problems previously, for example, when doing gardening. The pain usually lasted only a day or two and would go away. On this occasion, not only did the low back pain not go away, but she had left leg pain, which she had never had previously.

On examination, the patient was in severe distress. Her weight was 180 pounds, her height was 5 feet, 9 inches.

She indicated that her low back pain was not aggravated by coughing or sneezing; however, the pain occasionally was worse on sitting. She also indicated that her leg pain appeared simultaneously with the back pain, and that it went all the way to the foot. The patient exhibited a left limp, a left antalgic lean, and severe paravertebral muscle spasm.

Bechterew's test was normal. Minor's sign was positive on the left, and the Valsalva maneuver was negative. The Neri's bow test and Lewin's standing tests were normal.

Palpation revealed pain and tenderness on the spinous process of L4 with percussion positive. There was loss of lumbar lordosis.

Range of motion was limited to 60° flexion with pain.

Other motions were normal. Kemp's sign was positive on the left, with the right normal. Heel and toe walk were normal. Straight leg raise sign was left positive at 45° with a negative well leg raise sign. Patrick-Fabere sign was positive on the left and negative on the right.

Muscle testing revealed weak dorsiflexion of the foot, and great toe and foot eversion on the left. Milgram's sign was positive on the left low back. The deep reflexes at the patella and heel were +2 bilaterally and were equal. Sensory dermatome testing revealed a decrease of the left L5 dermatome as well as a slight decrease of the left S1 dermatome. Circulation of the lower extremities was normal. The clinical impression following work-up was an L4-L5 left subrhizal nuclear prolapse.

An initial MRI-CT combined study was made. It showed a degenerative L4-L5 disc and a posterior central and left-sided disc herniation measuring 6 mm (Figs. 12.61

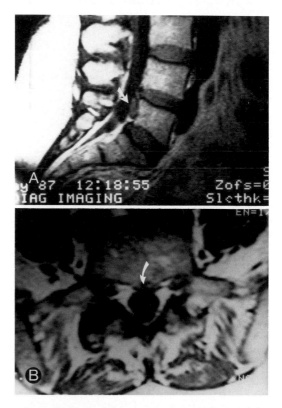

Figure 12.61. **A,** Sagittal and **B,** axial section MRI prior to manipulation shows decreased signal of the L4-L5 disc, indicating a degenerating disc. The L4-L5 disc extends 6 mm beyond the vertebral body end plate and compromises the cauda equina. A large free fragment of sequestered disc is seen to lie posterior to the L5 vertebral body, measuring 5 mm in diameter sagitally and over 1 cm craniocaudally (*straight arrow* on the sagittal and *curved arrow* on the axial view).

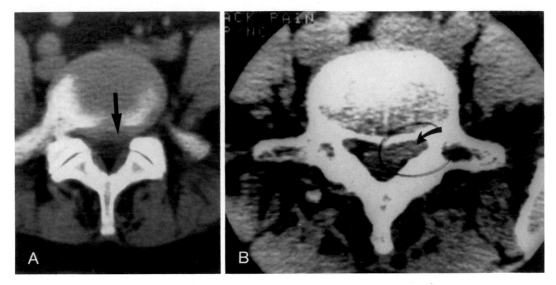

Figure 12.62. **A,** CT scan shows the large, left central disc protrusion (*straight arrow*); **B,** it is seen compromising the left lateral recess and thecal sac (*curved arrow*).

and 12.62). Also seen was a free sequestered fragment of disc material posterior to the L5 vertebral body, measuring 5 mm by over 1 cm in height. This had escaped from the L4-L5 space and migrated caudally behind the L5 body.

Treatment originally was for 2 weeks on the basis of daily care as the patient continued to work. On the day of the MRI-CT report, she was placed on disability and was treated twice a day for 9 days, at which time her pain decreased by 80% subjectively, and the straight leg raises were negative bilaterally. Prior to stopping work, she still had low back pain and a positive straight leg raise of 65°.

At the end of the 9th day of treating the patient twice daily while she was off work, she complained of only occasional leg numbness and tingling, which was felt to be compatible with residual healing of the disc lesions. The patient returned to work 1 month later and was totally asymptomatic. No neurological or orthopedic findings of a positive nature could be elicited from the patient at that time.

Follow-up MRI and CT scans (Figs. 12.63 and 12.64) were made 21 days following the initial study. The radiologist reported that the size of the sequestered fragment had decreased significantly since the initial study shown in Figures 12.61 and 12.62. In addition, there was an increase in the disc space height at L4-L5. Not only had the free fragment decreased in size, but also the L4-L5 posterior herniation had decreased in size, as shown on CT scan.

This was a severely sequestered disc fragment, and the patient had been told by a neurosurgeon to have sur-

gery for its removal. Seeking chiropractic care resulted in Cox closed reduction flexion distraction manipulation being administered, which enabled the patient to get well and resume her activities full-time with no partial disabilities.

Although there is still a disc bulge and a small sequestered fragment present on the second MRI, it certainly indicates and is concrete proof of the fact that the size of a patient's spinal canal is more important than the size of the disc lesion and must certainly be taken into consideration when there is a report of a sequestered fragment or a disc bulge.

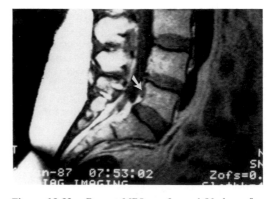

Figure 12.63. Repeat MRI, performed 21 days after the initial study shown in Figure 12.61, shows the disc sequestered fragment to be significantly smaller (*arrow*), and the patient now has no symptoms of low back or left leg pain.

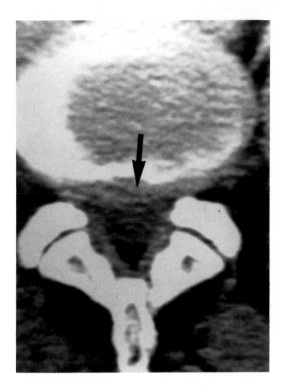

Figure 12.64. Repeat CT scan also shows marked reduction of the disc protrusion (*arrow*) as seen in Figure 12.62.

This was a unique case with "before and after" scans that demonstrated possible effectiveness of flexion distraction as applied and taught in this textbook. In the past, patients with fairly large disc herniations and ruptures of this nature had to resort to either conventional methods of chiropractic manipulative therapy or open surgery for relief of pain.

CASE 5

This 33-year-old white married female was seen for the chief complaint of low back, left leg, and more recent right leg pain. History revealed low back pain dating back 15 years, but 1 year ago, while doing aerobics, the patient developed more severe low back pain. She then developed numbness in the left leg, occurring in the posterior thigh to approximately the midthigh area. It then skipped to the lateral leg and dorsum of the foot, with numbness of the great toe. Approximately 4 weeks prior to seeing us, this pain worsened. It had been going down the right leg as well.

This patient had been seen by a neurosurgeon, who performed a CT scan and a myelogram. Surgery was recommended. She sought a second neurosurgical consultation and was advised against the surgery. She

then saw a chiropractor, who helped her a great deal utilizing flexion distraction manipulation. She also saw an orthopedic surgeon approximately 3 weeks before consulting us, when her low back symptoms worsened. She was placed on an antiinflammatory drug, which did give her relief. This patient also stated that she had gained approximately 40 pounds in the past 6 months, due largely to the fact that she could not exercise due to the low back pain.

This patient's low back and leg pain were aggravated by Déjérine's triad. She did not have night pain. Her Bechterew's sign was normal, but the recumbent straight leg raise was positive on the right at 45° creating low back pain, and positive on the left at 30°, creating leg pain. Ranges of motion of the thoracolumbar spine were normal. There was no striking pain on palpation of the lumbar spine, and the patient could heel-and-toe walk normally. The hip joints revealed no abnormal signs. The deep reflexes at the knee revealed diminished strength of the left patellar reflex. There was hypesthesia of the left L5 dermatome on pinwheel examination. We did not detect any weakness of the ankle, toe, or thigh muscles. The hamstring reflexes were bilaterally +2. Circulation of the lower extremities was adequate. Prone lumbar flexion, eliciting hyperextension, aggravated the low back pain. Plain radiographic examination is shown in Figures 12.65 and 12.66. There is thinning of the L4-L5 disc space, with traction spurs of the anterolateral margins at this level.

A myelogram reveals a large L4-L5 disc protrusion creating a waterfall sign of the dye-filled subarachnoid space. This is shown in Figures 12.67 and 12.68. The CT scan, shown in Figure 12.69, reveals a large L4-L5 midline disc protrusion.

Our impression was that this patient was suffering from a large L4-L5 nuclear disc protrusion that was now causing bilateral radiculopathy of the L5 nerve root into the lower extremities. However, we found no motor weakness signs. The left patellar reflex was diminished. However, the patient stated that this had been seen to be weaker approximately 1 year previously. She slept well and had no signs of cauda equina syndrome. She was obviously overweight and lacked good muscle tone.

Our suggestion was that this patient be placed on a strong program of flexion distraction manipulation for a 3- to 4-week period. If that did not provide at least 50% subjective and objective relief, then a surgical consultation should be strongly advised. The patient was told to avoid sitting, bending, lifting, and twisting at the waist. It was suggested that she go on a strong program of knee-chest exercise, abdominal tightening, and pelvic tilt exercises. As the sciatic pain abated, it was suggested that she begin stretching the hamstring muscles as well as strengthening the gluteus maximus muscles.

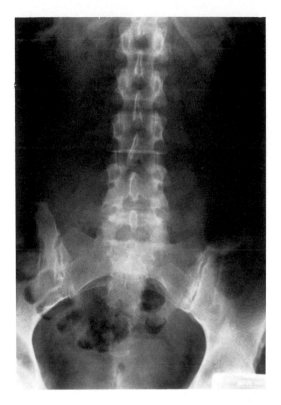

Figure 12.65. Normal lumbar posteroanterior x-ray study.

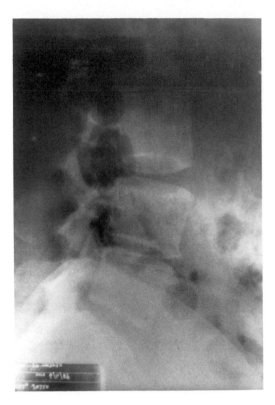

Figure 12.66. L4-L5 disc degeneration is seen.

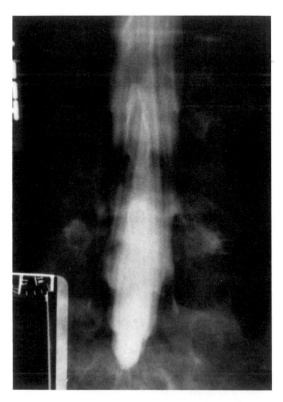

Figure 12.67. Myelogram shows an extradural filling defect at the L4-L5 level.

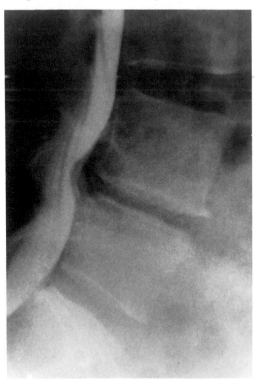

Figure 12.68. Lateral view of the myelogram shows an extradural filling defect at the L4-L5 level due to protrusion of the disc. Note the degenerative change of the L4-L5 disc.

This patient was referred to us by another chiropractor, and we did not carry out the treatment on this case or know the follow-up on it.

CASE 6

This case was given to us by Dr. M. D. Ville. The patient was a 29-year-old white male involved in an automobile accident. He later developed sciatica, and a CT scan was ordered by his surgeon. The CT scan revealed L4-L5 and L5-S1 annular bulging. Figures 12.70 through 12.73 reveal the lateral, neutroanteroposterior, and right and left lateral flexion studies of this patient. Note that in right lateral flexion we see a good Lovett positive rotation with the spinous process deviated into the right concavity. Left lateral flexion, however, sees that the spinous processes actually rotate to the right convexity of the curve. This is a typical finding often accompanying intervertebral disc protrusion as verified by CT scan in this case. We feel that this can be due to deep multifidus muscle spasm due to irritation of the dorsal ramus of the spinal nerve by the disc protrusion.

This case is presented to show the subtle findings of the Lovett reverse type of rotation accompanying known disc protrusion. This can be a very helpful finding in

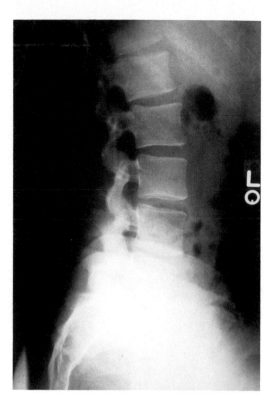

Figure 12.70. The L4-L5 and L5-S1 disc spaces show degenerative changes on lateral projection.

clinical practice to evaluate the possibility or the extent of involvement of an intervertebral disc protrusion.

CASE 7

A 24-year-old white married female was seen complaining of low back and left leg pain, occasionally into the right leg, in the distribution of the L5 and S1 dermatomes. Low back pain started following bowling and was aggravated by playing softball. She sought chiropractic care from two clinics, and then we had the opportunity to evaluate her.

Examination revealed marked limitation of ranges of motion, with flexion at 40°, 0° extension and the straight leg raising test positive at 35° on the left and 65° on the right, causing low back pain on the right and both low back and leg pain on the left. No muscle atrophy was noted. Hypesthesia of the left L5 and S1 dermatomes was noted. The deep tendon reflexes reveal an absent left Achilles reflex.

This patient walked with a right lean of the thoracolumbar spine, a limp of the left lower extremity, and a forward flexion posture.

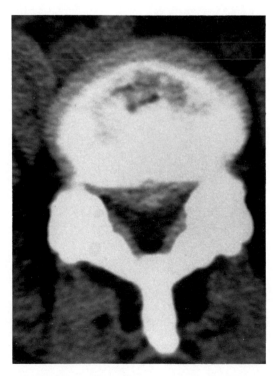

Figure 12.69. CT shows the L4-L5 central disc protrusion that is seen in the myelogram in Figures 12.67 and 12.68.

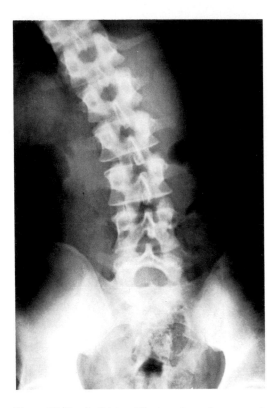

Figure 12.71. Left lateral flexion, shown here, reveals the spinous processes to rotate into the right convex side of the curve. Such reverse rotation of the spinous processes occurs in disc protrusion with multifidus muscle spasm. This patient had CT-verified L4-L5 and L5-S1 annular protrusions.

Our clinical impression was that this patient suffered from an L4-L5 or L5-S1 nuclear disc protrusion. Figures 12.74 and 12.75 show the posteroanterior and lateral projections of this patient's lumbar spine, which reveal a right lift of the thoracolumbar spine and a retrolisthesis subluxation of L5 on the sacrum. Figure 12.76 represents a CT scan at the L5-S1 level which shows a small midline disc protrusion.

This patient was given daily in-clinic treatment with approximately four treatments of flexion distraction, alternating hot and cold packs to the lumbar spine, and acupressure treatment until approximately 50% of the leg pain was relieved. The patient was then placed on a strong regimen of hamstring stretch, abdominal strengthening, and erector spinae muscle strengthening exercises. She attended low back wellness school in order to learn how to bend and lift with reduced irritation to the low back.

This patient returned to her job, working for a small number of hours at the beginning and gradually building up to a full day's work.

CASE 8

We are presenting here a case of L3-L4 and L4-L5 disc protrusion shown on axial and reformatted CT (Figs. 12.77, 12.78, and 12.79).

CASE 9

A 38-year-old man with an MRI revealing L3-L4, L4-L5, and L5-S1 disc bulges was seen (Fig. 12.80). His symptoms were low back pain and bilateral leg pain of nondermatomal isolation. There were no motor or reflex changes. We felt that his symptoms were due to annular disc tearing and early chemical irritation of the nerve root by nuclear leakage into the spinal canal. A course of in-clinic care consisting of flexion distraction manipulation, as well as home care consisting of exercise to return his muscle system to strength and flexibility, were refused; the patient preferred to take pain pills. Some patients require great pain before submitting to sensible treatment advice.

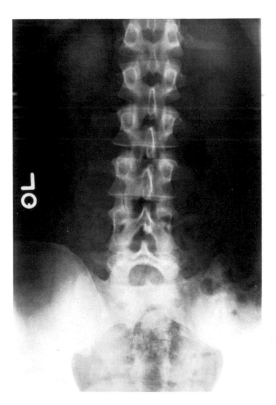

Figure 12.72. Neutral anteroposterior lumbar x-ray shows normal structure.

maintain constant care in the use of her low back to prevent more serious disc damage and nerve root compression irritation, which could necessitate surgery.

CASE 11

Spondylolisthesis of L5 is seen in the myelographic study shown in Figure 12.84 as well as the posterior herniation of the L4-L5 disc. The oblique view in Figure 12.85 shows the large extradural filling defect representing the L4-L5 disc herniation. It is not common to see spondylolisthesis with a disc protrusion at the cephalic level to it.

This 57-year-old truck driver was seen for low back pain and right L5 dermatome leg pain of 3 months duration. During that time, he had been scheduled for surgery three different times, but for various reasons it had been cancelled. One time, as the patient was taken into the surgical suite, the surgeon became ill and had to postpone the surgery.

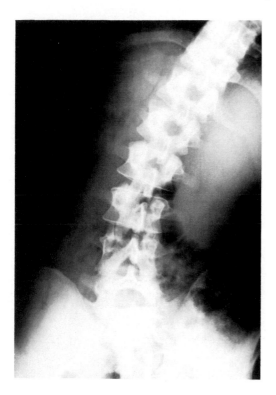

Figure 12.73. Normal right lateral flexion is seen, with the spinous processes rotating into the right concavity of the lateral flexion curve. Contrast this normal rotation motion with the reverse rotation of Figure 12.71.

CASE 10

A 40-year-old female with chronic low back pain and right knee pain was seen; her MRI studies are shown in Figures 12.81 to 12.83. Flexion distraction manipulation was given. The result, following 3 weeks of care, was absence of leg pain and isolation of pain to the right L5-S1 facet articulations. Treatment then consisted of full range of motion to the facet joints of the lumbar spine, with a vigorous home exercise program of stretching and Cox exercises. The patient was left with right L5-S1 facet joint pain upon prolonged sitting, bending, lifting, or twisting movements of the waist. She attended low back wellness school to learn ergonomic control of her low back pain.

This is an excellent case of a patient with an unstable disc at L4-L5 with annular tearing and herniation, as well as vertical stenosis by facet imbrication of the L5 superior facet into the upper aspects of the L4-L5 intervertebral foramen where the L4 nerve root exits the cauda equina and vertebral canal. This patient must

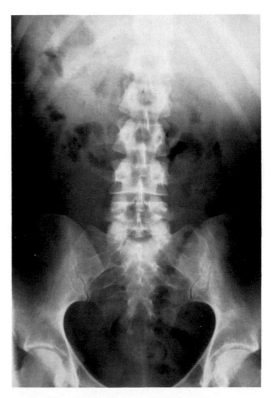

Figure 12.74. Anteroposterior lumbar spine x-ray of a patient with left L5 and S1 dermatome sciatica. The patient has a list to the right side, away from the side of sciatic pain.

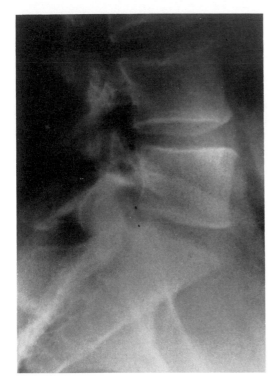

Figure 12.75. Lateral projection shows retrolisthesis subluxation of L5 on the sacrum.

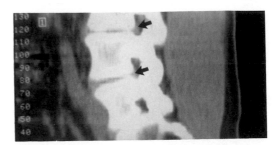

Figure 12.77. Reformatted CT scan shows nuclear disc protrusion at the L3-L4 and L4-L5 levels (*arrows*).

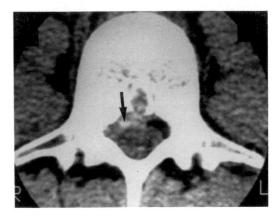

Figure 12.78. Axial CT shows the right central disc prolapse (*arrow*).

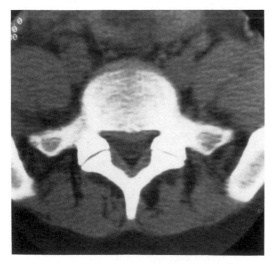

Figure 12.76. CT scan shows a small left central disc protrusion. Note that the left lateral recess is minimally stenosed by the first sacral facet.

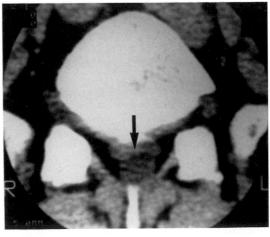

Figure 12.79. Axial CT shows the central disc prolapse (*arrow*).

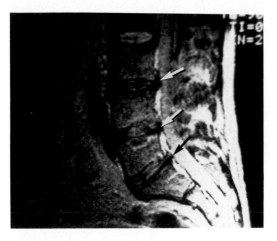

Figure 12.80. A 38-year-old man with L3-L4, L4-L5, and L5-S1 disc protrusions (*arrows*).

On examination, this patient had no sciatic scoliosis. The deep reflexes were +2 bilaterally and were equal. There is atrophy of the right calf and thigh compared with the left. The straight leg raises were positive bilaterally at 80°, creating pain into the anterior leg in the L5 dermatome.

With the diagnosis of an L4-L5 intervertebral disc herniation and possible prolapse, flexion distraction was administered twice daily. The other therapies, as described in this chapter, were administered. The patient slowly saw his pain diminish, and his homework of exercise and ergonomic training taught in low back wellness school resulted in slow healing and return to his usual work duties after 1 month of care.

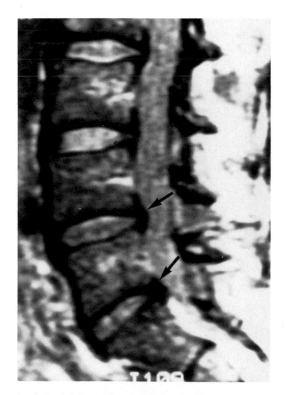

Figure 12.81. MRI sagittal study shows posterior bulging of the L4-L5 and L5-S1 discs, with degenerative changes of the discs noted (*arrows*).

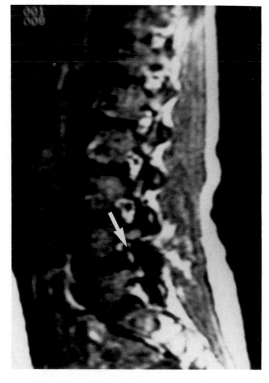

Figure 12.82. Note the foraminal narrowing (*arrow*) at the L4-L5 level and the compromised space for the L4 nerve root.

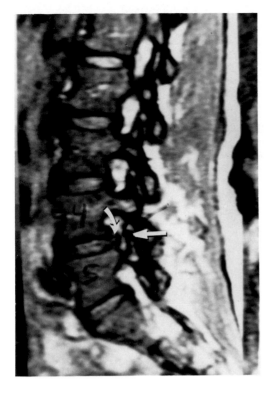

Figure 12.83. Observe the L4-L5 disc protrusion (*curved arrow*) and the vertical stenosis of the L4-L5 foramen by the telescoping of the L5 facet into the upper foraminal space (*straight arrow*).

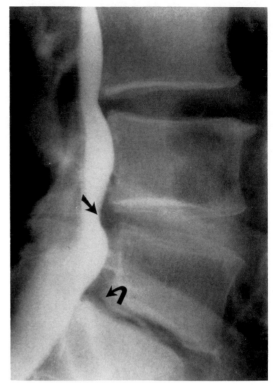

Figure 12.84. Myelographic study shows a large L4-L5 disc protrusion creating an extradural filling defect into the dye-filled subarachnoid space (*straight arrow*). Note the 15% true spondylolisthesis of L5 on the sacrum (*curved arrow*).

CASE 12

Always hesitate in accepting opinions from other physicians or institutions on patients who seek your opinion—regardless of where these other opinions have been sought or how numerous they are. The following case demonstrates that point.

This 40-year-old man was referred by his treating chiropractor to a neurosurgeon for symptoms of persistent low back and left leg pain into the first sacral dermatome. The hospital reports were negative for disc protrusion or noncontained disc material in the vertebral canal. The patient continued to be in pain, with loss of work duties and income due to the persistent pain. The chiropractor then referred the patient to our clinic for another chiropractic opinion. Our radiology department obtained the myelographic and myelographically enhanced CT scans shown in Figures 12.86, 12.87, and 12.88; as you can see, they were not negative. A large L5-S1 disc fragment is present within the lateral recess of the vertebral canal which prevents the metrizamide dye from filling the subarachnoid and dural root sleeve of the S1 nerve root on the left.

Surgery to remove this L5-S1 fragment gave immediate relief of pain and return to work duties.

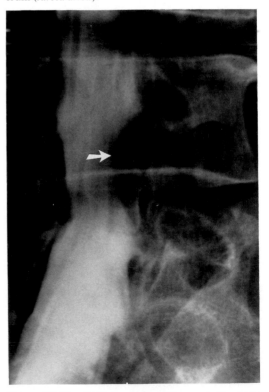

Figure 12.85. Oblique myelogram reveals the large right L4-L5 disc protrusion defect (*arrow*).

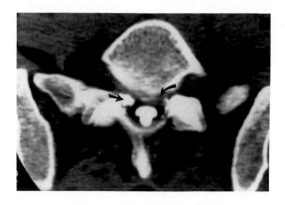

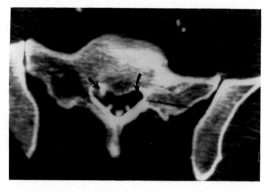

Figure 12.86. The *straight arrow* shows the right S1 nerve root to be opacified by the contrast medium on the myelographically enhanced CT scan. The *curved arrow* shows the left vertebral canal and lateral recess to be occupied by disc material, with failure of visualization and filling of the left S1 nerve root.

Figure 12.87. As in Figure 12.86, this figure is taken at a lower level of the spine, below the L5-S1 disc level; it shows failure of the left nerve root to fill (*curved arrow*), while the right nerve root is visualized with opaque myelographic medium (*straight arrow*).

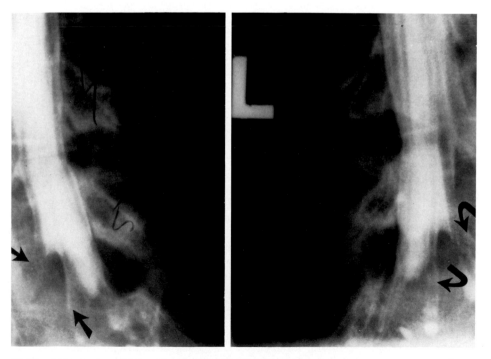

Figure 12.88. Oblique view of the myelographic study shows the right L5 and S1 nerve roots (*curved arrows*) to fill well, whereas the left L5 and S1 nerve roots (*straight arrows*) fail to fill as adequately. This, when coupled with the CT scan, enhances the opinion of compression of the left nerve root by discal material.

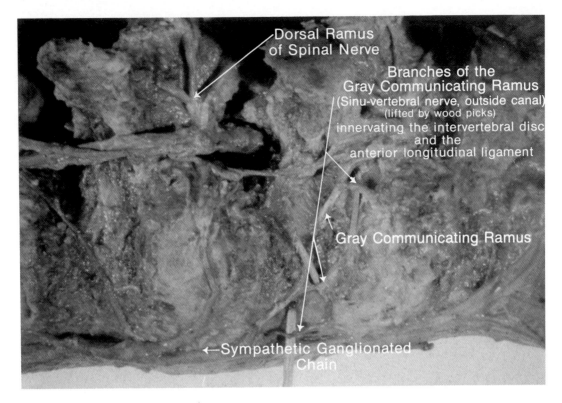

Figure 12.89. Dissection of the outside of the spine showing the sympathetic ganglionated chain giving rise to the gray rami communicantes that form the nerve supply to the circumference of the intervertebral disc and anterior longitudinal ligament. Note also the dorsal and ventral ramus of the spinal nerve.

CHAPTER CLIMAX

To end this chapter, an exciting dissection performed by Chae-Song Ro, M.D., Ph.D., of the anatomy department of the National College of Chiropractic is presented, followed by an algorithm of treatment selection dependent upon patient objective and subjective findings. I choose to end with this beautiful dissection (Figs. 12.89 and 12.90) since it so well capsulizes the probable pain pathways of the lumbar spine. It shows the spinal nerve within the intervertebral foramen and its divisions into the dorsal and ventral ramus. The dorsal ramus will supply the multifidi, sacrospinalis, aponeurosis of the latissimus dorsi, iliac crest, and buttock as cutaneous nerves (cluneal nerves L1, L2, L3), and the articular processes. The ventral ramus of the lumbar, sacral, and coccygeal nerves will form the lumbosacral plexus. This plexus will form the lumbar, sacral, and pudendal plexi. The lumbar plexus will form the iliohypogastric, ilioinguinal, genitofemoral, lateral femoral cutaneous, femoral, obturator, and accessory obturator nerves. The sacral plexus will form the sciatic nerve, and the pudendal plexus will form the pudendal nerve, perineal nerve, dorsal nerve, inferior hemorrhoidal nerve, and the scrotal branches.

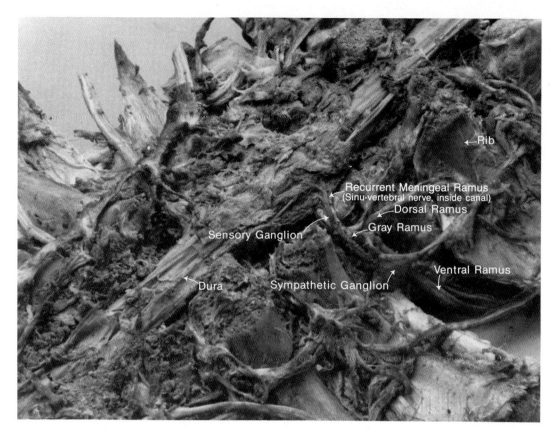

Figure 12.90. Here the vertebral bodies have been carefully removed to allow visualization of the recurrent meningeal ramus. The sympathetic ganglionated chain is seen, with the gray ramus from it joining the ventral ramus to form the recurrent meningeal nerve (sinuvertebral nerve) that will enter the vertebral canal to supply the structures within it.

The communicating ramus from the sympathetic ganglionated chain (gray ramus communicans) will join the ventral ramus, and the recurrent meningeal nerve will be formed, which will give off the nerve supply to the disc inside the vertebral canal, the posterior longitudinal ligament, the ligamentum flavum, the facet capsule, and the epidural vascular plexus of the medulla spinalis and its membranes.

The bottom line in care of the intervertebral disc patient is treatment selection and the proper chronology of such care. Physicians need to start with conservative care, being constantly aware of the changing faces of patient symptoms and findings that dictate and demand diagnostic action and treatment regimens. Table 12.2 summarizes this author's basic decision-making protocol in dealing daily with clinically positive low back disc cases. Hopefully it will aid in leading you through this often demanding and complex patient syndrome of low back pain and sciatica. Table 12.3 is a flow chart summarizing treatment selection procedures based on the diagnosis of the patient's complaint. This author (J.M.C.) uses Tables 12.2 and 12.3 as clinical decision-making parameters in daily practice.

Table 12.2.
Algorithm of Diagnostic and Treatment Protocol for Decision Making in the Sciatica Patient

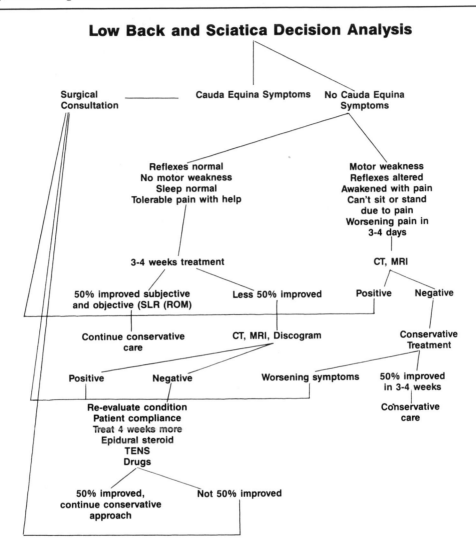

Low Back and Sciatica Decision Analysis

Surgical Consultation —————— Cauda Equina Symptoms   No Cauda Equina Symptoms

Reflexes normal
No motor weakness
Sleep normal
Tolerable pain with help

Motor weakness
Reflexes altered
Awakened with pain
Can't sit or stand
due to pain
Worsening pain in
3-4 days

3-4 weeks treatment   CT, MRI

50% improved subjective   Less 50% improved   Positive   Negative
and objective (SLR (ROM))

Continue conservative   CT, MRI, Discogram   Conservative
care   Treatment

Positive   Negative   Worsening symptoms   50% improved
in 3-4 weeks

Re-evaluate condition   Conservative
Patient compliance   care
Treat 4 weeks more
Epidural steroid
TENS
Drugs

50% improved,   Not 50% improved
continue conservative
approach

Table 12.3.
Flow Chart of Treatment for Low Back and Leg Pain Patients

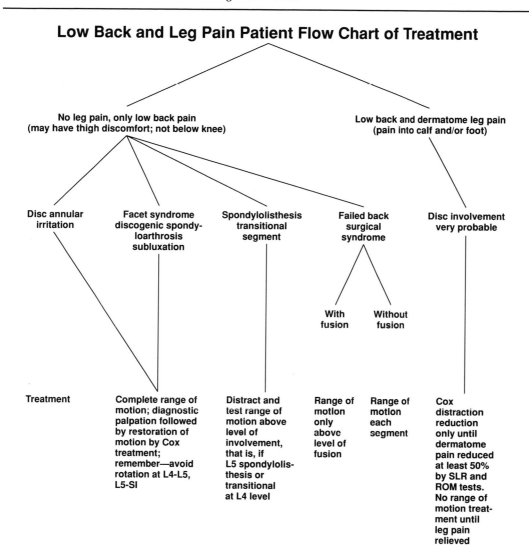

Low Back and Leg Pain Patient Flow Chart of Treatment

No leg pain, only low back pain
(may have thigh discomfort; not below knee)

Low back and dermatome leg pain
(pain into calf and/or foot)

Disc annular
irritation

Facet syndrome
discogenic spondy-
loarthrosis
subluxation

Spondylolisthesis
transitional
segment

Failed back
surgical
syndrome

Disc involvement
very probable

With
fusion

Without
fusion

Treatment

Complete range of
motion; diagnostic
palpation followed
by restoration of
motion by Cox
treatment;
remember—avoid
rotation at L4-L5,
L5-SI

Distract and
test range of
motion above
level of
involvement,
that is, if
L5 spondylolis-
thesis or
transitional
at L4 level

Range of
motion
only
above
level of
fusion

Range of
motion
each
segment

Cox
distraction
reduction
only until
dermatome
pain reduced
at least 50%
by SLR and
ROM tests.
No range of
motion treat-
ment until
leg pain
relieved

References

1. Pal B, Mangion P, Hossain MA, Diffey BL: A controlled trial of continuous lumbar traction in the treatment of back pain and sciatica. *Br J Rheumatol* 25:181–183, 1986.
2. Glover JR, Morris JG, Khosla T: Back pain: a randomized clinical trial of rotational manipulation of the trunk. *Br J Intern Med* 31:59–64, 1974.
3. Matthews JA: *Back Pain and Sciatica.* M.D. thesis, Cambridge, England, University of Cambridge, 1984.
4. Hoehler FK, Tobis JS, Buerger AA: Spinal manipulation for low back pain. *JAMA* 245:1835–1838, 1981.
5. Sims-Williams H, Jayson MIV, Young SMS, Baddeley H, Collins E: Controlled trial of mobilization and manipulation for patients with low back pain in general practice. *Br Med J* 2:1338–1340, 1978.
6. Doran DML, Newell DJ: Manipulation in treatment of low back pain: a multicentre study. *Br Med J* 2(April 26):161–164, 1975.
7. Paterson JK: A survey of musculoskeletal problems in general practice. *Manual Medicine* 3:40–48, 1987.
8. Robertson AM: Challenge of the painful back: rheumatism in industry. Report of Industrial Survey Unit of ARC. *Trans Soc Occup Med* 20:42–49, 1970.
9. Fisk JW: A controlled trial of manipulation in a selected group of patients with low back pain favouring one side. *N Z Med J* 90(645):288–291, 1979.
10. Fisk J: Manipulation in general practice. *N Z Med J* 74:172–175, 1971.
11. Rasmussen GG: Manipulation in treatment of low back pain—randomized clinical trial. *Manuelle Medizin* 17:8–10, 1979.
12. Farrell JP, Twomey LT: Acute low-back pain: comparison of two conservative treatment approaches. *Med J Aust* 1:160–164, 1982.
13. Evans DP, Burke MS, Lloyd KN, Roberts EE, Roberts GM: Lumbar spinal manipulation on trial: part I—clinical assessment. *Rheumatol Rehabil* 17:46–53, 1978.
14. Coxhead CE, Inskip H, Meade TW, North WRS, Troup JDG: Multicentre trial of physiotherapy in the management of sciatic symptoms. *Lancet* (May 16):1065–1068, 1981.
15. Kirkaldy-Willis WH, Cassidy JD: Spinal manipulation in the treatment of low-back pain. *Can Fam Physician* 31(March):535–540, 1985.
16. Nwuga VCB: Relative therapeutic efficacy of vertebral manipulation and conventional treatment in back pain management. *Am J Phys Med* 61:273–278, 1982.
17. Jayson MIV, Sims-Williams H, Young S, et al.: Mobilization and manipulation for low back pain. *Spine* 6:409–416, 1981.
18. Moritz U: Evaluation of manipulation and other manual therapy. *Scand J Rehabil Med* 11:173–179, 1979.
19. Zylbergold RS, Piper MC: Lumbar disc disease: comparative analysis of physical therapy treatments. *Arch Phys Med Rehabil* 62(April):176–179, 1981.
20. Kane R: Manipulating the patient: a comparison of the effectiveness of a physician and a chiropractor. *Lancet* 1:1333–1336, 1974.
21. Fonti M, Lynch D: Pain due to IVD syndrome and chiropractic care. In: *Abstracts of the World Chiropractic Conference, Venice, Italy, 1983.*
22. Deyo RA, Tsui-Wu Y: Descriptive epidemiology of low-back pain and its related medical care in the United States. *Spine* 12(3):264–268, 1987.
23. Cyriax JH: Manipulation in the treatment of low back pain. *Br Med J* 26:161–164, 1975.
24. Ebbetts J: Manipulation in the treatment of low back pain. *Br Med J* 2:393, 1975.
25. Donnelly WJ, Spykerboer JE, Thong YH: Are patients who use alternative medicine dissatisfied with orthodox medicine?. *Med J Aust* 142:539–541, 1985.
26. Swezey RL, Crittenden JO, Swezey AM: Outpatient treatment of lumbar disc sciatica. *West J Med* 145(1):43–46, 1986.
27. Snook SH: Cheap versus cost effective care. In: *Abstract Workbook, 7th Annual Challenge of the Lumbar Spine, Minneapolis, MN,* Challenge of the Lumbar Spine, 1985.
28. Deyo RA, Diehl AK, Rosenthal M: How much bedrest for backache? a randomized clinical trial. *Clin Res* 33(2):A228, 1985.
29. Hadler N, Curtis P, Gillings D, Stinnett S: Treatment—benefit of spinal manipulation as adjunctive therapy for acute low-back pain: a stratified controlled trial. *Spine* 12(7):703–706, 1987.
30. Arkuszeqski A: Involvement of the cervical spine in back pain. *Manual Medicine* 2:126–128, 1986.
31. Dommisse GF, Grabe RP: The failures of surgery for lumbar disc disorders. In Helfet AJ, Gruebel-Lee DM (eds): *Disorders of the Lumbar Spine.* Philadelphia, JB Lippincott, 1978, pp 202–203.
32. Ongley M, Dorman T, Hubert L, Klein R, Eek B: Treatment–a new approach to the treatment of chronic low back pain. *Lancet* (July 18):143–146, 1987.
33. Rupert RL, Wagnon R, Thompson P, Ezzeldin MT: Chiropractic adjustments: results of a controlled clinical trial in Egypt. *ICA Int Rev Chiro* (Winter):58–60, 1985.
34. Cox JM, Shreiner S: Chiropractic manipulation in low back pain and sciatica: statistical data on the diagnosis, treatment, and response of 576 consecutive cases. *J Manipulative Physiol Ther* 7:1–11, 1984.
35. Potter GE: A study of 744 cases of neck and back pain treated with spinal manipulation. *Journal of the CCA* (December):154–156, 1977.
36. Nyiendo J, Haldeman S: A critical study of the student interns' practice activities in a chiropractic

college teaching clinic. *J Manipulative Physiol Ther* 2:197–201, 1986.

37. Bronfort G: Chiropractic treatment of low back pain: a prospective survey. *J Manipulative Physiol Ther* 9:99–112, 1986.

38. Waagen GN, Haldeman S, Cook G, Lopez D, De-Boer KF: Short term trial of chiropractic adjustments for the relief of chronic low back pain. *Manual Medicine* 2:63–67, 1986.

39. Wooley FR, Kane RL: A comparison of allopathic and chiropractic care. In Buerger AA, Robis JS (eds): *Approaches to the Validation of Manipulation Therapy.* Springfield, IL, Charles C Thomas, 1977, pp 217–219, 223.

40. Chrisman OD, Mittnach R, Snook GA: A study of the results following rotatory manipulation in the lumbar intervertebral-disc syndrome. *J Bone Joint Surg* 46A:517–524, 1964.

41. Meade TW: Comparison of chiropractic and hospital outpatient management of low back pain: a feasibility study. *J Epidemiol Community Health* 40: 12–17, 1986.

42. Vernon HT, Dhami MSI, Howley TP, Annett R: Spinal manipulation and beta-endorphin: a controlled study of the effect of a spinal manipulation on plasma beta-endorphin levels in normal males. *J Manipulative Physiol Ther* 9:115–123, 1986.

43. Kuo PPF, Loh ZC. Treatment of lumbar intervertebral disc protrusions by manipulation. *Clin Orthop* 215:47–55, 1987.

44. Gillstrom P, Ericson P, Hindmarsh T: Computed tomography examination of the influence of autotraction on herniation of the lumbar disc. *Arch Orthop Trauma Surg* 104:289–293, 1985.

45. Li Y, Fei J, Zuliang L, Zhenqian L: Traction and manipulative reduction for the treatment of protrusion of lumbar intervertebral disc—an analysis of 1,455 cases. *J Tradit Chinese Med* 6(1):31–33, 1986.

46. McCarron RF, Wimpee MW, Hudkins PG, Laros GS: The inflammatory effect of nucleus pulposus, a possible element in the pathogenesis of low-back pain. *Spine* 12(8):760–764, 1987.

47. Fernstrom U: Discographical study of ruptured lumbar intervertebral discs. *Acta Chir Scand* (Suppl):258, 1960.

48. Harris W, Wagnon RJ: The effects of chiropractic adjustments in distal skin temperature. *J Manipulative Physiol Ther* 10:57–60, 1987.

49. Burton CV: Gravity lumbar reduction. In Kirkaldy-Willis WH (ed): *Managing Low Back Pain.* Edinburgh, Churchill Livingstone, 1983.

50. Hirschberg GG: Treating lumbar disc lesion by prolonged continuous reduction of intradiscal pressure. *Tex Med* 70:58–68, 1974.

51. Neugebauer J: Re-establishing of the intervertebral disc by decompression. *Med Welt* 27:19, 1976.

51a. Deyo RA: Conservative therapy for low back pain—distinguishing useful from useless therapy. *JAMA* 250(8):1058–1059, 1983.

52. Tien-You F: Lumbar intervertebral disc protrusion, new method of management and its theoretical basis. *Chin Med J* [Engl] 2(3):183–194, 1976.

53. Tsung-Min L, et al.: Vertical suspension traction with manipulation in lumbar intervertebral disc protrusion. *Chin Med J* 3(6):407–412, 1977.

54. Burton C: Gravity is now a useful tool in low back pain treatment. *Fam Treat Ctr* 7:4, 1977.

55. Tkachenko SS: Closed one-stage reduction of acute prolapse of the intervertebral disc. *Ortop Traumatal Protez* 34:46–47, 1973.

56. Mathews JA, Yates DAH: Treatment of sciatica. *Lancet* 1:352, 1974.

57. Pomosov DV: Treatment of slipped discs by a closed reduction method. *Voen Med Zh* 7(July): 76–77, 1976.

58. Edwards JP, et al.: A comparison of chiropractic technics as they relate to the intervertebral disc syndrome. *Dig Chiro Econ* (November/December):92–101, 1977.

59. Potter GE: A study of 744 cases of neck and back pain treated with spinal manipulation. *J Can Chiro Assoc* (December):154–156, 1977.

60. Sharubina I: Effectiveness of using medical gymnastics together with traction in a swimming pool in the overall treatment of discogenic radiculitis. *Vopr Kurortol Fizioter Lech Fiz Kult* 38:536–557, 1973.

61. Gupta RC, Ramarao SV: Epidurography in reduction of lumbar disc prolapse by traction. *Arch Phys Med Rehabil* (July):59, 1978.

62. Lind G: *Auto-Traction, Treatment of Low Back Pain and Sciatica, An Electromyographic, Radiographic and Clinical Study.* Linkoping, 1974.

63. Anonymous: Treatment of lumbar disc protrusion by automatic chiropractic traction instrument. Translated at the National College, 1982. (Available from library of author, J.M. Cox).

64. Raney FL: The effects of flexion, extension, Valsalva maneuver and abdominal compression of the large volume myelographic columns. Paper presented at *International Society of Study of the Lumbar Spine,* June 5–8, 1978.

65. Eagle R: A pain in the back. *New Scientist* (October 18):170–173, 1979.

66. Hukins DWL, Hickey DS: Relation between the structure of the annulus fibrosus and the function and failure of the intervertebral disc. *Spine* 6(2): 110, 1980.

67. Nachemson AL: The lumbar spine, an orthopaedic challenge. *Spine* 1(1):59–69, 1976.

68. Tindall GT: Clinical aspects of lumbar intervertebral disc disease. *J Med Assoc Ga* 70:247–253, 1981.

69. Cyriax J: *Textbook of Orthopaedic Medicine,* ed 3, vol 1, *Diagnosis of Soft Tissue Lesions.* Baltimore, Williams & Wilkins, 1969, pp 450–457.

69a. Levernieux J: *Les tractions vertébrales.* Paris, L'Expansion, 1960.

70. de Seze S: Les accidents de la détérioration structurale du disque. *Semin Hôp Paris* 1:2267, 1955.

71. de Seze S: Les attitudes antalgiques dans la sciatique discoradiculaire commune. *Semin Hôp Paris* 1:2291, 1955.

72. Graham CE: Lumbar discography: a prospective study designed to ascertain the frequency of precise pain reproduction during the discographic examination of the lumbar spines of 200 patients. *J Bone Joint Surg* 70B:162, 1987.

73. Kessler RM: Acute symptomatic disc prolapse: clinical manifestations and therapeutic considerations. *Phys Ther* 59(8):985, 1979.

74. McElhannon JE: Council on Chiropractic Physiological Therapeutics: Traction, a protocol. *ACA J* (October):82, 1985.

75. Gill K, Videman T, Shimizu T, Mooney V: The effect of repeated extensions on the discographic dye patterns in cadaveric lumbar motion studies. *Clin Biomed* 2(4):205–210, 1987.

76. Stoddard A: *A Manual of Osteopathic Technic*. New York, Harper & Row, 1969.

77. Trief P: Chronic back pain, a tripartite model of outcome. *Arch Phys Med Rehabil* 64)1\:53–56, 1983.

78. Malec J, Cayner JJ, Harvey RF, Timming RC: Pain management: long term follow-up of in-patient program. *Arch Phys Med Rehabil* 62:369–372, 1981.

79. Mensor MC: Non-operative treatment, including manipulation, for lumbar intervertebral disc syndrome. *J Bone Joint Surg* 37A:925–936, 1955.

80. Colonna PC, Friedenberg ZB: The disc syndrome, results of the conservative care of patients with positive myelograms. *J Bone Joint Surg* 31A: 614–618, 1949.

81. Wilson JN, Ilfeld FW: Manipulation of the herniated intervertebral disc. *Am J Surg* 83:173, 175, 1952.

82. Singer J, Gilbert JR, Hutton T, Taylor DW: Predicting outcome in acute low-back pain. *Can Fam Physician* 33(March):655–659, 1987.

83. Kostuik JP, Harrington I, Alexander D, Rand W, Evans D: Cauda equina syndrome and lumbar disc herniation. *J Bone Joint Surg* 68A:386–391, 1986.

84. Hellstrom P, Kortelainen P, Kontturi M: Late urodynamic findings after surgery for cauda equina syndrome caused by a prolapsed lumbar intervertebral disc. *J Urol* 135(February):308, 1986.

85. Myrseth E, Ganz JC, Petersen PH: The operative treatment of lumbo-sacral intervertebral disc prolapse. *Acta Neurochir* 84:3–4):144, 1987.

86. Fisher RG, Saunders RL: Lumbar disc protrusion in children. *J Neurosurg* 54:480–483, 1981.

87. Andersen KH, Mosdal C: Epidural application of cortico-steroids in low-back pain and sciatica. *Acta Neurochir* 84(3–4):145–146, 1987.

88. Bernini PM, Simeone FA: Reflex dystrophy. *Spine* 6(2):180–184, 1980.

89. Bogduk N: The anatomy of the lumbar intervertebral disc syndrome. *Med J Aust* 1:878, 1976.

90. Farfan HF: *Mechanical Disorders of the Low Back*. Philadelphia, Lea & Febiger, 1973, p 24.

91. Helfet AJ, Grubel-Lee DM: *Disorders of the Lumbar Spine*. Philadelphia, JB Lippincott, 1978, p 46.

92. Tsukada K: Histologische Studien über die Zwischenwirbelscheibe des Menschen. *Altersvanderugen Mitt Akad Kioto* 25:1–29, 207–209, 1932.

93. Malinsky J: The ontogenetic development of nerve transmissions in the intervertebral disc of man. *Acta Anat* 38:96, 1959.

94. Hirsch C, Inglemark BG, Miller M: The anatomical basis for low back pain. Studies on the presence of sensory nerve endings in ligamentous, capsular and intervertebral disc structures in the human lumbar spine. *Acta Orthop Scand* 1:33, 1963–1964.

95. Yoshizawa H, O'Brien J, Smith WT, Trumper M: The neuropathology of intervertebral discs removed for low-back pain. *J Pathol* 132:95–104, 1980.

96. Sunderland S: Anatomical paravertebral influences on the intervertebral foramen. In: *The Research Status of Spinal Manipulative Therapy*. Bethesda, MD, National Institute of Neurological and Communicative Disorders and Stroke, NINCDS Monograph No. 15, DHEW No. 76-998. 1975, p 135.

97. Edgar MA, Ghadially JA: Innervation of the lumbar spine. *Clin Orthop* 115:35–41, 1976.

98. Lazorthes G, Poulhes J, Espagno J: Etude sur les nerfs sinu-vertebraux lumbaires le nerf de roofe existe-t-il? *CR Assoc Anat* 34:317, 1948.

99. Shinohara H: A study on lumbar disc lesions. *J Jpn Orthop Assoc* 44:553, 1970.

100. Macnab I: Common vertebral joint problems. In GP Grieve (ed): *Mobilization of the Spine*, ed 3. London, Churchill Livingstone, 1979, p 63.

101. Farfan HF: A reorientation in the surgical approach to the degenerative lumbar intervertebral disc. *Orthop Clin North Am* 8(1):9–12, 1977.

102. Schultz AB:Mechanical factors in the etiology of idiopathic low back disorders. In: *American Academy of Orthopaedic Surgeons Symposium on Idiopathic Low Back Pain*. St. Louis, CV Mosby, 1982, pp 206–207.

103. Spurling R, Grantham E: Neurologic picture of herniations of the nucleus pulposus in the lower part of the lumbar region. *Arch Surg* 40:375–388, 1940.

104. Falconer M, McGeorge M, Begg A: Observations on the cause and mechanism of symptom-production in sciatica and low-back pain. *J Neurol Neurosurg Psychiatry* 11:13–26, 1948.

105. Hirsch C: An attempt to diagnose the level of a disc lesion clinically by disc puncture. *Acta Orthop Scand* 18:132–140, 1948.

106. Wiberg G: Back pain in relation to the nerve supply of the intervertebral disc. *Acta Orthop Scand* 19:211–221, 1941.

107. Smyth M, Wright V: Sciatica and the intervertebral disc. *J Bone Joint Surg* 40A:1401–1417, 1958.

108. Lindblom K: Technique and results of diagnostic disc puncture and injection (discography) in the lumbar region. *Acta Orthop Scand* 20:315–326, 1950.

109. Cloward R, Buzaid L: Discography technique, indications and evaluation of the normal and abnormal intervertebral disc. *AJR* 68:552–564, 1952.

110. Collis J, Gardner W: Lumbar discography: an analysis of one thousand cases. *J Neurosurg* 19: 452–461, 1962.

111. Holt E: Fallacy of cervical discography. *JAMA* 188:799–801, 1964.

112. Hudgins W: Diagnostic accuracy of lumbar discography. *Spine* 2:307–309, 1977.

113. Kellgren J: Observations on referral pain arising from muscle. *Clin Sci* 3:175–190, 1938.

114. Sinclair D, Feindel W, Weddell G, Falconer M: The intervertebral ligaments as a source of segmental pain. *J Bone Joint Surg* 30B:515–521, 1948.

115. LaMotte RH: Nociceptors in skin, joint, muscle and bone. In: *American Academy of Orthopaedic Surgeons Symposium on Idiopathic Low Back Pain.* St. Louis, CV Mosby, 1982, pp 417 and 427.

116. Torkildsen A: Lesions of the cervical spine roots as a source of pain simulating sciatica. *Acta Psychiatr Neurol Scand* 31:333–444, 1956.

117. Murphy F: Sources of pain in disc disease. *Clin Neurosurg* 15:343–351, 1968.

118. Herlin L: *Sciatic and Pelvic Pain due to Lumbosacral Nerve Root Compression.* Springfield, IL, Charles C Thomas, 1966, pp 79, 80, and 83.

119. Cole TC, Ghosh P, Taylor TKF: Arteparon modifies proteoglycan turnover in the intervertebral disc. *Bone Joint Surg* 70B:166, 1988.

120. Lowther DA: The effect of compression and tension on the behavior of connective tissues. In Glasgow EF, Twomey LT, Scull ER, Kleynhans AM Idezak RM (eds): *Aspects of Manipulative Therapy.* Edinburgh, Churchill-Livingstone, 1985, pp 16–20.

121. Wilhelmi G, Maier R: Experimental studies on the effects of drugs on cartilage. Basel, Switzerland, Ciba-Geigy Documents, 1982.

122. Naylor A, Happey F, Turner RL, Shentall RD, West DC, Richardson C: Enzymic and immunological activity in the intervertebral disc. *Orthop Clin North Am* 6:1, 1975.

123. Happey F, Wiseman A, Naylor A: Biochemical aspects of intervertebral discs in aging and disease. In Jayson M (ed): *Lumbar Spine and Back Pain.* New York, Grune & Stratton, 1976, p 318.

124. Robles J: Study of disc nutrition. *Rev Chir Orthop* 60:5, 1974.

125. Urban JPG, Holm S, Maraudas A: Diffusion of small solutes into the intervertebral disc: an in vivo study. *Biorheology* 15:203–223, 1978.

126. Ogota D, Whiteside L: Nutritional pathways of the intervertebral disc. *Spine* 6(3):211–216, 1981.

127. Brody JE: The origins of backache: studies begin to explain the crippling pain of millions. *New York Times,* January 12, 1982.

128. Kramer J: *Intervertebral Disc Diseases.* Chicago, Year Book, 1981, p 16.

129. Holm S, Nachemson A: Variations in the nutrition of the canine intervertebral disc induced by motion. *Spine* 8(8):866–874, 1983.

130. Eismont FJ, Wiesel SW, Brighton CT, Rothman RH: Antibiotic penetraction into rabbit nucleus pulposus. *Spine* 12(3):254–256, 1987.

131. Riggs BL, Melton LJ III: Involutional osteoporosis. *N Engl J Med* 314:1676–1686, 1986.

132. Riggs BL, Melton LJ III: Evidence of two distinct syndromes of involutional osteoporosis. *Am J Med* 75:899–901, 1983.

133. Heaney RP: Osteoporosis: the need and opportunity for calcium fortification. *Cereal Foods World* 5(May 31):349–353, 1986.

134. Walker ARP, Walker BF: Osteoporosis research— a new direction. *Lancet* (December), 1987.

135. Riggs L: Pathogenesis of osteoporosis. *Am J Obstet Gynecol* 155:1342–1346, 1987.

136. Heaney RP, Recker RR, Saville PD: Calcium balance and calcium requirements in middle-aged women. *Am J Clin Nutr* 22:85, 1977.

137. Heaney RP, Recker RR: Distribution of calcium absorption in middle-aged women. *Am J Clin Nutr* 43:299, 1986.

138. Heaney RP, Recker RR, Saville PD: Menopausal changes in calcium balance performance. *J Lab Clin Med* 92:953, 1978.

139. Finkelstein JS, Klibanski A, Neer RM, Greenspan SL, Rosenthal DI, Crowley WF: Osteoporosis in men with idiopathic hypogonadotropic hypogonadism. *Ann Intern Med* 106:354–361, 1987.

140. Mueleman J: Beliefs about osteoporosis. *Arch Intern Med* 147(April):762–765, 1987.

141. Lindsay R: Estrogen therapy in the protrusion and rearrangement of osteoporosis. *Am J Obstet Gynecol* 156:1347–1351, 1987.

142. Fatourechi V, Heath H: Salmon calcitonin in the treatment of postmenopausal osteoporosis. *Ann Intern Med* 107:923–925, 1987.

143. Block JE, Smith R, Black D, Genant HR: Does exercise prevent osteoporosis: *JAMA* 257: 3115–3117, 1988.

144. Genant HK, Block JE, Steiger P, Glueer CC, Smith R: Quantitative computed tomography in assessment of osteoporosis. *Semin Nucl Med* 17(4): 316–333, 1987.

145. Wahner HW: Single and dual photon absorptiometry in osteoporosis and osteomalacia. *Semin Nucl Med* 17(4):305–315, 1987.

146. Tohme JF, Lindsay R, Coleman TH: Letter to the editor. *N Engl J Med* (July 30):316, 1987.

13

Spondylolisthesis

James M. Cox, D.C., D.A.C.B.R.

There is a time in every man's education when he arrives at the conviction

that envy is ignorance; that imitation is suicide; that he must take himself for

better, for worse, as his portion; that though the wide universe is full of good,

no kernel of nourishing corn can come to him but through his toil bestowed on

that plot of ground which is given him to till. The power which resides in him

is new in nature, and none but he knows what that is which he can do, nor does

he know until he has tried.

—Emerson on "Self-Reliance"

Every time I see spondylolisthesis on the radiograph of a new patient, the question arises: how much of this person's pain is due to the defect and much is due to some other factor? As we will discuss in this chapter, age is a major determinant of the possible etiological role the spondylolisthesis may be playing. The degenerative versus the true etiologies are important. I have chosen to start this chapter with a relatively new diagnostic procedure to determine the role that spondylolisthesis may play in pain production, namely, the procedure developed by Friberg.

TRANSLATIONAL INSTABILITY OF A SPONDYLOLISTHETIC SEGMENT

In this author's (J.M.C.) clinical career, he has often heard the question of possible reduction of spondylolisthesis slippage discussed. It had always been considered that manipulative treatment of spondylolisthesis never altered the position of the anterior subluxation, whether the cause be a pars interarticularis stress fracture or a

degenerative spondylolisthesis. Today, the question of the motion instability present with the spondylolisthetic slip and the potential pain-producing qualities of this subluxation are important. We discussed the pain sensitivity of the intervertebral disc in Chapter 2 of this book, as well as the pain sensitivity of the facet capsule of the zygapophyseal articulations. The irritation of these structures must represent a pain source for the spondylolisthesis patient.

Concerning the question of movement of spondylolisthesis, Friberg (1) states, in a study of 117 patients with known spondylolisthesis or retrolisthesis displacement, that translatory segmental instability is provoked by successive axial traction and compression of the lumbar spine. The traction applied was vertical suspension from a horizontal bar, with the patient's lumbar spine parallel to the film plane (Fig. 13.1). This allowed a gravitational traction to be applied to the lumbar spine which represented approximately 40% of the total body weight (the percentage corresponding to the lower extremities and pelvis). Static lateral radiographs were made and com-

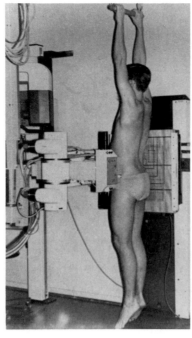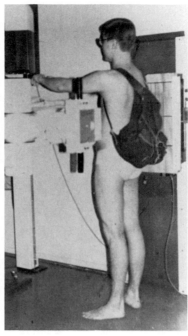

Figure 13.1. Positioning of the patient for traction-compression radiography. For traction, the patient hangs by hands from a horizontal bar. To prevent swaying, the toes slightly touch the ground. For compression, the patient stands with a 20-kg rucksack on the shoulders. During traction and compression, the hip is in contact with the cassette holder to keep the distance between the lumbar spine and film constant. The distance between the x-ray tube and the film was 1.5 m. (Reproduced with permission from Friberg O: Lumbar instability: a dynamic approach by traction-compression radiography. *Spine* 12(2):121, 1987.)

pared with vertical traction radiographs. The amount of forward or backward displacement of the segment in relation to the subjacent vertebra was measured in millimeters (Figs. 13.2 and 13.3). Also, the heights of the intervertebral disc spaces at the anterior and posterior points of the borders of the vertebral bodies were millimetrically measured.

Low Back Symptoms Increase with Motion Instability

Lateral spot radiography showed an anteroposterior translational movement of 5 mm or more in 24 of 45 patients with lytic spondylolisthesis of L5, in all of seven patients with degenerative spondylolisthesis of L4, and in 37 of 65 patients with a retrolisthesis displacement of L3, L4, or L5. In cases of spondylolisthesis or retrolisthetic instability, the upper vertebra moved posteriorly during traction and anteriorly during compression.

Specifically, the amount of translatory movement at the spondylolisthetic level differed signif-

icantly among groups complaining of different degrees of pain. The asymptomatic group of patients showed a mean amount of movement of 0.7 mm, while the group with moderate pain symptoms showed 5.2 mm of movement, and the group with severe pain symptoms showed 7.5 mm of movement (Fig. 13.4). Therefore, the frequency and severity of low back pain symptoms correlated significantly with the amount of translational movement.

The same is true in retrolisthesis (Fig. 13.5). As in the case of lytic spondylolisthesis, a correlation was found between the amount of translatory movement and the degree of low back pain symptoms in retrolisthesis. The difference between the asymptomatic group and the symptomatic groups with respect to the amount of instability was statistically significant.

Disc Changes under Traction

Friberg (1) also measured the height of the lumbar discs during distraction and compression. The height of the disc increased during traction.

In spondylolisthesis, traction not only decreased the anterior slippage but also increased the height of the disc significantly more than at normal or retrolisthetic segments. At an unstable retrolisthesis segment, the axial stretch of the disc was limited, probably by the posterior shear that occurs simultaneously.

Conclusions from Friberg's Work

Pertinent conclusions from Friberg's work are as follows:

1. Traction compression radiography of the lumbar spine offers a simple, practical method for assessment of translatory segmental instability.

2. *The degree of patient pain does not depend upon the slippage in spondylolisthesis or retrolisthesis, but rather, correlates significantly with the amount of translatory movement.* That means that a patient with one of these lesions who demonstrates less than 3 mm of translation is much less symptomatic than one who shows over 3 mm of translational motion.

3. One of the most important points of Friberg's work was that some patients with chronic low back pain of unknown etiology will show marked instability on axial traction of the spine and produce abnormal posterior movement at segments that appear quite normal on a static radiograph. An example of that is shown in Figures 13.2 and 13.3, which so well show the appearance of spondylolisthesis and retrolisthesis on traction and compression which appear less unstable in neutral radiographs.

Clinical Application of Friberg's Work

We installed a vertical traction device in our clinic to reproduce Friberg's work (Fig. 13.1). The patient hangs suspended from the horizontal bar with the toes slightly touching the floor in order to prevent sway during film exposure. We will now present studies we have performed under vertical distraction. The quality of the radiographs in these upright and suspended spondylolisthesis cases is deficient due to motion and

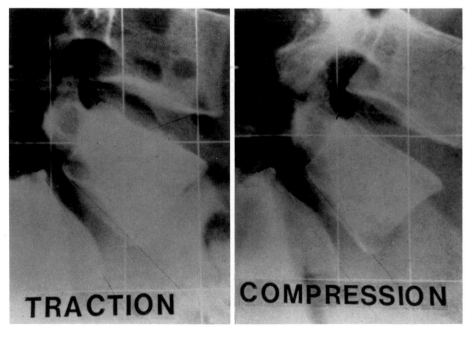

Figure 13.2. A patient with concurrent spondylolisthetic instability of L5 and retro-olisthetic instability of L4. During axial compression, the body of L5 presents an anterior slip of 8 mm, L4 being nearly in a normal vertebral alignment. During traction, the spondylolisthetic malalignment disappeared, but L4 presented a retro-olisthetic slip of 5 mm. (Reproduced with permission from Friberg O: Lumbar instability: a dynamic approach by traction-compression radiography. *Spine* 12(2):127, 1987.)

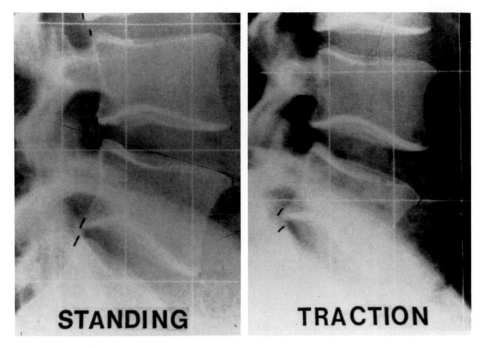

Figure 13.3. A lateral radiograph that looks normal during free standing (*left*), and a radiograph of the same patient during axial traction (*right*). On traction, a retro-olisthetic instability at both L4-L5 and L5-S1 segments was seen. (Reproduced with permission from Friberg O: Lumbar instability: a dynamic approach by traction-compression radiography. *Spine* 12(2):128, 1987.)

technical difficulties in taking upright films. Certainly, they are not the quality that would be obtained if the x-ray were taken in a table-top recumbent study. All cases were treated as shown later in this chapter.

Figure 13.6 shows a neutrolateral standing radiograph revealing a 10-mm spondylolisthesis slippage of L5 on the sacrum in a 31-year-old overweight white female. Figure 13.7 shows a vertical suspension lateral radiograph taken of this same patient which reveals total reduction of the spondylolisthetic slippage. This represents a 10-mm translational movement of the spondylolisthetic slip under vertical distraction. This patient's symptoms consisted of severe low back and radiating thigh pain, which interfered with her ability to sit, bend, lift, or twist at the waist. This case required considerably more days and manipulative treatments to attain relief than do less unstable cases.

A 61-year-old white male who complained of moderate low back pain was seen. His occupation was construction work involving much repetitive bending, lifting, and twisting at the waist. Figure 13.8 shows an 8-mm spondylolisthetic slippage of

L5 on the sacrum; this is a true spondylolisthesis. Vertical suspension distraction reveals that the spondylolisthesis slippage reduces to 4 mm, representing a 50% reduction of the total slippage under distraction (Fig. 13.9). This man responded to flexion distraction manipulation by becoming asymptomatic within 2 weeks of treatment.

A 16-year-old white female was seen with an 8-mm true spondylolisthesis slippage of L5 on the sacrum (Fig. 13.10). Under vertical distraction (Fig. 13.11), this 8-mm slippage reduces to 6 mm, representing a 25% reduction of the total subluxation. The response of this patient to flexion distraction was total relief within 1 month of treatment.

A 24-year-old white female developed back pain for the first time in her life following lifting a patient. Figure 13.12 reveals a 10-mm true spondylolisthetic slippage of L5 on the sacrum. Figure 13.13, under vertical distraction, shows us that the slippage is reduced to 4 mm, representing a 60% reduction of the anterolisthesis subluxation of L5 on the sacrum. This patient's response to treatment was very slow. She was not

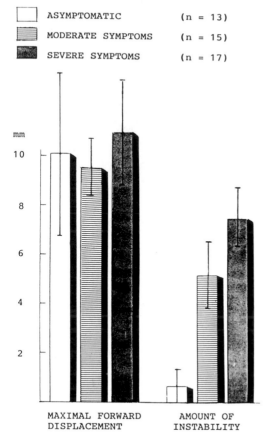

Figure 13.4. Means and standard deviations of the maximal anterior slip and of the amount of translatory instability provoked by axial traction and compression in 45 patients with lytic spondylolisthesis of L5. The patients were classified in three categories according to the severity and frequency of low back pain symptoms. (Reproduced with permission from Friberg O: Lumbar instability: a dynamic approach by traction-compression radiography. *Spine* 12(2):123, 1987.)

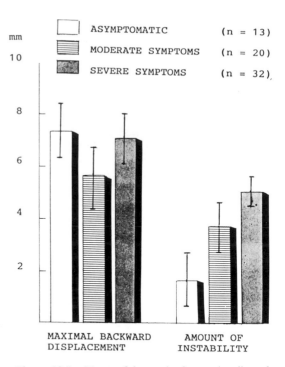

Figure 13.5. Means of the maximal posterior slip and of the translatory instability provoked by axial traction and compression of the lumbar spine in 65 patients with retro-olisthetic malalignment. The patients were classified in three categories according to the severity and frequency of low back pain symptoms as in Figure 13.4. (Reproduced with permission from Friberg O: Lumbar instability: a dynamic approach by traction-compression radiography. *Spine* 12(2):125, 1987.)

a patient in our clinic, but we did evaluate her progress under care by another chiropractor, and we do know that she had a prolonged treatment phase consisting of a surgical consideration for stabilization of the spondylolisthetic slip. Surgery was not needed, as relief was afforded by flexion distraction.

A 49-year-old white male, who had been seen as a patient at our clinic for the past 8 years, was seen complaining of marked low back pain. We knew from the past that he had a true spondylolisthesis of L5 on the sacrum, but it had never shown the degree of disc degeneration that is seen in Figure 13.14. You will note in Figure

13.14 that, in addition to the advanced degenerative disc disease at the L4-L5 and L5-S1 levels, this patient has a 12-mm anterior true spondylolisthetic slippage of L5 on the sacrum. Figure 13.15 is an anteroposterior view of this patient which reveals the typical appearance of L5 in spondylolisthetic slippage. The transverse processes sit low over the sacral ala, and a D line of Brailsford is seen over the sacrum, representing the anterior slippage and the vertebral body superimposed over the sacral promontory. Figure 13.16 represents vertical suspension of the patient, and we now note a 10-mm slippage reduction of L5 on the sacrum. This is a very small amount of motion as compared to the other cases shown, but here we have marked degeneration and stabilization of L5 on the sacrum. There is some attempt at buttressing of the anterior L5-S1 articulation. With this in mind, we can expect to see much less translation of a spondylolisthetic

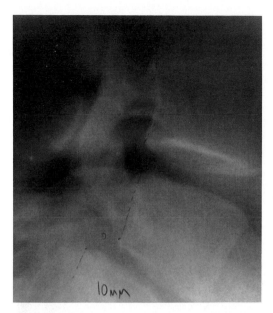

Figure 13.6. In the upright neutral posture, this 31-year-old female shows L5 to be 10 mm anterior on the sacrum.

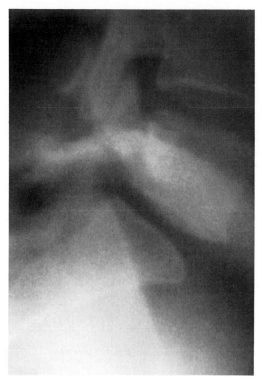

Figure 13.7. On vertical traction, the 10-mm slippage shown in Figure 13.6 is totally reduced to no slippage.

segment accompanied by advanced degenerative disc disease. It also is possible that the shifting of motion to the segment above, in this case L4-L5, results in pain at that level. In advanced true or degenerative spondylolisthesis, therefore, we may well be treating the segments cephalad of the spondylolisthetic slip, which are placed under an unstable stress condition due to the marked motion they are asked to perform.

A 25-year-old male was involved in a motorcycle accident and developed low back pain. Figure 13.17 shows a 5-mm anterior true spondylolisthetic slip of L5 on the sacrum, which reduces to 0 mm on vertical distraction, as shown in Figure 13.18. This patient was difficult to stabilize and required 6 weeks of manipulative care and the use of a stabilizing orthosis, as shown later in this chapter. We use this type of memory foam belt to stabilize our unstable spondylolisthesis patients, even having them wear the belt to bed at night until the pain is at least 50% reduced. We find that this stability hastens healing.

From the above studies, we see clinically that the greater the translation of the spondylolisthetic slippage on the sacrum, the more difficulty the case will have in responding to care. This is certainly in agreement with Friberg's work and represents a good clinical tool for the practicing

physician in determining the severity of a spondylolisthetic case and the prognosis to be expected under treatment.

HISTORICAL DATA

Herbinaux (2) in 1782 was the first to recognize spondylolisthesis as a cause of obstruction in his obstetric cases, but Killian (3) was the first to describe and name it, calling it a slow subluxation of the posterior facets. Robert (4) believed that some defect in the neural arch must be present, and Neugebauer (5) recognized that the slip could occur with or without a neural defect.

Figure 13.19 is an illustration of the normal L5-S1 locking mechanism of the intact intervertebral disc stabilizing the L5 vertebral body to the sacrum, of the neural arch solid bone stabilizing the anterior body to the arch, and of the articular facets locking the entire functional splint units of L5 and the sacrum. Figure 13.20 is an illustration of the progressive slippage that occurs in a person from birth through development.

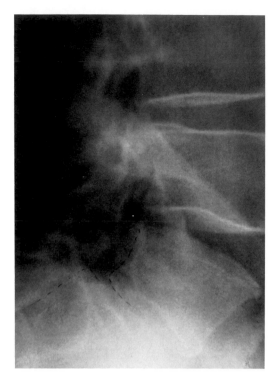

Figure 13.8. This 61-year-old male shows an 8-mm anterior slippage of L5 on the sacrum in the upright neutral lateral projection.

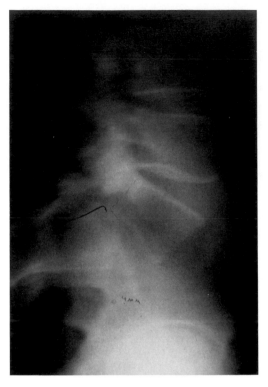

Figure 13.9. On vertical traction, the 8-mm slippage shown in Figure 13.8 is reduced 50% to 4 mm of slippage.

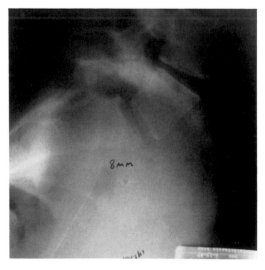

Figure 13.10. A 16-year-old female demonstrates an 8-mm true spondylolisthesis slippage of L5 on the sacrum.

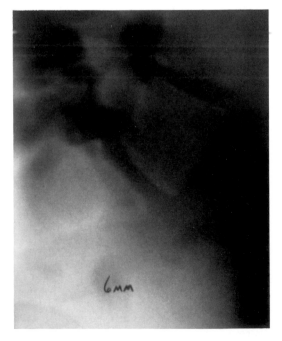

Figure 13.11. Under vertical traction, the 8-mm slippage reduces to 6 mm, a 25% reduction.

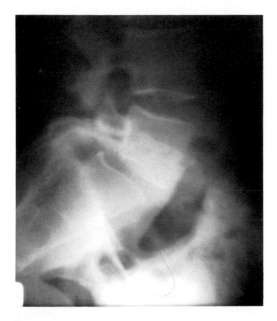

Figure 13.12. Here a 24-year-old female with low back pain reveals a 10-mm true anterolisthesis subluxation of L5 on the sacrum due to pars interarticularis fracture.

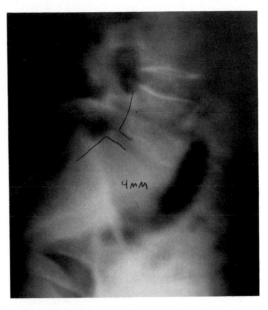

Figure 13.13. On vertical traction, the 10-mm slippage reduces to 4 mm, showing us a 60% motion of L5 on the sacrum. Remember that any motion in excess of 3 mm signifies instability.

CLASSIFICATION

In 1963, Newman (7) classified spondylolisthesis into five types. His classification, which follows, is still valid and useful today.

   I. Dysplastic (congenital). Congenital abnormalities of the upper sacrum or the arch of L5 permit the "olisthesis" to occur.

  II. Isthmic, in which the lesion is in the pars interarticularis. Three kinds can be delineated:
     a. Lytic, which is a fatigue fracture of the pars;
     b. Elongated but intact pars
     c. Acute fracture of the pars (not to be confused with "traumatic," see IV).

 III. Degenerative, due to a long-standing intersegmental instability.

 IV. Posttraumatic, due to fractures in areas of the bony hook other than the pars.

  V. Pathologic, i.e., generalized or localized bone disease.

Dysplastic Spondylolisthesis

Congenital or dysplastic spondylolisthesis occurs at L5-S1, with defects of fusion of the neural arch

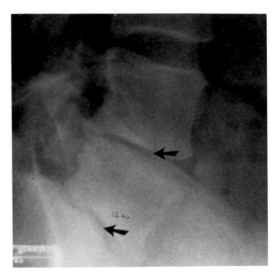

Figure 13.14. A 49-year-old male with a long history of intermittent low back pain shows advanced disc degenerative changes at the L4-L5 and L5-S1 levels (*arrows*), with a 12-mm anterior slippage of L5 on the sacrum representing true spondylolisthesis.

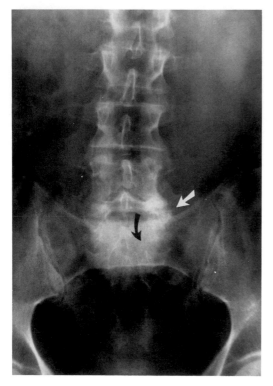

Figure 13.15. The anteroposterior view of the case shown in Figure 13.14 shows the overlapping of the L5 transverse processes over the sacral ala (*straight arrows*), with the body of L5 superimposed over the sacrum (*curved arrow*), giving the impression of loss of height of the L5 vertebral segment between L4 and the sacrum.

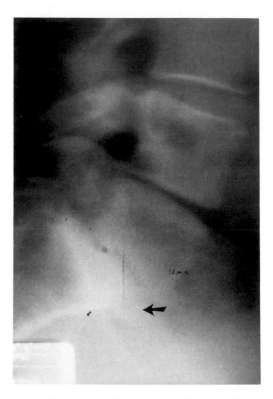

Figure 13.16. Vertical traction now shows the 12-mm slippage to reduce to 10 mm. There is marked L5-S1 disc degeneration, with attempts to buttress at the anterior plates of L5 and the sacrum to produce stability (*arrow*). In advanced spondylolisthetic changes, the arthrodesis formed by anterior buttress formation of hypertrophic changes acts to stabilize an unstable segment. The quality of the radiograph is poor because it is an upright suspended x-ray with motion.

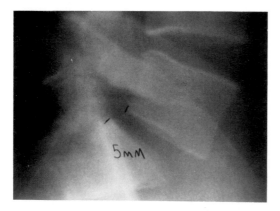

Figure 13.17. A 25-year-old male is shown with a 5-mm anterior true spondylolisthetic slip of L5 on the sacrum. The pain followed a motorcycle accident.

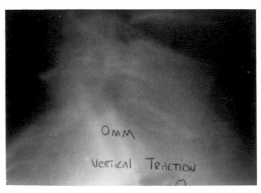

Figure 13.18. On vertical traction, the 5-mm anterior subluxation of L5 reduces to 0 mm.

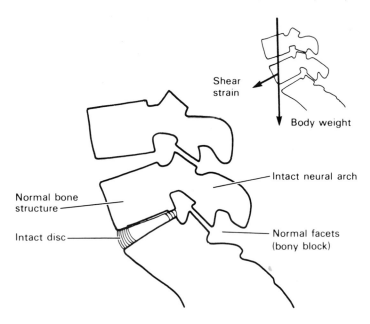

Figure 13.19. Illustration of normal locking mechanisms resisting forward displacement of the fifth lumbar vertebral body. (Reproduced with permission from Macnab I: *Backache*, p 45, ©1977, the Williams & Wilkins Co., Baltimore.)

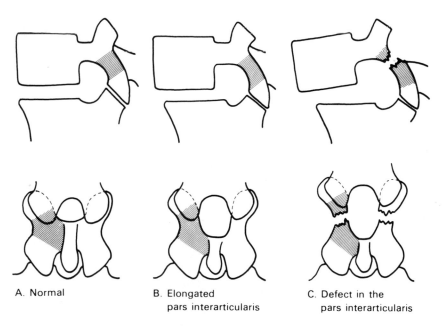

Figure 13.20. Illustration of isthmic spondylolisthesis. The pars interarticularis, which was normal at birth (**A**), becomes attenuated and elongated, allowing the vertebral body to slip forward in relation to the vertebral body below (**B**). Eventually, the elongated pars interarticularis may break (**C**). This defect in the pars interarticularis is, however, secondary to the slip and is not the cause of the forward displacement of the vertebral body. (Reproduced with permission from Macnab I: *Backache*, p 46, ©1977, the Williams & Wilkins Co., Baltimore.)

occurring in the upper sacral vertebrae as well as at L5. There is hypoplastic facet development of the sacrum which fails to provide sufficient resistance to the forward shear force of L5 on S1 (8). The L5 arch may reveal spina bifida, which occurs in girls twice as frequently as it occurs in boys. During the growth spurt between ages 12 and 16, the condition commonly manifests itself, probably due to increased weight bearing and stress. The pars interarticularis either elongates or separates (6). The dysplastic type of spondylolisthesis can be difficult to differentiate from the isthmic type on radiography. There is a strong genetic association in dysplastic spondylolisthesis (9), and a study by Wynne-Davies and Scott (10) showed that one in three (33%) of relatives of patients with dysplastic spondylolisthesis will be affected.

Isthmic Spondylolisthesis

Isthmic spondylolisthesis is the most common type of spondylolisthesis and is due to a defect in the ossifiction of the pars interarticularis. Three subdivisions of isthmic spondylolisthesis have been delineated: the lytic (subtype A), an elongated pars without separation (subtype B), and an acute pars fracture (subtype C).

Subtype A can be seen in Figure 13.21.

Spondylolysis

Spondylolysis is a term applied to the mechanical failure of an apparently normal isthmus. This occurs most frequently at the L5 level, less frequently at the L4 level, and rarely at levels above L4. It is no longer questioned that spondylolysis is a fracture that may or may not heal. These fractures are postulated to occur due to the assumption of the upright posture by the infant, allowing a fatigue type of fracture to occur when stress beyond the strength of bone occurs. Rosenberg (11) obtained radiographs of the lumbosacral spines of 143 patients who had never walked. The frequency of spondylolysis and spondylolisthesis as well as of other spinal abnormalities was determined. The average age of the patients was 27 years, with an age range from 11 to 93 years. The underlying diagnosis responsible for the nonambulatory status varied, but cerebral palsy predominated. No case of spondylolysis or spondylolisthesis was detected, and this is significant when it is compared with the 5.8% incidence in the general population. The incidences of

spina bifida (8.4%) and of transitional vertebra (10.9%) were similar to those found in the general population. Scoliosis was found in 49%, and vertebral body height was increased in 33%. Degenerative changes occurred in only 2.8%. These results support the theory that spondylolysis and isthmic spondylolisthesis represent fatigue fractures resulting from activities associated with ambulation.

According to Scoville and Corkill (12), King studied 500 normal school children whom he x-rayed at the ages of 6, 12, and 18. He also x-rayed 25 children with back problems. He found almost no progression or development of spondylolisthesis after the age of 6 years in any of these children. True spondylolisthesis rarely if ever progressed after the patient reached maturity. Pfeil (13) showed that the infant spine is susceptible to fatigue fracture in the isthmus.

The isthmus can be seen in Figure 13.22. There are two layers of cortical bone, the anterolateral and the posteromedial, which are joined by parallel thick trabeculae directed inferolater-

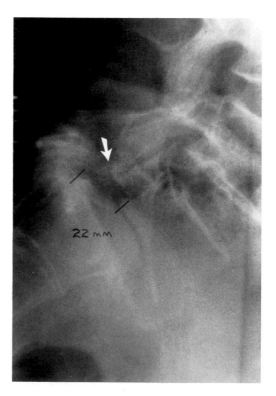

Figure 13.21. A lytic fatigue fracture defect of the pars interarticularis of L5 (*arrow*) is shown as the cause of this 22-mm slippage of L5 on the sacrum.

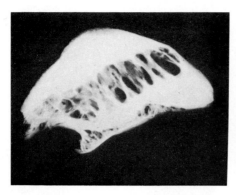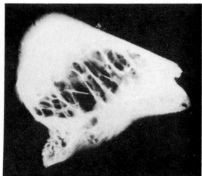

Figure 13.22. Photograph of two slices through the isthmus from the fifth lumbar vertebra of a 66-year-old man, which were cut parallel to the plane of the narrowest perimeter of the isthmus (i.e., the plane of a spondylolytic defect). This is typical of the normal appearance of the isthmus. The anterolateral layer of cortical bone can be seen in the *upper left* region of the slices. (Reproduced with permission from Krenz J, Troup JDG: The structure of the pars interarticularis of the lower lumbar vertebrae and its relation to the etiology of spondylolysis. *J Bone Joint Surg* 55B: 735, 1973.)

ally and anteriorly from the base of the superior articular process (14). The anterolateral layer is the thicker of the two and appears to be capable of resisting forces that tend to bend the inferior articular processes posteriorly or posteromedially, are induced whenever the effect of gravity is transmitted to a vertebra inclined below the horizontal anteriorly, and are induced when the vertebra is exposed to axial torque. Sullivan and Farfan (15) have studied the effect of axial torque, which tends to disrupt the inferior articular processes; they believe that such damage predisposes to spondylolysis.

INCIDENCE OF SPONDYLOLYSIS AND SPONDYLOLISTHESIS

In a study (16) reported by Wiltse, it was stated that if 100 children aged 5 were to be studied roentgenographically, there probably would not be one with a defect of the pars. If the same children were examined toward the end of the first grade (age 7), however, the incidence would be around 4.4%, which is just slightly below the national average. Baker [as reported in Finneson (17)] found that, as these children reached 18, only 1.4% more showed spondylolisthesis, with most of the increase occurring between ages 11 and 16, the time of greatest strenuous athletics which produce fatigue fractures.

One reason that forward slippage occurs most often in children 5 to 7 years old may be due to the increased activity or to the increased sitting in the lordotic posture done by children. It is known

that fracture never occurs in animals other than humans, and only humans have lordosis (19, 18–20).

The average age of onset of symptoms of spondylolisthesis is 14 in girls and 16 in boys (21). A sudden onset is termed the "listhetic crisis." The pelvis is rotated anteriorly, the sacrum is flat, and the hamstring is found to be in spasm, frequently making the patient walk with bent knees. The patient with an isthmic spondylolisthesis producing severs symptoms before age 21, with or without past symptoms, probably will not recover completely without surgery.

The severity of symptoms and the treatment of spondylolisthesis in the child vary greatly from that in the adult. Surgery may be more imperative in the child than in the adult because further slippage occurs more often in the child than in the adult. Furthermore, the outcome of fusion is better in the child than in the adult, with the adult being more willing to curtail activities, so as to prevent further aggravation of the condition, than the child would be. If is also known that, following surgery, there is a greater relief from pain for the child than there is for the adult. For the adult, the prime reason for surgical treatment is to relieve pain, not to prevent progression of slippage. Slippage rarely increases in the adult (17).

Semon (22) found that in a large group of college football players, spondylolysis was not a predisposing factor to low back pain. Furthermore, the mere indication of spondylolysis or spondylolisthesis on x-ray did not mean that spondylolysis or spondylolisthesis was the cause of the person's low back pain. Newman (2) observed that, despite the obvious displacement at the L5-S1 intervertebral joint, the symptomatology seems to derive from the L4-L5 joint. This would be logical, since the forward slippage of L5 does allow the superior facet of L5 to enter the intervertebral foramen in a telescoping effect at the L4-L5 level. Furthermore, at the time of the slippage, either or both discs, i.e., either the L4-L5 or L5-S1 discs, must break down, allowing annular stretching and tearing. Without this phenomenon, there could be no forward slippage of the vertebra. This would be true even if there were growth defects within the arch, namely, pars interarticularis fracture. The disc, being a very pain-sensitive structure, certainly creates symptomatology as the slippage occurs. Perhaps it is understandable why in the adult, after this slippage occurs and there is a healing of the annular fibers, the pain lessens or disappears.

Anatomy of the Partes Interarticularis Defect

A pars defect is visible on the x-ray and in a cadaver specimen (Fig. 12.23) and the actual specimen dissected out at necropsy can be seen in Figure 12.24.

In Figure 13.25, a discogram of the L4-L5 level, there certainly is disruption of the annular

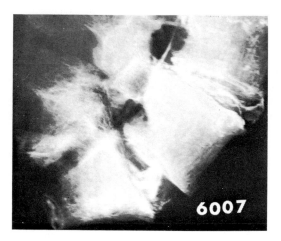

Figure 13.23. X-ray showing spondylolysis in a cadaver specimen. A defect of the inferior articular process is clearly visible. The lumbosacral disc shows degeneration, but this does not appear to be as advanced as that at the L4-L5 level. (Reproduced with permission from Farfan HF: *Mechanical Disorders of the Low Back.* Philadelphia, Lea & Febiger, 1973, chap 7, p 164.)

fibers, allowing escape of the dye from the nucleus into the perimeter of the disc. This certainly demonstrates the tearing that would occur in the annulus at the time of slippage.

In a study of facet joints with the use of arthrography, an abnormal communication be-

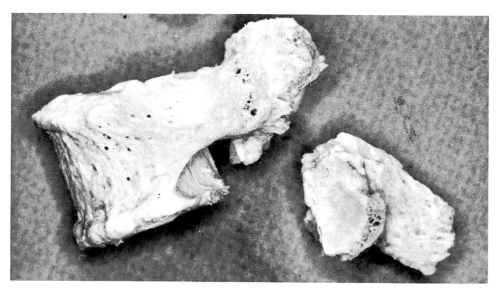

Figure 13.24. Photograph of L5 isolated from the same specimen as in Figure 13.23. (Reproduced with permission from Farfan HF: *Mechanical Disorders of the Low Back.* Philadelphia, Lea & Febiger, 1973, chap 7, p 165.)

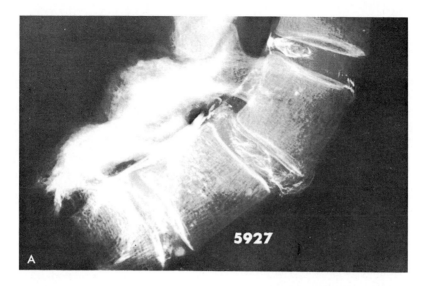

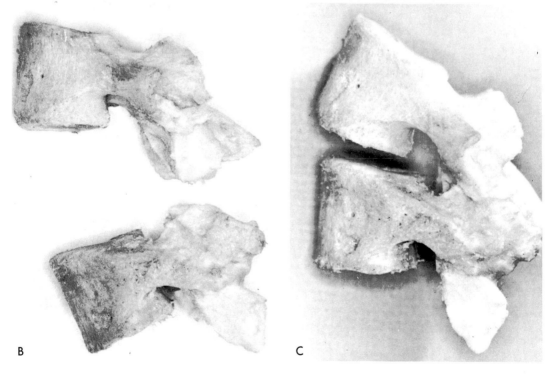

Figure 13.25. **A**, Discogram showing spondylolisthesis of L4 on L5 in a cadaver specimen. There is no defect in the pars interarticularis; however, there appears to be a prolonged inferior articular process. The disc is degenerated. **B**, Skeletal arrangement. The specimen does not show a true elongation. The apparent elongation is due to superimposition of subluxated superior and inferior articular facets and to the widening of the angle between the lamina and pedicle (**C**). (Reproduced with permission from Farfan HF: *Mechanical Disorders of the Low Back*. Philadelphia, Lea & Febiger, 1973, p 167.)

tween the two facet joints bordering the separated pars interarticularis was observed in nine of 11 patients. This communication occurred in the area of the defect. In one patient with bilateral spondylolysis of the L5 vertebra, both left adjacent apophyseal joints were observed to communicate not only with one another but also with the contralateral facet joints through a transverse channel joining the isthmic areas of L5 (23). Furthermore, it was found that spondylolysis considerably altered the soft tissues of the adjacent facet joints. Irritation of these structures might explain certain complaints such as low back and scleratogenous pain in patients with spondylolysis.

Among the causes of spondylolisthesis, the fifth lumbar vertebra, placed at the apex of the lumbar curve, is probably the recipient of the highest stress on flexion and rotation movement. If L5 is well anchored to the pelvis by enlarged transverse processes, the same findings may well be seen at the L4 level. According to Farfan (18), during forced rotation the neural arch is placed under such stress that a permanent sprain of the neural arch can occur. This sprain could take two forms:

1. The interarticular distance between the inferior facet articulations is reduced. This may allow the sprained neural arch to slip through the other.
2. The angle of these processes to the axis of the pedicle would be increased from a normal angle of about 90° to an abnormal angle of about 130°.

This produces an apparent lengthening of the pedicles, which in turn could allow the forward slip of the affected vertebra. Farfan further believes that the defect in the lamina is probably a fracture at the junction between the laminae and the pedicle, as the angle between these structures is opened up. Furthermore, the injury at the disc is an epiphyseal separation of the supper epiphysis of the sacrum.

Athletic Incidence of Spondylolisthesis

Competitive weightlifters seem to develop stress fractures of the pars interarticularis, unaccompanied by spondylolisthesis (24). In 47 subjects (27 Olympic lifters and 20 power lifters; average age, 30), 21 showed spondylolysis on x-ray examination (44% occurrence rate). It was felt that the hyperextension involved with lifting in such maneuvers as "clean and jerk" and "the snatch" in Olympic lifting and "the squat" and "the dead lift" in power lifting was the cause of the pars interarticularis fracture. The suggestion was made that weight training by physically immature athletes should be done, in most instances, in the sitting position while avoiding squats and overhead lifts.

Nineteen of 145 freshman football players who were radiographed were found to have spondylolysis (13.1%). All 145 were followed from 1978 through 1983, and 31 (21.3%) presented with low back pain. Ten of these had prior findings of spondylolysis. Of the remaining 21, three developed x-ray diagnosis of spondylolysis. This study concluded that the majority of affected players entered college with previously acquired spondylolysis, which seemed to indicate that their problem arose in the adolescent years during athletics or other stress situations. Linemen were felt to be more susceptible to development of this defect (25).

Troup (26) states that fatigue failure and fracture is the primary mechanism at the pars interarticularis causing spondylolysis, and that the increased incidence in athletes, gymnasts, wrestlers, and parachutists is not inconsistent with this concept. The intensity and repetitive nature of athletic training create situations involving a jerking motion, which is the most probable mechanism causing the fracture.

Semon (22) found that spondylolysis was not a predisposing factor in low back pain in a study of college football players. Thus we can see that it is questionable whether spondylolysis or spondylolisthesis is a cause of back pain.

Vibrational Effects in Spondylolisthesis

Helicopter pilots, due to vibrational forces, have been found to have a significantly higher incidence of spondylolisthesis than transport pilots or cadets (26). In a study of 21 pilots with spondylolisthesis followed for 12 to 131 months, 16 had follow-up examination. Only one was found to have significant progression of the displacement. Of the 12 pilots with spondylolisthesis who had back pain, all continued to fly. The other nine pilots did not develop pain. It was concluded that pilots with spondylolisthesis could continue to fly with minimal risk of morbidity and loss of flight time (27).

Spondylolysis Is Questionable as Cause of Back Pain

Hall (28) very interestingly points out that the incidence of spondylolysis was higher in asymptomatic persons (9.8%) than in those with low back pain (9.2%). He further concluded that preemployment x-ray examination does not have a high predictive value for future back problems and is not worth the radiation risk.

SPONDYLOLYSIS IN THE UPPER LUMBAR SPINE

Reports of spondylolysis in vertebrae other than those of the lower lumbar spine are rare. A report of 32 patients with upper lumbar spondylolysis found 20 to have bilateral lesions, and seven of those with unilateral lesions had structural changes or anomalies in the opposite posterior arch (29). This study suggested that local structural anomalies contributed to the abnormal loading of these upper lumbar vertebrae, resulting in the stress fractures. These anomalies were multiple-level lytic lesions in the lower lumbar levels, lumbosacral anomalies such as spina bifida in six cases, facet hypoplasia in seven cases, and hemisacralization in three cases. In all, 52 spondylolytic defects were found; seven lytic lesions at L1 in four patients, 13 at L2 in eight patients, and 32 at L3 in 20 patients. Twenty patients had bilateral spondylolytic defects: three at L1, five at L2, and 12 at L3.

Presentation of L3 Unilateral Spondylolytic Spondylolisthesis

A case of upper lumbar spondylolisthesis with unilateral spondylolysis from our clinic is presented here to illustrate this condition. Its clinical treatment and outcome are described.

CASE 1

This 52-year-old, 70-inch-tall, 180-pound white male was hospitalized in traction for 5 days for low back and right leg pain following unloading materials from his car. He stated that he had had low back problems off and on since he was 16 years old. Approximately 15 years previously, he had been told he had a ruptured disc following a sailboat accident and was treated with traction with good relief.

When first seen, he had completed a course of physical therapy consisting of traction, ultrasound, and massage with no relief. A neurosurgeon suggested surgery; he sought a second opinion at the Mayo Clinic, and they recommended a strong exercise program to him.

When we saw him, he was somewhat confused over what his problem really was and what to do about it. A prime symptom was testicle pain and frequent urination, up to hourly, as his pain persisted in the low back and right leg.

Examination revealed limited ranges of motion, with flexion at 30°, extension at 5°, lateral flexion of 5° and rotation of 5° bilaterally. The straight leg raises were bilaterally positive at 20°, creating marked low back pain. The patient had no spinal tilt but a marked loss of lumbar lordosis. The deep reflexes were +2 bilaterally at the ankle and patella. Sensory examination revealed hypesthesia of the right L5 and S1 dermatomes. Circulation of the lower extremities was normal. All attempts to test hyperextension, as in Nachlas', Ely's, or prone lumbar flexion, increased the low back pain.

Figures 13.26 to 13.29 reveal the anteroposterior, lateral, and oblique radiographs of this patient. They reveal L3 to be in right lateral flexion subluxation on L4 as well as in anterior subluxation of L3 on L4 with a unilateral pars interarticularis defect on the right side. The left appears to be intact. You will note the anterolateral lipping and spurring of the L3-L4 vertebral body plates with an attempt to buttress. Also note the alternation of the intervertebral foramen in its sagittal diameter at L3-L4. This would represent unilateral spondylolysis with degenerative disc disease at L3-L4. Therefore, this probably represents a combination of true spondylolisthesis due to the rotosubluxation caused by the unilateral spondylolysis as well as degenerative spondylolisthesis due to the degeneration of the L3-L4 disc.

Treatment was instituted, consisting of flexion distraction manipulation of the L3 anterolisthesis subluxation, as described at the end of this chapter. (A small flexion roll was placed under the L3 segment; the thenar contact of the treating hand was placed on the spinous process of L2 while gentle flexion distraction was applied to the L2-L3 segment. This was preceded by goading of acupressure points B22 through B49 and into the right extremity to B54.) He was placed on a very strong flexion type of exercise program consisting of knee-chest exercises, abdominal strengthening exercise, and hamstring stretching. We had him wear a 10-inch lumbosacral support in the acute phase. He was told to avoid sitting and rotation movements at the waist.

The result of this treatment was that, in 2 days, the testicular pain was almost totally relieved. The patient could stand upright and walk without the cane he needed when first seen. He slept well and felt much less low back pain, and the leg pain was totally relieved.

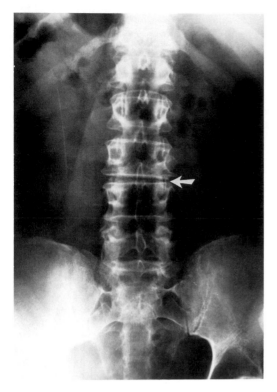

Figure 13.26. Note the L3-L4 disc space narrowing with right lateral flexion subluxation of L3 on L4 (*arrow*). There is also anterolateral lipping and spurring of the body plates at L3-L4.

MULTIPLANAR CT, MRI, AND DISCOGRAPHIC EXAMINATION IN SPONDYLOLISTHESIS

Seven hundred patients with various types of spondylolisthesis were evaluated with reformatted CT (30). Of these, 450 had pars interarticularis defects, 225 had degenerative spondylolisthesis, and 25 had iatrogenic subluxation. Of the 450 isthmic defects, 92% were at L5 and 7% were at L4. Unilateral clefts were demonstrated in 68 patients. The defect seen in the pars interarticularis is shown in Figure 13.30 from CT reformation.

Spondylolysis is seen to occur with two types of congenital clefts (31):

1. Retroisthmic defect (Fig. 13.31**A**), which occurs within the neural arch, behind the pars interarticularis and medial to the spinous process. It is probably of no consequence.
2. Retrosomatic cleft (Fig. 13.31**B**), which occurs anterior to the pedicle, in the fusion plane of

the pedicle with the vertebral body. This defect is associated with degeneration of the disc and spondylolisthesis.

One hundred and one disc levels in 36 patients with low back pain were studied with magnetic resonance imaging (MRI) sagittal images and conventional roentgenographic discography to detect early disc degeneration. In this study (32), the assessment of disc degeneration and discography in spondylolisthesis was given. Table 13.1 shows the MRI signal and discographic patterns found at the level of spondylolisthesis and adjacent levels.

Figure 13.32 shows the degenerative change of the L3-L4 disc, which is the level of degenerative spondylolisthesis of L3 on L4. Note how the nuclear material has dissipated throughout the entire annulus fibrosus of the disc and the signal intensity of the disc is decreased.

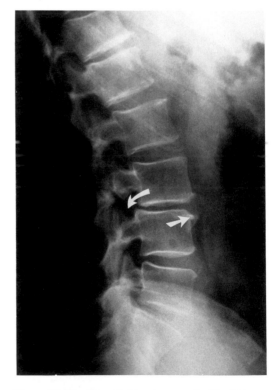

Figure 13.27. The third lumbar vertebral body is anterior on L4, with anterolateral traction spurring and attempted buttressing (*straight arrow*) of the anterior fourth lumbar vertebral body under the anterior slipped third lumbar body. Note the alteration (*curved arrow*) of the L3-L4 intervertebral foramen by the L3 slippage subluxation.

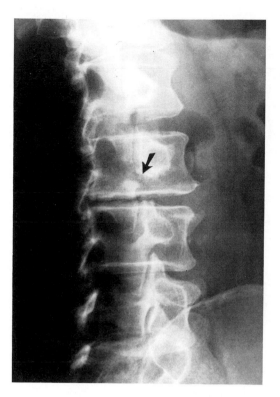

Figure 13.28. The right pars interarticularis at L3 (*arrow*) shows the stress fracture deformity of failed ossification.

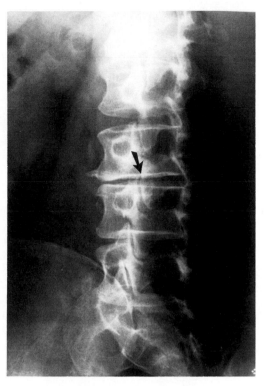

Figure 13.29. The left pars interarticularis at L3 (*arrow*) does not reveal pars interarticularis fracture. This represents, therefore, a unilateral spondylolysis and accompanying unilateral rotatory spondylolisthesis.

Table 13.1.
MRI Signal and Discographic Pattern of the Affected and Adjacent Levels in Patients with Spondylolisthesis[a]

Patient No.	Grade (1–4)	Level	MRI Signal	Disco	Adjacent Levels	MRI Signal	Disco
1	Lysis only	L5-S1	nl[b]	nl	L3-4	nl	nl
					L4-5	nl	nl
2	1	L5-S1	▼	hern	L3-4	nl	nl
					L4-5	nl	nl
3	2	L5-S1	▼	deg	L2-3	▼	deg
					L3-4		deg
					L4-5	↓	deg
4	1	L5-S1	▼	deg hern	L3-4	nl	nl
					L4-5	↓	deg hern
5	1	L3-4	▼	deg	L4-5	▼	deg
					L5-S1	nl	nl

[a]Reproduced with permission from Schneiderman G, Flannigan B, Kingston S, Thomas J, Dillin WH, Watkins RG: Magnetic resonance imaging in the diagnosis of disc degeneration: correlation with discography. *Spine* 12(3):280, 1987.

[b]Nl = normal; ▼ = marked loss or no signal; ↓ = intermediate signal loss; deg = degenerated; hern = herniated; deg hern = degenerated-herniated.

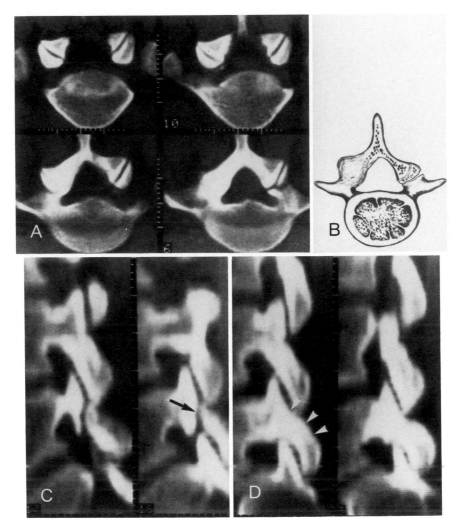

Figure 13.30. Unilateral pars interarticularis defect. **A,** Axial scan on a patient with unilateral right pars interarticularis defect. **B,** Diagram of **A**. **C,** Sagittal reformation through the right pars defect (*arrow*). **D,** Sagittal reformation through the thickened pars (*arrowheads*). (Reproduced with permission from Rothman SLG, Glenn WV: *Multiplanar CT of the Spine*. Baltimore, University Park Press, 1985, p 220.)

Figure 13.33 reveals the marked degenerative internal derangement of the nuclear material at L5-S1, with protrusion of the nuclear material posteriorly.

IS DISC DEGENERATION A SOURCE OF LOW BACK PAIN?

Can the discal degeneration accompanying spondylolisthesis be pain-producing? To answer that, let's look at the study of Vanharanta et al. (33), who found that as disc deterioration increases,

discography was found to be more painful. Painful discs were found to have higher degeneration and disruption scores than painless discs. However, as deteriorating discs become painful, the pain was not always similar to the patient's clinical back pain; it was sometimes graded as dissimilar. The number of discs with exactly the same or similar pain was found to increase consistently with the amount of deterioration. Therefore, increasing deterioration of lumbar discs is associated with increasing clinical pain. In answer to the question "does degeneration of discs explain

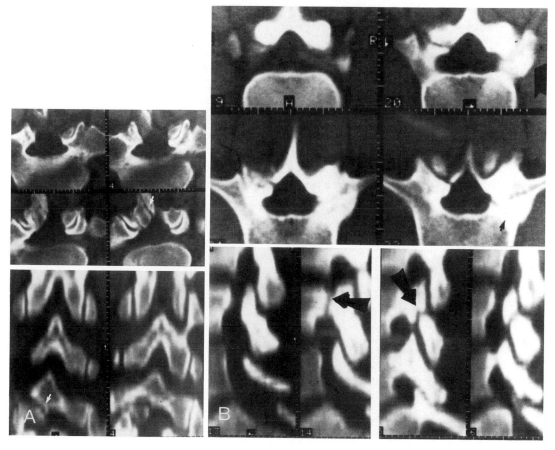

Figure 13.31. **A,** Retroisthmic cleft. Axial (*Top*) and coronal (*Bottom*) views reveal clefts within the left lamina (*arrows*). **B,** Retrosomatic clefts. **A,** (*Top*) Axial scan with pars defect on the left (*arrow*) and a retrosomatic cleft on the right. **B,** (*Bottom left*) Sagittal view through the retrosomatic cleft, which lies anterior to the pedicle (*arrow*). (*Bottom right*) Sagittal view of the opposite side through a typical pars defect (*arrow*). (Reproduced with permission from Rothman SLG, Glenn WV: *Multiplanar CT of the Spine*. Baltimore, University Park Press, 1985, pp 230, 231.)

back pain?'' Vanharanta stated that degeneration and disruption scores of these dissimilarly painful discs were high; these therefore would greatly affect the results and conclusions if combined with the no-pain group.

Results of this study (33) indicated that even small amounts of deterioration may be the cause of a disc being painful on discography.

Causes of Pain in Spondylolisthesis

Spondylolytic spondylolisthesis, i.e., a defect in the pars interarticularis allowing forward slippage, can and does occur without symptoms. It is

known that Eskimos have a 40% to 50% occurrence of spondylolisthesis but not that high an incidence of pain with it. Forward slippage of the body will not occur without degenerative changes occurring in the underlying disc; i.e., forward slippage is not possible without annular tearing or breakdown. The disc is not capable of withstanding the shearing stresses of the body above on the one below.

In a study comparing the incidence of pain in patients with spondylolisthesis by age, Macnab (21) divided patients into three age groups (under 26, 26 to 39, and 40 and older). In the 40-and-older group, the incidence of spondylolisthesis in patients with back pain was about the same as it was in the general population, whereas in the under-26 group, nearly 19% of back pain patients exhibited spondylolisthesis. Thus, if spondylotic spondylolisthesis is found in a patient under 26 years of age who does have back pain, it probably is the cause of the symptoms; if it is found in patients 26 to 39 years of age, it is a possible cause; and if it is found in patients 40 years of age or older, it rarely, if ever, is the sole cause of symptoms.

Figure 13.34 shows how L5 spondylolisthesis kinks the L5 nerve root passing under the L5 pedicles. This can be confused with root symptoms due to L4-L5 disc protrusion. In a patient with L5 nerve root symptoms, however, a negative myelogram at L4-L5 would lead to the suspicion that the L5 spondylolisthesis is kinking the L5 nerve root. An L4 spondylolisthesis could kink the L4 nerve root and cause femoral nerve paresthesia.

Clinical Findings in Children with Acute Spondylolysis Causing Low Back and Leg Pain

Three children with low back pain radiating to the leg and with spasm of the hamstring and paravertebral muscles were reported (34). All three showed x-ray findings of unilateral or bilateral spondylolysis, and localized positive bone scan pointing to spondylolysis as the cause of the pain. The ages of the three children were 10, 7½, and 14 years.

The authors felt that the symptoms of these

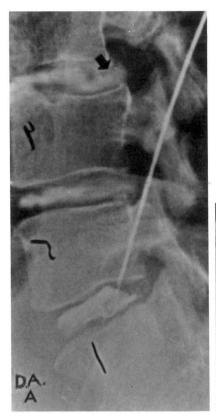
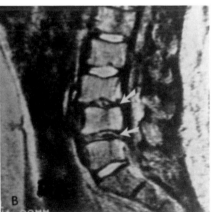

Figure 13.32. **A,** Lateral discogram examination demonstrates degenerated herniated discs at the level of L3-L4 and L4-L5. A normal disc is identified at L5-S1. There is a grade 1 spondylolisthesis L3 on L4 (*arrow*). **B,** Sagittal MR (SE 2000/56) demonstrates grade 1 spondylolisthesis L3 on L4 and marked loss of signal intensity at the levels of L3-L4 and L4-L5 (*arrows*). Note normal intensity at L2-L3 disc and L5-S1 disc. (Reproduced with permission from Schneiderman G, Flannigan B, Kingston S, Thomas J, Dillin WH, Watkins RG: Magnetic resonance imaging in the diagnosis of disc degeneration: correlation with discography. *Spine* 12(3):280, 1987.)

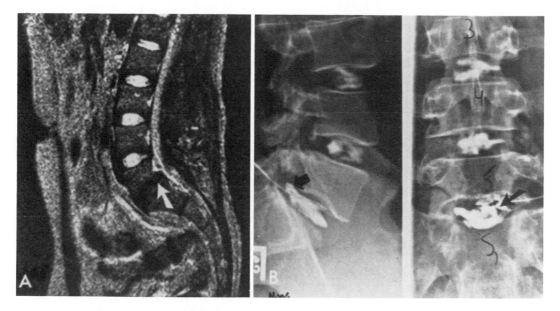

Figure 13.33. **A,** Sagittal MR (SE 2000/70) demonstrates grade 1 spondylolisthesis and disc degeneration at the L5-S1 level (*arrow*). Normal disc intensities are noted at the L4-L5 level. **B,** AP and lateral discography demonstrates normal disc levels at L3-L4, L4-L5, and a degenerated herniated disc at L5-S1 (*arrows*). (Reproduced with permission from Schneiderman G, Flannigan B, Kingston S, Thomas J, Dillin WH, Watkins RG: Magnetic resonance imaging in the diagnosis of disc degeneration: correlation with discography. *Spine* 12(3):281, 1987.)

three cases were due to referred pain from noxious stimuli affecting a branch of the posterior primary ramus in the facet joints, and the diagnosis of the cases was facet syndrome. The facet joint involvement was explained by a communication between the defective area of the pars interarticularis and the facets above and below it, as demonstrated by Ghelman and Doherty (35), and Maldague et al. (23). Irritation of these communicating joints and of the richly innervated periarticular tissues may account for the low back radiating pain of patients with spondylolysis.

Clinical Correlation with Severity of Spondylolisthesis Slippage

Saraste (36) did a 20-year follow-up study of 255 spondylolysis or spondylolisthesis patients to correlate the clinical and radiographic findings for their condition. Four millimeters was the mean value of progressive slippage of all cases; adolescents slipped 2.5 mm and adults 5 mm as a mean value. L4 showed a greater mean value of slippage, 7 mm, compared to 4 mm at L5.

Flexion-extension radiographs in the standing position as compared to recumbent films showed negligible positional changes. This author (J.M.C.) would contrast the use of flexion and extension failure to demonstrate motion at the spondylolisthetic segment to the Friberg work on vertical distraction translatory motion, showing marked motion. This author (J.M.C.) further feels that the sacral motion under the spondylolisthetic segment may be a far greater cause of the apparent motion on vertical traction than the movement of L5 on the sacrum or L4 on L5.

Saraste (36) found 20% of the spondylolytic patients to show severe disc degeneration at the L4 and L5 spondylolysis levels when originally seen, but at follow-up, 50% of the L5 and 70% of the L4 spondylolysis groups had progressed to severe degeneration of the disc. Interestingly, over half the cases showing more than 25% slippage at the time of diagnosis showed severe disc degeneration.

Pain is the most common symptom of spondylolysis and spondylolisthesis, with the peak onset of symptoms at the adolescent growth spurt (37–43). Most adolescents with spondylolysis are symptomless, although spondylolisthesis is the most common cause of low back pain and sciatica in children and adolescents (40).

In a study of 500 first-grade students, Fredrickson (44, 45) described the natural progression of spondylolytic patients as follows: at age 6, the incidence of spondylolysis and spondylolisthesis was 4.4% and 2.6%, respectively; the incidence at adulthood was 5.4% and 4.0%. He reported none of these children to be symptomatic, while Wiltse (45) found few symptomatic children between ages 10 and 15 years with spondylolisthesis, even though he felt that most slippage occurred between these ages. Wiltse also found a 5% incidence of spondylolysis in children 5 to 7 years old, with an increase to 5.8% by age 18. Most of the slippage occurred between ages 11 and 15, the time of growth spurt and vigorous exercise (41, 44, 46).

Effect of Hamstring Muscle Contracture

Patients with hamstring muscle contracture showed a higher degree of spondylolisthesis and greater disc degeneration than patients without hamstring contracture (36).

The age of symptom onset, in the patients with L5 spondylolisthesis, was 19 years, and the age at radiographic diagnosis was 23, while the L4 spondylolysis patients showed symptoms at 20 years and were radiographed for diagnosis at 30 years. Ninety-one percent had occasional low back pain, with chronic pain in 73%. Sixty percent found their pain constant, with 79% finding loading of the lumbar spine to be pain-producing.

Fifty-five percent of the 255 patients reported having had sciatica (36). Seventy percent had received treatment for low back pain. A comparison of surgically treated versus nonsurgically treated cases showed no statistically significant differences in frequency of symptoms and functional impairment, degree of spondylolysis at diagnosis, or progression of slippage.

Pregnancy showed no statistically significant differences in frequency of symptoms, functional impairment, or degree of progression of slippage when 63 pregnant women were compared to 21 women who had never been pregnant and to 171 men.

When the degree of slippage was compared to the occurrence of low back and sciatic pain, it was found that with greater than 15 mm of slippage, 83% of the patients had low back pain and 61% had sciatica, whereas with less than 15 mm of slippage, 50% had low back pain and 10% had sciatica (36).

MECHANISMS OF NERVE ROOT COMPRESSION IN SPONDYLOLISTHESIS

Macnab (21) described at least six mechanisms of compression of the L5 root in isthmic spondylolysis:

1. Disc herniation of L4-L5;
2. The free fragment of the L5 posterior neural arch rotating anteriorly and pivoting on the sacrum, with compression of the L5 root between the distal pars remnant and the sacrum;
3. Occasional kinking of the L5 root around the L5 pedicle in spondylolysis;
4. Encroachment by a degenerative, bulging annulus fibrosus at L5-S1;
5. Neuroforaminal stenosis;
6. Extraforaminal entrapment between the L5 corpotransverse ligament and the sacral ala.

Clinically, it is well to state here that pseudospondylolisthesis results in stenosis of the lumbar

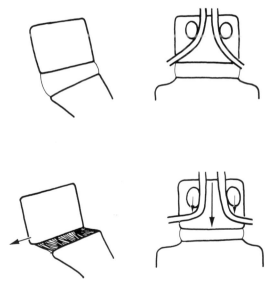

Figure 13.34. Illustration of kinking of the nerve roots by the pedicles as the body of L5 slips downward and forward. (Reproduced with permission from Macnab I: *Backache*, p 54. © 1977, the Williams & Wilkins Co., Baltimore.)

spinal canal and may impinge on the nerve roots of the cauda equina and induce neurogenic claudication (47).

CASES OF TRUE SPONDYLOLISTHESIS FROM THE CLINICAL PRACTICE OF THE AUTHOR

True Spondylolisthesis with Transitional Segment

CASE 2

Sacralization of L5 is four times more common in patients with degenerative spondylolisthesis than in the general population (31). However, this case presents an unusual finding of true spondylolisthesis at the L4 level and a bilateral pseudosacralization of L5 to the sacrum (Figs. 13.35, 13.36, 13.37). It is much more common to

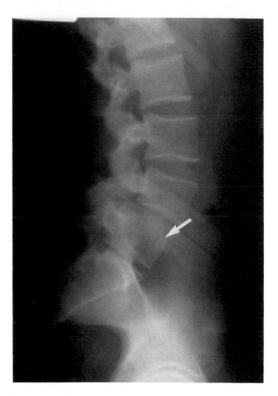

Figure 13.36. Lateral projection of Figure 13.35 showing the L4 spondylolisthesis on the fifth lumbar transitional pseudosacralized segment. Also note the failure of epiphyseal development of the anterior superior L5 vertebral body plate (*arrow*).

find intact pars interarticular with the spondylolisthetic slip above a transitional segment.

Dual Level Spondylolisthesis

CASE 3

A 31-year-old white male with low back and occasional buttock pain is shown in Figures 13.38, 13.39 and 13.40. His pain started after carrying tools as a carpenter. He consulted three chiropractors, all of whom gave him side-posture rotation adjustments. These treatments made him worse. He finally saw his family medical doctor, who referred him to a neurosurgeon in our city, who then referred him to our office for chiropractic manipulation.

His history revealed that this man first had low back pain in 1970, after he injured his back lifting furniture. He went to a chiropractor and the pain went away after a few treatments. In 1979, he hurt his back again and went to a chiropractor; two treatments helped him. In

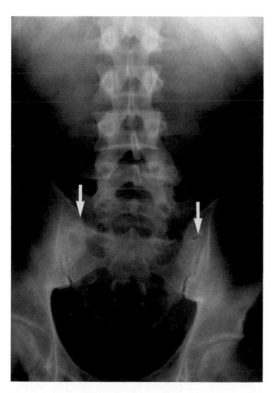

Figure 13.35. This is an unusual case of bilateral pseudosacralization (*arrows*) of both transverse processes with the sacrum with true spondylolisthesis above at the L4 level, as shown in Figure 13.36. (Courtesy of Alice E. Wright, D.C. Hatfield, Pennsylvania.)

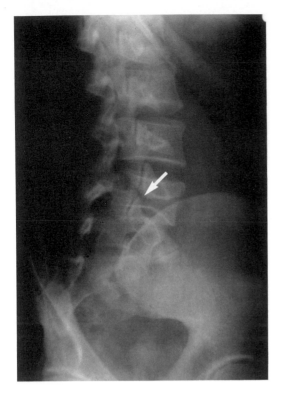

Figure 13.37. Note the pars interarticularis stress fracture deformity (*arrow*) on the oblique projection of Figures 13.35 and 13.36.

1982, he fell from a roof and went to a chiropractor and felt fine.

Examination now revealed no motor or sensory changes in the lower extremities. Ranges of motion were normal. The straight leg raise was negative. The diagnosis in this case was spondylolisthesis at the L4 and L5 levels, approximately 10% slippage at each level. There was failure of ossification of the pars interarticularis bilaterally at the L4 and L5 level.

This is a very interesting case in that it represents two spondylolistheses in one spine. Both of them slipped evenly. Please note the degenerative change of the L4-L5 disc and the anterolateral spurring, with perhaps some formation of buttress at the anterior superior plate of L5.

Our opinion is that the source of pain in this patient could be the disc tearing and strain at both the L4-L5 and L5-S1 disc levels. Remember that these discs are highly pain-sensitive, being supplied with mechanoceptors, nociceptors, and proprioceptors. The treatment consisted of flexion distraction manipulation as discussed in this chapter on spondylolisthesis. The

Dutchman roll was placed under the L4 and L5 vertebral bodies and flexion distraction manipulation given three times per week. In 3 weeks time, this patient had approximately 90% relief of his pain. He attended low back wellness school so as to learn how to control his back pain through proper ergonomics of lifting and bending. He also did strong abdominal strengthening exercises, and knee-chest exercise, and used the Nautilus super low back unit in our clinic for strengthening the erector spinae muscles. He minimized extension exercises, however, in performing these muscle-strengthening exercises.

This man obtained relief initially under the treatment described here, but following a physical altercation, his symptoms worsened and he did undergo surgical stabilization.

Unilateral Pars Interarticularis Defect (Spondylolysis)

Figure 13.30 describes sagittal reformation of a pars defect on the right side only at L5. A case from our clinic is presented here.

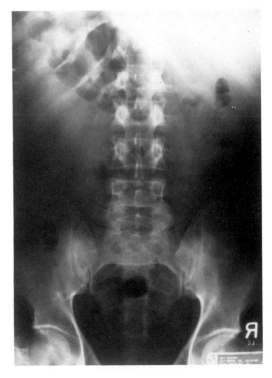

Figure 13.38. This is the posteroanterior study of a 31-year-old man with low back pain.

CASE 4

A 16-year-old boy was seen for low back pain.

Lateral x-ray (Fig. 13.41) revealed a 5% anterior slippage of L5 on the sacrum with a suspicion of a pars interarticularis defect. Oblique projection (Fig. 13.42) does reveal a defect at the right pars interarticularis, while Figure 13.43 on the left reveals that there is no pars defect, but there is hyperostosis of bone throughout the pars on this side.

Figure 13.44, an anteroposterior view, reveals a left lateral flexion of L4 on L5, and the lateral projection (Fig. 13.45) reveals that there is no facet syndrome or stenosis present in this spine. There is a hyperflexion subluxation of L3 on L4, however.

We feel that this is a good example of unilateral spondylolysis resulting in a slight spondylolisthesis of L5 on the sacrum with the resultant hyperostosis of bone on the intact pars interarticularis side in response to the stress placed upon it by the rotosubluxation created by the contralateral defect of the pars interarticularis.

Treatment of this case consisted of flexion distraction with a small flexion pillow under the L5 vertebral body. This patient was placed on strong knee-chest exercise,

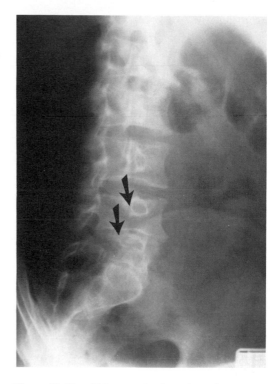

Figure 13.40. Oblique projections show the pars interarticularis stress fractures (*arrows*) at the L4 and L5 levels of case 3, also shown in Figure 13.39.

abdominal tightening exercises, and stretching of the hamstring muscles; he attended low back wellness school so as to learn how to avoid stress to his spine in daily living. He made a strong progressive recovery from his problem.

Eight-Year-Old Boy with Spondylolisthesis Following Trauma

CASE 5

Figures 13.46 and 13.47 are the lateral and oblique views of an 8-year-old boy who had had pain for approximately 2 weeks prior to seeing us. His parents related that 2 weeks prior to this, his brother had jumped on his low back while the boy was lying prone on the floor. He felt immediate low back pain and had suffered with it since.

We felt that there was a pars interarticularis fracture with an approximately 15% anterior slippage of L5 on the sacrum. We could not be certain that this pars defect occurred at the time of injury, but there was a strong clinical suggestion that it may have taken place

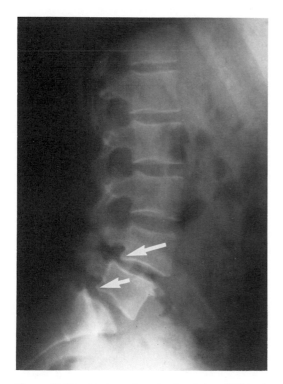

Figure 13.39. On lateral projection, L4 and L5 both show anterior displacement on their inferior segments (*arrows*).

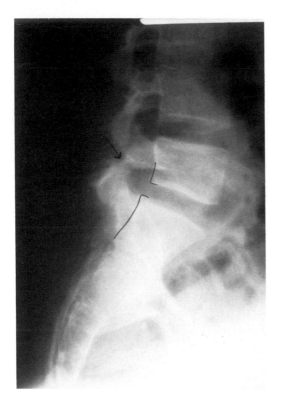

Figure 13.41. Lateral projection of a 16-year-old male with low back pain shows a 5% slippage of L5 on the sacrum with a pars interarticularis defect suspected (*arrow*).

when the brother jumped upon this segment with the boy lying on his stomach.

Treatment of this case consisted of flexion distraction with a small Dutchman roll under the L5 vertebral body while the contact hand was placed upon the L4 spinous process. This boy made a rapid recovery and had no pain after 2 weeks of treatment.

Instability at Spondylolisthesis

CASE 6

A 45-year-old male was seen complaining of low back and right leg pain following twisting at work. He remembered that at age 20 he had injured his back while on the track team throwing a discus. Since then he had had periodic low back pain. In the past, he had exercises prescribed, pain killers, and muscle relaxants for his back problem. He had polio as a child, but there was no paralytic residual problem. He had been a jogger for many years. This was the first time he had ever had leg pain; in the past, he had only had low back pain.

The pain went down the right lateral leg, middle calf, to the outside of the foot. It awakened him during the night.

Radiographs (Figs. 13.48, 13.49, and 13.50) reveal that this patient had an approximately 20% anterior slippage of L5 on the sacrum with a pars interarticularis defect present. Extension (Fig. 13.50) reveals that L5 translates posteriorly on the sacrum, while flexion (Fig. 13.49) reveals that there is increase in the intervertebral disc space at L5-S1 and that L5 translates anteriorly on the sacrum. With this instability of L5 on S1, we offered the patient a 3-week course of flexion distraction manipulation with the expectation of 50% relief or we would not continue such conservative manipulative care. In addition to the flexion distraction manipulation, this patient was placed on hamstring stretching exercises with proprioceptive neuromuscular facilitation, abdominal strengthening exercises, and knee-chest exercises; he also attended low back wellness school. After 5 weeks of care, this patient was approximately 95% subjectively improved.

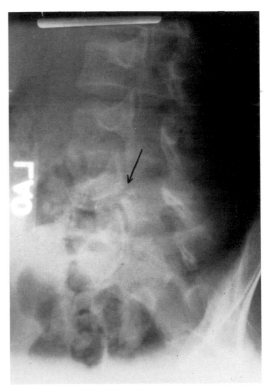

Figure 13.42. Oblique view shows a unilateral spondylolysis at L5 (*arrow*).

Stability of Spondylolisthesis

CASE 7

Figures 13.51 through 13.53 represent neutrolateral, flexion, and extension views of a 50% spondylolisthetic slip, true variety, of L5 on the sacrum. We note that there is only 1 mm of movement on flexion of L5 on the sacrum and no movement on extension. Please note the increased facet syndrome change at the L4-L5 level on extension. We feel that this is a good example showing the stability of a 50% spondylolisthetic slip, and we also note that there is minimal visible buttressing of the L5-S1 anterior disc space. Such stable spondylolisthetic slips seem to respond best to conservative care, as in this case.

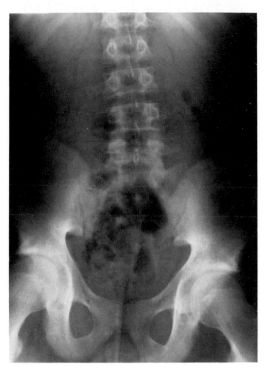

Figure 13.44. Left lateral flexion subluxation of L4 on L5 is noted in case 4.

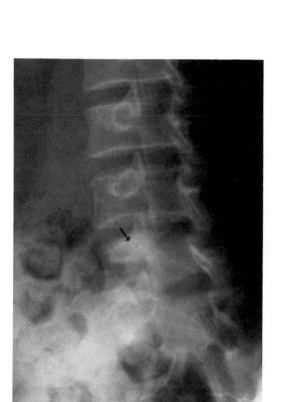

Figure 13.43. The opposite oblique view shows no spondylolysis defect but rather hyperostosis of bone at the pars (*arrow*). This is felt to be a reaction (Wolff's law) to the stress placed on this intact pars by the rotatory stress created by the opposite failed pars fusion.

DEGENERATIVE SPONDYLOLISTHESIS

Lumbar Degenerative Spondylolisthesis

Degenerative spondylolisthesis (DS) is the slipping of one vertebral segment on the one below in the presence of an intact neural arch. It occurs secondary to arthritis of the facet joints and degeneration of the disc (7, 48–51). DS usually affects people older than 50, being more common in blacks; women are more often affected than men. The L4-L5 level is most often involved (7, 49, 51–53), with L3 next in order of frequency (53). Approximately 10 to 15% of patients with DS require surgery for relief of pain (7, 51–53). The severe pain is radicular, not relieved by conservative therapy, and usually associated with cauda equina symptoms secondary to stenosis of the canal by the hypertrophic subluxating facet joints (7, 50–53). Twenty-five percent of spondylolisthesis is of DS etiology (7).

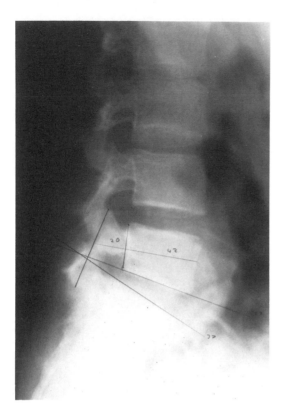

Figure 13.45. Lateral view of patient shown in Figure 13.44 shows that stenosis is not present by Eisenstein's measurement at the L5 level.

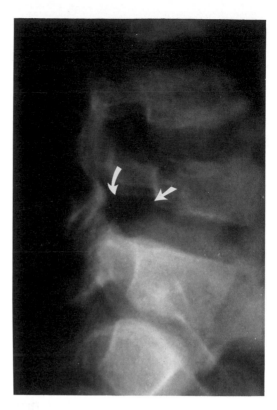

Figure 13.46. Lateral view shows true spondylolisthesis of L5 on the sacrum (*straight arrow*), with a suspected pars interarticularis fracture (*curved arrow*).

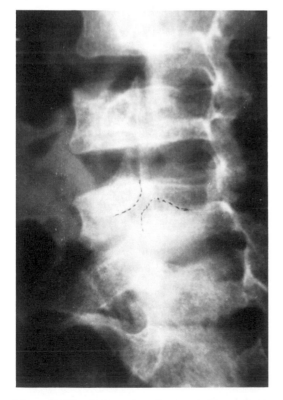

Figure 13.47. Oblique view of patient in Figure 13.46 shows the outlined pars interarticularis fracture.

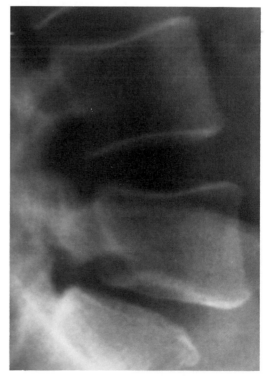

Figure 13.48. Neutral lateral view shows a 20% slippage of L5 on the sacrum in a 45-year-old male with low back and right leg pain following a twisting injury.

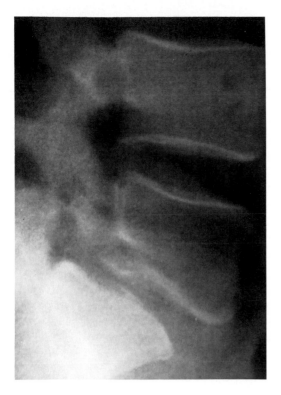

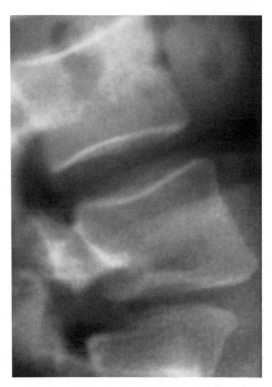

Figure 13.49. Flexion study of patient shown in Figure 13.48 shows increased anterior translation of L5 on the sacrum.

Figure 13.50. Extension again shows posterior motion of L5 on the sacrum.

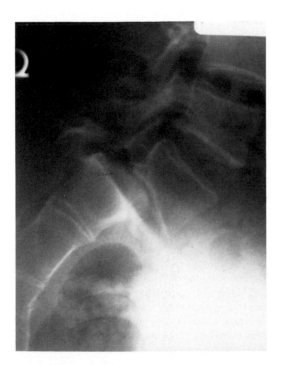

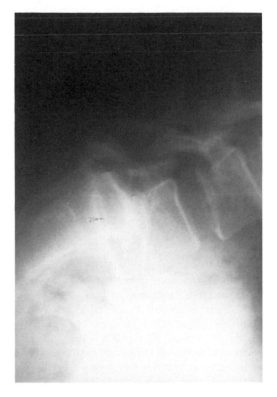

Figure 13.51. Neutral lateral view shows a 20-mm anterior slippage of L5 on the sacrum.

Figure 13.52. Flexion reveals only 1 mm of increased translation of L5 on the sacrum.

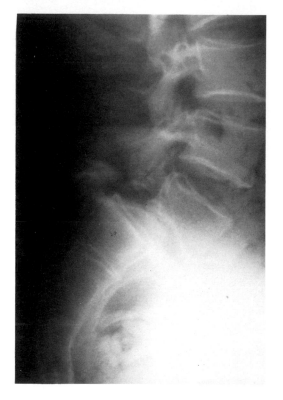

Figure 13.53. Extension does not indicate any increased translation of L5; therefore, instability of L5 on the sacrum is not present. This type of stability is shown to be clinically easier to manage than unstable movement.

The etiology (7, 18, 50, 51, 54), pathology (18, 52, 53, 55–57), symptoms (50–53), and diagnosis (7, 18, 51–53) of DS have been discussed in the literature.

The degenerative lesion is due to long-standing intersegmental instability (50, 58, 59). Farfan believes that there are multiple small compressive fractures of the inferior articular processes of the vertebra that slip forward (18). Because of this, the bone of the articular processes has a peculiar appearance grossly resembling the bone in Paget's disease. As the slip progresses, the articular processes change direction and become more horizontal. One side virtually always slips down more than the other, and rotation at the level of olisthesis is an integral characteristic.

In the patients who come to the doctor with clinical symptoms, degenerative spondylolisthesis occurs six times as frequently in females than males, six to nine times more frequently at the L4 interspace than the adjoining levels, and four times more frequently when L5 is sacralized than when it is not (53). When the lesion is at L4, the L5 vertebra is more stable and in less lordosis than average. Finneson states that he has never seen DS in a patient under age 40 (17).

Slipping in DS never seems to exceed 33% unless there has been surgical intervention. The predisposing factor is thought to be a straight, stable lumbosacral joint that sits high between the ilia. This arrangement puts increased stress on the joints between L4 and L5, leading to decompensation of the ligaments, hypermobility and degeneration at the articular processes, and multiple microfractures of the inferior articular processes of L4, allowing forward slipping (53).

Finneson (17) states that the appropriate treatment is symptomatic therapy, with surgery used only for severe pain. Most patients have little or no neurological deficit, but a very few have rather severe changes. The myelogram is characteristically dramatically abnormal. Circulatory change in the legs is not part of the syndrome. It is the L5 nerve root that is compressed in an L4-L5 olisthesis. The nerve is compressed between the inferior articular process of L4 and the upper margin of the body of L5.

Many structures may be stressed and irritated in DS. In discussing pain mechanisms in DS, it is well to remember the innervation of the facet joints (60–66), intervertebral disc (18, 62, 65–78), posterior longitudinal ligament (18, 62, 68, 71, 74, 76, 79), anterior longitudinal ligament (62, 66, 68, 71, 74, 79), dura mater (66, 68, 71, 79, 80), and vertebral periosteum and bone (62, 66, 71, 79). It is not well understood just how the pain in spinal stenosis due to DS is produced. Probably the best explanation is that the nerves are denied adequate nourishment because of pressure on the tiny blood vessels that supply them (81, 82). The perineurium of the spinal nerves themselves is richly supplied with tiny nerve fibers. Perhaps ischemia of these may cause the pain (83).

Naked nerve endings of the sinuvertebral nerve have been identified in the granulation tissue ingrowth of reparative healing in the annulus fibrosus (77). There may be pain receptors, which would explain discogenic pain in the absence of herniation. Certainly tearing of disc fibers occurs in DS. Souter and Taylor (84) state that branches of the sinuvertebral nerve supply the outer layer of the annulus fibrosus, most of the terminations being naked nerve endings, probably mediating pain sensation. Fine nerve fibers were also found by them in the granulation tissue in the deeper layers of the annulus fibrosus of a degenerative disc.

Bogduk (68) states that the lumbar intervertebral discs are innervated posteriorly by the sinuvertebral nerve, and the lateral and anterior aspects of the annulus fibrosus as well as the anterior longitudinal ligament are innervated by a series of nerves derived from the ventral rami and the sympathetic nervous system. The posterior lateral aspect of each intervertebral disc receives branches from the ventral ramus at each level and/or the terminal portion of the grey ramus communicans. The lateral aspects of the intervertebral disc receive ascending or descending branches from the grey rami communicantes, which reach the annuli fibrosi by passing between and then deep to the attachments of the psoas major. Three recent studies (68, 77, 78) have corroborated earlier reports of nerve fibers up to as far as a third of the way into cadaveric annuli fibrosi, and nerve endings as deeply as halfway into annuli fibrosi obtained during posterior and anterior fusion operations.

Degenerative spondylolisthesis (DS) is also termed *pseudospondylolisthesis* and is a cause of stenosis at the vertebral canal due to compensatory hypertrophy and sclerosis of the superior facets, which consequently encroach on the lateral recesses, causing an hourglass deformity seen on myelography (80, 85). Anterior slippage of this superior vertebra compresses the dural sac between its anteriorly migrated inferior facets and the superior border of the lower vertebra (Figs. 13.54 and 13.55). The slippage has a natural tendency to increase (86), but the severity of symptoms cannot always be correlated with the severity of the slip because there may be a severe slip without marked degenerative change, and vice versa. Backache of several years duration, most commonly increased by exercise or by getting up from bed rest, is common. Sciatic pain usually follows months or years or back pain. Weakness and numbness of the legs as well as absent ankle reflexes may be seen in DS.

Nerve entrapment is the most important feature of degenerative spondylolisthesis. This can

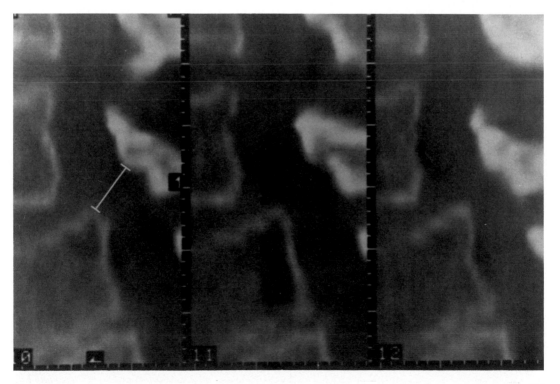

Figure 13.54. Degenerative spondylolisthesis, L4-L5. Sagittal reformations reveal 8-mm forward subluxation of L4 on L5. The diameter of the spinal canal is reduced to 8 mm. This is measured from the posterior lip of the superior end plate of L5 to the undersurface of the L4 lamina. (Reproduced with permission from Rothman SLG, Glenn WV: *Multiplanar CT of the Spine*. Baltimore, University Park Press, 1985, p 235.)

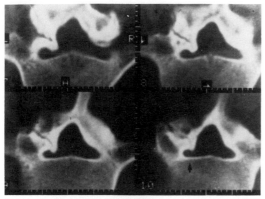

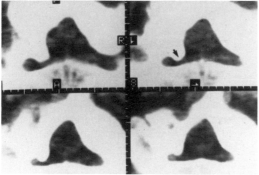

Figure 13.55. Lateral recess stenosis. **Top four panels**, Bone window axial scans demonstrate lateral recess stenosis at the level of a pars interarticularis defect (*arrow*). **Bottom four panels**, Soft-tissue axial views on the same patient. (Reproduced with permission from Rothman SLG, Glenn WV: *Multiplanar CT of the Spine.* Baltimore, University Park Press, 1985, p 234.)

occur in any of four ways (79): (*a*) pressure on the L4 nerve at the foramen by osteophytes arising from the posteroinferior surface of the vertebral body of L4; (*b*) pressure on the L5 nerve from posterior displacement of L5 on L4, forming a bony ridge in the region of the lateral recess; (*c*) pressure on the L5 nerve root in a narrow lateral recess at the lower border of the L5 vertebra; (*d*) pressure on the L5 nerve by the anteriorly inferior articular process of L4.

Treatment of DS should be conservative as long as the pain is tolerable (83, 87), as only rarely do patients with lumbar spine stenosis have neurological changes that in themselves warrant surgery.

FACET ROLE IN DEGENERATIVE SPONDYLOLISTHESIS

Facet orientation plays a significant role in the advancing slippage in degenerative spondylolisthesis. Sagittally oriented facets offer less bony resistance to the forward and downward force of the L5 vertebral body than do oblique or coronally faced facet joints (Fig. 13.56). Facet tropism is extremely common in these patients and is likely a very important predisposing factor leading to dislocation (50).

Facet joint arthrosis (severe erosion and degeneration) is a hallmark of spondylolisthesis with intact neural arches (degenerative spondylolisthesis) (31). These changes are seen in Figure 13.57. The joint space seems unusually widened because of severe erosion of the articular surfaces.

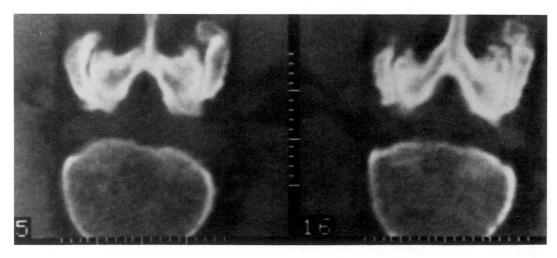

Figure 13.56. Degenerative spondylolisthesis, L4-L5. Axial views demonstrate saggitally oriented facets that have dislocated. Cartilaginous surfaces are irregular and eroded. (Reproduced with permission from Rothman SLG, Glenn WV: *Multiplanar CT of the Spine.* Baltimore, University Park Press, 1985, p 235.)

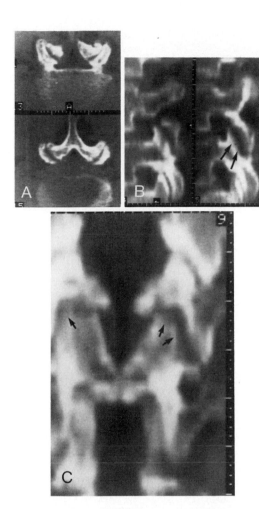

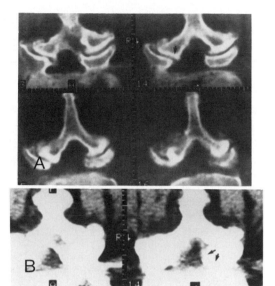

Figure 13.57. Arthropathy in degenerative spondylolisthesis. **A,** Axial scan demonstrates severe erosive arthritis of the facet joints, especially on the left. There is erosion of the cartilage, and the joint space is widened. **B** and **C,** Sagittal and coronal views similarly show a widening of the joint, with destruction of the articular surfaces (*arrows*). (Reproduced with permission from Rothman SLG, Glenn WV: *Multiplanar CT of the Spine.* Baltimore, University Park Press, 1985, p 241.)

Figure 13.58. Lateral subluxation. Axial scans windowed for **A,** bone and **B,** soft tissue reveal coronally oriented facets. There is considerable lateral subluxation of the facets, causing prominent compression of the left lateral recess. The space available for the theca and cauda equina is remarkably reduced. (Reproduced with permission from Rothman SLG, Glenn WV: *Multiplanar CT of the Spine.* Baltimore, University Park Press, 1985, p 247.)

SUBLUXATION AT THE LEVEL OF SPONDYLOLISTHESIS

The most severe clinical symptoms may occur when there is unrestricted anterior dislocation of the inferior facet of the upper vertebral body, beyond the confines of the anterior limb of the superior facet. This may occur bilaterally, causing forward dislocation, or unilaterally, causing rotatory or lateral subluxation (Fig. 13.58).

REVERSE SPONDYLOLISTHESIS (RETROLISTHESIS)

Reverse spondylolisthesis (retrolisthesis) is an instability occurring at usually the L3-L4 and L4-L5 levels due to disc degeneration (disc narrowing, spur formation, sclerosis, erosion of the end plates, and facet joint laxity). Foraminal stenosis is an important feature due to upward displacement of the superior facet of the lower vertebra into the neural foramen. Figure 13.59 reveals retrolisthesis above a spondylolisthesis subluxation.

AUTHOR'S CASE PRESENTATIONS OF DEGENERATIVE SPONDYLOLISTHESIS

Advancing Degenerative Spondylolisthesis

CASE 8

Figures 13.60 through 13.66 are studies of a 52-year-old black female who developed low back pain and ulcerative colitis in 1982. She required a colon resection

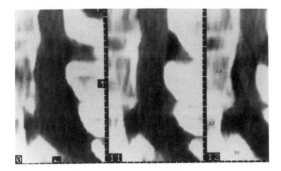

Figure 13.59. Retrolisthesis above spondylolisthes.s A series of sagittal reformations reveals that there is 9-mm forward spondylolisthesis of L5 on the sacrum and 9-mm retrolisthesis of L4 on L5. Note that there is only minimal compression of the spinal canal in this patient. (Reproduced with permission from Rothman SLG, Glenn WV: *Multiplanar CT of the Spine*. Baltimore, University Park Press, 1985, p 251.)

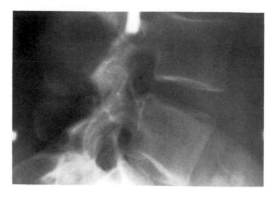

Figure 13.60. A neutral lateral lumbar spine x-ray taken in 1982 shows normal bone, disc, and soft tissue at all levels.

in 1983. The progressive nature of her degenerative spondylolisthesis is unusually revealed by progressive x-ray studies. Figure 13.60 is a neutral lateral radiograph taken in 1982 which does not show disc degeneration or spondylolisthesis at L4. Figure 13.61, taken in 1984, does show disc degeneration of the L4-L5 disc, with anterior subluxation of L4 on L5 by about 8 mm. Figure 13.62, made in 1987, shows advanced degenerative changes of the L4-L5 disc, with total loss of disc space and permanent stabilization of L4 on L5 as shown on extension and flexion studies (Figs. 13.63 and 13.64, respectively). Figures 13.65 and 13.66 are the axial and sagittal reformation showing the extensive L4-L5 discal degeneration and the L4 pseudospondylolisthesis. Note the rotatory subluxation of the inferior facets with narrowing of the lateral recesses and sagittal diameter of the vertebral canal.

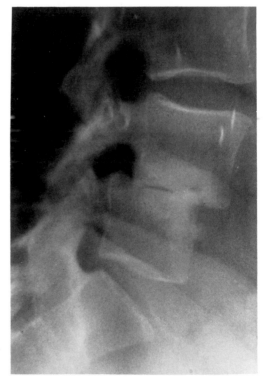

Figure 13.62. Repeat lateral x-ray of the spine seen in Figures 13.60 and 13.61 shows advanced degenerative disc disease at L5-S1, with total loss of the disc space and extreme hyperostosis of the opposing vertebral body plates of L4 and L5.

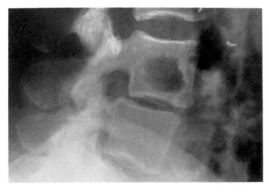

Figure 13.61. Repeat lateral x-ray taken in 1984 reveals degenerative disc disease at L4-L5, with degenerative spondylolisthesis of L4 on L5.

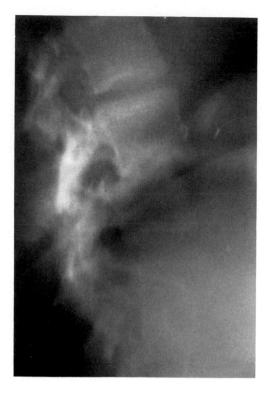

Figure 13.63. Extension reveals no motion of L4 on L5; thus, stability is further verified.

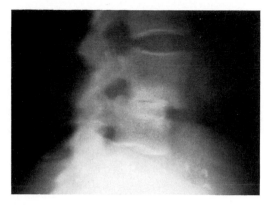

Figure 13.64. On flexion, there is no translation of L4 on L5, indicating stabilization.

Stable Pseudospondylolisthesis of L4 on L5

CASE 9

A 60-year old white male was seen complaining of low back and bilateral leg pain, which was worse following walking. There was no pain on sleeping or sitting, except that when he stood after sitting he again felt the discomfort in the legs. The Doppler examination of the lower extremities revealed no evidence of vascular claudication.

Figures 13.67 and 13.68 are the anteroposterior and lateral radiographs of this case, which reveal an anterolisthesis of L4 on L5. Figure 13.69, an oblique view of

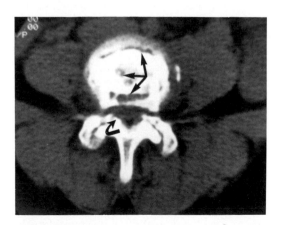

Figure 13.65. Axial CT scan at the L4-L5 disc level reveals osteochondrosis vacuum phenomenon of the disc (*straight arrows*) as well as facet degeneration. The lateral recesses are narrowed, with rotosubluxation of the vertebral arch and the right inferior facet rotating anteriorly (*curved arrow*).

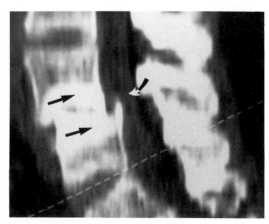

Figure 13.66. Sagittal reformatting shows the degenerative spondylolisthesis of L4 on L5 with the marked bone hyperostosis of the opposing bone plates (*straight arrows*). Note the stenosis at the vertebral canal between the posterior superior L4 vertebral body arch (*curved arrow*).

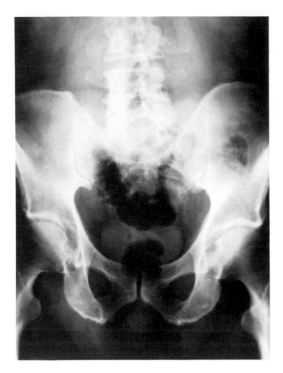

Figure 13.67. Anteroposterior view of case 9, a 60-year-old male with symptoms of intermittent claudication.

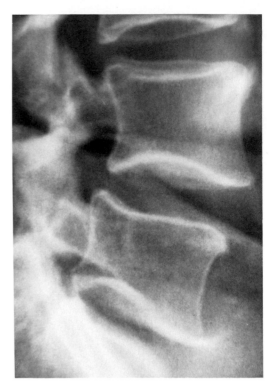

Figure 13.68. Lateral projection of Figure 13.67 shows anterior displacement of L4 on L5, with traction spurring of the anterior lateral body plates of L3, L4, and L5.

the lumbar spine, shows us that there is no pars interarticularis defect. This is a degenerative spondylolisthesis of L4 on L5. We do note the marked loss of the L5-S1 disc space with nuclear invagination of the L5 disc into the inferior plate of L5. There are marked anterolateral hypertrophic changes at the L3-L4, L4-L5, and L5-S1 levels. There is a left lean of the lumbar spine with a levorotation subluxation of the L3-L5 segments.

Figure 13.70, a lateral projection with Eisenstein's measurements made, does show that this patient has stenosis at the L5 level. Remember that any time the sagittal diameter of the vertebral canal is less than 12 mm, stenosis is present, and 12 to 15 mm is an impending stenosis. We also note that there is a 4:1 ratio of the 41-mm vertebral body sagittal diameter to the 10-mm vertebral canal sagittal diameter.

Figures 13.71 and 13.72 are the flexion and extension studies of this case. We note that flexion (Fig. 13.71) shows a 2-mm anterior translation of the L4 vertebral body on L5, while extension reveals a 0.5-mm posterior translation of L4 on L5 compared to the neutrolateral view. We feel that 3 mm of movement is within stability at a disc level, so that this L4-L5 disc is not markedly unstable at this time.

Treatment of this case consisted of flexion distraction

with a small Dutchman pillow under the L4 vertebral body while the contact was made on the L3 spinous process to allow flexion distraction to be applied. This patient was placed on knee-chest exercises, a strong course of hamstring stretching, abdominal strengthening exercises, and gluteus maximus strengthening exercises as well.

This resulted in a slow, yet progressive, relief of the patient's symptoms until, after approximately 6 weeks of care, he was approximately 75% relieved of his problem.

Tandem Lumbar and Cervical Spinal Stenosis

The triad of intermittent neurogenic claudication, progressive gait disturbance, and the findings of mixed myelopathy and polyradiculopathy in both the upper and lower extremities is the symptom complex of mixed cervical and lumbar spondylotic degeneration resulting in stenosis (88). Nineteen such patients were operated on for relief of symptoms, and none of them showed

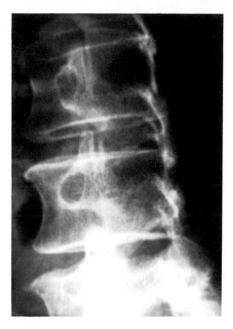

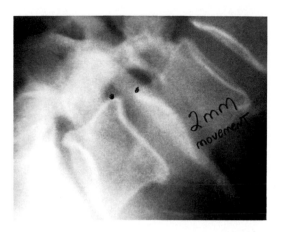

Figure 13.71. Flexion x-ray of patient seen in Figure 13.68 shows only 2 mm of motion of L4 on L5, indicating stability of the functional spinal segments.

Figure 13.69. Oblique view shows no pars interarticularis fracture at L4.

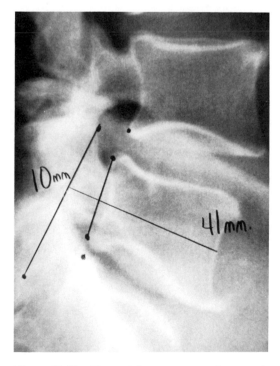

Figure 13.70. Eisenstein's measurement for stenosis reveals a 10-mm vertebral canal at the L5 level, with a 4:1 ratio of the vertebral body to the canal sagittal diameter.

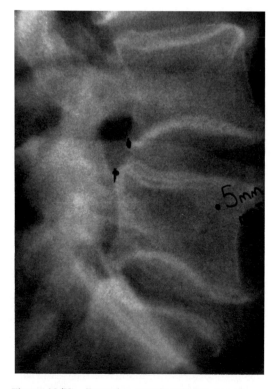

Figure 13.72. Extension reveals only 0.5 mm of motion of L4 on L5.

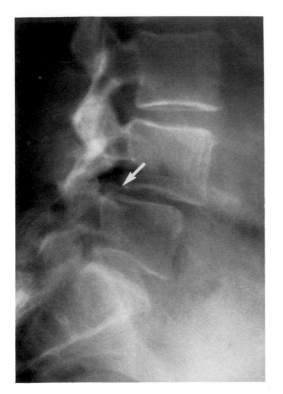

Figure 13.73. Neutral lateral projection of a 64-year-old female with signs of stenosis of the lumbar canal shows degenerative spondylolisthesis of L4 on L5 (*arrow*).

Case Presentation of Tandem Spinal Stenosis

CASE 10

The following is a study of tandem lumbar and cervical stenosis from the author's practice. Figure 13.73 shows a neutral lateral projection of a 64-year-old female with gait disturbance, muscle weakness of the lower extremities, reduced ankle and patellar reflexes, pain into the lower extremities of a nonspecific dermatome nature, and equilibrium disturbance. L4 shows a degenerative spondylolisthesis on L5. Figure 13.74, a flexion study, reveals the instability of the lesion as evidenced by the marked anterior translational subluxation of L4. Figure 13.75 was taken in extension and shows marked posterior translation. Figures 13.76 and 13.77 show that the partes interarticularis are bilaterally intact. Figure 13.78 reveals a degenerative spondylolisthesis of C7 on T1. Also note the kyphotic curvature at the C4, C5, and C6 levels. Spondylolisthesis at both the L4 and C7 levels is capable of inflicting stenosis on the canal and its spinal contents.

prognostically significant sphincter disturbance, radiculopathy, myelopathy, cerebrospinal fluid analysis, or electrophysiological testing result.

Except for the intermittent claudication, the clinical presentation of tandem spinal stenosis is similar to that of classic cervical spondylotic myelopathy (82, 89, 90, 90a). The insidious onset and the duration of symptoms are comparable. Although the prominence of radicular pain, spasticity, and sphincter disturbance is relatively diminished in tandem spinal stenosis, the extent of posterior column dysfunction is virtually identical. Like spondylotic myelopathy, tandem stenosis appears to be a diffuse rather than a segmental condition (91, 92).

Most patients with tandem stenosis complain of "numb, clumsy legs" analogous to the feelings reported with high cervical spine lesions. Complex gait disturbances are also seen due to proprioceptive disturbance, lower extremity weakness, unbalanced stooped posture adopted to relieve the back and lower extremity pain, and compensatory hyperextension of the neck in order to see (88).

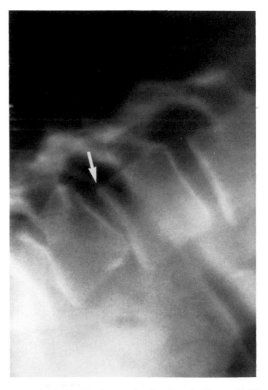

Figure 13.74. Flexion study of patient in Figure 13.73 shows marked instability of the L4-L5 disc, as evidenced by the great increased translation of the L4 vertebral body on L5 (*arrow*).

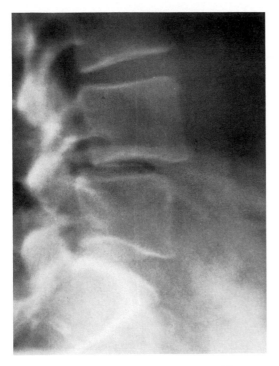

Figure 13.75. Extension shows several millimeters of posterior translation of L4, indicating marked instability.

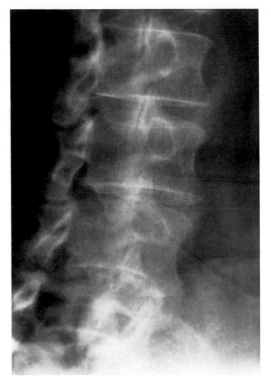

Figure 13.76. Left anterior oblique view shows no pars interarticularis defect.

Myelographic Finding in Degenerative Spondylolisthesis

CASE 11

This was a 52-year-old white female who complained of low back pain radiating into the right lower extremity for approximately the past 2 years. She sought consultation from a surgeon, and surgery was recommended to her.

Figure 13.79 is a lateral lumbar view revealing a minimal anterolisthesis subluxation of L4 on L5. Figure 13.80 is a lateral myelographic study showing mild bulging of the disc at the L4-L5 and L5-S1 levels. Figure 13.81 represents oblique studies of this patient's lumbar spine, and you will note that there is no break in the pars interarticularis, meaning that the anterolisthesis represents a pseudospondylolisthesis of L4 on L5.

Figure 13.82 shows a posteroanterior myelogram revealing a filling defect posterior to the L4-L5 disc space representing the traction deformity at the pseudospondylolisthesis dye-filled subarachnoid space. Treatment of this case consisted of flexion distraction manipulation with a small flexion pillow placed under the L4 vertebral segment. The contact hand was placed on the spinous process of L3 while gentle flexion dis-

traction was applied. This resulted in a slow but progressive relief of the patient's low back and right leg pain, and during this time she attended low back wellness school, where she was taught how to bend and lift in daily living so as to minimize stress to this low back. The treatment resulted in approximately 75% relief of her symptoms.

Typical Case of Degenerative Spondylolisthesis

CASE 12

This 42-year-old white male was seen for low back and buttock pain.

Figure 13.83 reveals a degenerative spondylolisthesis of L4 on L5, and the oblique views shown in Figures 13.84 and 13.85 reveal that the pars interarticularis is intact with no fracture present. Figure 13.86 is an anteroposterior view that reveals a suggestion of tropism at the L5-S1 level, with the right being sagittal and the left coronal. The facets at the remaining lumbar segments are sagittally oriented throughout. The oblique views do show degenerative arthrosis at the L4-L5 and L5-S1 facet joints.

This is a good example of a patient who has vague low back and buttock pain. There is no pain into the lower extremities. It is to be remembered that degenerative spondylolisthesis can often create muscle weakness and even diminished ankle jerks in the lower extremities.

This patient responded well to flexion distraction with a small Dutchman roll placed under the L4 vertebral body while flexion distraction was applied with the contact hand on the L3 spinous process. Both the clinicians and the patient were satisfied with an approximately 75% relief of pain. As usual, this patient had short hamstring muscles. We see this so commonly in degenerative spondylolisthesis. The appropriate proprioceptive neuromuscular facilitation was utilized in stretching these hamstrings. The patient was given knee-chest exercise and abdominal strengthening exercises; he attended low back wellness school.

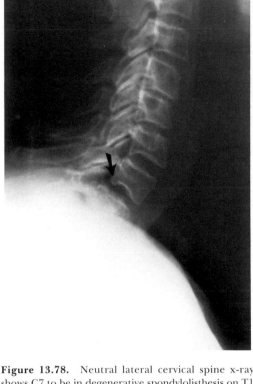

Figure 13.78. Neutral lateral cervical spine x-ray shows C7 to be in degenerative spondylolisthesis on T1 (*arrow*). There is also a kyphosis of the sagittal cervical curve.

Pseudosacralization with Pseudospondylolisthesis

CASE 13

Degenerative spondylolisthesis at L4 is much more common in females than males. However, this case represents a 74-year-old white married male who has low back and occasional bilateral leg pain, which is aggravated upon ambulation. Figure 13.87 reveals the degenerative spondylolisthesis, approximately 10%, of L4 on L5. Oblique projections (Fig. 13.88) reveal that there is no fracture of the pars interarticularis; however, there is marked degenerative change of the articular facets at the L4-L5 and L5-S1 levels bilaterally. Compare these facets with those of the upper lumbar spine. Note the transitional segment at L5, realizing that pseudospondylolisthesis occurs four times more frequently with transitional segment (50) (Fig. 13.89). Treatment of this case consisted of flexion distraction over a small flexion roll. The response of the patient was very dramatic in that his low back pain eased, and he was able to walk without the discomfort previously encountered.

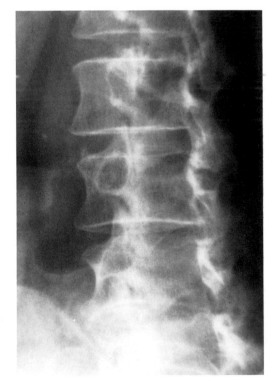

Figure 13.77. Right anterior oblique view shows no pars interarticularis fracture.

UNCOMMON VARIETIES OF SPONDYLOLISTHESIS

Traumatic Spondylolisthesis

Traumatic spondylolisthesis is a fracture of any part of the vertebral arch other than the pars, which allows forward displacement to occur. This type of spondylolisthesis is rare.

Pathological Spondylolisthesis

If the bony hook mechanism (articular facet, pedicle, pars) fails to hold the body of the articulation in place because of local or generalized bone disease, pathological spondylolisthesis can occur. Since pathological spondylolisthesis is rare, only one variant, spondylolisthesis adquista, is mentioned here. In this type, there is a fatigue fracture of the pars at the upper end of a lumbar surgical fusion that allows forward slipping.

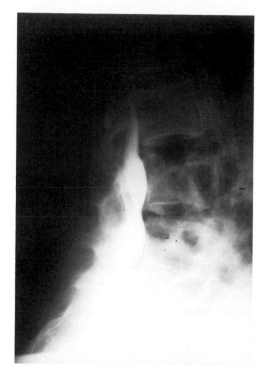

Figure 13.80. Lateral myelogram reveals mild protrusion of the L4-L5 and L5-S1 discs.

CONSERVATIVE TREATMENT OF SPONDYLOLISTHESIS

Testing Patient Tolerance for Distraction

Prior to the application of flexion distraction manipulation, always test the patient's ability to tol-

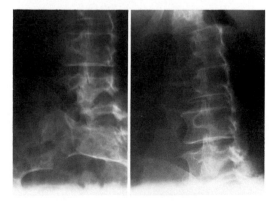

Figure 13.81. Oblique views show no break in the pars interarticularis on either side.

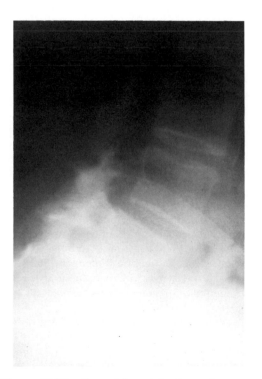

Figure 13.79. Neutral lateral lumbar spine x-ray shows minimal anterolisthesis subluxation of L4 on L5.

erate this form of care. This is done by having the patient lie prone on the table without the ankle cuffs applied. While contacting the spinous process at the level of the problem, as well as above and below this level, apply a mild downward tractive force with the caudal table section. Feel for muscle spasm, and ask the patient if the manipulation causes pain in the back or lower extremity. If pain is produced, this type of treatment is contraindicated until such time as this test procedure proves to be nonpainful. We recommend that therapies in the form of positive galvanism, alternating ice and heat, treatment of acupressure or trigger points, rest in recumbency, and mild exercises be performed if pain is found on testing for tolerance to flexion distraction. It may be hours or days before the patient is adequately relieved of acute pain and inflammation of nerve roots and flexion distraction can be applied. *Always do this preliminary test for adverse effects to flexion distraction prior to its application.*

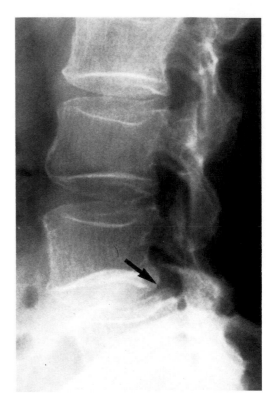

Figure 13.83. Neutral lateral view of a 42-year-old male with low back and buttock pain reveals an anterolisthesis of L4 on L5 (*arrow*).

Flexion-Distraction Treatment of Spondylolisthesis

The treatment of both true lytic and pseudo-degenerative spondylolisthesis is performed with Cox® flexion distraction manipulation. Figure 13.90 shows the flexion Dutchman roll under the spondylolisthetic segment. With this flexion roll in place, all facet motions will be performed as long as the patient does not experience sciatica, which is uncommon with spondylolisthesis.

The contact hand, as shown in Figure 13.91, is placed under the spinous process of the vertebra directly above the spondylolisthetic slip. The thenar pad is the contact with the spinous process so as to minimize pressure against a commonly tender spinous process (Fig. 13.91).

Figure 13.92 shows the contact hand on the spinous process lifting the spine cephalad as the caudal section of the table is placed into downward distraction. We now open the dorsal arch of the spine at the level of contact. This author suggests that *no more than 1 to 2 inches* of downward

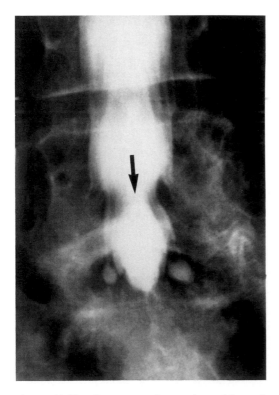

Figure 13.82. Posteroanterior myelographic study reveals narrowing of the dye-filled subarachnoid space at the L4-L5 level (*arrow*).

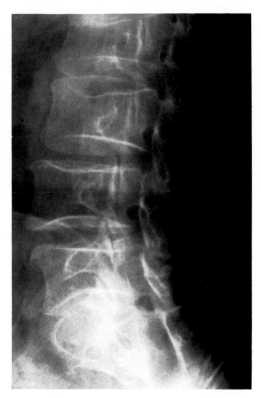

Figure 13.84. Right anterior oblique view shows L4-L5 and L5-S1 facet arthrosis but no pars interarticularis defect.

and gain free flexion mobility. Between 20-second periods, the traction force is released, a new contact made on the spine, and the procedure repeated.

Lateral Flexion Manipulation

Following flexion application, lateral bending of the spinal segment is performed. A contact is made in which the spinous process of the vertebra to be manipulated is grasped between the thumb and index finger (Fig. 13.93). The caudal section is then placed into lateral flexion to test the motion of each facet level (Fig. 13.94). During this motion, the spinous process is resisted by the thumb or index finger on the side to which the table is laterally flexed. If restriction to motion is felt, this facet articulation is not fully executing its physiological motions, and we will continue motion manipulation until mobility is free.

caudal distraction of the table be utilized in this treatment. This 1- to 2-inch downward tractive force is applied after bringing the spine to tautness: that is, while holding the spinous process with the thenar contact of the hand on the spine, the caudal section of the table is lowered until the hip, knee, and spinal joints are taut. This means that these joints are distracted to their limits of joint play, and any further traction will place them beyond normal joint space relief. From this point, we will place the joint under our contact hand into distraction by limiting the downward force on the table to 1 to 2 inches. This minimizes the leverage force applied and prevents excessive tractive force.

We apply flexion distraction until a gentle separation and opening of the spinous processes is felt. This may require only one or two pumps of the caudal table section or several repetitions of five or six such pumping actions in a 20-second period. Up to three 20-second distraction sessions may be necessary to open the vertebral arch

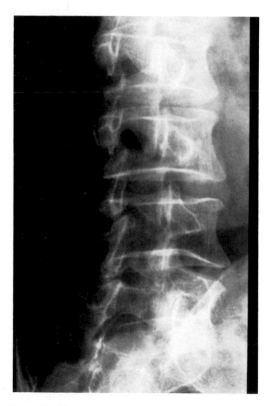

Figure 13.85. Left anterior oblique view shows L4-L5 and L5-S1 facet arthrosis but no pars interarticularis defect.

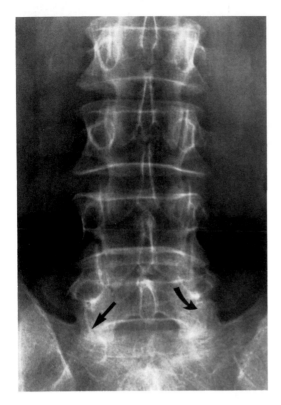

Figure 13.86. Anteroposterior view shows that tropism is suspect at L5-S1, with sagittal facet facings on the right (*straight arrow*) and coronal on the left (*curved arrow*).

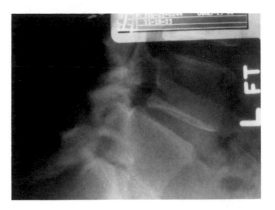

Figure 13.87. Lateral projection shows a 10% slippage of L4 on L5.

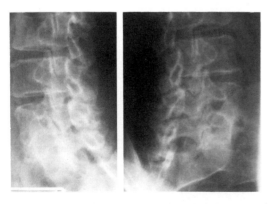

Figure 13.88. Oblique views of patient in Figure 13.87 show no fracture of the pars interarticularis. There is arthrosis of the facet articulations at the lower two levels.

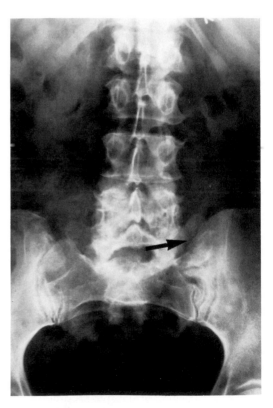

Figure 13.89. Anteroposterior study of patient in Figure 13.87 shows a right pseudosacralization of L5 (*arrow*). Here is a good example of a transitional fifth lumbar segment with degenerative spondylolisthesis of L4 on L5.

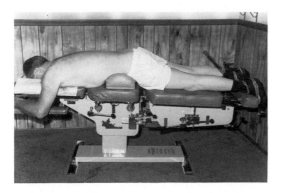

Figure 13.90. With the patient lying prone, a flexion roll is placed under the abdomen at the level of the spondylolisthesis slip. This provides a flexion of the lumbar spine at the level of spondylolisthesis and prepares for application of flexion distraction.

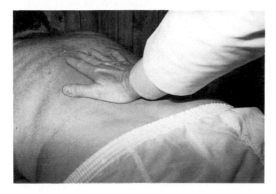

Figure 13.91. Contact is made by the thenar eminence of the doctor's hand under the spinous process of the vertebra above the level of spondylolisthesis.

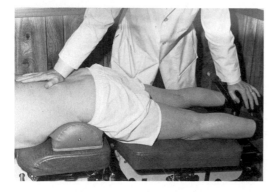

Figure 13.92. While lifting cephalad with the thenar eminence under the spinous process, the caudal section of the table is gently placed into flexion. We recommend that no more than 1 to 2 inches of downward motion be applied with the caudal section of the table.

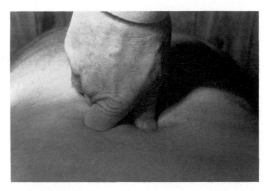

Figure 13.93. To apply lateral flexion, the spinous process at the level of the facets to be manipulated is contacted between the thumb and index finger.

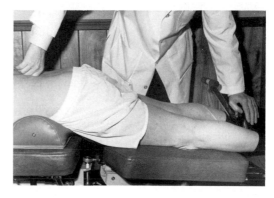

Figure 13.94. Flexion and lateral flexion are applied to the spinal segment while the spinous process is stabilized with the thumb and index finger. This combination of flexion and lateral flexion is called circumduction; it represents the strongest combination for restoring full range of motion to an articular facet.

Foramen Magnum Pump

The foramen magnum pump, or full spine distraction, as demonstrated in Figure 13.95**A** and **B**, is administered. By grasping the occiput in the hand, flexion distraction can be applied from the occiput to the level of spondylolisthesis. Full spine traction is applied to each segment cephalad to the spondylolisthetic segment (Fig. 13.96).

The desired effect of this treatment is to create minimal flexion of the segments, with the Dutchman roll acting as a reduction force on the forward slippage of the spondylolisthesis. The frequency of distraction at each session is as follows: the distraction is applied for an average of three 20-second periods while the contact hand is

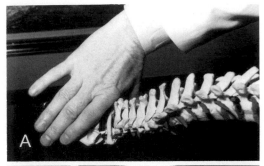

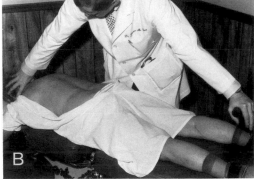

Figure 13.95. **A,** Demonstration of how the occiput is held in the palm of the distracting hand as a cephalad lifting pressure is applied to the occiput while a downward distractive force is applied with the caudal section of the treatment table. This relaxes the suboccipital musculature and tension. **B,** The actual application of the foramen magnum pump is shown on a patient. In applying this technique, be sure to lift cephalad with the tractioning hand on the occiput, and take care not to apply a downward force to the head which causes too much facial pressure into the cushion of the table. Remember, it is not nice to cause the patient pain on top of pain!

on the spinous process directly above the forward slipped segment. During this 20-second distraction, a "milking" action is applied to the segment by maintaining a firm spinous process contact while slowly moving the caudal section of the table up and down, thus achieving a push-pull effect on the posterior elements and intervertebral disc space. This can be sensed under the treating hand, and the relaxation of the patient during this application can be felt. It is important not to fight any resistance of the paravertebral muscles or the voluntary or involuntary contraction of these muscles by the patient. At the outset of care, it is important to gain the patient's confidence so that the patient can relax and allow this manipulation.

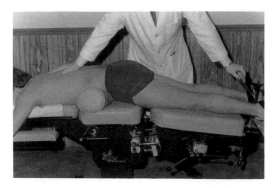

Figure 13.96. By contacting the spinous process of each segment above the spondylolisthetic segment, distraction can be applied at each spinal level.

Side-Lying Application When Pain Prevents Prone Treatment

Figure 13.97 shows the patient lying on his or her side to be given flexion distraction. We do this when the patient cannot lie prone due to discomfort. Also, pregnant women are treated in this manner, especially in the last trimester. The spinous processes are held and palpated while the segments are placed into flexion distraction. Lateral flexion can also be applied in this side-lying posture by moving the caudal section up and down from the neutral position.

Figure 13.98 shows side-lying treatment for reverse spondylolisthesis (retrolisthesis).

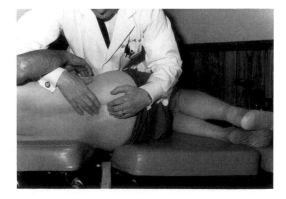

Figure 13.97. With the patient lying on his side, flexion distraction manipulation is applied for spondylolisthesis. This is especially useful for treating patients who have too much pain to lie prone, or pregnant women.

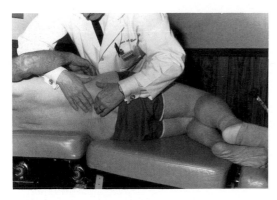

Figure 13.98. Retrolisthesis is shown being treated with the patient lying on the side. The caudal section is brought into extension as pressure is exerted on the spinous process of the segment that the doctor wishes to place into extension. Here we see pressure placed on the L5 spinous process as the caudal section is brought into the extension movement.

Further Technique and Treatment Description

Note: A 1- to 2-inch downward movement on the caudal section of the table is maximum in the treatment of spondylolisthesis. This is not the time to be a "macho" clinician. It is recommended that the pressure of one finger on the caudal section is adequate. The Dutchman roll acts as a fulcrum that reduces the need for strong distractive force.

Lateral flexion is applied to check for hypomobility of the articular facets; if hypomobility is found, the facets are put through their full range of motion so as to bring them back to their physiological mobility.

The paravertebral muscles can then be treated with physical modalities if needed. These modalities might well include positive galvanism to reduce inflammation and sedate irritated tissues or sinosoidal currents to return normal tone to the musculature (Figs. 13.99 and 13.100).

A belt support may be worn if the patient is in acute pain, but this is only a temporary measure (Fig. 13.101). Exercises for the spondylolisthesis patient are extremely important. We most often use the first three Cox exercises in the treatment of spondylolisthesis. Hamstring-stretch exercises (Fig. 13.102) are very important to regaining normal lumbopelvic rhythm.

In a study of 47 patients with symptomatic back pain secondary to spondylolisthesis who were treated with flexion and extension exercises of the lumbar spine, it was found that patients

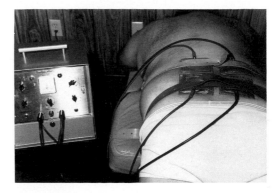

Figure 13.99. Application of positive galvanism or tetanizing current.

treated with flexion type exercises were less likely to require back supports, require modification of their jobs, or limit their activities because of pain (93). In this study, 19 patients were treated with extension type exercises in addition to flexion exercises, and 28 patients were treated with only flexion exercises of the lumbar spine. At follow-up evaluation, treatment results from the two groups were compared. Eighty-two percent of those who underwent flexion exercises stated that they had less pain, whereas 37% of those who did only extension exercises stated that they had less pain. The flexion group was found to have less pain, less need to modify their work, less need for continued use of bracing, and a greater chance of recovery. The type of spondylolisthesis had no effect on the response to flexion exercises.

Figures 13.103 and 13.104 reveal the effects

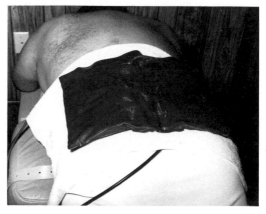

Figure 13.100. Cryotherapy is added to relieve inflammatory effects of low back pain.

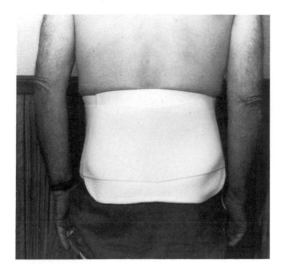

Figure 13.101. A lumbosacral support is worn in unstable spondylolisthesis cases.

of flexion exercises on the lumbar spine in a patient performing abdominal strengthening exercises. Please note that extension exercises are to be avoided in spondylolysis and spondylolisthesis, as they have been shown to increase the pain not only in gymnasts but also in the general public.

RESULTS OF TREATMENT FOR SPONDYLOLISTHESIS

Analysis of the Results of Chiropractic Treatment of Spondylolisthesis

In 1981, Lenz (95) reported on the results of chiropractic treatment of spondylolisthesis. The following notes are given from his report.

Using the "time-honored" specific side posture technics, we treated 10 cases of "olisthesis" (3 males, 7 females) and achieved the following results: 4 of the 10 (40%) showed excellent, good, or fair results and 6 of the 10 (60%) either showed no change or, unfortunately, were made worse.

Since learning the lumbar flexion distraction technic as taught by J.M. Cox, D.C., Fort Wayne, Indiana, we can now report a more favorable outcome in 15 cases of olisthesis and 1 case of "oloptosis": 86.6% showed a favorable outcome (excellent, good, or fair results) and only 13.4% showed poor outcome.

The age of these patients ranged from 20 years (8 years since onset of symptoms) to 62 years (30 years since onset of symptoms). Of these 15, 4 were men and

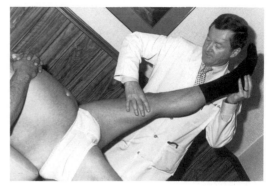

Figure 13.102. Proprioceptive neuromuscular facilitation is used to stretch the hamstring muscles in spondylolisthesis cases.

11 were women. The sex or age of the patient did not affect the results.

In only 2 cases could we detect any measurable difference in the olisthetic movement following treatment and that was only a 3% and a 5% improvement in position. In all of the other cases, there was no measurable difference. In the 1 case of oloptosis, there was also no detectable change of position.

The procedure used was mild lumbar flexion distraction with the use of a Dutchman roll under the abdomen. After distraction, any severe lateral misalignment of adjacent bony structures was specifically corrected (as much as possible) by a mild side posture technique. The patient was then instructed in a simple exercise to do at home to loosen the hamstring muscles.

The patient was then placed in a supine position with both the hips and the knees flexed at 90°, with the calf of the leg supported in that position. While in this position the patient was given a 20- to 30-minute period of very mild short-wave diathermy, with one pad under the cervical area and the other under the lumbar area. Only one patient required the use of an orthopedic lumbar restraint, and that was used more for abdominal support than for lumbar support.[a]

Effectiveness of Spinal Adjustment for Spondylolisthesis

The effectiveness of spinal manipulation therapy for low back pain was compared in two groups of patients: 25 patients with lumbar spondylolisthesis and 260 patients without spondylolisthesis. The result of manipulative treatment was not significantly different in those patients with or without lumbar spondylolisthesis (96). The authors of

[a] From Lenz W: Spondylolisthesis and spondyloptosis of the lower lumbar spine: a microstudy. *ACA J Chiropractic* 15: S107–S110, 1981.

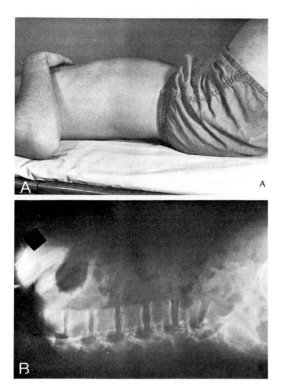

Figure 13.103. **A**, Photograph showing a decrease in lumbar lordosis while the subject is lying supine with the knees bent. **B**, Roentgenogram of spinal column while the subject is lying supine with the knees bent and is performing the pelvic-tilting exercise. (Reproduced with permission from Gramse RR, Sinaki M, Ilstrup DM: Lumbar spondylolisthesis—a rational approach to conservative treatment. *Mayo Clinic Proceedings* 55: 681–686, 1980.)

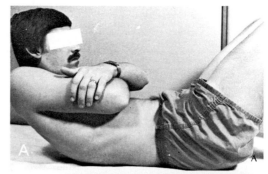

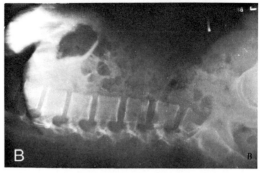

Figure 13.104. **A**, Photograph of the subject performing abdominal strengthening exercise. **B**, Roentgenogram of spinal column while the subject performs abdominal strengthening exercise. (Reproduced with permission from Gramse RR, Sinaki M, Ilstrup DM: Lumbar spondylolisthesis—a rational approach to conservative treatment. *Mayo Clinic Proceedings* 55: 681–686, 1980.)

this study chose to manipulate the level of the spine above or below the demonstrated level of spondylolisthesis. They found that 80% of the spondylolisthesis group had a good result with manipulation, versus 77% in the overall study. They concluded that spondylolisthesis does not contraindicate spinal manipulation, and in fact manipulation is an appropriate treatment for this condition.

Effectiveness of Surgical Treatment for Spondylolisthesis

This chapter concludes with a comment on surgical outcome in grade 3 and 4 spondylolisthesis. Eleven patients in this category were treated nonsurgically, as compared with 21 patients in whom

the same degrees of spondylolisthesis were treated by posterior interlaminar fusion. Of the nonsurgical group, at an average follow-up of 18 years, four (36%) were nonsymptomatic, six (55%) had mild symptoms, and only one had significant symptoms. Five (45%) had one or more neurological findings, but none were incontinent. All of the patients in this group led an active life, and all had required only minor adjustments in their lifestyle.

Of the 21 surgical patients, at an average follow-up of 24 years, 12 (57%) were asymptomatic, eight (38%) had mild symptoms, and only one had significant symptoms. Nine (50%) of the 18 patients who had a physical examination had one or more neurological findings (97).

As stated earlier in this chapter, Saraste (36) found no statistically significant differences between surgically and conservatively treated spondylolisthesis patients with respect to frequency of symptoms, functional impairment, degree of spondylolysis, or progression of slippage.

In summation, spondylolisthesis is an entity well controlled by conservative measures such as manipulation, and few cases require surgical fusion. Remember, gentle manipulation as described in this chapter produces the best clinical result.

References

1. Friberg O: Lumbar instability: a dynamic approach by traction-compression radiography. *Spine* 12(2):119–129, 1987.
2. Newman PH: Spondylolisthesis: its cause and effect. *Ann Coll Surg Engl* 16:305, 1955.
3. Kilian HF: Schilderungen neuer Beckenformen and ihres Verhalten im leben Bassermann und Mathy. Mannheim, 1854 (cit da Brocher).
4. Robert (zu Koblenz): Eine eigentumliche angeborene Lordose, wahrseheinlich bedingt eine Verschiebung des Korpers des letzten Lindenwirbels auf die vordere Flaches des ersten Kreuzheinwirbels (Spondylolisthesis Kilian), nebst Bermerlsungen über die Mechanik dieser Beckenenformation. *Monatsschr Geburtskunde Frauenkrank* 5:81–94, 1855.
5. Neugebauer F: Die Entschung der Spondylolisthesis. *Zentrable Gynaekol* 5:260–261, 1881.
6. Wiltse L, Newman PH, Macnab I: Classification of spondylosis and spondylolisthesis. *Clin Orthop* 117:23–29, 1976.
7. Newman PH: The aetiology in spondylolisthesis. *J Bone Joint Surg* 45B:39–59, 1963.
8. Newman PH: Spondylolisthesis. *Physiology* 60:14, 1974.
9. Wiltse LL: Spondylolisthesis and its treatment. In Finneson BE: *Low Back Pain*. Philadelphia, JB Lippincott, 1980.
10. Wynne-Davis R, Scott JHS: Inheritance and spondylolisthesis: a radiographic family survey. *J Bone Joint Surg* 61B:301–305, 1979.
11. Rosenberg NJ, Bargar WL, Friedman B: The incidence of spondylolysis and spondylolisthesis in non-ambulatory patients. *Spine* 6(1):35–38, 1981.
12. Scoville WB, Corkill G: Lumbar spondylolisthesis with ruptured disc. *J Neurosurg* 40:529–534, 1974.
13. Pfeil E: Experimentelle Untersuchunngen zur Frage der Entstehung der Spondylolyse. *Z Orthop* 109:231, 1971.
14. Krenz J, Troup JDG: The structure of the pars interarticularis of the lower lumbar vertebrae and its relation to the etiology of spondylolysis: with a report of a healing fracture in the neural arch of a fourth lumbar vertebra. *J Bone Joint Surg* 55B:735, 1973.
15. Sullivan JD, Farfan HF: The crumpled neural arch. *Orthop Clin North Am* 6:199, 1975.
16. Rowe GG, Roche MB: The etiology of separate neural arch. *J Bone Joint Surg* 35A:102, 1953.
17. Finneson BE: *Low Back Pain*, ed 2. Philadelphia, JB Lippincott, 1980, pp 453, 456–491.
18. Farfan HF: *Mechanical Disorders of the Low Back*. Philadelphia, Lea & Febiger, 1973.
19. Troup D: Paper read at the meeting of the International Society for the Study of the Lumbar Spine, London, 1975.
20. Hutton WC, Cyron BM: Spondylolysis: the role of the posterior elements in resisting the intervertebral force. *Acta Orthop Scand* 49:604–609, 1978.
21. Macnab I: *Backache*. Baltimore, Williams & Wilkins, 1977.
22. Semon RL, Spengler D: Significance of lumbar spondylolysis in college football players. *Spine* 6(2):172–174, 1981.
23. Maldague B, Mathurin P, Malghem J: Facet joint arthrography in lumbar spondylolysis. *Radiology* 140:29–36, 1981.
24. Duda M: Elite lifters at risk for spondylolysis. *Physicians and Sports Medicine* 15(10):57–59, 1987.
25. McCarroll J, Miller J, Ritter M: Lumbar spondylolysis and spondylolisthesis in college football players. *Am J Sports Med* 14(5):404–405, 1986.
26. Troup JDG: Mechanical factors in spondylolisthesis and spondylolysis. *Clin Orthop* 117(June): 62–63, 1976.
26a. Froom P, Froom J, Van Dyk D, Caine Y, Rabik J, Margaliot S, Floman Y: Lytic spondylolisthesis in helicopter pilots. *Aviat Space Environ Med* 55: 556–557, 1984.
27. Froom P, Ribak J, Tendler Y, Cyjon A, Kriwisky M, Gross M: Spondylolithesis in pilots: a follow-up study. *Aviat Space Environ Med* (June):588–589, 1987.
28. Hall FM: *Controversies in Lumbosacral Spine Radiography: Indications, Projections, and Clinical Implications*. Boston, MA, Beth Israel Hospital, Department of Radiology.
29. Lowe J, Libson E, Ziv I, Nyska M, Flaman Y, Bloom RA, Rohin GC: Spondylolysis in the upper lumbar spine: a study of 32 patients. *J Bone Joint Surg* 69B:582–589, 1987.
30. Rothman SLG, Glenn WV Jr: CT multiplanar reconstruction in 253 cases of lumbar spondylolysis. *AJNR* 5:81–90, 1984.
31. Rothman SLG, Glenn WV: *Multiplanar CT of the Spine*. Rockville, MD, Aspen, 1985.
32. Schneidermer G, Flannigan B, Kingston S, Thomas J, Dillin WH, Watkins RG: Magnetic resonance imaging in the diagnosis of disc degeneration: correlation with discography. *Spine* 12(3): 276–281, 1987.
33. Vanharanta H, Sachs BL, Spivey MA, Guyer RD, Hochschuler SH, Rashbaum RF, Johnson RG, Ohnmeiss D, Mooney V: The relationship of pain

provocation to lumbar disc deterioration as seen by CT/discography. *Spine* 12(3):295–298, 1987.

34. Halperin N, Copeliovitch L, Schachner E: Radiating leg pain and positive straight leg raising in spondylolysis in children. *J Pediatr Orthop* 3: 486–490, 1983.

35. Ghelman B, Doherty JM: Demonstration of spondylolysis by arthrography of the apophyseal joint. *Am J Radiol* 130:986–987, 1978.

36. Saraste H: Long-term clinical and radiological follow-up of spondylolysis and spondylolisthesis. *Pediatr Orthop* 7:631–638, 1987.

37. Boxall D, Bradford DS, Winter RB, Moe JH: Management of severe spondylolisthesis in children and adolescents. *J Bone Joint Surg* 61A:479–495, 1979.

38. Bunnell WP: Back pain in children. *Orthop Clin North Am* 13:587–604, 1982.

39. Dandy DJ, Shannon MJ: Lumbosacral subluxation (group I spondylolisthesis). *J Bone Joint Surg* 53B: 578–595, 1971.

40. Laurent LE, Osterman K: Operative treatment of spondylolisthesis in young patients. *Clin Orthop* 117:85–91, 1976.

41. Newmann PH: A clinical syndrome associated with severe lumbosacral subluxation. *J Bone Joint Surg* 47B:472–481, 1965.

42. Newman PH: Stenosis of the lumbar spine in spondylolisthesis. *Clin Orthop* 115:116–121, 1976.

43. Osterman K, Lindholm TS, Laurent LE: Late results of removal of the loose posterior element (Gill's operation) in the treatment of lytic lumbar spondylolisthesis. *Clin Orthop* 117:121–128, 1976.

44. Fredrickson BE, Baker D, McHolick WJ, et al.: The natural history of spondylolysis and spondylolisthesis. *J Bone Joint Surg* 66A:699–707, 1984.

45. Wiltse LL, Jackson DW: Treatment of spondylolisthesis and spondylolysis in children. *Clin Orthop* 117:92–100, 1976.

46. Wiltse LL: Spondylolisthesis: classification and etiology. In *Symposium on the Spine, American Academy of Orthopaedic Surgeons*. St. Louis, CV Mosby, 1969, pp 143–168.

47. Swenson M: Neurogenic claudication due to pseudospondylolisthesis. *Am Fam Physician* 28(4): 250–252, 1983.

48. Dall, BE, Rowe DE: Degenerative spondylolisthesis, its surgical management. *Spine* 10(7):668–672, 1985.

49. Junghann SH: Spondylolisthesis Ohne spalt in Zwischengelen Kstuck. *Arch Orthop Unfall-chir* 29: 118–127, 1930.

50. Macnab I: Spondylolisthesis with an intact neural arch—the so-called pseudo-spondylolisthesis. *J Bone Joint Surg* 32B:325–333, 1950.

51. Newman PH: Surgical techniques for spondylolisthesis in the adult. *Clin Orthop* 117:106–111, 1976.

52. Rosenberg NJ: Degenerative spondylolisthesis, surgical treatment. *Clin Orthop* 117:112–120, 1976.

53. Rosenberg NJ: Degenerative spondylolisthesis, predisposing factors. *J Bone Joint Surg* 57A: 467–474, 1975.

54. Rissanen RM: Comparison of pathologic changes in intervertebral discs and interspinous ligaments of the lower part of the lumbar spine in light of autopsy findings. *Acta Orthop Scand* 34:54–65, 1964.

55. McAfee PC: Computed tomography in degenerative spinal stenosis. *Clin Orthop* 161:221–234, 1981.

56. Potter RM, Norcross JR: Spondylolisthesis without isthmic defect. *Radiology* 643:678–684, 1954.

57. Verbiest H: A radicular syndrome from developmental narrowing of the lumbar vertebral canal. *J Bone Joint Surg* 36B:230–237, 1954.

58. Junghanns H: Spondylolisthesis, 30 pathologischanatomisch Untersuchte. *Klin Chir* 158:554, 1929.

59. Neugebauer FI: *Zentrabl Gynaekol* 5:260, 1981.

60. Arnoldi CC: Intervertebral pressure in patients with lumbar pain: a preliminary communication. *Acta Orthop Scand* 43:129, 1972.

61. Arnoldi CG, Linderholm M, Musselbechler M: Venous engorgement and interosseous hypertension in osteoarthritidy. *J Bone Joint Surg* 54B:409, 1972.

62. Hirsch C, Inglemark BC, Miller M: The anatomical bases for low back pain: studies on the presence of sensory nerve endings in ligamentous, capsular and intervertebral disc structure in the human lumbar spine. *Acta Orthop Scand* 1:33, 1963–1964.

63. Kaplan EB: Recurrent meningeal branch of the spinal nerves. *Bull Hosp Joint Dis* 8(1):108, 1947.

64. Lewin T, Moffet B, Viidilo A: Morphology of the lumbar synovial intervertebral joints. *Acta Morpho Neerl Scand* 4:299, 1962.

65. Pederson ME, Blunck CFJ, Gardner E: The anatomy of lumbosacral posterior primary rami and meningeal branches of spinal nerves (sinu-vertebral nerves) with an experimental study of their functions. *J Bone Joint Surg* 38A:377, 1956.

66. Stilwell DL Jr: The nerve supply of the vertebral column and the associated structures in the monkey. *Anat Rec* 125:139, 1956.

67. Bernini PM, Simmeone FA: Reflex sympathetic dystrophy associated with low lumbar disc herniation. *Spine* 6(2):180–185, 1981.

68. Bogduk N: The innervation of the lumbar spine. *Spine* 8(3):286–290, 1983.

69. Ehrenhaft JL: Development of the vertebral column as related to certain congenital and pathological changes. *Surg Gynecol Obstet* 76:282, 1943.

70. Flerlic DC: The nerve supply of the cervical intervertebral disc in man. *Johns Hopkins Hosp Bull* 113: 347, 1963.

71. Jackson HC, Winkelmann RK, Beck WM: Nerve endings in the human lumbar spinal column and related structures. *J Bone Joint Surg* 48A:1272, 1966.

72. Lindblom K: Technique and results of diagnostic disc puncture and injection. *Acta Orthop Scand* 20: 315, 1951.

73. Luschka H: Die Nerves des menschlichen Wirbelkanales. Verlag der H Lapschen Buchhandellung P.V. 4850:8:1, 1850.

74. Malinsky J: The antogenetic development of nerve terminations in the intervertebral discs of man. *Acta Orthop* 38:96, 1959.

75. Nachemson A: The lumbar spine, an orthopaedic challenge. *Spine* 1(1):59, 1976.

76. Roofe PG: Innervation of annulus fibrosus and posterior longitudinal ligaments, fourth and fifth lumbar level. *Arch Neural Psychiat* 44:100, 1940.

77. Shinohara H: A study on lumbar disc lesions. *J Jpn Orthop Am* 44:553, 1970.

78. Tsukada K: Histologische Studien über die Zwischenwirbel scheibe des menschen. *Altersvander ungena Mitt. Adak. Kioto* 25:1–29, 207–209, 1939.

79. Reilly J, Yong-Ying K, MacKay RW, Kirkaldy-Willis WH: Pathological anatomy of the lumbar spine. In Helfet AJ, Gruebel Lee D, (eds): *Disorders of the Lumbar Spine.* Philadelphia, JB Lippincott, 1978, pp 42–47.

80. Edgar MA, Nundy S: Innervation of the spinal dura mater. *J Neurol Neurosurg Psychiatr* 29:530, 1966.

81. Jaffe R, Appleby A, Arjona V: Intermittent ischemia of the cauda equina due to stenosis of the lumbar canal. *J Neurol Neurosurg Psychiatr* 29:315, 1966.

82. Nelson MS: Lumbar spinal stenosis. *J Bone Joint Surg* 55B:506–512, 1973.

83. Wiltse LL, Kirkaldy-Willis WH, McIvor GWD: The treatment of spinal stenosis. *Clin Orthop* 115: 83–91, 1976.

84. Souter WA, Taylor TKF: Sulphated mucopolysaccharide metabolism in the rabbit intervertebral disc. *J Bone Joint Surg* 52B:371, 1970.

85. Sheldon JJ, Russin LA, Gargans FP: Lumbar spinal stenosis, radiographic diagnosis with special reference to transverse axial tomography. *Clin Orthop* 115:59, 1976.

86. Cauchoix J, Benoist M, Chassaing MD: Degenerative spondylolisthesis. *Clin Orthop* 115:122–129, 1976.

87. Ailsby RL, Wedge JH, Kirkaldy-Willis WH: Managing low back pain. *C.M.E. News, Union of Saskatchewan* 2:81, 1971.

88. Dagi TF, Tarkington MA, Leech JJ: Tandem lumbar and cervical spinal stenosis: natural history, prognostic indices, and results after surgical decompression. *J Neurosurg* 66:842–849, 1987.

89. Crandall PH, Batzdorf U: Cervical spondylotic myelopathy. *J Neurosurg* 25:57–66, 1966.

90. Lunsford LD, Bissonette DJ, Zorub DS: Anterior surgery for cervical disc disease. Part 2. Treatment of cervical spondylotic myelopathy in 32 cases. *J Neurosurg* 53:12–19, 1980.

90a. Epstein NE, Epstein JA, Carras R: Coexisting cervical and lumbar spinal stenosis: diagnosis and management. *Neurosurgery* 15:489–496, 1984.

91. Nugent GR: Clinicopathologic correlations in cervical spondylosis. *Neurology* 9:273–281, 1959.

92. Nurick S: The natural history and the results of surgical treatment of the spinal cord disorder associated with cervical spondylosis. *Brain* 95: 101–108, 1972.

93. Granse RR, Mehrsheed S, Ilstrup DM: Lumbar spondylolisthesis: a rational approach to conservative treatment. *Mayo Clin Proc* 55:681–686, 1980.

94. Jackson DW, Wiltse LL, Cerincione RJ: Spondylolysis in the female gymnast. *Clin Orthop* 117: 68–73, 1976.

95. Lenz W: Spondylolisthesis and spondyloptosis of the lower lumbar spine: a microstudy. *ACA J Chiropractic* 15:S107–S110, 1981.

96. Mierau D, Cassidy JD, McGregory M, Kirkaldy-Willis WH: A comparison of the effectiveness of spinal manipulative therapy for low back pain patients with and without spondylolisthesis. *J Manipulative Physiol Ther* 10:49–55, 1987.

97. Harris IE, Weinstein SL: Long-term follow-up of patients with grade-III and IV spondylolisthesis. *J Bone Joint Surg* 69A:960, 1987.

14

A Neurosurgeon Looks at Low Back Pain

Rudy Kachmann, M.D.

Sometimes one has to say difficult things, but one has to say them as simply as possible.

—G.P. Hardy

Editor's Note: This chapter was requested of Rudy Kachmann, M.D., to detail his daily routine in dealing with the low back pain patient. It is my opinion that Dr. Kachmann's keen clinical ability as a diagnostician and surgeon will help practitioners reach correct opinions in dealing with low back pain patients. I have worked with Dr. Kachmann for 15 years in Fort Wayne in the area of surgical opinion and treatment. Dr. Kachmann's views are his own in this chapter, developed by his successful neurosurgical practice. While some physicians may have differing views, the value of putting the abilities of such an erudite physician and surgeon in print is undeniable.

The best results from a neurosurgical approach to back problems are attained, first of all, when the patient clearly has the problem; when there is a correct diagnosis of the problem; when the patient is psychologically normal, with no obvious secondary gain; and then when the operation is performed by an experienced surgeon. This also assumes that some conservative approach to the problem, if possible, has been followed.

HISTORY

The history is extremely important in instituting correct treatment. If one can pinpoint the initial symptom in the disease process, that can be ex-

tremely helpful. Even in this day of advanced testing equipment, a good history and a good physical examination are really much more important than any diagnostic tests in the great majority of situations, with some exceptions.

It is very important to determine whether the patient is just having back pain or whether, in addition to back pain, there is leg numbness, leg weakness, rectal or vaginal numbness, and/or difficulty walking. The description of the gait by the patient and observation of the patient's walk are extremely important. Of course, it is very important to have the patient remove his or her clothing, except for the underwear and bra, so that one can observe the musculature in motion, as well as determining weight loss or atrophy.

Patients with a spinal cord problem generally will walk with a broad-based, spastic type of gait, with their legs seeming very stiff and far apart. Patients who have lumbar spine problems, ruptured discs, or tumors will describe pain typically in the sciatic distribution, through the buttocks, going down to the whole leg or part of the leg. This usually involves only one extremity, but in advanced cases it can involve both extremities. Patients with spinal tumors will classically complain of bilateral leg pain and bilateral leg numbness. As you are watching them on the examining table, the advanced cases generally will tend to flex their legs to try to relieve their pain. I always ask them what seems to make the pain better or worse, and they quite commonly will state that flexing the leg, curling up in the fetal position, or flexing the body will improve the pain. I remember having a gymnast as a patient. When I walked into the room, I found her lying on the floor, totally curled up in a ball, as she stated that this gave her complete relief. When she straightened out, her terrible sciatic pains returned. Of course, anything that will increase intraspinal pressure, for example, coughing, sneezing, and retching, all accentuate nerve root irritation symptoms. Also, I have found that patients with a problem in their spine, especially in the thoracic and cervical area, have great difficulty raising their body off the bed and will tend to splint themselves and get up with jerking movements, holding their head with both their hands; this can be a useful question or observation.

With disc problems, you classically will have low back pain, which then progresses into buttock pain and eventually pain all the way down the leg, but there is tremendous variation between different patients. A reasonable number of them will have only leg pain and have no back pain at all. When you try to tell them that they are having a back problem and not a leg problem, they tend to be skeptical.

Persistent intolerable thoracic spine pain always makes me concerned about cancer. If this is accompanied by any type of weight loss, of course, this is extremely suspicious. The patient's past history of illnesses is, of course, extremely significant. One needs to know if they have been recently operated on for a tumor or cancer. Invariably, if there is a history of any cancer within the last 5 years or of breast cancer in the last 20 to 30 years, the most common cause of intolerable spinal pain is recurrent cancer. This is especially so in some forms of cancer such as breast, lung, or renal. The probability of that being the cause of a patient's intolerable pain is high; if that is in the history, I think over 90% of the time, a metastatic lesion would be found. So the history of past illnesses is extremely important.

Also, whether the patient smokes a great deal is very important. The incidence of metastasis from lung cancer is extremely high in the brain and spinal column. I probably see a case of metastasis from the lung to the brain or spinal column every 2 weeks. The history of smoking is very important to obtain.

Spinal Disaster

Obviously, if the patient comes in with severe back and leg pain and has alteration of his or her gait, accompanied by complaints of numbness in the legs, rectum, or vagina, that is an extremely important symptom complex and indicates an advanced case of spinal compression. If the patient has a history of back pain progressing to numbness, weakness, and difficulty with urination and bowel control, I generally call this a potential spinal disaster. The reason I name it such is because over the years I have seen this complex of progression enough times, and it occurs uncommonly enough for the average practitioner, chiropractic or medical, that delayed diagnosis or misdiagnosis can occur. For the above reasons, I would like to spend a few moments discussing what I consider to be the potential spinal disaster syndrome.

Spinal disaster generally presents, at first, strictly with back pain: lumbar, thoracic, or cervical. Generally, the patient has sought the help of a chiropractor or medical doctor, and he or she is treated specifically for the back pain because there are no other accompanying symptoms. The pain tends to persist and recurs, and the patient contacts the treating doctor multiple times.

I will digress for a moment and bring this point up. With a patient who repeatedly returns to see or telephones the physician, one must pay some special attention, as something much more serious than expected may be occurring. We all have patients sometimes who seek too much medical attention, but I am much more afraid of the person with the serious illness that might be missed. Repeated contacts made by that patient should always arouse suspicion in the personnel in the office and the treating professional. As a matter of fact, I have a rule in my office, generally, that if a patient makes a second contact within a few days, we just don't handle it on the phone but must see him or her personally in the emergency room or in the office. This will save a number of mistakes. Pain is a subjective complaint and, without accompanying symptoms, one can easily make an error in judgment if one does not know the patient very well.

If the patient has been calling about repeated back pain and has had examinations, but now is calling back and stating that he or she cannot urinate, a possible spinal cord compression is indicated. That patient must be seen immediately and a complete workup instituted. Sometimes the next symptoms can be numbness, or difficulty in walking or in moving the extremities. I have noticed, over the years, that when a patient tells you his or her legs are numb, this can sometimes include some paralysis of the legs. Instead of calling it paralysis, the patient will call it numbness. This is especially true in nonambulatory settings such as hospital beds or nursing homes, where the nurse will have called to tell me that the patient's legs are numb, but when I examine them, I find that in reality what the patient meant is that they are paralyzed. I have personally seen situations where a number of practitioners are involved in treating a condition with this progressive spinal disaster syndrome. This also reduces the likelihood of correct diagnosis because of vacation schedules and on-call situations, and unless one sits down and puts the whole history together, an incorrect diagnosis could be made.

In summary, the history of repeated and progressive cervical, thoracic, and lumbar pain syndrome, progressing into numbness, gait difficulty, paralysis, and bladder, rectal, or bowel symptoms, indicates progressive spinal cord compression and possibly the development of permanent paralysis, if appropriate and rapid medical intervention is not instituted.

I must say, in my area, we have had very little problem with this because of an excellent relationship I have with the chiropractors in my immediate area. They know who to call and who will respond to their concerns. I think it is very important that, if you are practicing in an area, you have a good relationship with a neurologist or neurosurgeon because of the potential severe neurological residuals if immediate treatment is not carried out.

Case in Point

I most recently examined a case that is quite interesting. It involved a persistent low back pain accompanied by elevated temperature. This patient went to the local emergency room a number of times, and laboratory studies of his blood and urinalysis were negative. He then called the offices of the treating professionals a number of times, and after a 10-day period he finally came back to the emergency room with numbness in his legs, difficulty in walking, stiffness in his cervical spine, and a temperature of 105°. This turned out to be a spinal epidural abscess with staphylococcal meningitis. With appropriate surgical drainage of this abscess and intravenous antibiotics for 7 weeks, the patient has made a full recovery. The main lesson, in this case, is that repeated visits to the emergency room, repeated phone calls, and of course a temperature should have been of greater-than-normal concern. Spinal abscesses are not common, but they do occur, and in almost every case there is a history of some infection such as a cat scratch, a dog bite, cutting one's fingers, or a heart infection, lung infection, or septicemia. In this case, the patient had a pilonidal cyst, which had been drained by his wife without the supervision of his physician.

In summary, the history, as you can see, is extremely important: the initial event, the progression of the difficulty, the number of visits the patient makes to your office, or the number of phone calls you receive all might possibly indicate a progressive spinal problem.

My last point regarding the history is that, of course, one has to try to differentiate between organic and functional problems. In this day and age of workmen's compensation, whiplash syndromes, and secondary gain from lawsuits, this complicates the history a great deal. One gets a feeling at times that one has to be a mind reader to determine whether the patient's symptoms are real or not. The ability to separate out hysterical symptoms, functional symptoms, and organic symptoms is a real art. In the end, it may determine how good a professional you really are—the reason being, of course, that you can only determine the correct treatment if you have the accurate diagnosis. Treating patients who have a whiplash syndrome, for example, can worsen the patient's condition and impress on their minds that in reality something is very seriously wrong. Then again, ignoring these patients, and telling them it is all in their head, has not been found to be of any value either. There is a happy medium here which I think each practitioner must determine from years of experience. Of course, in my field of surgery, this situation can be a great deal more serious, as operating on one of these patients in error, when in reality they are having a psychological problem, can be a grave error and may result in life-long disability.

PHYSICAL EXAMINATION

Once I am satisfied with the history, I proceed in the examination. Many times, while examining the patient, I ask questions at the same time to try to extract every bit of information regarding the disease process. I think it is quite important to have the patient undress at least to the underwear and bra, when examining. This may require, in a number of circumstances, that a nurse also be present.

Observation

The first thing I generally do is to observe the musculature, looking for weight gain or loss and trying to observe any possible atrophy. I then will proceed with some range of motion tests of the cervical, thoracic, and lumbar spine to try to estimate any limitations of motion; at the same time, I am also looking for severe muscular spasm or spinal curvature. In severe ruptured disc problems, one can clearly feel that the paravertebral musculature is in severe spasm. The patient generally leans away from the side of the ruptured disc to try to get some pressure off the nerve. Also, the patient generally does not like posterior extension to the side of the main part of the ruptured disc. The straight leg raising test can be done in a sitting position and the supine position. For L3-L4 disc problems, one also can flex the leg with the patient prone, and this sometimes will accentuate the pain. Generally, watching the patient move around on the examining table and in the room, as well as the position he or she is in when you enter the room, can be of great value in diagnosing spinal conditions. Some patients with large, ruptured discs may even have negative straight leg raising tests, and others won't let you raise the leg even 15° without complaining of pain. Dorsiflexing the foot generally accentuates the pain, although not in every case.

Hip Examination

At that point, I also examine both hips. To confuse hip disease with spine disease is quite common. I will talk about this more later. Generally, having the patient place his or her heel on the opposite knee will tell you a great deal about the hip and the patient. I can't help but reiterate that a hip examination is extremely important. I see many patients in my office whose primary problem is hip disease and not a spinal problem. This can be quite confusing, because everybody thinks that, when they have a hip problem, the pain will be in the area of the hip, which it is not. Their pain generally tends to be in the groin on the anterior part of the leg, and a third of the patients

have buttock pain. For those reasons, one can see that these conditions can be very easily confused.

Then I also feel the patient's pulses in his or her feet. Arterial insufficiency in the lower extremities also can present as spinal problems, and I have diagnosed vascular insufficiency in the lower extremities as the cause of a patient's complaint of leg pains on numerous occasions. I remember an occasion when I saw this in a 32-year-old female who came to see me with right leg pain. It never entered my mind that she had a vascular insufficiency syndrome. I saw her again the following week, and she had some blue and black toes, indicating advanced circulatory insufficiency, needing immediate vascular intervention. Even in young people, it is important to check for the dorsalis pedis, popliteal, and femoral pulses.

Motor System

I then proceed to a motor examination, carefully checking the quadriceps, and the flexors and extensors of the hips, knees, and ankles. Of course, the most common weakness in disc problems is weakness in dorsiflexion of the feet. Plantar flexion of the feet seems to be spared in a great number of nerve root compressions and is not of as great a value. Quadriceps weakness is much more predictable. If the patient cannot extend his or her leg properly against resistance, that can indicate with high probability L4 nerve neuritis or compression by a disc or tumor. Diabetic neuropathy may also present with intolerable leg pain and quadriceps weakness, as well as a foot-drop. I will discuss this further in the next section.

Sensory Testing

Sensory examination is done to see if the area of numbness matches reflex changes, weakness, or the patient's symptoms. The problem with sensory examination is that it takes the input of the patient to determine the abnormality. This can result in a hysterical or functional overlay. In other words, detailed extensive sensory examinations in some patients are valueless and can lead one astray. In reality, if there is nothing wrong with the patient, and you do a detailed sensory examination, and the patient claims all sorts of numbness, you are going to have a difficult time explaining to him or her that there is nothing really seriously wrong. This has occurred to me enough times over the years that I have become very selective and careful about sensory exams. I try to do them in the right situation and don't hang my hat on them. If sensory abnormality is your only finding, be very careful, because in the majority of cases you will not have much to go on. When doing spinal testing, say for a spinal cord tumor, and one runs a pin on the patient and reaches a certain level at which you can see him wince and jump and the pain is worse, generally that is quite reliable. To do dermatomal analysis of sensory examination in patients is very tricky, and it takes a physician of great experience to interpret the results. Generally, new practitioners fall for this, and it takes a number of years before one finally realizes that the sensory examination has its place but one generally doesn't like to hang one's hat on it, if that is the only finding. As mentioned above, if one is suspicious of a spinal tumor, the thing to do is to undress the patient, take a safety pin, start on the heels and run it all the way up the patient's extremity. If the patient can clearly show you the level where the sensation becomes much sharper, this can be of clear value. Observing the patient can be of more value than what he is telling you because, as you reach the critical area, he may jump or pull up or have some reflex to indicate the true, organic nature of what you suspect.

Reflex Examination

The reflex examination is very important in the lower extremities. A general rule to follow is that, if both reflexes are absent, for example, at the ankles, it may or may not mean anything. Bilaterally absent ankle reflexes do occur in the population and may not be of diagnostic value. If the patient has pain down his or her leg, with an absent ankle reflex on that side and a normal one on the opposite leg, the odds of that being significant, I would think, would run 99% or higher. Previous ankle surgery in the area may affect the reflexes. If the patient is a diabetic, he or she may have no reflexes whatsoever in the knees or ankles to begin with. That may be a confusing point. Absent reflexes can mean diabetic neuropathy. With a history of diabetes, it can be of significance.

In spite of all that, the patient may have a ruptured disc, and one has to be careful making a diagnosis. An absent knee reflex, with a normal one on the opposite side, can be of great value in indicating a ruptured L3-L4 disc or an L4 nerve root neuritis such as diabetic femoral neuropathy. If both ankle reflexes are present and both knee re-

flexes are absent, this probably is a meaningful finding, indicating some problem at the L3-L4 level. If the reflexes are hyperactive, that could indicate spinal cord involvement of the thoracic or cervical area from myelopathy related to spinal cord compression from arthritis, spinal tumor, or demyelinating diseases of the spinal column.

Multiple sclerosis presents with hyperactive reflexes in the arms and legs, spastic gait, and not uncommonly, numbness in the feet. These patients generally do not have any spinal pain, and this is a good differentiating symptom.

Observing the patient's walk is extremely important; sometimes I sit across the hall and watch the patient walk into the examining room or will ask him or her to walk down the hall or in the examining room. This can be of great value. Also, specific tests will sometimes have to be done to determine rectal tone, and it may take an experienced proctologist and his equipment to make a judgment. A urologist also may have to be called in to do a cystometric testing of the bladder to determine whether the patient has a neurogenic bladder or not. These tests can be of great importance and significance in individual cases.

CONFUSING CAUSES OF BACK PAIN, LEG PAIN, AND NUMBNESS

Diabetic Neuropathy

In obtaining the history from the patient, the history of diabetes can be extremely significant. Over 50% of diabetics will develop some form of neurological complication from the diabetes. For the above reasons, just like the history of cancer, diabetes is very important to keep in mind. The pain of diabetic neuropathy can be so severe that it can simulate cancerous pain or a ruptured disc. It is quite common to face a diagnostic dilemma when attempting on the basis of history and physical examination to distinguish a disc or tumor from a diabetic neuropathy. Sometimes a patient will come in with bilateral symptoms of arms and legs, accompanied by numbness and muscular atrophy, and the differentiation of diabetic neuropathy from more advanced debilitating neurological diseases will be necessary.

Amyotrophic Lateral Sclerosis

Occasionally one sees a patient with a severe curvature and back pain and the problem is Lou Gehrig's disease (amyotrophic lateral sclerosis).

This disease is characterized by severe muscular weakness, severe muscular atrophy, and constant fasciculation of the musculature. The muscles will be jumping throughout the shoulders and lower extremities. These patients have no numbness whatsoever. This disease can start in the legs, in the arms, or at times even in the throat. In the latter case, the patient will have difficulty talking as the initial symptom. I remember seeing one patient come in with a severe kyphosis, and it turned out that he had amyotrophic lateral sclerosis.

Discitis

Disc space infections are an unusual, uncommon entity, but when they occur they are quite interesting. The pain from a disc space infection is extremely severe and probably is one of the severest pain syndromes that I have seen. These patients generally object to anyone even walking into the room, touching their bed, manipulating them, or moving them about the room. They find any sort of movement or vibration to be extremely painful. They generally look ill. They may have a temperature or they may not. The clue in disc space infections generally is that the patients look quite ill and have intolerable pain. As a matter of fact, the thought may cross your mind that they have cancer in the spine, because they look that ill. Causes of disc space infections include urinary tract infections, septicemia, and rarely, previous recent disc surgery. The diagnosis is generally made by history, examination, and x-ray. The blood sedimentation rate is extremely elevated in every case and can sometimes be the only clearly positive diagnostic test. X-ray changes may not occur for a period of time.

Cancer

The diagnosis of cancer as a cause of spinal pain is quite common. Every treating professional must be aware at all times of the patient harboring a known or hidden cancer as the cause of his or her pain. If the history of cancer is elicited, then one of course may have a fairly easy time making a diagnosis based on plain x-rays, bone scans, and possibly CT or MRI scanning. Plain x-rays may not reveal the cancer every time, and a bone scan can be much more diagnostic. Clues of this condition generally are persistent, progressive pain resulting in repeated phone calls, repeated examinations, and treatments without success. If this situation arises, be aware of the possibility of

cancer. I have seen a number of cases, over the years, in which these patients have been going from doctor to doctor, or from chiropractor to chiropractor, and possibly seeing both. The diagnosis is not made until the disease is very advanced, and much unhappiness can result for the treating professional and, most importantly, for the poor patient.

SPECIFIC LOW BACK SYNDROMES

I would like to, at this point, discuss disc and spinal syndromes at specific levels. Generally, 85% of all ruptured discs occur between the L4-L5 and L5-S1 level. About 15% occur at the L3-L4 level; perhaps 1 or 2% occur at the L2-L3 and, very rarely, at the L1-L2 level. I have seen ruptured discs at those levels, but they are extremely rare and present generally as cauda equina syndromes such as a spinal tumor.

Stenosis

Spinal stenosis narrowing of the spinal column from arthritis and degeneration of the spine has become an extremely common diagnosis in the last few years. With an aging population, this will increase in frequency even further. These patients usually do not present with an acute problem, such as might be seen with a severely ruptured disc, but occasionally this will occur. Stoic patients, especially, may come in acting completely like patients with a ruptured disc but in reality will have severe spinal stenosis. The majority of these patients' symptoms are chronic, being progressive over many years. Classically, they will have what is called spinal claudication. This is pain on ambulation, which will attenuate itself. If the patient stops and flexes forward and stands there for a few minutes, the pain tends to improve. This, of course, can be confused with vascular claudication, as patients with the latter condition also present with bilateral leg pain when walking, which is improved by resting. Many times, a spinal stenosis case will present with unilateral leg pain but some are bilateral, and act like an acute disc because the progression has become so severe that specific nerve root syndromes present themselves. I have seen cases where spinal stenosis is so severe that the patient will come in with atrophy of the lower extremities. I recall one case where the patient came to the office in a wheelchair. She had severe atrophy of the lower extremities to the point that she looked like a stork. The patient had severe bilateral leg pain and had been seen by many different practitioners, but no one really ever came up with a diagnosis. When a patient sees many different practitioners, I find that he or she is much more likely to have an incorrect diagnosis because no one is consistently looking at the same problems. One must be aware of this also.

Lumbar stenosis can be diagnosed by a combination of history, physical examination, good CT scanning, and lastly a myelogram.

Herniated Disc

L2-L3 ruptured discs tend to present with bilateral leg pain, gait difficulty, bilateral leg numbness, bladder involvement, and sometimes ileus. If there is compression of the cauda equina, patients many times will develop neurogenic bladder and sympathetic involvement of the bowels, and the bowels will distend and not contract. The latter condition is called ileus and does occur in advanced spinal cord or cauda equina compression.

The L3-L4 disc rupture will present with anterior leg pain, weakness in the quadriceps muscle, absent knee reflexes, numbness in the distribution of the L4 nerve root, and difficulty in walking. The patient may state that his or her knee gives out when walking up the stairs. Occasionally, I have seen these patients come in and complain of problems with their knees when in reality the problem was that they didn't have the musculature to support their knees.

Ruptured L4-L5 discs, which are quite common, present as sciatica with pain through the buttocks and down the leg, numbness in the large toe, and weakness in dorsiflexion of the foot. If these conditions are not treated fairly rapidly, sometimes the patient will indeed come in with a complete foot-drop. I have seen patients, over the years, who have been treated for 6 months with therapy or manipulation; they then come to see me with a complete foot-drop, dragging the foot when they walk, and there is really nothing at that point that I can do about it. This must be kept in mind, and these patients must be treated surgically, fairly rapidly. Sometimes it is difficult, on basic clinical examination, to determine who these patients are, but intolerable leg pain, with weakness on dorsiflexion of the foot, generally are the symptoms and findings.

The ruptured L5-S1 disc, compressing the S1 nerve root, will present with typical sciatic pain

through the buttock and down the leg, numbness in the side of the foot, the bottom of the foot, and the lateral plantar surface of the foot, and an absent ankle reflex. This can, on occasion, be the easiest condition to diagnose because of the obvious reflex change.

Spinal Cord Lesions

In involvement of the spinal cord, the patients generally present with numbness in both arms, both legs, or parts of the above; difficulty with their gait; and neurogenic bladder or ileus. Sometimes they will not have pain, although in spinal cord compression, these are the tricky cases. If the patient has a spinal cord tumor, especially in the spine itself (intramedullary tumor), this may be a totally painless situation presenting as arm and leg numbness, difficulty in walking, or neurogenic bladder changes. The confusing diagnosis then could be multiple sclerosis, which is not uncommon, and generally multiple sclerosis patients have no pain and the patients tend to be younger. Occasionally a benign tumor or meningioma in the foramen magnum can be very confusing, with the patient having numbness, reflex changes, and gait problems with no pain of a chronic nature; the patient may even have the history of a negative myelogram, when someone didn't put the dye through the foramen magnum to pick up this rare cause of these symptoms.

Generally, patients with compression of the cervical spinal cord from arthritis will have pain, but not in every case. The thoracic spinal syndromes to watch out for are metastasis from cancer to the thoracic spine. Many of these patients I have seen over the years have been treated with therapy or manipulation and misdiagnosed because nothing is visualized clearly on x-ray and they have no other symptoms. I think the clue here is progressive, eventually severe, pain; and if this patient states that he or she has numbness in the legs or cannot urinate, he or she may have the typical spinal neurogenic disaster syndrome. Tumors of a benign nature, such as neurofibromas, in the lower thoracic and upper lumbar spine can be very difficult to diagnose. There have been many cases over the years where the diagnosis was confused and the correct diagnosis was not made, causing a great deal of disability for the patient. These patients may have chronic back pain, and previous studies may have been negative. Then finally someone does a detailed myelogram over this area and makes the diagnosis. A myelogram done only to the L1 level might miss a neurofibroma sitting at the T9 area. This must be kept in mind, and sometimes this type of study needs to be repeated.

There is no harm in repeating a workup in a patient periodically, for instance, 6 months or 1 or 2 years later, if the initial workup was not productive. This must be kept in mind and the patient referred back to the neurologist or neurosurgeon for repeat workup.

In females one has an additional problem of cancer of the pelvic organs. These patients will tend to present to the practitioner with low back pain; of course, if they have low abdominal pain, one should be quite suspicious of a cancer or endometriosis. A good pelvic examination, accompanied by CT scanning of the retroperitoneal space and abdominal content, can be of great value. These cases also tend to be diagnostic puzzles, and they fairly commonly get misdiagnosed because persistent low back and pelvic pain are found without other symptoms in a female patient who may possibly be nervous and neurotic-appearing. I have seen this numerous times over the years, and have concluded that one has to be very suspicious to avoid making a mistake, and repeat the examinations periodically and/or adjust one's thinking or diagnosis about the patient as different situations arise. The crux of the problem in these cases is to try to determine what is functional and what is organic, and proceed accordingly. This can, of course, be extremely difficult.

DIAGNOSTIC TESTS

As mentioned previously, I still feel that the history and examination are the most important factors in the correct diagnosis. This, in today's era of modern diagnostic tests, is forgotten by many professionals. Taking the history and performing an examination are the cheapest things you can do, and the most valuable. Repeated, excellent, complete examinations have more value than repeated multiple diagnostic tests in the majority of cases. Generally, the next step after the above is to take good plain x-rays. This should include AP, lateral, and oblique views, as well as possibly some taken in flexion and in extension. I think that good quality x-rays at this point are very important.

CT and MRI

In the lumbar spine, the next test of greatest value is a CT scan. Computerized tomography gives you an excellent view of the skeleton and can be quite diagnostic for fractures and spinal stenosis; it probably will detect intraspinal tumor in about 75% of the cases. Magnetic resonance imaging scanning (MRI scanning) is not as reliable as CT scanning at this time. This was the opinion of our last National Association Neurosurgical Meeting in Dallas. I find that magnetic resonance imaging scanning is ordered much too often by treating physicians and leads to false-negative and false-positive tests. How often I see a patient in the office with a "positive MRI scan," when in reality the patient doesn't even have a pain down his leg, and the scan probably should not have been ordered in the first place. These are very expensive scans, and I think are much overprescribed. CT scanning also is not necessary in every case, but it can be an intermediate test if no neurosurgical consultation is planned. Certainly, in obvious cases, where the patient has a clear-cut sciatica, severe pain, numbness, weakness, and/or reflex changes, the surgeon may decide to operate on the basis of a CT scan or on the basis of a myelogram. I don't think both tests would have to be ordered; I think one would be sufficient. Hopefully, the treating professional has CT scanning available at a local hospital, as we have in Fort Wayne; it can be of great help in his or her practice. As mentioned, MRI scanning should generally be reserved for spinal tumors at this time. This suggestion probably will change in the next few years.

Electromyography (EMG)

Electromyographic examination can sometimes be of value. Hopefully, this is available through a local neurologist. The specialist in that field can generally differentiate muscular disease from nervous disease and indicate to you whether there is muscular or neuritic involvement. I would not operate completely on the basis of an EMG finding unless it is accompanied by CT or myelographic confirmation. The neurologist performing EMGs can, for example, differentiate diabetic neuropathy from a ruptured disc for you.

With my experience and in my hands, at least, I still find the myelogram to be extremely important. I don't feel that we are anywhere near the stage where a CT or MRI scan could replace the myelographic test. I find that the myelogram really is a physiological test in addition to a pure x-ray test. In other words, if I see a complete block to the dye on the myelogram, there is a very high probability that the patient's symptoms are related to that block. On the other hand, just because I see narrowing on a CT scan does not prove significant compression of the spinal column. I would never operate just on the basis of a stenosis present on the CT scan. I know of some surgeons who do, and I think they will make a lot of mistakes, do unneeded surgery, and have questionable results.

Bone Scan

The importance of obtaining a bone scan when one is suspicious of infectious or carcinomatous diseases must be stressed. Laboratory tests for blood sugars, blood counts, and sedimentation rates are also very important. Occasionally, chronic leukemia, like multiple myeloma, will present with constant back pain. Multiple myeloma is a carcinoma of the bone marrow, patients suffering from it generally complain of pain, pain, pain. They have a very severe pain problem, and on x-ray many times will have multiple compression fractures. If this happens in an elderly person, it may be diagnosed as osteoporosis, and sometimes osteoporosis and multiple myeloma are difficult to differentiate. Generally, the patients with myeloma look quite ill and are losing weight, and the diagnosis is fairly obvious, although in the early stages, obviously, this is not the case.

Anyone with multiple compression fractures on x-ray must be considered and worked up for myeloma. This should include a Bence Jones protein and urine test, bone scan, sedimentation rate, and possibly even a bone marrow test. Interpretation of the myelogram can be difficult. Patients with a ruptured disc at the L5-S1 level sometimes don't show a large defect, or any defect at all, because of the coning of the dura at this level. The dye just doesn't cover that interspace well, and the test may be negative or may show only minimal nerve root impingement. At the L4-L5 level, there may be only minimal defect over the nerve root although the patient is having intolerable leg pain, numbness, and foot-drop. At the L3-L4 level, sometimes there is only a small lateral defect although the patient has an absent knee reflex, weak quadriceps muscle, and numbness in the L4 nerve root, and has difficulty in walking. Occasionally the disc ruptures are so large that on the myelogram there are complete blocks, with no dye going past the appropriate level. At times, we will pick up a benign or meta-static spinal tumor to account for the pain and numbness when it had been felt the patient could be having a disc problem. Spinal tumors of any type are uncommon compared to benign disc problems.

THE WHIPLASH PROBLEM

The problem of patients complaining of spinal pain following injury due to accidents can be a perplexing one for the treating professional. These patients are very commonly seen in practice. Generally, these patients have been rear-ended by someone going anywhere from 10 to 100 mph. Others have been hit head-on and from the side. From my experience, it is difficult to determine how much of the pain is functional and what percentage is organic.

I am not in the business of reading people's minds, and have developed a stepwise approach, which, I feel, has been useful in treating these problem patients.

I have found that arguing with these patients, and trying to tell them that their symptoms are not quite as severe as they would seem on the basis of x-rays, examination, and history, is useless. The patients will only become belligerent, and you are not going to help them. I think that the best approach is to obtain a good, thorough history; do a good, thorough examination; obtain some x-rays; and recommend some conservative form of treatment. Good flexion-extension views, plain x-rays of the cervical, thoracic, and lumbar spines are important. This examination may need to be repeated.

A word of caution about x-raying cervical spines might be indicated at this point. Plain x-rays don't discover every fracture of the cervical spine. I think one should be able to examine C1 through T1. If these cannot be visualized properly, then a computerized scan should be obtained. I am convinced that in really severe trauma, CT scanning of the cervical spine is indicated because the plain x-rays of the cervical spine, even of good quality, can miss a significant number of these fractures. I find that good cervical spine examination and CT scanning after the initial injury, perhaps repeated during the hospitalization before discharge, and perhaps repeated again on an outpatient basis, will pick up most of these fractures. If this is not done, they can be missed. Dislocations can occur hours after supposedly normal cervical spine x-rays. Fractures in the C1 and C2 area, especially, can be missed. When you obtain x-rays 1 or 2 weeks later, because the patient continues to complain of neck pain, you may discover dislocation that was not present on the original films. I highly recommend repeat x-rays, including CT scanning, in patients who have had major trauma. If you don't do this, you are going to miss some additional fractures or dislocations over the years, and they can be costly to the patient. Paralysis can set in in a delayed fashion in some of these patients. I think most chiropractors in their lifetime have experienced seeing patients who had previously been treated by physicians and who had, 1, 2, or 3 years later, obtained further x-rays and discovered dislocations that were not present on the original x-rays.

Also, you must keep in mind that the fact that an x-ray is read as negative by a radiologist does not guarantee that it is negative. Occasionally, I have seen that radiologists have missed dislocations. All this proves is that they are human beings like the rest of us, and x-ray reports and readings are not always 100% accurate. Therefore, personal inspection of x-rays is very important if the patient has continuing, repeated complaints.

I generally prefer to treat whiplash or flexion-extension injury symptoms with hot showers, exercises, mild weight-lifting, physical therapy, and chiropractic treatments. These are mainly musculoligamentous types of injury and should be treated conservatively.

The emotional aspect of the case can have an influence on these symptoms, and I think one has to be careful in judging or responding to the patient's complaints. I think that some of the patients get out of hand with their symptoms when there is not that much evidence of injury, yet the symptoms seem to be devastating their lives. There is very little doubt in my mind that they believe they have these symptoms, but their basis in reality probably is marginal in some cases. I generally have found that pointing this out to the patient, or arguing with him or her about it, is most often useless. Occasionally I see a patient get totally out of hand with these symptoms, and generally I will become quite frank with them because they might ruin their lives completely—quit their jobs or break up their marriages over minimally significant medical problems. These patients are difficult to deal with, but occasionally one has to bite the bullet and carry out the job.

I think the best treatment, as mentioned, is exercise, mild weight-lifting, physical therapy, and chiropractic treatments. I do not recommend medications because the patient may well become addicted to muscle relaxants or pain medication. Chronic, benign pain is best treated with exercise, physical therapy, and chiropractic treatment, not with medication. Patients with these types of injuries also are more likely to develop arthritis. Follow-up x-rays years later will many times indicate a post-traumatic arthritic condition. Helping the patient settle these cases from a legal standpoint can also be of value. I find that some patients are not interested in this at all, and legal settlement really doesn't help the patient, so I think it is part of the doctor's general obligation, as unpleasant as the situation may be at times, to help settle such matters.

In summary, I think you have to gauge the injury, the x-rays, and the examination and get some idea about the mental aspect of the patient to treat these problems successfully. I think that if one is very rigid in treating people without understanding the human nature of the medical problem, one could be very unhappy treating these patients; frankly, one probably would be incapable of helping them. Medicine is not quite as predictable as a mathematical problem might be because of the mental aspect of each and every medical problem.

SPONDYLOLYSIS AND SPONDYLOLISTHESIS

Six percent of the population has at least one defect in the pars interarticularus. This is also called spondylolysis. This can be seen in very young people. I remember that, when the Vienna Boys' Choir passed through town, I saw a young choir member in the emergency room at our hospital with a bilateral spondylolysis producing severe muscular spasm and back pain due to riding the bus across the country. If the patient has a bilateral spondylolysis, of course, over the years this may dislocate and develop a typical spondylolisthesis.

The unilateral spondylolysis I generally suggest be treated conservatively with exercises, braces, physical therapy, and chiropractic treatments. These generally are not surgical lesions except in rare situations. If spondylolysis continues to progress over a period of years and causes significant, repeated, untreatable back pain, surgical fusion may be indicated. Certainly the great majority of these cases are best treated with exercises, bracing, physical therapy, and chiropractic treatments. Certainly if the patient develops significant nerve root irritation with bilateral leg pain indicating that the spondylolisthesis is compressing the cauda equina, this is a surgical case. Fusions in general have been in disrepute in the last 10 years because of miserable results in the past.

In the last 3 or 4 years, I have been carefully recommending and performing some fusions in patients with spondylolisthesis and secondary spinal stenosis or compression of the cauda equina. I must say I have been very happy with the results in these carefully selected cases. This seems to indicate that my opinion has been too harsh about the fusions, and that the combination of a good surgical decompression followed by good lateral mass fusion can give you reasonable results in over 90% of cases. The crux of the whole thing, I think, is good patient selection. This means that one must be certain that the patient indeed has this medical condition, and an experienced surgeon must perform the fusion. Certainly, fusions should not be done for low back pain with no evidence of nerve root irritation unless one is dealing with a progressive, intolerable problem. Fusions should never be performed just for low back pain without spondylolysis or spondylolisthesis. Years ago, there were many fusions that were performed just for low back pain in patients without spondylolysis or a dislocation, and the results in general from these operations were very poor.

SURGICAL RESULTS, TECHNIQUES, AND COMPLICATIONS

There are a number of methods of surgically treating an acute lumbar disc condition. Using the micro technique with an incision no longer than an inch, and removing the majority of the disc under magnification, has given me the best results. If the patient clearly has the symptoms, the physical findings, and x-rays to confirm the diagnosis, then I feel I have a 95 to 98% chance of giving the patient good relief with a very low incidence of complications.

I have performed about 5000 disc operations and have had less than six postoperative infections, which all responded to treatment. I have seen two disc space infections with serious complications, which involve bedrest for 1 month and some back bracing for another month. Both of these eventually cleared up, but that is a serious complication. The incidence of disc space infections is extremely low, but it can occur. I have had no incidences of paralysis or foot-drop necessitating the use of bracing. On two occasions, I injured the iliac artery, necessitating surgery on that vessel with full recovery of the patient. Considering the location at which I was operating, one can expect that complication, if one does a great deal of surgery, about every 8 to 10 years. This, of course, can be a fatal complication, but fortunately this did not occur in my patients.

Injecting the disc space with a lytic substance such as chymopapain was extremely popular a few years ago. I and my partners trained in this method for 10 days in Chicago and at Georgetown University, but after going through the course decided it was too risky. It turned out that we were the only city in the United States of our size where no chymopapain injection was ever carried out during this period. We felt that the allergic reaction, resulting in one death per 1000 procedures, was just too risky, considering that I had done 5000 disc operations with no fatalities. Interestingly enough, when I was at our national meeting last year and they asked for a show of hands of how many people were still doing it actively, I could count no more than 15 hands. I must say that there are still some very skilled people in this country, and a number of them also in Canada, who still use this technique and I think use it very well. The complications included death, paralysis, and injury to the nerves and the cauda equina. Also, the disc space itself is so destroyed by the chymopapain that many of these patients have chronic backache. I saw no reason to use this technique when the majority of my patients were going home in 2 to 4 days with smiles on their faces, and I felt personally that I could not improve on that. There are some physicians constantly attempting to change the technique of back surgery based on poor results with the present system of treatment, but I think that the poor results that they cite are the result of poor surgeons, poorly-selected patients, and poor surgical technique.

I think the well-trained neurosurgeon using the micro-technique can have 98% excellent results with a very low complication rate. I think it is very difficult to improve on this technique. I don't think we should just jump at every new thing that comes along and change our way of treating this condition, accepting any new technique because someone is trying to get his name on an article or on television. I think that, unless someone comes along with a very well-studied technique that provides a lower complication rate and better results, we shouldn't attempt to change our method of treatment. In my experience, if the patient really has the diagnosed problem and is in the hands of an experienced surgeon, the results are excellent in the majority of patients.

15

Care of Other Specific Low Back Conditions

James M. Cox, D.C., D.A.C.B.R.

Have the courage to be ignorant of a great many things, in order to avoid the calamity of being ignorant of everything.

—Sidney Smith

DEGENERATIVE SCOLIOSIS OF THE SPINE

The incidence of back pain is no greater in those with adult idiopathic scoliosis than in those persons without scoliosis, but the severity of the pain is greater. Pain increases with age and degree of scoliotic curvature, and patients with major lumbar curves have the worst pain. The pain comes primarily from the concavity of the scoliotic curve; it includes pain of discogenic, facet, and radicular origins (1).

In a study of 50 women with proven osteoporosis and back pain, 48% were found to have at least 10° of structural scoliosis. Compression fractures occurred within these curves but were not felt to be a cause of the scoliotic curve (2). Scoliosis in elderly women may indicate osteoporosis. Negative calcium balance has been documented in one-half of ambulatory, untreated, adolescent idiopathic scoliosis patients (3). Osteoporosis should be aggressively treated for scoliosis prevention in adult women. Fluoride, calcium, physiological vitamin D supplementation, and physical therapy augments bone mass, reduces symptoms, and prevents vertebral fractures in osteoporotic women (4). Scoliotic adults without objective evidence of osteoporosis should receive calcium supplements. Young scoliotic women should take calcium to prevent osteoporosis and fractures (4).

It was thought, until recently, that significant scoliotic progression did not occur after bone epiphyseal growth ceased. Now we know that 1° to 3° per year of progression occurs in 55 to 70% of adult scoliotics (5, 6, 7, 8). Of 20 patients with painful adult idiopathic scoliosis, 12 (60%) progressed an average of 3.8° per year. Pain severity increased with curve progression (1).

Back pain in scoliosis is felt to be primarily discogenic in nature and along the apex of the major curve. This is supported by discographic studies (9, 10, 11).

Scoliosis is found in 8.3% of adults in the United States aged 25 to 74 years. The incidence in women is twice that in men, and there is lower bone density among scoliotics. Delayed menarche was more common in scoliotic women, and they had a lower mean age of menstruation termination than nonscoliotic women (12).

Pain Patterns in the Lumbar Spine in Adult Scoliosis

Since most idiopathic lumbar curves are left-sided, left-sided convexity pain is commonly present; it is muscular pain in type. The concavity pain is caused by degenerative facet changes, and may lead to radicular pain due to foraminal stenosis created by facet hypertrophy (13). Anterior and lateral thigh pain is possible due to L2 and L3 nerve root compression.

Surgical Treatment of Adult Scoliosis

Progression of pain or deformity is an indication for surgical intervention. A 50 to 80% incidence of surgical complications is seen, with pseudoarthrosis predominating (14).

Surgery has been found to result in a reduction in the levels of peak and constant pain, but no change in the frequency of peak pain (15). No patients were pain-free after surgery. Improvement in the ability to perform the daily activities of living was seen, but no change in occupational or recreational activity. Sixty percent had a surgical complication, and patients should be made aware of such limitation prior to surgery (15).

Surgery can require staged procedures—for example, one surgery to release arthritically fused joints, then traction to align the segments, followed by fusion. Twenty to twenty-five percent of all treated scoliotic patients are adults (16). The object of adult scoliosis surgery is to obtain a well-balanced, painless spine with a solid fusion. The lowest rate of complication was found in single-stage posterior fusion with Luque instrumentation. Pseudoarthrosis was higher with Harrington than with Luque instrumentation.

Two-stage anterior and posterior fusion for rigid-curve adult scoliosis has been recommended to obtain maximum correction and to allow the head, shoulders, and torso to be centered over the pelvis (17). Internal skeletal fixation uses intrapedicular screw fixation of a threaded rod to stabilize vertebral segments in scoliosis. This is a procedure in the prototype stage (18).

Nonoperative Adjustment Treatment of Adult Scoliosis

Always remember that scoliosis and pain do not have to occur together. They can be two totally different findings, with the pain coming from a cause other than the scoliosis. Therefore, diagnosis demands consideration of what these other causes might be.

Chiropractic adjustments can be applied with expectation of pain relief and increased mobility. The techniques must be applied very carefully, with complete awareness of patient discomfort, while applying low-force levered manipulative adjustments to the intervertebral disc and facet joint spaces. It is to be remembered that, the greater the arthrotic change present, the less force must be used in the application of the adjustment. The facets are tested individually as they are moved through their physiological ranges of motion. The presence of pain will preclude the use of that particular levered motion with the instrument. Let's study the application of such manipulative adjustive techniques to an actual case treated by this author.

CASE 1

A 71-year-old white female was seen complaining of pain in the lumbar spine primarily, with some radiation into the thoracic spine in the T6 to T12 area bilaterally. The chief pain was at the L3-L4 level and was more severe on the right side of the spine. To complicate the pain scenario, this patient had gallbladder dysfunction that caused her pain in the right abdomen and spine, for which she was under treatment. Her spinal pain had progressed to awaken her at night after she was asleep for about 4 hours. Examination revealed normal vital signs, normal urine analysis, the abdomen negative for masses or pain at this time, and no other cause for her spinal discomfort aside from the degenerative scoliosis.

Radiographic examination (Figs. 15.1 and 15.2) shows a levorotatory degenerative scoliosis of the lumbar spine with the apex at the L3-L4 level and an L3-L4 vacuum phenomenon present. The lateral view (Fig. 15.2) reveals the extensive degenerative state of the L3-L4 disc. The extensive atherosclerosis of the abdominal aorta was noted; this always makes a manipulating physician beware of applying any pressure to this abdomen.

Our impression was that we were dealing with a degenerative levoscoliosis of the lumbar spine which was a major cause of this patient's pain. She remembered having been told of a minor curve in her younger years.

Now, again we want to stress that total relief of this patient's pain is impossible. Our goal was to attain some measure of relief and improved quality of life. To that end, we applied the following chiropractic adjustments.

Figure 15.3 shows the use of the thoracic rotatory movement applied to the lumbar segments. Grasping the spinous process of the lumbar segment, we *very gently* placed the vertebral segment into right and left rotation. Here we used more rotation to the left in an attempt to very gently derotate the left posterior rotatory subluxation of the vertebral body. We certainly realized that Wolff's law had done its work so that no permanent correction of the subluxation was possible. Our goal was to regain maximal motion to this segment. We repeated this movement as shown in Figure 15.3 to each lumbar segment from L1 to L4.

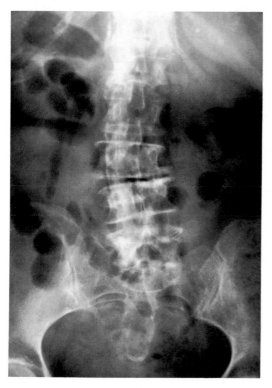

Figure 15.1. Degenerative levoratatory scoliosis of the lumbar spine with the apex at the L3-L4 level and osteochondrosis of this disc space noted. Atherosclerosis of the abdominal aorta is seen.

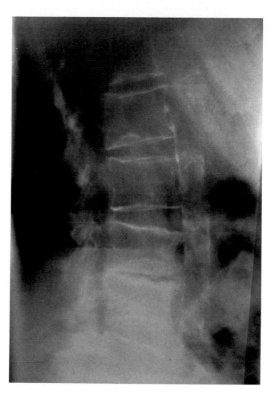

Figure 15.2. Lateral projection of the patient seen in Figure 15.1 shows the L3-L4 advanced degenerative disc disease with loss of lordotic curve. The intervertebral foramina at the midlumbar levels appear narrowed sagittally and vertically compared to the upper lumbar levels. The aortic arteriosclerosis is seen.

Figure 15.4 shows that we maintained the left derotation movement of the thoracic section on which we had just derotated the lumbar segments. Then we made a contact well above the rotatory scoliosis, in this case at the lower thoracic segments, and applied a very gentle distraction to the spine by taking the caudal section of the table downward slowly while we lifted the spinous process of the thoracic segment with thenar contact of our right hand. We moved down, one vertebra at a time, to the L4 segment while carefully and gently applying this slight distraction.

Figure 15.5 shows that we lateral flexed the caudal section of the table to the left side so as to very gently stretch the lumbar scoliosis into its left convexity. Here, therefore, we were using three movements—flexion, left derotation, and left lateral flexion—to the lumbar levoscoliotic curve. (Note: if the patient felt any discomfort to any such motion, the adjustment would be stopped and only motion applied that caused no discomfort.)

If the patient felt too much discomfort to lie prone, or if the treatment caused discomfort when lying on the ab-

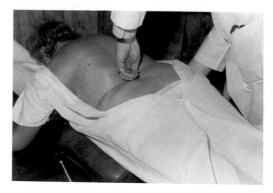

Figure 15.3. The left posterior lumbar vertebral body rotations are adjusted by rotating the thoracic section of the table so as to allow the left vertebral body rotation to rotate anteriorly as the spinous process of the segment being manipulated is held in the midline.

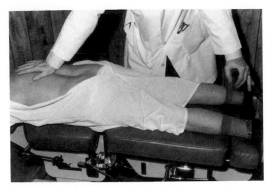

Figure 15.4. The left posterior lumbar vertebral body rotation subluxations are held in derotation by locking the midsection of the adjusting table in the position of derotation. Distraction is then applied by placing the thenar contact of the right hand under the spinous process of the vertebrae above the scoliotic curve. The caudal section of the table is then placed into downward distractive position. This figure shows a coupled adjustment of left derotation and traction being supplied.

domen, we applied the treatment with the patient lying on the side.

Figure 15.6 shows the patient lying on the side with the convexity—in this case, the left side—down on the table. This was done to allow us to reduce the levorotation component of the curve, to a slight degree and depend-

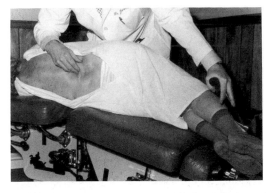

Figure 15.6. For patients who feel pain when treated lying on the abdomen, the adjustment can be delivered with the patient lying on the side, as shown here. When treating the spine shown in Figures 15.1 and 15.2, we would have the patient lie on the left side so as to allow the levorotation of the lumbar segments to be reduced by posture alone. A small pillow may also be placed under the lumbar spine to enhance the effect of reducing the left lumbar spinal curvature. *Note:* By placing the caudal section of the table into flexion, you can see that lateral flexion of the lumbar spine is applied.

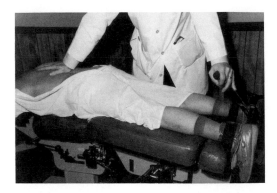

Figure 15.5. With left derotation and traction applied, gentle left lateral flexion of the spine is introduced by placing the caudal section of the instrument into left lateral flexion. This is done very gently, with patient comfort monitored at all times.

ing on patient tolerance, by lowering the caudal section of the table as shown in Figure 15.6. We now contacted the spinous process of the lumbar vertebra, as shown in Figure 15.7, and brought the table into forward lateral motion so as to apply a mild flexion to the lumbar spine while we palpated the interspinous space for fanning (opening of the interspinous space). Figure 15.8 shows us placing the lumbar spine into mild, carefully controlled extension while again feeling the interspinous spacing for motion. We could also place the lumbar spine in flexion or extension by moving the caudal section of the table laterally, and while in this position we could apply downward motion with the caudal section so as to laterally flex and derotate the lumbar spine. *All*

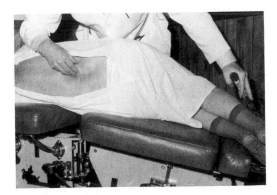

Figure 15.7. Traction is applied by forward bending of the caudal section of the table so as to open the lumbar spinous processes. The doctor's right hand palpates the spinous processes to detect fanning (opening of the spinous processes) while this maneuver is carried out. Please also note that, in patients with atherosclerosis of the abdominal aorta, this form of care prevents pressure on the arterial system.

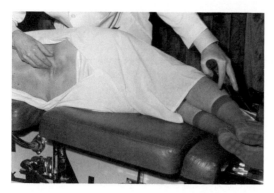

Figure 15.8. Extension can also be applied by lateral bending the caudal section posteriorly while again monitoring the interspinous spaces with the palpating hand.

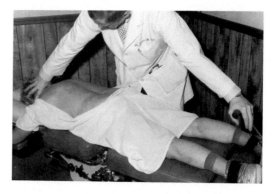

Figure 15.9. Foramen magnum pump technique applied for full spine distraction adjustment. Here the basiocciput is cradled in the doctor's right hand. Downward caudal traction is applied while the occiput is gently lifted cephalad. Upper cervical tension, headaches, cervical muscle spasm, zygapophyseal degeneration and subluxation, discal degeneration, and cephalgic tension are helped by this technique.

such adjustments are done very slowly and carefully while monitoring patient comfort or complaint.

Figure 15.9 shows the foramen magnum pump technique applied. Here we cradled the basiocciput in our hand and applied full spine distraction. This applies a very mild full spinal tractive force. Patients often state that they feel as though it would feel good if someone pulled them apart. I think they are stating that the effects of gravity in compression of the spine are painful to their disc, facets, and supporting elements. The foramen magnum pump is used in many conditions, one of which is degenerative scoliosis, but always very slowly and gently, as patient tolerance allows. Figure 15.10 demonstrates how we continued this distraction down into the thoracic spine by tractioning the thoracic segment spinous process cephalad, grasping it in the web of the contact hand between the thumb and first finger. Downward distraction was applied gently with the caudal section of the table as the spinous contact was lifted cephalad.

Other treatment of this case included home exercises consisting of *gentle* knee-chest procedures. The patient was told to precede these exercises with 15 minutes of heat to the low back, followed by 10 minutes of cold application, which was followed again by 15 minutes of heat. We find that this relaxes the spinal muscles and makes the exercises less irritating. In this type of case, knee-chest is the only maneuver we recommend for home exercise. Too many exercises tend to aggravate this type of spine. We followed the chiropractic adjustment with positive galvanic current into the L3-L4 area and then mild tetanizing currents to the paravertebral muscles from L1-L2 to L4-L5, with moist heat applied while this 15 minutes of electrical stimulation is applied. This patient attended low back wellness school to learn the proper ways to lift, bend, and twist in daily living, so as to reduce strain to her spine. She also was given 1000 mg of nonphosphorous calcium per day to take orally

and encouraged to walk as much as her stamina allowed.

This combination of therapy was applied three times weekly for 3 weeks and then two times weekly for 2

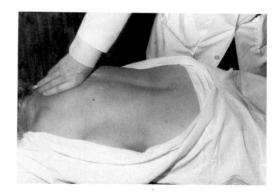

Figure 15.10. The traction shown in Figure 15.9 is continued down the cervical spine by contacting the spinous processes and laminae of each cervical vertebra and repeating the distractive pull until separation of the interspinous space is felt. As you continue down the cervical spine, the thoracic spinous processes are felt to press into the web between the thumb and index finger. At that time, firmly contact the thoracic spinous processes between the web of the thumb and index finger, and continue to apply the cephalad distraction throughout the thoracic spine. This can be carried out throughout the scoliotic curve. Always be mindful of patient comfort when applying the technique. Monitor patient comfort at all times.

weeks, with the result that the patient felt about 50% relief and certainly felt positive about having undergone this conservative approach to her problem. In the end, success has been achieved when the patient feels that the relief obtained is greater than the expense or inconvenience of therapy attendance.

DISCOGENIC SPONDYLOARTHROSIS

The most common condition seen in a manipulative practice may be the degenerative disc with resultant facet weight-bearing increase which results in the clinical entities of facet arthrosis and disc spondylosis—a condition termed discogenic spondyloarthrosis. Middle-aged to elderly people are extremely prone to this condition as the nucleus pulposus dehydrates; the opposing vertebral body plates approximate one another, with loss of disc space height and subchondral end plate sclerosis. The person becomes shorter in stature and may become stooped if stenosis of the canal accompanies these changes. Such stooped posture affords a greater sagittal diameter of the vertebral canal. These patients often state that it would feel good if somehow they could be "pulled apart" or tractioned. This condition, therefore, can be effectively treated by using flexion distraction adjustments while monitoring patient tolerance.

By working within patient tolerance, the doctor can distract the specific disc space and facet joints while placing the facet joints through their normal ranges of motion, which are *flexion, extension, lateral flexion, circumduction, and rotation*. A vertebra capable of performing its physiological ranges of motion is less encumbered with subluxation and the resulting nerve root irritations accompanying it. This technique can increase the range of motion of an articulation previously considered degenerated and nonmobile until the patient is pain-free, or at least in less pain, and realizes a range of motion which was not enjoyed previously.

Figures 15.11, 15.12, and 15.13 show a typical case seen in clinical practice every day. Figure 15.11 and 15.12 are the anteroposterior and lateral views showing degeneration of the lower three lumbar discs, with the oblique view in Figure 15.13 revealing the facet imbrication that follows disc degeneration and the resultant increased weight-bearing on the facet. This causes the facet joint to imbricate upward into the intervertebral foramen, resulting in lateral recess stenosis. You will also notice that the inferior facet

of the vertebra tends to contact the lamina of the vertebra below, which results in periosteal reaction with sclerosis. This has been termed facet-lamina syndrome and is considered a source of pain. You will also note how the superior facet tends to telescope upward to contact the pedicle of the vertebra above, resulting in periosteal sclerosis as well.

Treatment of Discogenic Spondyloarthrosis

In Figure 15.14, flexion is being applied to each lumbar disc space and facet facing. By maintenance of hand contact with the spinous process of each lumbar and thoracic vertebra, the downward pressure on the caudal section of the table allows stretching and spreading apart of each functional spinal unit.

Testing for patient tolerance of traction, as demonstrated in Figure 15.15, is performed before the cuffs are applied. This is done by grasp-

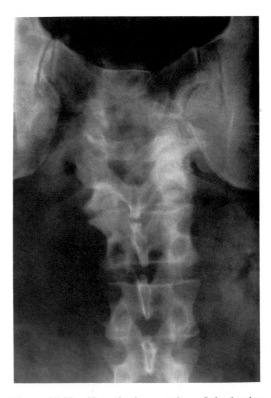

Figure 15.11. Note the levorotation of the lumbar segments, the loss of disc space and hypertrophic changes of the anterior lateral body plates at L3-L4 and L4-L5, and the transitional changes of the L5 segment.

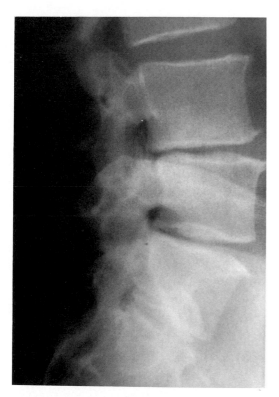

Figure 15.12. Lateral view of Figure 15.11 shows degenerative L3-L4 and L4-L5 disc disease with stenosis of the intervertebral foramina at these levels. The rudimentary disc of L5-S1 is seen at this level of transitional segment. This is Bertolotti's syndrome, i.e., a transitional L5 segment with degenerative disc disease at the disc level above.

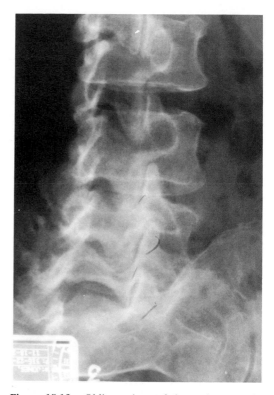

Figure 15.13. Oblique views of the patient seen in Figures 15.11 and 15.12 show the L3-L4 and L4-L5 facet joints to have loss of joint space with subchondral sclerosis, and to imbricate superiorly into the intervertebral foramen to create stenosis of the osteoligamentous canal. With this imbrication, we find that the superior tip of the superior facet contacts the pedicle of the vertebra above and the inferior tip of the inferior facet contacts the lamina of the vertebra below. This creates some periosteal reaction, which could be a source of back pain. This is termed the facet-lamina or facet-pedicle syndrome.

ing the ankle and applying traction while asking whether the patient feels any pain in the low back. Muscle resistance can be felt in patients who cannot tolerate traction. If there is no pain, the cuffs are attached, and flexion, as demonstrated in Figure 15.14, is carried out.

Lateral flexion is demonstrated in Figure 15.16 and is performed by grasping the spinous process of each lumbar segment individually between the thumb and index finger (Fig. 15.17). Motion palpation is elicited by testing the ability of the articular facets to lateral bend during movement of the caudal section of the table in lateral flexion. Hypomobility is evidenced by resistance to movement laterally, pain to the patient, or both.

Circumduction, which is a combination of lateral flexion and plain flexion, is demonstrated in Figure 15.18. This coupled movement of the ta-

ble allows full range of motion of the facet and is very effective in restoring mobility to the facet.

Rotation, as demonstrated in Figure 15.19, is applied by rotating the caudal section of the table while the vertebral segment is held in resistance. Traction can be applied prior to this movement and maintained during rotation by leaving the ankle cuffs on the patient and opening the caudal section of the table. Keep in mind that L4-L5 and L5-S1 have very restricted ranges of motion in rotation and should not be forced into rotation. The upper lumbar and thoracic segments are capable of rotation.

Rotation and flexion as applied simultaneously to the upper lumbar and thoracic seg-

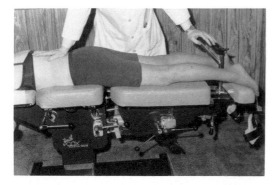

Figure 15.14. Flexion distraction manipulation.

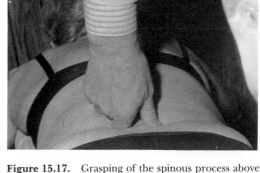

Figure 15.17. Grasping of the spinous process above the facets to be motion-palpated and manipulated.

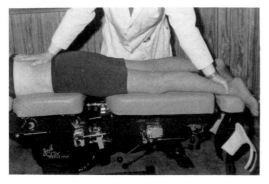

Figure 15.15. Testing patient tolerance to distraction before applying distraction cuffs.

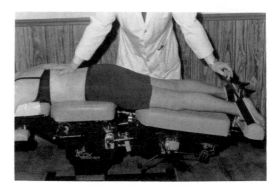

Figure 15.18. Circumduction manipulation.

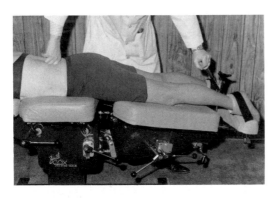

Figure 15.16. Lateral flexion being applied to the articular facets.

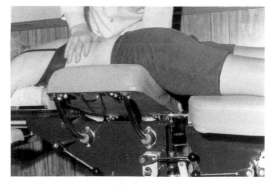

Figure 15.19. Rotation being applied to the thoracolumbar spine.

ments are demonstrated in Figure 15.20. This coupled mobilization is powerful and must be done to patient tolerance.

Goading of acupressure bladder meridian points B24 and B35, as demonstrated in Figure 15.21, is performed prior to and after distraction.

Deep pressure into the belly of the gluteus maximus muscle and bladder meridian point B49, as demonstrated in Figure 15.22, is used to relieve the pain of sciatica.

Pressure being applied to the adductor and gracilis tendons at their origins is demonstrated in Figure 15.23; pressure being applied to the

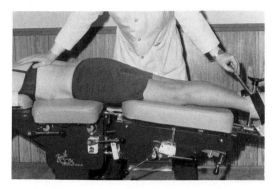

Figure 15.20. Rotation and flexion distraction being applied simultaneously.

their insertions on the medial femur and medial condyle of the tibia is demonstrated in Figure 15.24.

Application of the "foramen magnum pump" is demonstrated in Figure 15.25 and is performed by grasping the occiput while applying traction to the full spine with caudal distraction.

The application of heat and sinusoidal muscle stimulation or ultrasound with sinusoidal currents, either before or after manipulation, also provides relief from pain for patients with discogenic spondyloarthrosis.

Other considerations in the treatment of patients with the degenerative low back are important.

1. Nutrition. Osteoporosis is a common accompanying factor with the older spine. There-

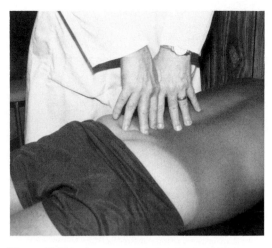

Figure 15.21. Acupressure points B24 to B35 being goaded.

fore, amino acids to build osteoid tissue and calcium to aid in bone ossification are recommended and prescribed. Manganese (500 to 800 mg/day), which is an ingredient of Discat, a nutritional supplement containing glucosaminoglycan, is also prescribed. Niacin (200 mg/day) and vitamin B_6 (150 mg/day) are also recommended. The alkalinity of the bowel depresses the absorption of calcium. This is due to the low output of HCl and enzymes in the elderly and may account for the etiology of osteoporosis along with endocrine hyposecretion. Thus, digestive enzymes are also prescribed.

2. Exercise. Walking improves the circulation

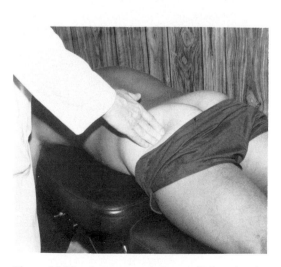

Figure 15.22. Acupressure being applied to the gluteus maximus and bladder meridian point B49.

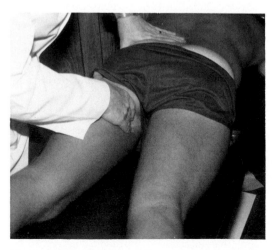

Figure 15.23. Goading of the adductor and gracilis tendons at their origins.

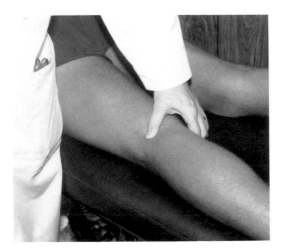

Figure 15.24. Insertion of the gracilis tendon being goaded at the medial tibial condyle.

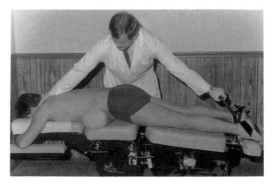

Figure 15.25. Application of the "foramen magnum pump" in full-spine occipital distraction.

and increases the muscular activity of the paravertebral musculature, thereby enhancing the flow of nutrients to the bone tissue as well as the removal of waste materials. Thus, it is recommended for patients with discogenic spondyloarthrosis.

3. The gracilis tendon should be checked and strengthened to enhance the adrenal output and, thereby, the general well-being of the patient. This is shown later in this chapter.

4. Low back wellness school is presented to these patients so that they learn the proper methods of lifting, bending, and twisting in daily living. They are shown how to perform the Cox exercises. We find that if the patients are not drilled on these exercises, or if they are merely given a sheet of exercises and told to do them, they will either not do them, or even worse, do them incorrectly. A videotape of the entire exercise program is given to the patient to follow and perform at home.

COMPRESSION FRACTURE OF THE THORACIC OR LUMBAR VERTEBRAL BODIES

The treatment described here is intended for the compression-type fractures resulting in trapezoid-shaped vertebral bodies. Pathological compression fractures are not treated with a manipulative adjustment approach. Figures 15.26 and 15.27 show serial studies of a compression fracture of the ninth thoracic vertebral body fol-

lowing a fall. The x-ray in Figure 15.27 was taken 4 months following the x-ray in Figure 15.26, thus showing the progressive nature of the compression fracture. Remember that the severity of fracture can increase in the weeks following the initial injury and the discovery of the fracture.

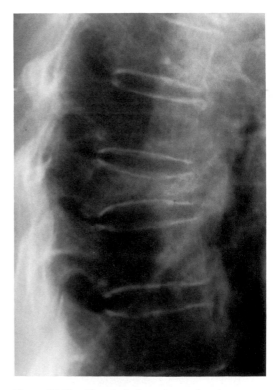

Figure 15.26. The ninth thoracic vertebra shows compression fracture and about 60% loss of the normal height. This is the result of a fall.

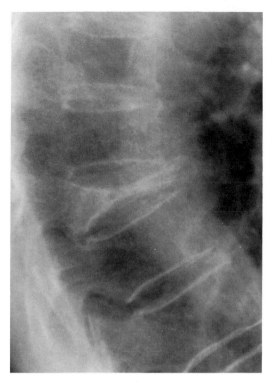

Figure 15.27. The fracture shown in Figure 15.26 is again shown 4 months later; it now shows progressive trapezoid-shaped collapse, with about 90% loss of the normal vertebral body height.

This is especially true in the osteoporotic elderly female spine.

Treatment of compression fracture of the thoracolumbar spine, which is so common at the T12-L1 level, is shown in Figures 15.28 and

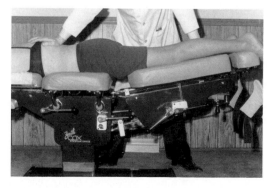

Figure 15.29. Mild extension manipulation being applied.

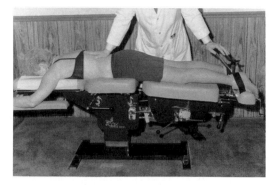

Figure 15.28. Mild flexion distraction being applied.

15.29. The treatment of the fracture seen in Figures 15.26 and 15.27 is shown in Figure 15.30.

Long-Term Results of Conservative Care of Thoracolumbar Fractures

A long-term study of 216 patients without neurological complications who sustained thoracolumbar compression fractures was carried out for an

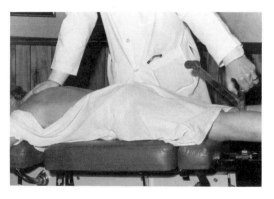

Figure 15.30. Treatment of the fracture seen in Figures 15.26 and 15.27 is shown here. The compression defect is placed over the split sections of the adjustment table. With a gentle anterior pressure applied to the spinous process of the compressed segment, the caudal section of the table is gently brought into extension. This places the flexion deformity created by the compression fracture to be brought into extension. This treatment is applied to patient tolerance and until the spine is felt to gain some measure of extension motion. This patient, as is true with all compression fractures, is advised to hold the spine in extension by wearing an extension support, lying over a small pillow under the thoracic segment, and performing extension exercises of the thoracic spine.

average of 9 years. The functional results of single versus multiple fractures were no different, nor was the degree of spontaneous fusion found to cause any statistical difference in the functional outcome. There was no correlation between reduction in vertebral height, encroachment upon the spinal canal, and persistent kyphotic deformities. It was concluded that nonoperative treatment of these fractures was a sound method and that attempts at surgical reduction were not justifiable. None of the 216 patients required surgical reduction due to persistent symptoms (19).

Weinstein et al. (20) also found that nonoperative treatment of thoracolumbar burst fractures was a viable alternative to surgery in patients without neurological deficit and that such conservative care resulted in acceptable long-term results.

FAILED BACK SURGERY SYNDROME

Recurrent herniated disc and symptomatic hypertrophic scar can produce similar low back symptoms and radiculopathy. Gradually increasing symptoms beginning a year or more after discectomy are considered more likely to be due to scar radiculopathy, while a more abrupt onset at any interval after surgery is more likely due to recurrent herniated disc (21).

Failed back surgery syndrome is seen in 10 to 40% of patients who undergo back surgery. It is characterized by intractable pain and varying degrees of functional incapacitation occurring after spine surgery (22).

Epidural adhesions may occur with no previous treatment of low back pain or sciatica in some patients. Primary formation of epidural adhesions in the epidural space could explain why treatments sometimes fail and why surgery should be avoided in patients whose CT or myelograms are negative for nerve root compression (23).

Differentiation of Recurrent Disc Herniation from Scar Formation

Epidural scarring and adhesions can be differentiated from recurrent disc herniation by intravenous contrast-enhanced CT scan of the postoperative spine (21). Gd-DTPA (gadolinium-diethylenetriaminepentaacetic acid/dimeglumine) enhanced MRI imaging is also used (22). Scar tissue is enhanced by the contrast agent, whereas the disc material is not enhanced. A study (22) showed that precontrast and early postcontrast T1-weighted spin-echo studies are highly accurate in separating epidural fibrosis from herniated disc.

Repetitive back surgery is the unfortunate consequence of persistent pain, although the improvement from additional operations is very slight. De La Porte (24) states that Ohio Workmen's Compensation reported than no patients are cured by a second low back operation, 20% are improved, 20% are made worse, and 60% are essentially unchanged. With additional operations the outcome worsens, and after four operations, 5% are improved and 50% are made worse.

The clinical features of lumbosacral spinal fibrosis are polymorphic. Lumbar pain and sciatica that become worse, even with minimal physical activities (seen in 60% of patients) are the main complaints. Nocturnal cramps and distal paresthesia are common. Twenty-five percent of patients have low back pain without radiculopathy. Ten percent show cauda equina syndrome with sphincter dysfunction and saddle hypesthesia. Lasègue's sign is positive only in 20% of the cases, but the absence of knee and ankle reflexes is frequent. The syndrome of spasm in the legs, muscular cramps, increasing radicular pain, elevated temperature, and shivering occur within the first 3 days following surgery and may signify the first signs of spinal fibrosis (24).

In patients with epidural scar fibrosis, additional surgery can only magnify the scarring and resultant disability. One approach, used when all other conservative measures fail, is the application of epidural stimulation with an electrode lead wire anchored deeply into the epidural space. A percutaneous wire extends out through the skin and is attached to a small (pocket watchsized) pulse generator implanted beneath the skin. A gentle buzzing sensation is imparted to the dorsal columns to produce a stimulus that acts as a signal jamming the chronic pain sensations that occur with nerve damage (25).

Case Presentation of a Postsurgical Failed Back

CASE 2

A 43-year-old white single male was seen for the chief complaints of low back and right leg pain, occasionally some pain into the left leg as well. The patient had had back surgery performed twice, the first time in 1967 for a laminectomy and in 1968 for a spinal fusion. He noted that his back pain returned immediately following the surgeries. He had been seen at many clinics without help.

This patient also complained of neck pain and pain in the right shoulder, arm, and hand. Neck pain had started approximately 20 years previously following an injury, at which time he was told he had a cervical disc problem.

Examination of the low back at this time revealed marked restriction of range of motion, with flexion at 40°, extension at 5°, right and left lateral flexion at 10°, and rotation at 20°, all of which were accompanied by pain. Straight leg raising was bilaterally painful at 50°, creating leg pains. The muscle power of the lower extremities was grade 5 of 5 bilaterally. The right ankle reflex was absent, while the remaining deep reflexes of the lower extremities were +2 bilaterally. No sensory changes were noted on pinwheel examination. The circulation of the lower extremities was good.

Radiographic examination revealed the following: Figure 15.31 shows an extensive interlaminar fusion at the L4-S1 levels. Figure 15.32 is a lateral projection that reveals advanced degeneration of the L4-L5 and L5-S1 disc spaces with the posterior fusion in place. Figure 15.33 is an oblique projection, again outlining the bone fusion between the laminae at L4-L5 and the sacrum.

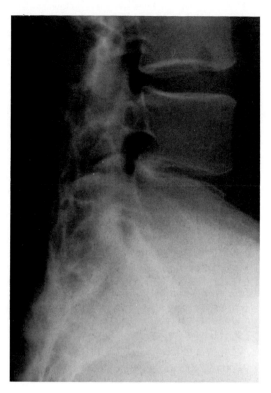

Figure 15.32. Lateral view of Figure 15.31 showing the spinal fusion with the extensive L4-L5 and L5-S1 discal degeneration.

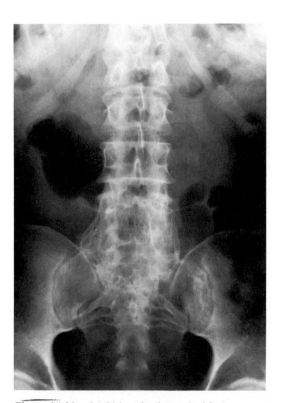

Figure 15.31. L4-S1 interlaminar spinal fusion, anteroposterior view.

Figure 15.34 shows a lateral cervical x-ray of this patient, revealing extensive degenerative disc disease at the C5-C6 and C6-C7 levels. The oblique view in Figure 15.35 reveals the right C5-C6 intervertebral foramen to be somewhat narrowed due to the degenerative disc disease at that level.

Examination of the cervical spine, physically, orthopedically, and neurologically, revealed reduction of ranges of motion on rotation to approximately 70°, with otherwise normal ranges of motion. Palpation revealed pain over the C4 through C7 levels bilaterally, with cervical compression being positive at the C5, C6, and C7 levels, radiating pain into the right shoulder and arm. There were no signs of thoracic outlet syndrome. The deep reflexes of the upper extremities were +2 bilaterally, with no sensation changes to pinwheel examination. No motor weakness was noted in either upper extremity.

Our impressions of this case were as follows: (a) degenerative disc disease at the C5-C6 and C6-C7 levels, creating some foraminal stenosis and a resultant right brachial radiculopathy; (b) spinal fusion, interlaminar, at L4-L5 and the sacrum with advanced degenerative disc disease at the L4-L5 and L5-S1 levels; (c) possibility of postsurgical stenosis at the L4-L5 and L5-S1 levels.

This patient was given flexion distraction of the C5-C6 and C6-C7 levels, followed by ultrasound with mild tetanizing current.

The lumbar spine was treated by goading of acupressure points B22 through B49 and flexion distraction to the L3-L4 segment. The reason for this is that, with the fusion of L4 to the sacrum, all of the flexion, extension, and lateral bending motions have been transferred to the L3-L4 level. We feel that maintaining complete ranges of motion with minimal stress can help to alleviate and prevent future degenerative change at the L3-L4 level. This will be the level of motion of this patient's spine for the rest of his life.

In addition to the above, we utilized tetanizing current to the paravertebral muscles of the lumbar spine and pelvis, with alternating hot and cold packs. The treatment of postsurgical backs can be extremely difficult, especially when sciatic pains are present. In this case, the patient became discouraged by slow relief of pain and discontinued treatment before meaningful clinical treatment could be administered.

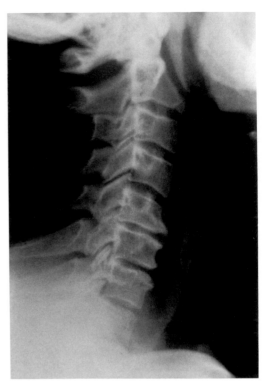

Figure 15.34. Lateral cervical spine x-ray of the patient in Figures 15.31 through 15.33. This shows C5-C6 and C6-C7 degenerative disc disease. This author notes that disc degenerative changes occur in those spinal segments where rotation is a minimal motion and flexion and extension are primary motions. Such areas occur at the L4-L5, L5-S1, C5-C6, and C6-C7 levels.

Treatment of Failed Back Surgery Syndrome

Spinal manipulative therapy for the patient with the failed back surgery syndrome is applied under strict parameters:

1. Never is the caudal section of the table lowered over 2 inches.
2. Rotation is never applied to the lower lumbar spine.
3. No electrical intermittent traction is used—only hand-controlled manual manipulation.
4. Any lateral flexion is restricted to facet capability; lateral bending should never be forced.
5. The primary motion used is flexion.
6. Traction is applied above the fused segments.

Flexion to the spinous process is applied

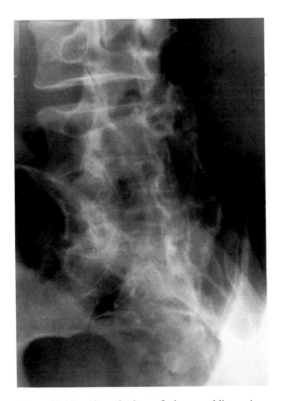

Figure 15.33. Note the bone fusion on oblique view.

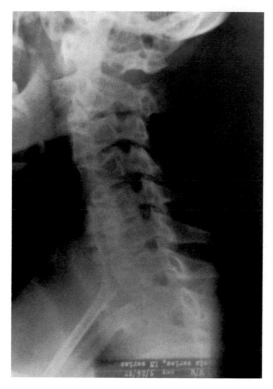

Figure 15.35. Oblique view of patient seen in Figure 15.34 does show some narrowing of the C5-C6 intervertebral foramen due to discal degeneration and loss of vertical height of the foramen.

above the fusion, as is demonstrated in Figure 15.36. The rules for application of traction, which were given previously, are followed. In Figure 15.37, lateral flexion of the segments is demonstrated.

Sinusoidal currents are applied to the paraver-

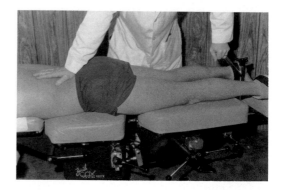

Figure 15.36. Contact is maintained on the spinous process above the surgical fusion shown in Figure 15.31.

tebral muscles as demonstrated in Figure 15.38. Hydrocollator packs are applied over the sinusoidal current pads for 10 minutes (Fig. 15.39). Cold packs are then applied for 5 minutes (Fig. 15.40). Hot and cold packs, beginning and ending with heat, are applied alternately.

In Figure 15.41, unilateral traction being applied without the ankle cuffs is shown; the ankle is held while distraction is being applied. By the holding of each lower extremity, the facets can be more strongly tractioned unilaterally.

Figures 15.42 and 15.43 are x-rays of a patient with hip arthroplasty. Commonly, these patients also have degenerative disc disease and are best treated unilaterally, as shown in Figure 15.41, in

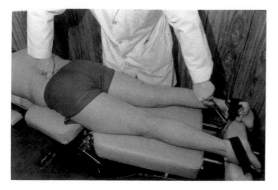

Figure 15.37. Lateral flexion being applied to the same patient as in Figure 15.31.

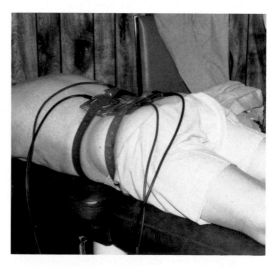

Figure 15.38. Sinusoidal current being applied to the same patient as in Figure 15.24.

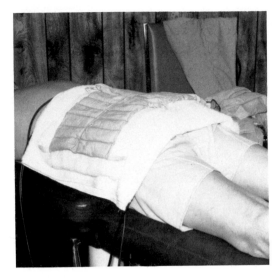

Figure 15.39. Moist heat being applied.

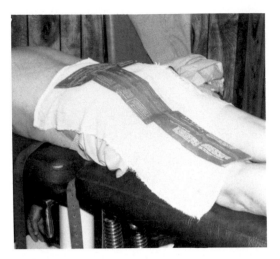

Figure 15.40. Cold packs being applied to the low back and sciatic distribution.

order to control traction on the involved replaced hip socket.

Patients with the failed back surgery syndrome are treated by goading of acupressure kinesiology points, as shown in Chapter 12, "Care of the Intervertebral Disc." Treatments are given daily until the pain subsides in the lower extremities; then they are reduced to three visits weekly until 50% relief is obtained. We tell these patients that 50% relief is an excellent clinical response.

EFFECTS OF CHRONIC LOW BACK PAIN ON FUNCTIONAL STATUS

Patients suffering from chronic low back pain evidence significant impairment in physical, psychosocial, work, and recreational activities.

The greatest impairment is in the area of work, but disability ratings for recreation, home management, social interaction, emotional behavior, and sleep and rest were also comparatively high. In persons with chronic low back pain, the use of a sickness impact profile, which is a global measure of disability, is valid as a measure of functional status. The results of this test assist in the

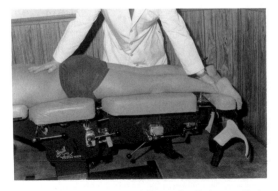

Figure 15.41. Unilateral distraction being applied.

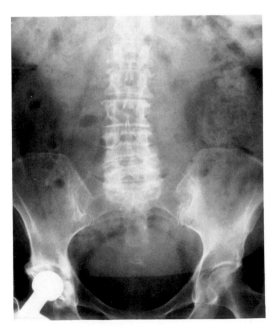

Figure 15.42. Anteroposterior view of the lumbar spine and pelvis of a patient with hip arthroplasty.

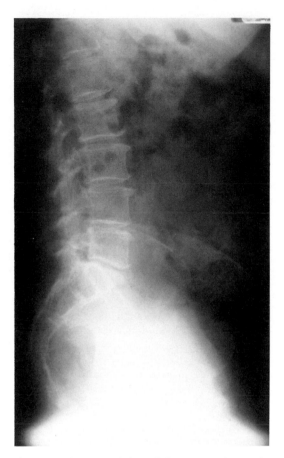

Figure 15.43. Lateral view of the same patient as in Figure 15.42.

evaluation of the efficacy of multidisciplinary pain units (26).

MUSCLE EVALUATION AND TREATMENT

It seems reasonable to trace the development of disc weakness and protrusion to early muscle weakness or spasm causing altered motoricity of the low back. In treatment of a disc protrusion, we must first concern ourselves with the extreme pain of the patient due to the nerve root compression. This necessitates the use of the Cox technique for reduction. Following reduction, we retrace the etiology by evaluating the muscles for weakness or spasticity and correct the muscles in order to establish a stable low back and to avoid future disc problems.

General Muscular Condition

Following reduction of the protruded nuclear material via Cox technique, we proceed with the evaluation of the musculature. The patient is asked to stand with his feet 4 inches apart. As we examine the patient, we look for the following:

1. Height of the ilia. Mark the high and low side. We are primarily interested in the side of pain.
2. Forefoot or hindfoot valgus or varus deformity of the feet; note pes planus or cavus deformity.
3. Relative internal or external flare rotation of the ilia.
4. Height of occiput. Mark the high side.
5. Anteroposterior lumbar curvature for lordotic decrease or increase.
6. Lean of the lumbar spine laterally.

We, of course, admit that congenital anomalies of the low back precipitate instability and lead to altered motoricity. We assert, however, that muscle balancing can afford the stability needed to render these anomalies asymptomatic.

Next, the patient is asked to walk across the room. We look for changes of the feet and observe gait.

Then we study the individual muscles and groups of muscles, such as the adductor, piriformis, gluteal, psoas, multifidus, and rotatores, quadriceps, and abdominal muscles.

Adductor Muscles

GRACILIS MUSCLE

The gracilis or "tie-down" muscle of the pelvis permits anterior and posterior rotation of the ilium. Its origin is in the pubic bone near the symphysis pubis (Fig. 15.44). Its insertion is in the medial tibia below the condyle. Its nerve supply is the L3 and L4 nerve roots.

Functional alterations result in extreme tenderness and weakness of muscles in patients with sciatica. Ilium rotation often accompanies sciatica, and weakness of the gracilis allows the pelvis to rotate posteriorly.

Treatment of gracilis weakness consists of 10 to 20 seconds of deep goading at its origin and insertion.

According to Goodheart (27), the gracilis and sartorius muscles are indicators of the condition of the adrenal gland. In all cases of repeated posterior ilium subluxations, consider adrenal

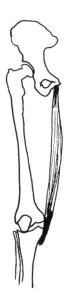

Figure 15.44. Illustration of gracilis muscle.

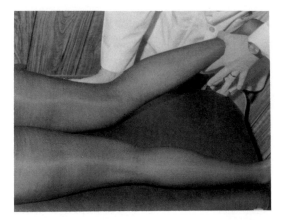

Figure 15.45. Testing for gracilis muscle strength.

depletion from stress as the etiology. The use of the neurolymphatic reflexes or adrenal protomorphogen is helpful in the treatment of this condition.

Remember these factors about the gracilils muscle:

1. Weakness of the gracilis muscle results in a posterior ilium.

2. Adrenal insufficiency causes weakness of the gracilis and sartorius muscles. Stress, therefore, is involved.

3. The inguinal ligament is sore over its lower half in cases of sciatica and posterior ilium.

Test for gracilis weakness by pressing downward and outward on the patient's leg at the ankle while stabilizing the thigh as shown in Figure 15.45.

ADDUCTOR GROUP INCLUDING LONGUS, BREVIS, AND MAGNUS MUSCLES

We have found that the adductor group is the specific key treatment area in patients with sciatic neuralgia caused by disc protrusion. Treatment of these muscles allows relief of pain much as acupressure provides control of pain. Therefore, the adductor group is the most important and the first muscle group we treat in controlling sciatica in patients with a disc lesion.

Its origin is in the pubis, ischium, and ramus (Fig. 15.46). Its insertion is in the medial femur in the linea aspera and femoral condyle. Its nerve supply is the third and fourth lumbar nerve roots and a branch of the *sciatic* nerve. (*This is my idea of the reflex pattern allowing the relief of sciatica.*)

I have never treated a patient with sciatica caused by disc protrusion without finding some degree of adductor soreness. I test for this in the following way:

1. Palpation of the muscle will reveal adductor soreness.

2. Weakness can be evaluated by having the

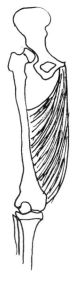

Figure 15.46. Illustration of the origin and the insertion of the adductor muscle group.

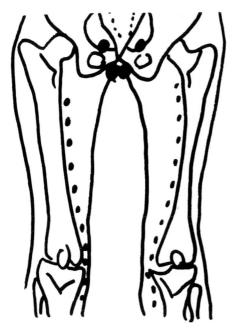

Figure 15.47. Illustration of origin and insertion points of the adductor muscles, which are used for goading.

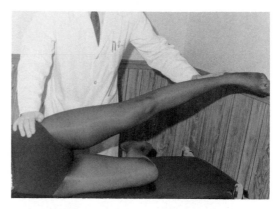

Figure 15.48. Testing for weakness of the gluteus medius muscle. Push the thigh forward and down.

patient lie supine, holding the legs tightly together. The patient is asked to keep his legs together while I grasp both legs just below the knee and try to force one leg apart (the other leg is being stabilized with my other hand). Due to pain, often the test cannot be performed in any other patient position.

Treatment of the adductor group consists of firm rotatory pressure being applied at its insertion along the medial femur for 20 to 30 seconds (Fig. 15.47). This pressure may bruise someone with capillary fragility, but this is of no significance. Constant pressure with the index area of the hand is applied to the pubic and ischial origins for 15 to 20 seconds while pressure over the inguinal ligament is maintained.

Gluteal Muscles

The gluteus maximus arises from the ilium behind the ilial gluteal line, the posteroinferior sacrum, and the sacrotuberous ligament to insert into the iliotibial band. It acts to extend and laterally rotate the thigh.

The gluteus medius arises from the ilium crest to insert into the greater trochanter. It acts as an internal rotator and abductor of the thigh.

The gluteus minimus arises from the outer ilium and sciatic notch to insert into the greater trochanter. It acts as a medial rotator and abductor of the thigh. Figures 15.48, 15.49, and 15.50 show muscle testing for the gluteal muscles.

Gluteus maximus spasm causes the ilium to externally rotate and posteriorly deviate (posterior ilium). Gluteus maximus spasm causes the foot to rotate outward.

Sixty percent of patients with a L5-S1 disc lesion have weakness and visible atrophy of the gluteus maximus muscle on the side of these lesions: this is called the gluteal skyline sign (28).

Gluteus medius and minimus weakness allows external rotation of the leg and foot as well as elevation of the ilium. Spasm of the gluteus medius and minimus causes internal rotation of the feet. *Therefore, external rotation of the leg and foot repre-*

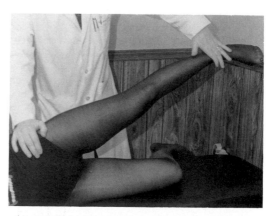

Figure 15.49. Testing for weakness of the gluteus minimus muscle. Push the thigh backward and down.

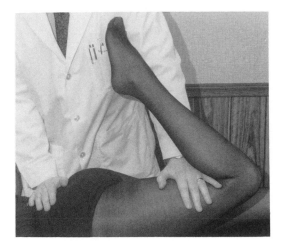

Figure 15.50. Testing for the strength of the gluteus maximus muscle.

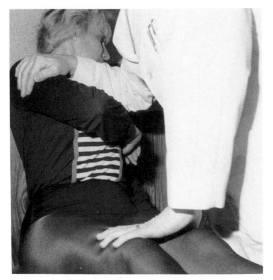

Figure 15.51. Testing for abdominal muscle strength. The patient sits upright to 70° and rotates at the waist while pressure is applied on the chest to push the patient supine. Stabilize the patient at the thighs so that the patient's legs don't rise from the table.

sents gluteus maximus spasm and/or gluteus medius and minimus weakness.

Elevation of the ilium represents weakness of the gluteus medius and minimus muscles, as is seen in posterior ilium.

Treatment for gluteus maximus spasm and/or gluteus medius and minimus weakness consists of the following:

Treatment for gluteus maximus spasm and/or gluteus medius and minimus weakness consists of the following:

1. Apply deep pressure into the belly of the gluteus maximus muscle for relaxation.
2. Goad the origins and insertions of the gluteus minimus and medius muscles.
3. Check for weak abdominalis muscles as shown in Figure 15.51. These muscles are antagonists to the gluteals. Treat by pressure to the origin and insertions.
4. Goodheart (72) neurolymphatic reflexes can be used in strengthening these muscles.

A typical anterior ilium pattern may be seen with gluteus maximus weakness and/or medius and minimus spasm.

Treatment consists of the following:

1. Goad the origin and insertion of the gluteus maximus muscles.
2. Apply pressure to the belly of the medius and minimus muscles.

The anterior and posterior ilium patterns may be seen with sciatic conditions. These two specific entities have been discussed in detail previously. They are treated after the disc protrusion has been reduced.

Piriformis Muscle

This flat muscle originates at the front of the sacrum, inserting it into the greater trochanter and acting as an external rotator of the thigh. It is intimate with the gluteus medius at its anatomical insertion.

Testing of the piriformis muscle is accomplished by grasping the patient's leg and ankle as shown in Figure 15.52 with the thigh externally rotated. Medial ankle pressure is applied laterally while the thigh is stabilized.

Weakness of the piriformis muscle results in internal rotation of the thigh and foot and a "knock knee" appearance. Strengthening of this muscle is usually accomplished by applying pressure on its insertion at the greater trochanter.

Spasm of the piriformis muscle externally rotates the thigh and foot and is relieved by pressure in the belly of the muscle from outside or by pressure applied from inside by rectal entrance.

The piriformis muscle is capable of sacral motion independent of the innominate by causing the sacrum to be inferior and posterior on the

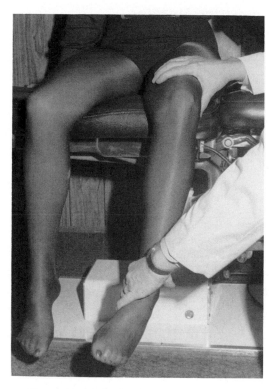

Figure 15.52. Piriformis muscle strength test.

chemical irritation properties explain the possible role of this muscle more adequately than mechanical theories.

OCCIPUT HEIGHT

We wish to stress that weakness of the posterior and anterior cervical spine muscles occurs with low back and pelvic weakness. A high occiput can occur on the side of gluteus medius and minimus muscle weakness and/or piriformis muscle weakness.

The cervical muscles should be balanced and any weakness in the low back should be strengthened.

Psoas Muscle

In acute sciatica, treatment of the psoas muscle is not helpful in controlling pain (Fig. 15.53). Later, after the pain has lessened, it can be treated for weakness by firm pressure at its insertion at the lesser trochanter and for spasm by lateral side-bending and flexion on the Zenith®-Cox® table. Goodheart (27) reflexes are utilized in the treatment of any kidney pathology.

side of spasticity and relatively anterior and superior on the weak side.

Steiner et al. (29) found the piriformis, when inflamed, to release a biochemical agent that irritates the sciatic nerve, and he felt it could cause sciatic neuritis. He found the symptoms identical to lumbar disc syndrome. Diagnosis was done by palpation of the myofascial trigger points within the piriformis muscle. Treatment included local anesthetic, manipulation, muscle spasm reduction, maintenance of range of motion, and ambulation.

In its anatomical location, contraction of the piriformis muscle produces abduction and external rotation of the thigh, and in 20% of the population, the sciatic nerve is found to pass through the belly of the piriformis.

Neuritis of the sciatic nerve due to piriformis chemical irritation causes no neurological deficits but only point tenderness over the muscle.

It is interesting to note that contraction of the piriformis has been argued as a cause of sciatic irritation for a long time, and it may be that the

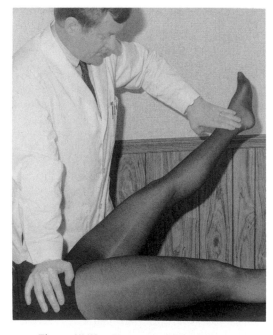

Figure 15.53. Psoas muscle strength test.

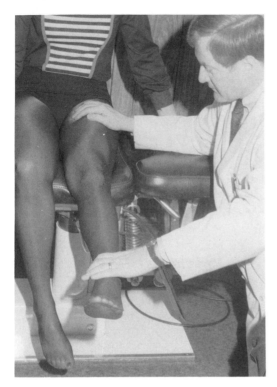

Figure 15.54. Testing of the quadriceps muscles. Press down on the leg at the ankle while stabilizing the thigh. (The quadriceps muscles may also be tested by flexing the knee and having the patient attempt extension of the knee joint.)

Quadriceps Muscles

Treatment of the quadriceps muscles is not important in cases of acute disc lesions. Treatment of these muscles is important, however, in cases of anterior and posterior innominate lesions.

In cases of anterior ilium lesions, the quadriceps are spastic; in cases of posterior ilium lesions, they are weak.

Testing for weakness of the quadriceps muscles is accomplished as shown in Figure 15.54. Press down on the ankle while stabilizing the thigh.

Treatment of the quadriceps muscles is accomplished as follows: If there is spasm, pressure is applied into the belly of the rectus femoris and vastus lateralis, medialis, and intermedius muscles. If there is weakness, goading of the origin and insertions is done. Remember: it is weakness of the vastus group that leads to cartilage problems of the knee joint.

Hamstring Muscles

The hamstring muscles are important in cases of disc lesion, as weakness of the hamstring muscles occurs along with the gluteus maximus and calf muscles with S1 dermatome involvement.

Testing for hamstring muscle weakness is accomplished as shown in Figure 15.55. The medial hamstrings (semitendinosus and semimembranosus) are tested by having the patient resist a force applied laterally on the ankle. The lateral hamstring (biceps femoris) is tested by having the patient resist a force applied medially on the leg.

Treatment of the hamstrings is accomplished as follows: If there is spasm, pressure is applied into the belly of the muscles for 20 seconds. If there is weakness, goading of the origins and insertions is done for 15 seconds.

Multifidus and Rotatores Muscles

Multifidus muscles are important in extension and rotation of the vertebral column. Their origin is in the mammillary processes in the lumbar region. Their insertion is in the spinous processes of one, two, three, or four vertebrae above.

Rotatores muscles are important in rotation of the vertebral column. Their origin is in the transverse process. Their insertion is in the lamina of the vertebra above.

Treatment of the multifidus and rotatores muscles is accomplished with deep Nimmo-type goading or application of pulsating sinusoidal

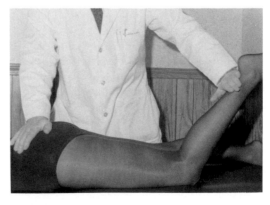

Figure 15.55. Testing of the hamstring muscle group. Have the patient forcefully resist extension of the knee joint as a force is applied on the leg at the ankle. Also ask the patient to attempt flexion of the knee joint while forced resistance is placed on the leg at the ankle.

current which brings about relaxation of these deep spinal muscles.

In all cases of sciatica, these muscles are checked and treated accordingly. Specific conditions of the low back may be found in conjunction with sciatica, and each will necessitate correction following reduction of the disc protrusion by the Cox technique in order to insure stability of the low back in the future and to prevent a recurrence.

TEACHING CASES FROM THE AUTHOR'S CLINICAL PRACTICE

These cases are presented to illustrate interesting concepts for the physician dealing with low back pain patients every day.

Figures 15.56 and 15.57 contrast the plain film and MRI findings on changes within the disc. Figure 15.56 shows the common finding of loss of disc height with anterior plate hypertrophy accompanying degenerative disc disease. The MRI

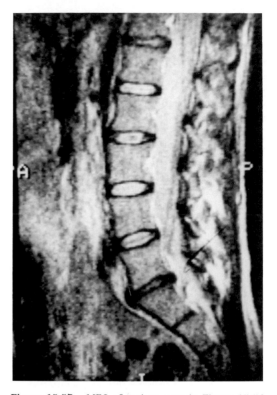

Figure 15.57. MRI of patient seen in Figure 15.56 reveals loss of signal intensity of the L5-S1 disc compared to the upper lumbar segments. Also note the extensive anterior and posterior bulging of the disc. This patient had a lengthy recovery time until he could return to his job as a carpenter. He was off work for 4 months and was seen by a neurosurgeon and an orthopedic surgeon. No surgery was recommended due to the fact that he did not have sciatic pain with appropriate objective findings to warrant surgery. I feel that the progressive degenerative change of the disc maintained his low back pain. This meant that the pain was of discal origin. Ultimately, the degeneration progressed to the point of stabilization and dehydration of the nucleus, to the extent that the intradiscal pressure was reduced enough to stop annular fiber irritation. Thus the pain diminished.

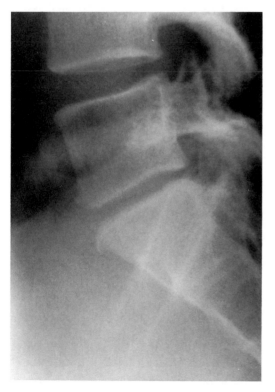

Figure 15.56. Plain lateral x-ray shows narrowing of the L5-S1 disc space with anterior and lateral hypertrophic changes of the vertebral body plates. L5 is minimally posterior on the sacrum.

in Figure 15.57 shows the loss of disc space and the loss of signal intensity from the L5-S1 disc. The disc is seen to protrude posteriorly and anteriorly, which is not appreciated on the plain film study.

Kambin (30) wrote that there was a direct correlation between the size of an annular bulge and the degree of narrowing of the disc space. Thus, annular protrusion is an integral part of the degeneration process. Kambin developed a measurement of the degree of annular protrusion by dividing the anteroposterior diameter of the intervertebral disc by the anteroposterior diameter of the vertebral plate as determined on radiographic studies. This was called the *A/V index*. Patients with greater disc degeneration exhibited a statistically higher annular/vertebral diameter ratio (A/V index) than patients with normal discs.

The physician can imagine the possible disc protrusion that may be creating stenosis in the vertebral canal when such degenerative disc disease is present. This must be tempered with the fact that oftentimes we see such degenerative change without the presence of disc protrusion.

The Postural Complex

The feet are responsible for low back pain when ankle pronation and lower extremity mechanical aberrations result in sagittal lumbar curve exaggeration. Figure 15.58 shows subtalar valgus change with ankle pronation. Figure 15.59 shows the genu valgus deformity that is aggravated by pronation of the ankles. This patient was hyperlordotic, and the MRI (Figs. 15.60 and 15.61) shows the bulging and fragmentation of the L4-L5 disc. Treatment here entailed orthotics to control the ankle pronation and subtalar valgus while flexion distraction was applied to the L4-L5 disc degeneration and fragmentation. This was a case we felt would have little chiropractic treatment relief until we corrected the foot aberrations that had been causing pain since this 33-year-old female was a teenager. We felt that the ankle pronation and genu valgus deformities caused the hyperlordosis, and this resulted in

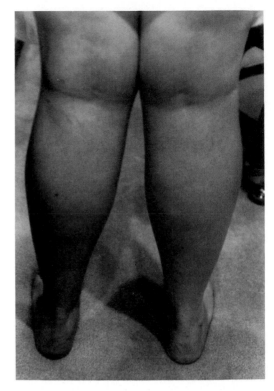

Figure 15.59. Note the genu valgus deformity of the knees.

progression of discal tearing and eventual prolapse.

Mellin (31) alludes to this type of case by stating that the pelvis and lower limbs form the basis

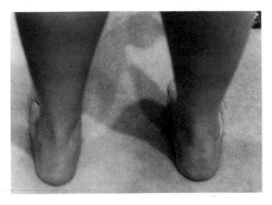

Figure 15.58. Note the subtalar valgus changes of the heels and the planus change of the longitudinal arches.

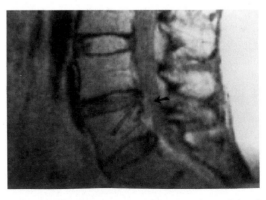

Figure 15.60. The lower two discs show loss of signal intensity due to degenerative changes. The L4-L5 disc shows posterior protrusion and a free fragment within the vertebral canal posterior to the L4 vertebral body (*arrow*).

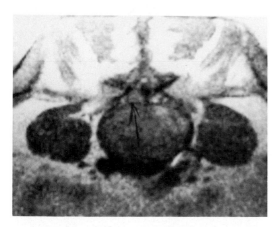

Figure 15.61. Axial view shows the large free fragment within the right lateral recess and vertebral canal (*arrow*).

for the spine, implying that their posture and movements affect those of the spine. Gait alterations are related to spinal movement, and osteoarthritis of the hip joint is found to increase spinal and pelvic movements when walking. He discussed hip mobility and low back pain relationships and stated the following possible contributing factors between them. Due to the intricate relationship between Mellin's ideas and this case, I would like to discuss his ideas on hip and low back pain interrelationships:

1. Back pain may cause restriction of hip movements because of a decrease in general physical activity.

2. Back pain and spinal pathology, through neurological reflexes, may cause spasm in the muscles and changes in movement patterns of the spine, pelvis, and hips. Painful stimulation of spinal structures has been shown experimentally to cause spasm in the hamstring muscles.

3. Back pain may provoke spasm of the psoas muscle followed by shortening and hip flexion, which may contribute to a strong correlation of extension with low back pain.

4. Restriction of hip mobility may put excessive load on the spine, as has been described for arthrosis of the hip.

5. Hip stiffness may be associated with development of low back pain.

This case of postural complex from feet to lumbar spine illustrates all of Mellin's ideas and strengthens the need for clinical intervention as

used in this case to delay or prevent further mechanical deterioration.

Spondylolisthesis Advancement

Figure 15.62 shows a lateral lumbar spine film with minimal slippage of L5 on the sacrum. Figure 15.63 shows further slippage following a fall, and Figure 15.64 shows the CT scan with the pars interarticularis fracture defects. This patient had extreme low back and left leg pain following the fall, requiring epidural block injections, which did afford relief.

L5-S1 Disc Prolapse with Lateral Bending Changes

Figure 15.65 shows a large midline L5-S1 disc prolapse. Figure 15.66 is a neutral posteroanterior view showing L5 in left lateral flexion on the sacrum, and Figure 15.67 shows attempted left lateral flexion of the lumbar spine, in which we note how the spinous processes rotate to the right convexity of the curve instead of into the left con-

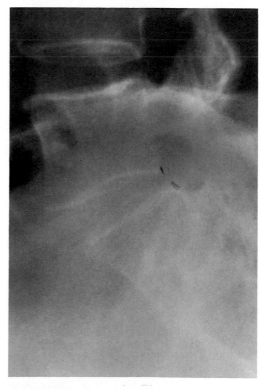

Figure 15.62. L5 shows minimal anterior subluxation on the sacrum.

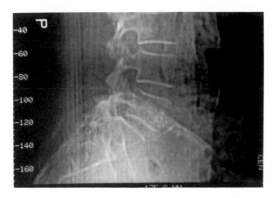

Figure 15.63. Following a fall, the patient in Figure 15.62 is radiographed again and now shows a greater degree of slippage of L5 on the sacrum. Also, her symptoms are much worse, consisting of low back and left first sacral nerve root radiculopathy.

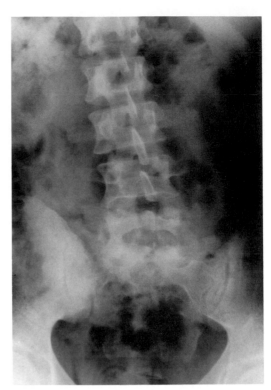

Figure 15.66. L5 is in left lateral flexion subluxation on the sacrum in this neutral posteroanterior lumbosacral x-ray of the patient seen in Figure 15.65.

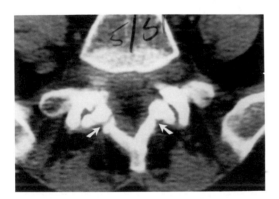

Figure 15.64. CT axial cut shows the spondylolisthesis pars interarticularis fractures (*arrows*). Probably the fall irritated this fibrous tissue healed pars defect and allowed some further slippage that resulted in nerve root and discal irritation.

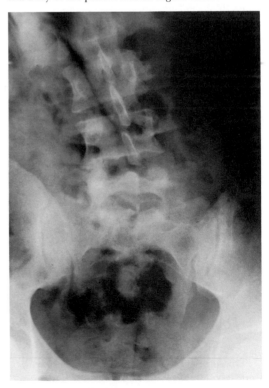

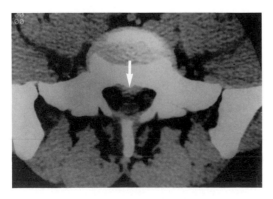

Figure 15.65. A large midline disc prolapse (*arrow*) is seen at the L5-S1 disc level.

Figure 15.67. Left lateral flexion sees the spinous processes rotate into the convexity of the curve on the right side instead of into the left concavity, as is normally seen.

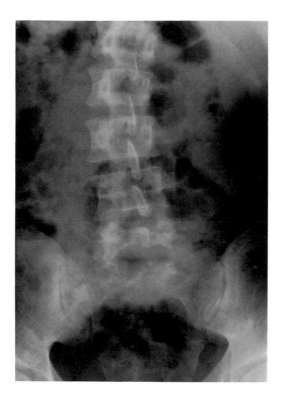

Figure 15.68. Right lateral flexion sees the spinous processes rotate to the right into the concavity of the curve. This is normal lateral flexion- and rotation-coupled movement. The L4 and L5 segments, however, do not rotate to the right. All movement takes place at the L3 level and above. Remember, this patient has pain down the left first sacral dermatome.

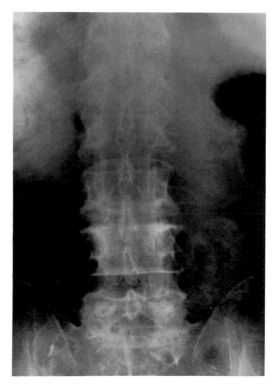

Figure 15.69. This study shows L3-L4 intervertebral disc degeneration. There is sclerosis of the L4 superior vertebral body plate.

cavity as normally seen. Figure 15.68 shows right lateral flexion; the spinous processes rotate into the concavity of the curve on the right, which is the normal finding for lumbar rotation. This patient had pain into the left first sacral dermatome.

Normal Plain X-ray of L2 Vertebral Body with Abnormal MRI of L2

Figure 15.69 shows degenerative L3-L4 disc changes. Figure 15.70 shows the same L3-L4 disc degeneration, while the inferior L2 vertebral plate reveals some nuclear invagination of its inferior body plate. Figure 15.71 shows a bone scan that was ordered since this patient continued to have night pain and unremitting low back pain.

Here we see that the L2 vertebral body has increased uptake, as well as two areas on the left paralumbar area that are felt to be within rib tissue. Figure 15.72 is an MRI that shows the L2 vertebral body to have low T1-weighted signal intensity in comparison to the adjacent vertebrae. The superior plate of L4 has a superior compression defect, a probable Schmorl's node. Also seen is an abdominal aneurysm with a large hematoma within it anterior to the L3-L4 vertebral bodies.

At the time of writing this chapter, the diagnosis of this case was not final, but malignant disease was the primary impression.

This case again demonstrates the lack of diagnostic detail from plain x-ray and supports the need for further detailed imaging in cases having unremitting pain under conservative care, especially when clinical findings are present.

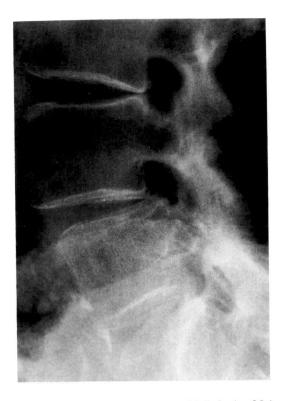

Figure 15.74. Degenerative spondylolisthesis of L4 on L5 is seen, with degeneration of the discs above and below this level as well.

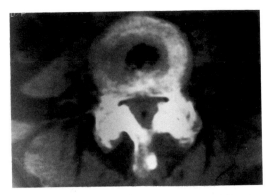

Figure 15.75. Thickening hypertrophy of the ligamentum flavum is noted, as well as hypertrophy of the facet joints at the L4-L5 level, resulting in lateral recess stenosis. The facet joints are markedly arthrotic. Note the vacuum phenomenon of the disc. There is also disc protrusion into the canal. Overall marked stenosis of the vertebral canal is present, creating thecal sac compression.

References

1. Jackson RP, Simmons EH, Stripinis D: Incidence and severity of back pain in adult idiopathic scoliosis. *Spine* 8(7):749–756, 1983.
2. Healey JH, Lane JM: Structural scoliosis in osteoporotic women. *Clin Orthop* 195(May):216–223, 1985.
3. Bronner F, Richelle LJ, Savelli PD, Nicholas JA, Cobb JR: Quantitation of calcium metabolism in postmenopausal osteoporosis and scoliosis. *J Clin Invest* 42:898, 1963.
4. Lane JM, Healey JH, Schwartz E, Vigorita VJ, Schneider R, Einhorn TA, Suda M, Williams R: Treatment of osteoporosis with sodium fluoride and calcium: effects on vertebral fracture incidence and bone histomorphometry. *Orthop Clin North Am* 15(4):729, 1984.
5. Collins DK, Ponseti IV: Long term follow-up of patients with idiopathic scoliosis not treated surgically. *J Bone Joint Surg* 51A:425–445, 1969.
6. Coonard RW, Feierstein MS: Progression of scoliosis in the adult. *J Bone Joint Surg* 58A:738, 1976.
7. Keim HA: Scoliosis can progress in the adult. *Orthopaedic Review* 3:23–28, 1974.
8. Kostuik JP, Isreal J, Hall JE: Scoliosis surgery in adults. *Clin Orthop* 93:225–234, 1973.
9. Ghavamian T: Future of minor scoliotic curves of the spine. Exhibit presented at American Academy of Orthopedic Surgeons, Washington, DC, 1972.
10. Kostuik JP: Assessment of painful adult scoliosis using discography: a prospective study. Presented at the Scoliosis Research Society, Boston, MA, 1978.
11. Kostuik JP: Decision making in adult scolisis surgery. Presented at the Canadian Orthopaedic Association, Montreal, Canada, 1979.
12. Carter OD, Haynes SG: Prevalence rates for scoliosis in U.S. adults: results from the first national health and nutrition examination survey. *Int J Epidemiol* 16(4):537–544, 1987.
13. Winter RB, Lonstein JE, Denis FD: Pain patterns in adult scoliosis. *Orthop Clin North Am* 19(2):339–345, 1988.
14. Nuber GW, Schafer MF: Surgical management of adult scoliosis. *Clin Orthop* 208(July):228–237, 1988.
15. Sponseller PD, Cohen MS, Nachemson AL, Hall JE, Wohl MEB: Results of surgical treatment of adults with idiopathic scoliosis. *J Bone Joint Surg* 69A(5):667, 1987.
16. Floman Y, Micheli LJ, Penny JN, Riseborough EJ, Hall JE: Combined anterior and posterior fusion mass in seventy-three spinally deformed patients. *Clin Orthop* 164:110, 1982.
17. Byrd JA, Scoles PV, Winter RB, Bradford DS, Lonstein JE, Moe JH: Adult idiopathic scoliosis treated by anterior and posterior spinal fusion. *J Bone Joint Surg* 69A:843, 1987.

18. Aebi M: Correction of degenerative scoliosis of the lumbar spine. *Clin Orthop* 232(July):80–86, 1988.

19. Taylor TKF, Ruff SJ, Alglietti PL, DiMuria GV, Marcucci M, Novenbri A, Innocenti M: The long term results of wedge and compression fractures of the dorsolumbar spine without neurological involvement: proceedings and reports of universities, colleges, councils, associations and societies. *J Bone Joint Surg* 69A:334, 1987.

20. Weinstein JN, Collalto P, Lehmann TR: Thoracolumbar burst fractures treated conservatively: a long term follow up. *Spine* 13(1):33, 1988.

21. Teplick JG, Haskin ME: Intravenous contrast-enhanced CT of the postoperative lumbar spine: improved identification of recurrent disc herniation, scar, arachnoiditis, and diskitis. *Am J Neuroradiol* 5(4):373–385, 1984.

22. Hueftle MG: Lumbar spine: postoperative MR imaging with Gd-DTPA. *Radiology* 167(3):817, 1988.

23. Revel M, Amor B, Mathiew A, Wybier M, Vallee C, Chevrot A: Sciatica induced by primary epidural adhesions. *Lancet* (March 5):527–528, 1988.

24. De La Porte C, Siegfried J: Lumbosacral spinal fibrosis (spinal arachnoiditis): its diagnosis and treatment by spinal cord stimulation. *Spine* 8(6):593–599, 1983.

25. Ray CD: *Treating the Failed Back Patient with Epidural Stimulation.* Minneapolis, MN, Medtronic Company, 1987.

26. Follick MJ, Smith TW, Ahern DK: The sickness impact profile: a global measure of disability in chronic low back pain. *Pain* 21:67–76, 1985.

27. Goodheart G: *Applied Kinesiology (the Neurolymphatic Reflex and Its Relationship to Muscle Balancing),* ed 3. Private publication, 1970, pp 15–18, 36, 37, 45.

28. Katznelson A, Nerubay J, Lev-el A: The gluteal skyline sign. *Spine* 7(1):74, 1982.

29. Steiner C, Staubs C, Ganon M, Buhlinger CD: Piriformis syndrome: pathogenesis, diagnosis, and treatment. *J Am Osteopath Assoc* 87(4):318–322, 1987.

30. Kambin P, Nixon JE, Chait A, Schaffer JL: Annular protrusion: pathophysiology and roentgenographic appearance. *Spine* 13(6):671–675, 1988.

31. Mellin G: Correlations of hip mobility with degree of back pain and lumbar spinal mobility in chronic low back pain patients. *Spine* 13(6):668–670, 1988.

Index

Page numbers in *italics* denote figures; those followed by "*t*" denote tables.